# Mechanisms and Therapeutic Approaches of Antimicrobial Resistance

# Mechanisms and Therapeutic Approaches of Antimicrobial Resistance

Editor: Leona Ahrens

AMERICAN
MEDICAL PUBLISHERS
www.americanmedicalpublishers.com

AMERICAN
MEDICAL PUBLISHERS
www.americanmedicalpublishers.com

**Cataloging-in-Publication Data**

Mechanisms and therapeutic approaches of antimicrobial resistance / edited by Leona Ahrens.
p. cm.
Includes bibliographical references and index.
ISBN 979-8-88740-246-8
1. Drug resistance in microorganisms. 2. Microorganisms--Effect of drugs on.
3. Anti-infective agents. 4. Antibiotics. 5. Immunology. I. Ahrens, Leona.
QR177 .M43 2023
616.904 1--dc23



American Medical Publishers,
41 Flatbush Avenue,
1st Floor, New York,
NY 11217, USA

ISBN 979-8-88740-246-8 (Hardback)

# Contents

# Preface

The main aim of this book is to educate learners and enhance their research focus by presenting diverse topics covering this vast field. This is an advanced book which compiles significant studies by distinguished experts in the area of analysis. This book addresses successive solutions to the challenges arising in the area of application, along with it; the book provides scope for future developments.

Antimicrobial resistance (AMR) occurs when microbes develop mechanisms to defend themselves from the impact of antimicrobials. Infections occurring due to resistant microbes are not easy to treat as they require high doses of antimicrobial drugs or other alternative medicines which are more toxic. The microbes resistant to various antimicrobials are referred to as multidrug resistant (MDR). Every class of microbes may evolve resistance, which may develop naturally through genetic mutation or through acquisition of resistance from one another. Antimicrobial resistance is majorly caused by the excessive use of antimicrobials, which supports the mutations and results in making the antimicrobials ineffective. The control of antimicrobial resistance requires intelligent combination of approaches for various complimentary therapies. These combination therapies should extend beyond biologically active molecules for controlled delivery of strategies. This book includes some of the vital pieces of work being conducted across the world, on various topics related to antimicrobial resistance. It includes contributions of experts and scientists which will provide innovative insights to the readers on the mechanisms and therapeutic approaches to combat antimicrobial resistance.

It was a great honour to edit this book, though there were challenges, as it involved a lot of communication and networking between me and the editorial team. However, the end result was this all-inclusive book covering diverse themes in the field.

Finally, it is important to acknowledge the efforts of the contributors for their excellent chapters, through which a wide variety of issues have been addressed. I would also like to thank my colleagues for their valuable feedback during the making of this book.

**Editor**

1

# Gas Plasma Pre-Treatment Increases Antibiotic Sensitivity and Persister Eradication in Methicillin-Resistant *Staphylococcus aureus*

*Li Guo[1]*, Ruobing Xu[2], Yiming Zhao[2], Dingxin Liu[1], Zhijie Liu[1], Xiaohua Wang[1], Hailan Chen[3] and Michael G. Kong[1,3,4]**

*[1] State Key Laboratory of Electrical Insulation and Power Equipment, Center for Plasma Biomedicine, Xi'an Jiaotong University, Xi'an, China, [2] School of Life Science and Technology, Xi'an Jiaotong University, Xi'an, China, [3] Frank Reidy Center for Bioelectrics, Old Dominion University, Norfolk, VA, United States, [4] Department of Electrical and Computer Engineering, Old Dominion University, Norfolk, VA, United States*

***Correspondence:**
*Li Guo*
*guoli35@mail.xjtu.edu.cn*
*Michael G. Kong*
*mglin5g@gmail.com*

Methicillin-resistant *Staphylococcus aureus* (MRSA) is a major cause of serious nosocomial infections, and recurrent MRSA infections primarily result from the survival of persister cells after antibiotic treatment. Gas plasma, a novel source of ROS (reactive oxygen species) and RNS (reactive nitrogen species) generation, not only inactivates pathogenic microbes but also restore the sensitivity of MRSA to antibiotics. This study further found that sublethal treatment of MRSA with both plasma and plasma-activated saline increased the antibiotic sensitivity and promoted the eradication of persister cells by tetracycline, gentamycin, clindamycin, chloramphenicol, ciprofloxacin, rifampicin, and vancomycin. The short-lived ROS and RNS generated by plasma played a primary role in the process and induced the increase of many species of ROS and RNS in MRSA cells. Thus, our data indicated that the plasma treatment could promote the effects of many different classes of antibiotics and act as an antibiotic sensitizer for the treatment of antibiotic-resistant bacteria involved in infectious diseases.

**Keywords: cold atmospheric-pressure plasma, antibiotics resistance, methicillin-resistant *Staphylococcus aureus*, reactive oxygen species, reactive nitrogen species**

## INTRODUCTION

Antibiotics are the primary treatment for infectious bacterial diseases (Li et al., 2017). Antibiotic resistance typically emerges several years after the development and use of a new antibiotic, usually within an average of 8 years after introduction (Schmieder and Edwards, 2012). Furthermore, infections with multidrug-resistant bacteria are occurring more frequently, and few or no drugs are available to combat them (Boucher et al., 2009; Wright, 2016; Gonzalez-Bello, 2017). One of the major multidrug-resistant bacteria is methicillin-resistant *Staphylococcus aureus* (MRSA), which is recognized as a leading cause of nosocomial infections (Shahsavan et al., 2012; Emaneini et al., 2017). Persisters are a small non-growing population of bacteria which could also escape from different antibiotics (Levin and Rozen, 2006). Persisters extend the duration of antibiotic treatment, cause the recurrence of infectious diseases, and the generation and ascent of antibiotic resistance (Levin and Rozen, 2006). Increased antibiotic resistance and the shortage of new antibiotics threaten global public health (Boucher et al., 2009; Dwyer et al., 2014). Therefore, strategies to combat antibiotic resistance, such as the development of new antibiotics or prolonging the lifespan of current antibiotics, are in high demand (Melander and Melander, 2017).

One strategy that has been explored recently is developing approaches that induce bacterial killing via the same mechanism as existing antibiotics. Antibiotics with different targets have been proposed to share a common mechanism of bactericidal activity—enhancing intracellular reactive oxygen species (ROS) in bacterial cells (Kohanski et al., 2007, 2010). Although ROS could be developed as antimicrobials to treat infectious diseases, treatment with these highly reactive molecules is problematic because ROS react non-selectively with such a range of critical, macromolecular targets, which could lead to "off-target" effects (Dharmaraja, 2017). Given that oxidative stress is also associated with antibiotic treatment, low levels of ROS could be used as an adjuvant to potentiate the antibacterial activity of commercial antibiotics (Brynildsen et al., 2013; Morones-Ramirez et al., 2013; Shen et al., 2016). A previous study showed that $^{\bullet}OH$ induced in $Ag^+$-treated bacteria potentiated the bactericidal activity of antibiotics against bacterial persisters and biofilms (Morones-Ramirez et al., 2013). Furthermore, fosfomycin, which acts by generating $O_2^{\bullet-}$, was used to successfully treat MRSA infections when combined with many commercial antibiotics (Shen et al., 2016). These strategies relied on the addition of inorganic or organic chemicals, which would bring residues after the treatment.

Cold atmospheric-pressure plasma (referred to as "plasma") generates many reactive oxygen and nitrogen species (ROS and RNS), such as $H_2O_2$, $^1O_2$, $O_3$, $^{\bullet}NO$, and $^{\bullet}OH$ as well as electrons, ions, and photons. This form of plasma is atmospheric-pressure and near room temperature, thus it treats cells and tissues without thermal damage, making it attractive for a range of biomedical applications, such as bacteria inactivation (Fridman et al., 2008; Moreau et al., 2008; Kong et al., 2009; Kang et al., 2014). The FDA has authorized the use of at least three gas plasma-based products using "plasma biomedicine" technology, such as blood coagulation. In addition, there have been several phase-II clinical trials for plasma-based therapies, such as chronic wound healing, which is the promising applications of plasma in medicine (Isbary et al., 2010, 2012; Heinlin et al., 2013). In the treatment of wounds, the reactive species of plasma could not only kill the microorganisms in the infectious wounds and burns but also increase proliferation of fibroblasts and other cells (Lloyd et al., 2010). Bayliss et al. (2013) found that treating MRSA with sublethal doses of plasma restored the sensitivity of MRSA to trimethoprim, kanamycin, and oxacillin, but the utility of plasma treatment with other types of antibiotics was not studied.

In the present study, in order to further our understanding of the effect of plasma treatment on antibiotic sensitivity, MRSA was treated with both plasma and plasma-activated saline prior to exposure to multiple antibiotics. Sublethal treatment of MRSA with plasma increased the sensitivity of MRSA to seven antibiotics whilst also reducing the numbers of persisters. These results support the use of plasma as an antibiotic sensitizer for the treatment of antibiotic-resistant bacteria involved in infectious diseases.

# MATERIALS AND METHODS

## Plasma Device and Plasma Treatments

As shown in **Figure 1A**, the surface discharge structure of the plasma consisted of a high-voltage plane electrode, a liquid-facing grounded mesh electrode of a hexagonal shape and a dielectric layer (made of polytetrafluoroethylene) sandwiched between the two electrodes. The surface plasma was generated when a sinusoidal high voltage was applied and the discharge power density was 0.2 $W/cm^2$ with good mesh-to-mesh homogeneity (showed in the front view of the plasmas in **Figure 1A**). One milliliter MRSA suspension or saline in a Petri dish (diameter 35 mm) with the depth of 1 mm was placed under the plasma, whereas the air gap between the plasma and the liquid surface was about 8 mm. The gas plasma system was housed in a sealed organic glass box with a gas flow of helium and 1% artificial air (79% $N_2$ + 21% $O_2$) at a constant rate of 4 L/min. The artificial air was used as the source of ROS and RNS, while the helium was used to enhance the production efficiency of those species as well as their fluxes on the treated samples via diffusion.

## Measurement of ROS and RNS Generated by the Plasma

The concentrations of $H_2O_2$ and $NO_2^-/NO_3^-$ in 0.9% NaCl were measured using hydrogen peroxide/peroxidase assay kit (Thermo Fisher Scientific) and nitrite/nitrate colorimetric assay kit (Cayman), respectively. $^{\bullet}OH$, $^1O_2$, $^{\bullet}NO$, $O_2^{\bullet-}$, $^{\bullet}NO_2$, and $ONOO^-$ were measured using an electron spin-resonance (ESR) spectroscopy (Bruker) together with relevant spin traps. The latter include: 100 mM DMPO (5,5-Dimethyl-1-pyrroline N-oxide, Dojindo), 5 mM MGD (N-(Dithiocarbamoyl)-N-methyl-D-glucamine, Dojindo), 10 mM TEMP (2,2,6,6-Tetramethylpiperidine, TCI), and 10 mM TEMPONE-H (1-Hydroxy-2,2,6,6-tetramethyl-4-oxo-piperidine, Enzo).

## Treatment of *Staphylococcus aureus* With Plasma or Plasma-Activated Saline

A single *S. aureus* ATCC33591 colony was grown in 4 ml of Mueller-Hinton (MH) broth (Oxoid) at 225 r.p.m. at 37°C overnight, and the resulting overnight culture was diluted 1:100 in MH and incubated at 37°C at 225 r.p.m. until an $OD_{600}$ of 0.6 was reached. The bacterial cells were collected by centrifugation, washed once with saline (0.9% NaCl) and resuspended in saline at an $OD_{600}$ of 2.0. *S. aureus* suspensions were treated with plasma directly, or the suspensions were centrifuged and resuspended in plasma-activated saline (saline treated with plasma for the indicated time), saline with 250 μM $H_2O_2$ + 125 μM $NO_2^-$ + 375 μM $NO_3^-$, or saline with 500 μM $H_2O_2$ + 250 μM $NO_2^-$ + 750 μM $NO_3^-$ and then incubated for 30 min at room temperature. Samples were serially diluted with 0.9% NaCl, and 10 μl of each dilution was spotted onto MH agar plates and incubated overnight at 37°C and the numbers of surviving bacteria were determined by counting the resulting CFUs.

## Determination of Antibiotic Sensitivity

The *S. aureus* suspensions prepared as described above were either untreated, treated with plasma directly for 30 or 40 s, or

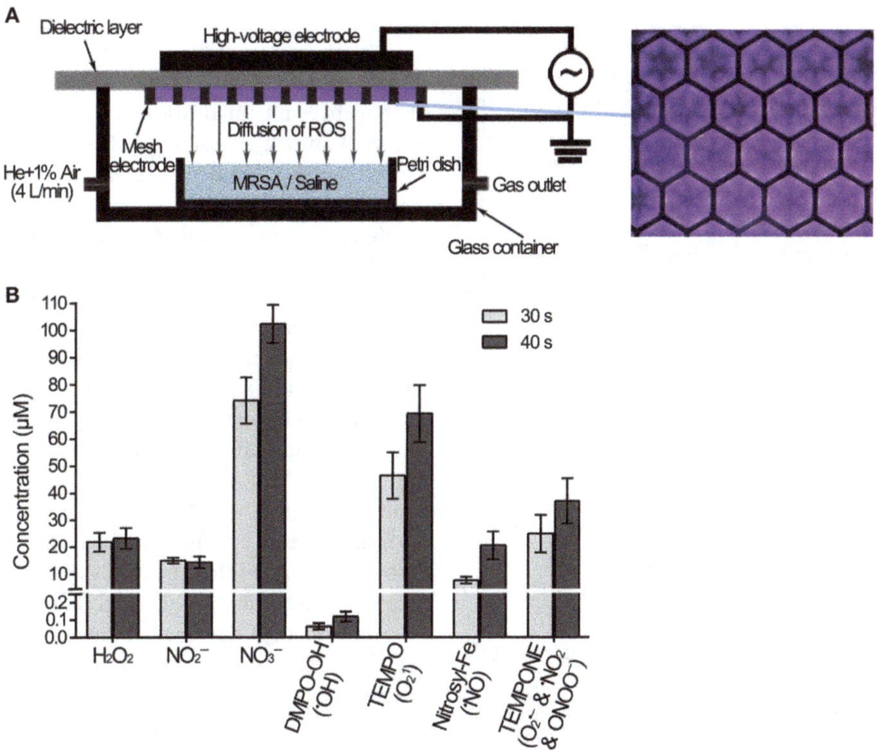


**FIGURE 1 |** Measurement of the ROS and RNS diffused into the saline treated with plasma. **(A)** Diagram of MRSA suspension or saline treated with plasma. **(B)** The concentrations of ROS, RNS and spin trap adducts diffused into the saline treated with plasma for 30 and 40 s.

centrifuged and resuspended in plasma-activated saline (saline treated by plasma for 30 or 40 s), followed by incubation for 30 min at room temperature. Untreated *S. aureus*, or cells treated with either plasma or plasma-activated saline (100 µl), were plated on MH agar plates. Next, antibiotic susceptibility tests were performed using Etest paper (Biomerieux) for tetracycline (0.016–256 µg/ml), gentamycin (0.016–256 µg/ml), clindamycin (0.016–256 µg/ml), chloramphenicol (0.016–256 µg/ml), ciprofloxacin (0.02–32 µg/ml), rifampicin (0.02–32 µg/ml), and vancomycin (0.016–256 µg/ml) or the Kirby-Bauer method for clindamycin (250, 500, 1,000, and 2,000 µg). Then the plates were cultured overnight at 37°C and bacteriostatic rings were analyzed. The MICs of antibiotics were measured by the microdilution assay using 8–0.016 × MIC of untreated MRSA as described (Lepe et al., 2014).

## Quantification of Persister Survival

*S. aureus* treated with plasma or plasma-activated saline was diluted six times with MH medium containing antibiotics. The final antibiotic concentrations, corresponding to 10× the minimum inhibitory concentration (MIC), were as follows: tetracycline, 500 µg/ml (MP Biomedicals); gentamycin, 200 µg/ml (Sigma); clindamycin, 5,000 µg/ml (TCI); chloramphenicol, 500 µg/ml (MP Biomedicals); ciprofloxacin, 50 µg/ml (Sigma); rifampicin, 4 µg/ml (Sigma); and vancomycin, 50 µg/ml (Sigma). The numbers of surviving bacteria were determined at the time points indicated by harvesting 100 µl of bacterial culture, which was centrifuged at 10,000× g for 1 min. The resulting pellet was resuspended in 100 µl 0.9% NaCl. Samples were serially diluted, and 10 µl of each dilution was spotted onto MH agar plates and incubated overnight at 37°C and the numbers of surviving bacteria were determined by counting the resulting CFUs.

## Detection of Reactive Species in MRSA

The probes 3′-(p-aminophenyl) fluorescein (APF, Sigma), 3′-(p-hydroxyphenyl) fluorescein (HPF, Sigma), and MitoSOX™ Red mitochondrial superoxide indicator (ThermoFisher) were incubated with *S. aureus* cultures, at a final concentration of 5 µM, and trans-1-(2′-methoxyvinyl)pyrene (tMVP, J&K Scientific) was used at a final concentration of 10 µM at 37°C for 30 min. Cultures were collected by centrifugation, washed with saline (0.9% NaCl) three times and resuspended in saline at an $OD_{600}$ of 2.0. *S. aureus* suspensions were untreated, treated with plasma directly for 40 s, or the suspensions were centrifuged and resuspended in plasma-activated saline (saline treated with plasma for 40 s). Immediately after the treatments, the fluorescence intensities were detected using a microplate reader (Thermo Scientific Varioskan Flash) at the excitation and emission wavelengths [APF and HPF: 490/515 nm; superoxide indicator: 510/580 nm; trans-1-(2′-methoxyvinyl)pyrene: 405/460 nm] of each probe.

# RESULTS

## Plasma-Induced Aqueous ROS/RNS

MRSA or saline treated with the plasma device was shown in **Figure 1A**. Gaseous ROS and RNS were generated by the surface discharge, and some of them would diffuse across the air gap and then dissolved into the liquids. The plasma-induced aqueous ROS and RNS dissolved into saline were measured after the plasma treatment for 30 s and 40 s. Long-lived species $H_2O_2$, $NO_2^-$, and $NO_3^-$, as well as the short-lived species $^{\bullet}OH$, $^1O_2$, $^{\bullet}NO$, and $ONOO^-$, were detected in the saline. The concentrations of aqueous $H_2O_2$, $NO_2^-$, and $NO_3^-$ after the plasma treatment for 40 s were 23, 14, and 102 μM, respectively (**Figure 1B**). Electron spin resonance (ESR) spectroscopy was used for the measurement of short-lived species, in which the results were the concentrations of spin adducts, only reflecting the relative concentrations of the specific ROS and/or RNS. The concentrations of spin adducts DMPO-OH, TEMPO, Nitrocyl-Fe, and TEMPONE after the plasma treatment for 40 s were 0.1, 69, 21, and 37 μM (**Figure 1B**). The spin adducts concentrations after the plasma treatment for 30 s were lower, such as TEMPO was 30% lower than that after the plasma treatment for 40 s. These results suggested that the concentration of aqueous $^{\bullet}OH$ was very low, and the concentration of aqueous $^1O_2$ should be much larger. The plasma generated many species ROS and RNS, which were thought to play a crucial role in the biological effects.

## Sublethal Treatment With Plasma Increased the Sensitivity of MRSA to Antibiotics

The sublethal dose (reduction about 50% viability of MRSA) of plasma and plasma-activated saline were determined by exposing the bacteria to plasma for increasing times or incubating with saline treated with plasma for increasing times and subsequently determining bacterial viability. The treatment of plasma for 40 s or the saline activated by plasma for 40 s lead to about 50% death of MRSA cells (Figure S1). For safety, a lower dose was also employed, so a slightly lower dose (plasma treatment for 30 s) that lead to about 40% death of MRSA cells and the $LD_{50}$ dose (plasma treatment for 40 s) were both used to detect the effects on antibiotic sensitivity.

To study the effect of plasma on the sensitivity of MRSA to the antibiotics, MRSA were sublethally pre-treated with plasma or plasma-activated saline followed by incubation with a range of antibiotics including tetracycline, gentamycin, clindamycin, chloramphenicol, ciprofloxacin, rifampicin, and vancomycin. The minimal inhibitory concentration (MIC) of tetracycline for untreated MRSA measured by Etest paper was ~32 μg/ml, whilst the MIC of tetracycline for MRSA treated with plasma for 30 or 40 s was 10-fold lower, at ~3 μg/ml (**Figure 2A**). In the second approach, the MICs were measured by the microdilution assay, and the MIC of tetracycline against MRSA treated with plasma for 40 s was 8-fold lower than that against untreated MRSA (**Table 1**). The effects of plasma pre-treatment on MRSA sensitivity to antibiotics were independent of the particular antibiotic used, and the increase in sensitivity was observed for most of the antibiotics tested. The MICs of gentamycin against untreated MRSA and MRSA treated with plasma for 30 and 40 s measured by Etest paper were ~1.5, 1.0, and 0.5 μg/ml, respectively, and the MIC of gentamycin against MRSA treated with plasma for 40 s was 16-fold lower than that against untreated MRSA as indicated by the microdilution assay (**Figure 2A**; **Table 1**). The MICs of chloramphenicol, ciprofloxacin, rifampicin, and vancomycin against MRSA treated with plasma also decreased in varying degrees (**Figure 2A**; **Table 1**). Plasma-treated MRSA did not appear to be susceptible to treatment with clindamycin at the tested concentration (**Figure 2A**). Two possible explanations for this were that either the plasma treatment did not change the antibiotic sensitivity of MRSA to clindamycin or the MIC of clindamycin against MRSA was beyond the range of the Etest. Thus, MRSA susceptibility to clindamycin was measured at a higher antibiotic dose using the Kirby-Bauer method. The diameter of the bacteriostatic ring of untreated MRSA to 2,000 μg clindamycin was about 16 mm, and that of the MRSA treated for 30 and 40 s were 23 and 26 mm, respectively (Figures S2A,B). The microdilution assay also demonstrated that the MICs of clindamycin against MRSA treated with plasma for 30 and 40 s was 2- and 4-fold lower, respectively, than that against untreated MRSA (**Table 1**). These data indicated that sublethal plasma treatment to MRSA restored the sensitivity to five different classes of antibiotics.

Next, the effects of plasma-activated saline upon changing the sensitivity of MRSA to these antibiotics were detected. The minimal inhibitory concentration (MIC) of tetracycline against untreated MRSA was ~32 μg/ml, whilst that for MRSA treated with saline activated by plasma for 30 or 40 s was 10-fold lower, at ~3 μg/ml (**Figure 2B**). The MIC of tetracycline against MRSA treated with saline activated by plasma for 40 s was also 8-fold lower than that against untreated MRSA as indicated by the microdilution assay (**Table 1**). The MICs of gentamycin, clindamycin, chloramphenicol, ciprofloxacin, rifampicin, and vancomycin against MRSA treated with plasma-activated saline were also lower than those against the untreated MRSA, demonstrating that plasma-activated saline exhibited the same effect in increasing the sensitivity to five different classes of antibiotics (**Figures 2B**, Figures S2C,D; **Table 1**).

## Plasma Pre-treatment Promoted Eradication of MRSA Persisters

Given that pre-treatment of MRSA with plasma or plasma-activated saline decreased the MIC of multiple antibiotics, we next asked whether either of these pre-treatment conditions could also promote the killing of persisters. To test this, untreated and sublethal dose plasma-treated MRSA were incubated with different antibiotics, as indicated (**Figure 3A**). Incubation of untreated and double-diluted untreated MRSA with the different antibiotics generally exhibited typical killing curves, with bacterial numbers decreasing from $2 \times 10^8$ to $10^4$-$10^6$ CFUs, with a small fraction of persisters detected after 3 days of antibiotic exposure. Of note, the numbers of untreated MRSA and double-diluted untreated MRSA that incubated with rifampicin increased after 1 day. These results indicated that the decrease of the initial MRSA numbers did not greatly influence the killing

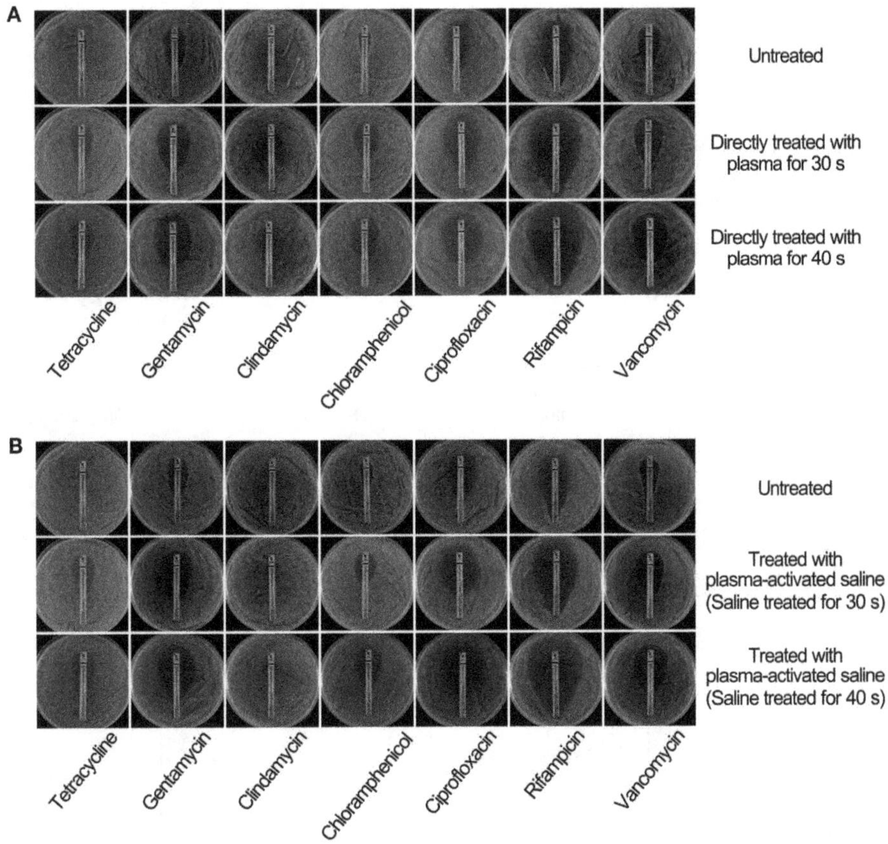


**FIGURE 2** | Treatment with sublethal doses of plasma or plasma-activated saline increased the sensitivity of MRSA to antibiotics. **(A)** Direct plasma treatment. **(B)** Plasma-activated saline treatment. Plasma treated, plasma-activated saline treated and untreated MRSA were plated on MH agar with Etest strips and cultured at 37°C overnight.

**TABLE 1** | Antibiotic susceptibilities of *Staphylococcus aureus* treated with plasma and plasma-activated saline.

| Antibiotics | MIC[a] (mg/liter) of indicated antibiotic | | | | |
|---|---|---|---|---|---|
| | Untreated | Directly treated with plasma for 30 s | Directly treated with plasma for 40 s | Treated with plasma-activated saline (Saline treated for 30 s) | Treated with plasma-activated saline (Saline treated for 40 s) |
| Tetracycline | 50 | 12.5 | 6.25 | 12.5 | 6.25 |
| Gentamycin | 20 | 2.5 | 1.25 | 1.25 | 1.25 |
| Clindamycin | 500 | 250 | 125 | 250 | 250 |
| Chloramphenicol | 50 | 25 | 12.5 | 25 | 25 |
| Ciprofloxacin | 5 | 1.25 | 0.31 | 1.25 | 0.625 |
| Rifampicin | 0.4 | 0.025 | 0.0125 | 0.025 | 0.0125 |
| Vancomycin | 5 | 5 | 2.5 | 5 | 2.5 |

[a] *MICs were determined by broth microdilution method. The results were read after 24 h of incubation at 37°C.*

curves of antibiotics. In contrast, plasma-treatment reduced the number of MRSA persisters to below the limit of detection when incubated with tetracycline, gentamycin, clindamycin, chloramphenicol, and rifampicin within only 1 day of exposure (**Figure 3A**). A similar decrease was also observed within 2 and 3 days of incubation with ciprofloxacin and chloramphenicol, respectively (**Figure 3A**). For vancomycin, plasma treatment for 30 and 40 s effectively reduced the numbers of remaining MRSA recovered during exposure to this antibiotic to $10^4$ and $10^3$ CFUs, respectively, though these did not drop below the detection limit (**Figure 3A**). Treatment with plasma-activated saline exhibited the same effect of inactivating persisters as observed by direct plasma treatment (**Figure 3B**). The numbers of plasma-activated saline treated MRSA recovered upon

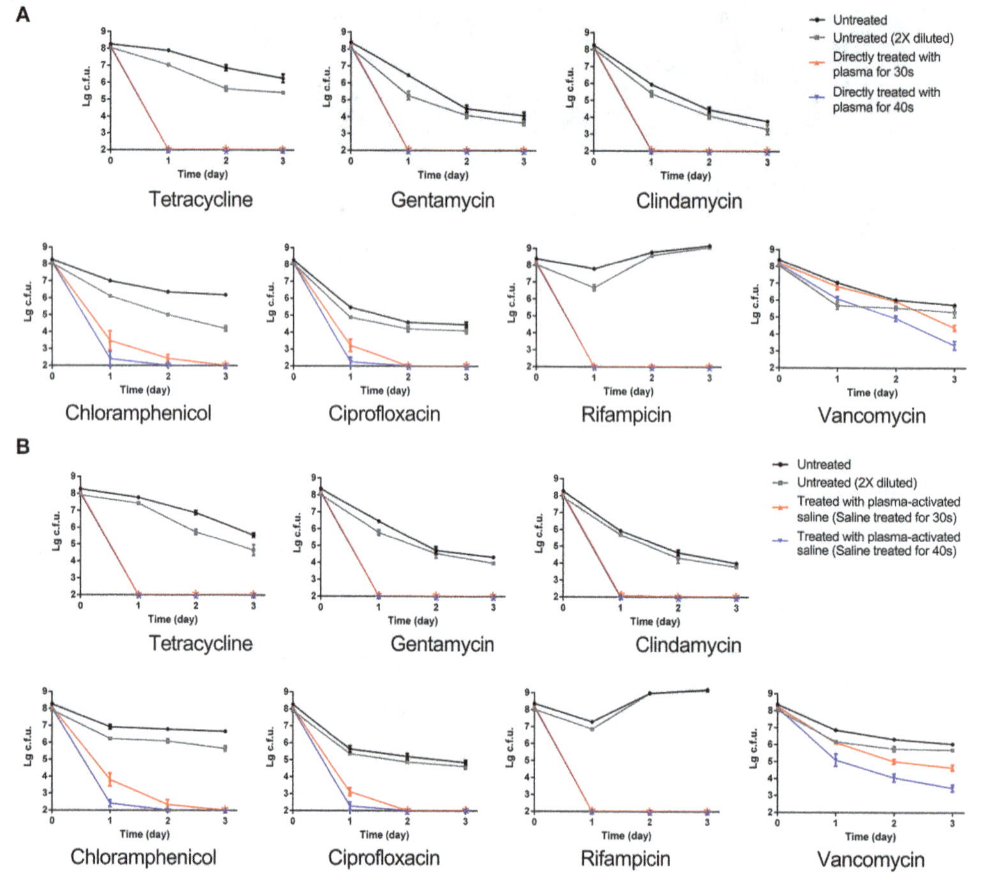


**FIGURE 3 |** MRSA sublethally treated with plasma or plasma-activated saline increased the eradication of persisters by antibiotics. **(A)** Direct plasma treatment. **(B)** Plasma-activated saline treatment. Plasma treated, plasma-activated saline treated and untreated MRSA were grown in MHB with 10 × MIC of the indicated antibiotics, and aliquots of the cultures were taken at the times indicated, serially diluted and plated. Then the plates were cultured at 37°C overnight and the numbers of bacteria were counted. The asterisks represented eradication to the limit of detection.

exposure to antibiotics tetracycline, gentamycin, clindamycin, and rifampicin dropped to below the detection limit, but plasma-activated saline similarly only decreased the numbers of MRSA to $10^3$ CFUs upon exposure to vancomycin (**Figure 3B**). These results indicated that both plasma and plasma-activated saline treatment promoted the eradication of MRSA persisters by antibiotics.

## Reactive Species in MRSA

Plasma-treated solutions contain many active species, such as the long-lived species $H_2O_2$, $NO_2^-$, and $NO_3^-$ as well as the short-lived species $^{\bullet}OH$, $^1O_2$, $^{\bullet}NO$, $O_2^{\bullet-}$, and $ONOO^-$ (**Figure 1B**). To evaluate the impact of long-lived species, a mixture of $H_2O_2$ (500 µM), $NO_2^-$ (250 µM), and $NO_3^-$ (750 µM) was used to treat the MRSA. $H_2O_2$, $NO_2^-$, and $NO_3^-$ treatment did not change the antibiotic susceptibility of MRSA and the inactivation of persisters by antibiotics, indicating that the three long-lived species are not likely the direct and driving factor (Figure S3). Hence, short-lived species were considered more important, and the ROS and RNS in MRSA cells were measured. MRSA were incubated with 3′-(p-aminophenyl) fluorescein (APF) for $^{\bullet}OH$, $ClO^-$, and $ONOO^-$, HPF for $^{\bullet}OH$ and $ONOO^-$, MitoSOX™ Red mitochondrial superoxide indicator for $O_2^{\bullet-}$ and trans-1-(2′-methoxyvinyl)pyrene (tMVP) for $^1O_2$, then exposed to plasma or plasma-activated saline for 40 s, and the levels of different ROS/RNS determined by changes in the fluorescence intensities (**Figure 4**). After plasma treatment, the fluorescence intensities of the four probes increased. The fluorescence intensities of MRSA incubated with APF and HPF increased slightly after 30 min of plasma treatment, by 28 and 25%, respectively, which indicates an increase in the levels of $^{\bullet}OH$, $ClO^-$, and $ONOO^-$ (**Figures 4A,B**). Fluorescence of MRSA incubated with MitoSOX™ Red mitochondrial superoxide indicator increased by 77%, and the trans-1-(2′-methoxyvinyl)pyrene (tMVP) for $^1O_2$ increased by 130% after 30 min of plasma treatment (**Figures 4C,D**). The fluorescence intensities of the probes which incubated with plasma-activated saline-treated MRSA were slightly weaker than those of the direct plasma-treated samples. These data suggested that the plasma and plasma-activated saline treatment induced the increases of many species of ROS and RNS in MRSA cells.

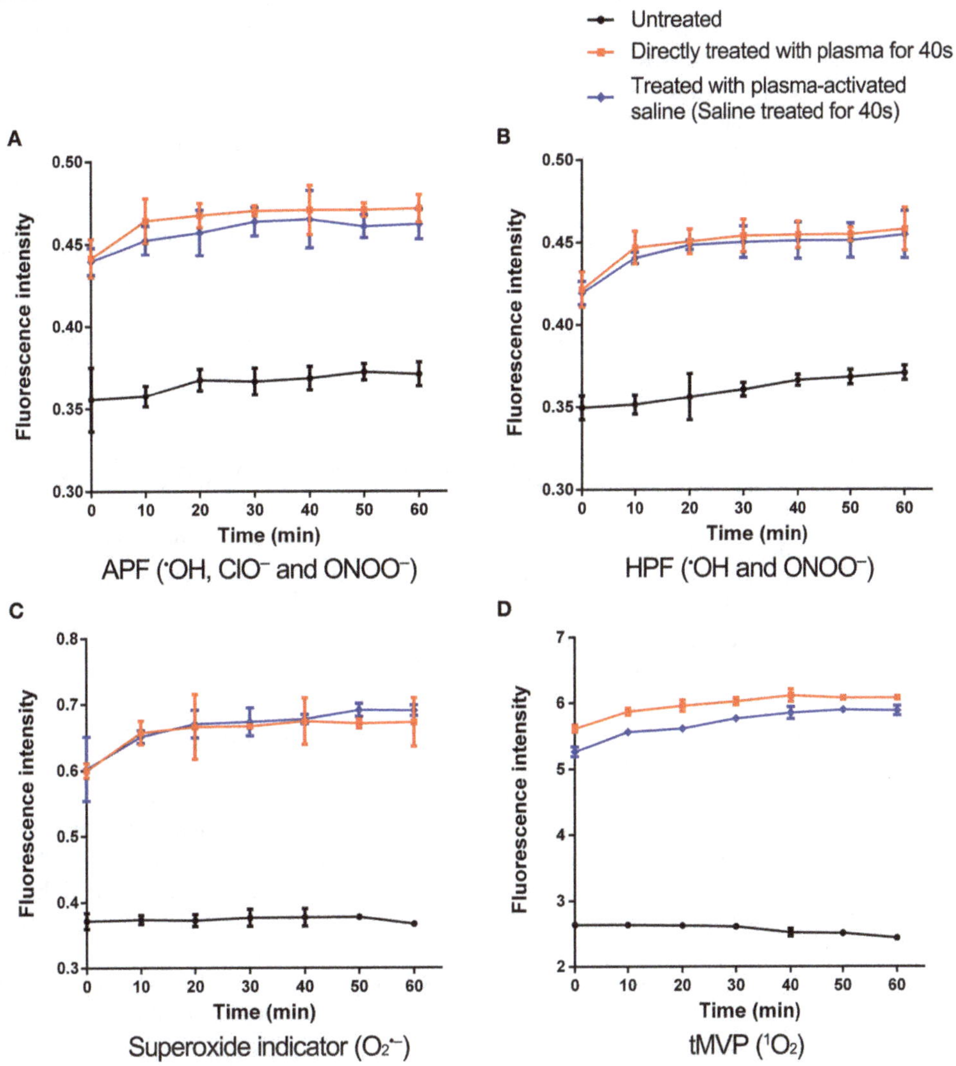


**FIGURE 4 |** ROS and RNS levels increased in plasma-treated and plasma-activated saline-treated MRSA. MRSA incorporated with APF **(A)**, HPF **(B)**, superoxide indicator **(C)**, and tMVP **(D)**, which measured the ROS or RNS as indicated, treated with plasma for 40 s or saline treated with plasma for 40 s. Then the fluorescence intensities of were measured in plasma-treated, plasma-activated saline-treated, and untreated MRSA. Data are representative of three independent experiments. Error bars represent s.d.

## DISCUSSION

In this study, we demonstrated that treating MRSA sublethally with plasma-generated ROS and RNS decreased the MICs of several antibiotics and increased persister eradication, along with increases in the levels of ROS and RNS in MRSA cells. Plasma-activated saline had the same effect upon the antibiotic sensitivity of MRSA and persister inactivation as direct plasma treatment, suggesting that the plasma-generated ROS and RNS could be applied in both gaseous or aqueous form depending on the mode of application. The short-lived species in the plasma-activated saline had short half-lives, but they could react and generate long-lived species, which also could generate to short-lived species reversibly, such as $ONOO^-$ generated from $NO_3^-$ (Oehmigen et al., 2011; Liu et al., 2017). Plasma generated various ROS, which are involved in a great many chemical reactions (Oehmigen et al., 2011). The underlying reactions and detailed mechanisms of plasma-activated saline are still not well understand and require further study.

Unlike other treatments that have previously been used as antibiotic adjuvants to enhance ROS production in bacterial cells, plasma induces the production of a wider range of ROS species (Morones-Ramirez et al., 2013; Shen et al., 2016). The ROS and RNS generated by the plasma constitute a complex mix of products, including $^\bullet OH$, $^1O_2$, $O_2^{\bullet -}$, $ONOO^-$, and $ClO^-$ (Liu et al., 2016). Subsequently, these many different ROS or RNS species were also detected in plasma-treated bacterial cells. The intracellular ROS and RNS could induce oxidative stresses, such as damaging lipids, proteins and DNA by $^\bullet OH$, $^1O_2$, and $O_2^{\bullet -}$, as well as protein damages by

$ONOO^-$ and $ClO^-$ (Davies, 2016). $O_2^{\bullet-}$ could be detoxified by endogenous antioxidants of the oxidative response, but no enzyme can detoxify $^{\bullet}OH$ or $^1O_2$, and MRSA could not detoxify all the multiple reactive species induced by plasma (Vatansever et al., 2013). It was speculated that the compound damages stimulated multiple response pathways and kept MRSA busy with repairing, which contributed to the effects of antibiotics.

Reactive species generated by plasma could also induce damages in eukaryotic cells, subsequently, the safety and toxicity of this application should be considered. The $CC_{50}$ of the plasma treatment used in this study for human primary dermal fibroblasts was about 40 s treatment, which was close to the $LD_{50}$ on MRSA (Figure S4A). Comparing with bacterial cells, the cultured cells are more easily to be inactivated *in vitro* because of the lack of cell wall. However, the plasma treatment did not increase micronuclei formation in fibroblast cells (Figures S4B,C). Coincidently, a newly published paper found similar results on lymphocyte TK6 cells (Bekeschus et al., 2018). Further, the olive tail moment of plasma-treated cells exhibited little difference with that of untreated cells (Figures S4D,E). So the plasma treatment did not remarkably increase the mutagenicity of fibroblasts as demonstrated by both micronucleus assay and comet assay. Besides, Maisch et al. (2012) showed that gas plasma could efficiently inactivate *S. aureus* and *Escherichia coli* on pig skin without inducing morphological changes or damage-related apoptosis. Clinical trials also demonstrated that 5 min daily treatment with plasma decreased bacteria in chronic wounds of patients without side effects (Isbary et al., 2010). These studies demonstrated the safety of plasma treatment under limited conditions. Many topical biocides are toxic, and the plasma could be developed as alternative, especially the plasma-activated saline could be the save alternative (Wales and Davies, 2015). When used as a sensitizer with antibiotics as was done in this study, the doses of plasma were much lower than that used for bacteria inactivation, which would reduce the risk of toxicity and improve the safety.

In conclusion, sublethal treatment with plasma-generated ROS and RNS decreased the MICs of several antibiotics and increased persister eradication, along with increases in the levels of ROS and RNS in MRSA. Plasma and plasma-activated saline could be explored as a novel antibiotic sensitizer to generate oxidative stress to combat the increasing problem of antibiotic resistance. Further studies are needed to test these methods against other multidrug-resistant bacteria and to elucidate the underlying mechanism.

## AUTHOR CONTRIBUTIONS

LG, RX, and YZ designed and executed most of the experiments and analyzed the data. ZL assisted in the execution of some experiments. LG, DL, and MK wrote the manuscript. MK, LG, DL, XW, and HC reviewed and approved the final version of the manuscript.

## ACKNOWLEDGMENTS

This work was supported by National Natural Science Foundation of China (51477136 and 51521065), Doctoral Fund of Ministry of Education of China (2017M613106), Doctoral Fund of Ministry of Education of Shaanxi Province, State Key Laboratory of Agricultural Microbiology (AMLKF201705), State Key Laboratory of Electrical Insulation and Power Equipment (EIPE14123), and Fundamental Research Funds for the Central Universities.

## REFERENCES

Bayliss, D. L., Shama, G., and Kong, M. G. (2013). Restoration of antibiotic sensitivity in meticillin-resistant *Staphylococcus aureus* following treatment with a non-thermal atmospheric gas plasma. *Int. J. Antimicrob. Agents* 41, 398–399. doi: 10.1016/j.ijantimicag.2012.12.005

Bekeschus, S., Schmidt, A., Kramer, A., Metelmann, H. R., Adler, F., von Woedtke, T., et al. (2018). High throughput image cytometry micronucleus assay to investigate the presence or absence of mutagenic effects of cold physical plasma. *Environ. Mol. Mutagen.* doi: 10.1002/em.22172. [Epub ahead of print].

Boucher, H. W., Talbot, G. H., Bradley, J. S., Edwards, J. E., Gilbert, D., Rice, L. B., et al. (2009). Bad bugs, no drugs: no ESKAPE! An update from the infectious diseases society of America. *Clin. Infect. Dis.* 48, 1–12. doi: 10.1086/595011

Brynildsen, M. P., Winkler, J. A., Spina, C. S., MacDonald, I. C., and Collins, J. J. (2013). Potentiating antibacterial activity by predictably enhancing endogenous microbial ROS production. *Nat. Biotechnol.* 31, 160–165. doi: 10.1038/nbt.2458

Davies, M. J. (2016). Protein oxidation and peroxidation. *Biochem. J.* 473, 805–825. doi: 10.1042/BJ20151227

Dharmaraja, A. T. (2017). Role of Reactive Oxygen Species (ROS) in therapeutics and drug resistance in cancer and bacteria. *J. Med. Chem.* 60, 3221–3240. doi: 10.1021/acs.jmedchem.6b01243

Dwyer, D. J., Belenky, P. A., Yang, J. H., MacDonald, I. C., Martell, J. D., Takahashi, N., et al. (2014). Antibiotics induce redox-related physiological alterations as part of their lethality. *Proc. Natl. Acad. Sci. U.S.A.* 111, E2100–E2109. doi: 10.1073/pnas.1401876111

Emaneini, M., Beigverdi, R., van Leeuwen, W. B., Rahdar, H., Karami-Zarandi, M., Hosseinkhani, F., et al. (2017). Prevalence of methicillin-resistant *Staphylococcus aureus* isolated from burn patients: a systematic review and meta-analysis. *J. Glob. Antimicrob. Resist.* 12, 202–206. doi: 10.1016/j.jgar.2017.10.015

Fridman, G., Friedman, G., Gutsol, A., Shekhter, A. B., Vasilets, V. N., and Fridman, A. (2008). Applied plasma medicine. *Plasma Process. Polym.* 5, 503–533. doi: 10.1002/ppap.200700154

Gonzalez-Bello, C. (2017). Antibiotic adjuvants - a strategy to unlock bacterial resistance to antibiotics. *Bioorg. Med. Chem. Lett.* 27, 4221–4228. doi: 10.1016/j.bmcl.2017.08.027

Heinlin, J., Zimmermann, J. L., Zeman, F., Bunk, W., Isbary, G., Landthaler, M., et al. (2013). Randomized placebo-controlled human pilot study of cold atmospheric argon plasma on skin graft donor sites. *Wound Repair Regen.* 21, 800–807. doi: 10.1111/wrr.12078

Isbary, G., Heinlin, J., Shimizu, T., Zimmermann, J. L., Morfill, G., Schmidt, H. U., et al. (2012). Successful and safe use of 2 min cold atmospheric argon plasma in chronic wounds: results of a randomized controlled trial. *Br. J. Dermatol.* 167, 404–410. doi: 10.1111/j.1365-2133.2012.10923.x

Isbary, G., Morfill, G., Schmidt, H. U., Georgi, M., Ramrath, K., Heinlin, J., et al. (2010). A first prospective randomized controlled trial to decrease bacterial load using cold atmospheric argon plasma on chronic wounds in patients. *Br. J. Dermatol.* 163, 78–82. doi: 10.1111/j.1365-2133.2010.09744.x

Kang, M. H., Hong, Y. J., Attri, P., Sim, G. B., Lee, G. J., Panngom, K., et al. (2014). Analysis of the antimicrobial effects of nonthermal plasma on fungal spores in ionic solutions. *Free Radic. Biol. Med.* 72, 191–199. doi: 10.1016/j.freeradbiomed.2014.04.023

Kohanski, M. A., Dwyer, D. J., and Collins, J. J. (2010). How antibiotics kill bacteria: from targets to networks. *Nat. Rev. Microbiol.* 8, 423–435. doi: 10.1038/nrmicro2333

Kohanski, M. A., Dwyer, D. J., Hayete, B., Lawrence, C. A., and Collins, J. J. (2007). A common mechanism of cellular death induced by bactericidal antibiotics. *Cell* 130, 797–810. doi: 10.1016/j.cell.2007.06.049

Kong, M. G., Kroesen, G., Morfill, G., Nosenko, T., Shimizu, T., Dijk J. V., et al. (2009). Plasma medicine: an introductory review. *New J. Phys.* 11:115012. doi: 10.1088/1367-2630/11/11/115012

Lepe, J. A., Domínguez-Herrera, J., Pachón, J., and Aznar, J. (2014). Determining accurate vancomycin MIC values for methicillin-resistant *Staphylococcus aureus* by the microdilution method. *J. Antimicrob. Chemother.* 69, 136–138. doi: 10.1093/jac/dkt308

Levin, B. R., and Rozen, D. E. (2006). Non-inherited antibiotic resistance. *Nat. Rev. Microbiol.* 4, 556–562. doi: 10.1038/nrmicro1445

Li, J., Xie, S., Ahmed, S., Wang, F., Gu, Y., Zhang, C., et al. (2017). Antimicrobial activity and resistance: influencing factors. *Front. Pharmacol.* 8:364. doi: 10.3389/fphar.2017.00364

Liu, D. X., Liu, Z. C., Chen, C., Yang, A. J., Li, D., Rong, M. Z., et al. (2016). Aqueous reactive species induced by a surface air discharge: heterogeneous mass transfer and liquid chemistry pathways. *Sci. Rep.* 6:23737. doi: 10.1038/srep23737

Liu, Z. C., Guo, L., Liu, D. X., Rong, M. Z., Chen, H. L., and Kong, M. G. (2017). Chemical kinetics and reactive species in normal saline activated by a surface air discharge. *Plasma Process. Polym.* 14:1600113. doi: 10.1002/ppap.201600113

Lloyd, G., Friedman, G., Jafri, S., Schultz, G., Fridman, A., and Harding, K. (2010). Gas Plasma: medical uses and developments in wound care. *Plasma Process. Polym.* 7, 194–211. doi: 10.1002/ppap.200900097

Maisch, T., Shimizu, T., Li, Y. F., Heinlin, J., Karrer, S., Morfill, G., et al. (2012). Decolonisation of MRSA, *S. aureus* and *E. coli* by cold-atmospheric plasma using a porcine skin model *in vitro*. *PLoS ONE* 7:e34610. doi: 10.1371/journal.pone.0034610

Melander, R. J., and Melander, C. (2017). The challenge of overcoming antibiotic resistance: an adjuvant approach? *ACS Infect. Dis.* 3, 559–563. doi: 10.1021/acsinfecdis.7b00071

Moreau, M., Orange, N., and Feuilloley, M. G. (2008). Non-thermal plasma technologies: new tools for bio-decontamination. *Biotechnol. Adv.* 26, 610–617. doi: 10.1016/j.biotechadv.2008.08.001

Morones-Ramirez, J. R., Winkler, J. A., Spina, C. S., and Collins, J. J. (2013). Silver enhances antibiotic activity against gram-negative bacteria. *Sci. Transl. Med.* 5:190ra181. doi: 10.1126/scitranslmed.3006276

Oehmigen, K., Winter, J., Hähnel, M., Wilke, C., Brandenburg, R., Weltmann, K., et al. (2011). Estimation of possible mechanisms of *Escherichia coli* inactivation by plasma treated sodium chloride solution. *Plasma Process. Polym.* 8, 904–913. doi: 10.1002/ppap.201000099

Schmieder, R., and Edwards, R. (2012). Insights into antibiotic resistance through metagenomic approaches. *Future Microbiol.* 7, 73–89. doi: 10.2217/fmb.11.135

Shahsavan, S., Emaneini, M., Noorazar Khoshgnab, B., Khoramian, B., Asadollahi, P., Aligholi, M., et al. (2012). A high prevalence of mupirocin and macrolide resistance determinant among *Staphylococcus aureus* strains isolated from burnt patients. *Burns* 38, 378–382. doi: 10.1016/j.burns.2011.09.004

Shen, F., Tang, X., Cheng, W., Wang, Y., Wang, C., Shi, X., et al. (2016). Fosfomycin enhances phagocyte-mediated killing of *Staphylococcus aureus* by extracellular traps and reactive oxygen species. *Sci. Rep.* 6:19262. doi: 10.1038/srep19262

Vatansever, F., de Melo, W. C. M. A., Avci, P., Vecchio, D., Sadasivam, M., Gupta, A., et al. (2013). Antimicrobial strategies centered around reactive oxygen species - bactericidal antibiotics, photodynamic therapy, and beyond. *FEMS Microbiol. Rev.* 37, 955–989. doi: 10.1111/1574-6976.12026

Wales, A. D., and Davies, R. H. (2015). Co-Selection of resistance to antibiotics, biocides and heavy metals, and its relevance to foodborne pathogens. *Antibiotics* 4, 567–604. doi: 10.3390/antibiotics4040567

Wright, G. D. (2016). Antibiotic adjuvants: rescuing antibiotics from resistance. *Trends Microbiol.* 24, 862–871. doi: 10.1016/j.tim.2016.06.009

2

# Emergence of a Clinical *Escherichia coli* Sequence Type 131 Strain Carrying a Chromosomal $bla_{KPC-2}$ Gene

*Dairong Wang[1,2†], Xinli Mu[1,3†], Ying Chen[1,3], Dongdong Zhao[1,3], Ying Fu[3,4], Yan Jiang[1,3], Yiwei Zhu[1,3], Jingjing Quan[1,3], Xiaoting Hua[1,3], Guofeng Mao[5], Xi Li[6]* and Yunsong Yu[1,3]**

*[1] Department of Infectious Diseases, Sir Run Run Shaw Hospital, College of Medicine, Zhejiang University, Hangzhou, China, [2] Blood Center of Zhejiang Province, Hangzhou, China, [3] Key Laboratory of Microbial Technology and Bioinformatics of Zhejiang Province, Zhejiang Institute of Microbiology, Hangzhou, China, [4] Department of Clinical Laboratory, Sir Run Run Shaw Hospital, College of Medicine, Zhejiang University, Hangzhou, China, [5] Department of Laboratory Medicine, Shaoxing People's Hospital, Shaoxing, China, [6] Centre of Laboratory Medicine, Zhejiang Provincial People's Hospital, People's Hospital of Hangzhou Medical College, Hangzhou, China*

***Correspondence:**
*Xi Li*
*lixi_0611@163.com*
*Yunsong Yu*
*yvys119@zju.edu.cn*

*†These authors have contributed equally to this work and share first authorship*

**Objectives:** Bacteria carrying the *Klebsiella pneumoniae* carbapenemase genes have rapidly spread worldwide and have become a great threat to public health. The $bla_{KPC-2}$ gene has been primarily located on plasmids cocirculating in various strains. However, chromosomal integration of the $bla_{KPC-2}$ gene in *Escherichia coli* has not been reported. In the present study, we report the detection of the first clinical strain of *E. coli* ST131 with a $bla_{KPC-2}$ gene, which integrated in the chromosome. *E. coli* strain EC3385 was identified and subjected to susceptibility testing and genotyping. The complete genome sequences of this strain and four *Proteus mirabilis* strains were obtained. Chromosomal integration of the $bla_{KPC-2}$ gene was confirmed using a combination of short- and long-read sequencing. Comparative genetic analyses were performed and the origin of the chromosomal location of the $bla_{KPC-2}$ gene was further analyzed. Whole-genome sequencing revealed that strain EC3385 belonged to the ST131 type and possessed various resistance and virulence genes. Sequence analysis showed that the $bla_{KPC-2}$ gene was carried in a 24-kb insertion sequence on the chromosome. This insertion sequence possessed high sequence similarity to previously reported $bla_{KPC-2}$-habouring plasmids of *P. mirabilis* in China. To the best of our knowledge, this is the first report of a clinical ST131 *E. coli* strain carrying $bla_{KPC-2}$ on the chromosome. The $bla_{KPC-2}$ gene was probably horizontally transferred from the *P. mirabilis* plasmid to the *E. coli* chromosome by the *IS*26 element, indicating that *P. mirabilis* might be an important reservoir of $bla_{KPC-2}$ gene for *E. coli*. Furthermore, the *E. coli* ST131 strain carrying the chromosomal $bla_{KPC-2}$ gene could be further spread due to its carbapenem resistance and high virulence. It is imperative to perform active surveillance to prevent further dissemination of KPC-2 type carbapenemase-producing isolates.

**Keywords: *E. coli*, KPC-2, cre, resistance mechanism, whole genome sequencing**

## INTRODUCTION

Bacteria carrying the *Klebsiella pneumoniae* carbapenemase genes (*$bla_{KPC}$*) have rapidly spread worldwide and have become a great threat to public health because these bacteria are often associated with high morbidity and mortality (Wang et al., 2016; An et al., 2018). KPC-2 is the main type of KPC carbapenemase and is most common in *K. pneumoniae* bacteria. In China, clonal spreading is a main mode of transfer of KPC-2 type carbapenemase-producing *K. pneumonia*. Our previous research demonstrated that multilocus sequence type 11 (ST11) originated from a successful lineage of KPC-2 type carbapenemase-producing *K. pneumonia* in China (Qi et al., 2011).

In contrast to *K. pneumoniae*, *E. coli* strains have rarely been reported to carry the *$bla_{KPC-2}$* gene. However, recent reports found that the number of *E. coli* strains carrying the *$bla_{KPC-2}$* gene has increased. In addition, unlike *K. pneumoniae*, clonal spread has not been found for the *$bla_{KPC-2}$* gene of *E. coli* (Chen et al., 2014). These strains also have different clone types, such as ST131, ST410, ST2281, ST43, ST721, ST4385, and ST8 (Kim et al., 2012; Mavroidi et al., 2012; Tian et al., 2020). Notably, among these clone types, *E. coli* ST131, an international multidrug-resistant high-risk clone, has gained a further selective advantage as a result of acquiring carbapenem resistance (Rogers et al., 2011; Kim et al., 2012) and *E. coli* ST131 may become a successful lineage of KPC-2 type carbapenemase-producing *E. coli*.

In addition, *K. pneumoniae* carbapenemase genes have been primarily located on plasmids cocirculating with various strains (Nordmann et al., 2011). They are considered a major mechanism responsible for the dramatic increase in the prevalence of carbapenem-resistant *Enterobacteriaceae* isolates. Plasmid DNA can act as a temporary "lending library" allowing vital genes to survive various selective pressures (Harrison et al., 2015). Notably, *in vitro* data demonstrated that once a gene is incorporated into a chromosome, it is maintained through replication without being subject to selective pressures, and gene loss from bacterial populations is rare (Bergstrom et al., 2000; Bahl et al., 2009; Carraro et al., 2015). Interestingly, the earliest observed chromosomal *$bla_{KPC}$* gene integration events have been sporadic in gram-negative bacteria, such as *Pseudomonas aeruginosa* in 2006 (Villegas et al., 2007), *Raoultella spp.* in 2008 (Castanheira et al., 2009) and *Acinetobacter baumannii* in 2009 (Martínez et al., 2014). Recently, chromosomal integration has been described in four *K. pneumoniae* ST258 isolates (Conlan et al., 2014; Chen et al., 2015; Mathers et al., 2017). However, *$bla_{KPC-2}$* gene chromosomal integration events in *E. coli* have not been reported.

In the present study, we report the detection of the first clinical strain of *E. coli* ST131 with a chromosomal *$bla_{KPC-2}$* gene integrated in the chromosome. In addition, the genetic origin of this gene was further analyzed using whole-genome sequencing.

## MATERIALS AND METHODS

### Patient and Strain Data

A patient was admitted to the hospital for a craniocerebral infarction in 2017. A carbapenem-resistant strain of *E. coli* EC3385 was isolated from sputum because the patient developed hospital-acquired pneumonia (HAP) secondary to postoperative intubation during the hospitalization. In addition, four *P. mirabilis* strains isolated at the same period (**Table 1**) as *E. coli* EC3385 in the ICU department were analyzed retrospectively. These strains were preliminary identified by the VITEK 2 system (Sysmex-bioMérieux, Marcy l'Etoile, France) and further confirmed by 16S rRNA sequencing.

### Antibiotic Susceptibility Test

Antibiotic susceptibility was determined using the VITEK 2 system and broth microdilution method and the results were interpreted according to the Clinical and Laboratory Standard Institute (CLSI) guidelines (CLSI, 2017) except for tigecycline and colistin, which were interpreted according to the European Committee on Antimicrobial Susceptibility Testing breakpoints for *Enterobacteriaceae*[1].

### Whole-Genome Sequencing and Assembly

Total genomic DNA extraction and analysis were performed as previously described (Li et al., 2018). Briefly, *E. coli* strain EC3385 and four *P. mirabilis* strains were cultured to mid-logarithmic phase in 50 ml of MH medium at 37°C. The

[1]http://www.eucast.org/clinical_breakpoints

**TABLE 1** | Strains collection date and Vitek-2 antibiotic susceptibility.

| Isolates | Collection day | MICs (mg/L) | | | | | | | | | | | |
|---|---|---|---|---|---|---|---|---|---|---|---|---|---|
| | | AMK | CZA[a] | CRO | CST[a] CIP | ETP | GEN | IPM[a] | LEV | TGC[a] | SXT | TGC | TZP |
| *E. coli* EC3385 | 10-03-2017 | ≤2 | 0.25 | ≥64 | 0.25 ≥ 4 | ≥8 | ≤1 | 64 | ≥8 | 0.125 | ≤1/19 | ≤0.5 | ≥128 |
| PM380 | 10-03-2017 | ≤2 | 0.125 | ≥64 | - ≥ 4 | ≥8 | ≥16 | 64 | ≥8 | - | ≥16/304 | - | 64 |
| PM906 | 21-03-2017 | ≤2 | 0.125 | ≥64 | - ≥ 4 | ≥8 | ≥16 | 64 | ≥8 | - | ≥16/304 | - | 64 |
| PM431 | 11-03-2017 | ≤2 | 0.125 | ≥64 | - ≥ 4 | ≥8 | ≥16 | 64 | ≥8 | - | ≥16/304 | - | 64 |
| PM187 | 08-02-2017 | ≤2 | 0.125 | ≥64 | - ≥ 4 | ≥8 | ≥16 | 64 | ≥8 | - | ≥16/304 | - | 64 |
| *E. coli* ATCC 25922 | NA | ≤2 | ≤0.125 | ≤1 | 0.125 ≤0.25 | ≤0.5 | ≤1 | ≤1 | ≤0.25 | 0.125 | ≤1/19 | ≤0.5 | ≤4 |

[a] *Drug susceptibility was determined with broth microdilution method according to the Clinical Laboratory Standards Institute (CLSI) guidelines. NA, not applicable. AMK, amikacin; CZA, Ceftazidime-avibactam; CRO, ceftriaxone; CST, colistin; CIP, Ciprofloxacin; ETP, ertapenem; GEN, gentamicin; IPM, imipenem; LEV, levofloxacin; SXT, trimethoprim-sulfamethoxazole. TGC, Tigecycline, TZP, piperacillin-tazobactam.*

**TABLE 2 |** Genome and plasmids of *E. coli* EC3385.

| Genomic structure | Size (bp) | GC content(%) | CDS no. | rRNA no. | tRNA no. | Accession no. | Resistance genes | Virulence genes | Incompatibility |
|---|---|---|---|---|---|---|---|---|---|
| EC3385 chromosome | 4,910,422 | 50.9 | 4749 | 66 | 267 | CP029420 | $bla_{KPC-2}$ | *iss, gad,lpfA,chuA fyuA,irp2,kpsMII_K5 ompT,sitA,terC,traT, Usp,yfcV* | – |
| EC3385-P1 plasmid | 101,340 | 46.3 | 121 | – | 9 | CP029421 | – | – | incFIB |
| EC3385-P2 plasmid | 89,323 | 50.5 | 132 | – | – | CP029422 | $bla_{TEM-1B}$ | – | incFIA |

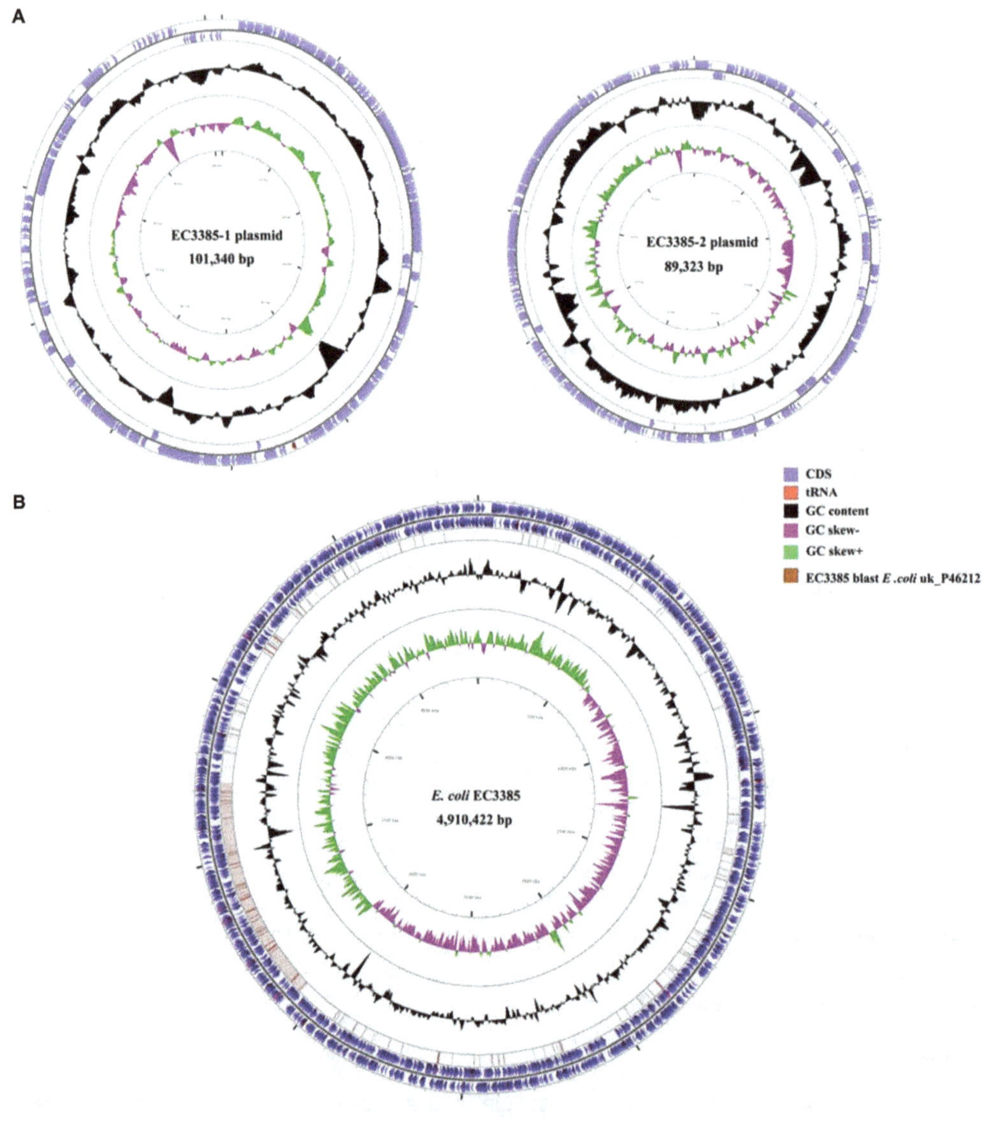


**FIGURE 1 |** Circular maps of the *E. coli* EC3385 genome and its plasmids. **(A)** Circular graphs of two plasmids. **(B)** Circular graph of the EC3385 genome sequence and genome alignment. Blue arrows denote coding sequences, red arrows denote tRNA genes, and replication genes are denoted by green arrows. Genome alignment between EC3385 and *E. coli* uk_P46212 is shown in the outer circle in pink, and the GC content is shown in the inner circle in black. The region surrounding the $bla_{KPC-2}$ gene is highlighted with a red frame.

genomic DNA of these strains was extracted using a QIAamp DNA MiniKit (Qiagen, Valencia, CA, United States) following the manufacturer's recommendations. The DNA library was prepared using a Nextera XT DNA library preparation kit (Illumina, Inc., Cambridge, United Kingdom), and genomic DNA was sequenced on an Illumina HiSeq 4000 instrument with a 150-bp paired-end approach at a depth of approximately 200 × . The raw reads of the strains were assembled into draft genomes using the CLC Genomics Workbench 10.0.

In addition, *E. coli* EC3385 strain sequencing was further performed via a single molecule real-time (SMRT) technique using a PacBio RS II platform and the resulting sequences were assembled *de novo* using the hierarchical genome assembly process (HGAP) with the default settings of the SMRT Analysis v2.3.0 software package (Shen et al., 2017).

## Genome Annotation and *in silico* Analyses

The Rapid Annotation using Subsystems Technology (RAST) annotation website server[2] was used to annotate the genomes. Multi-locus sequence typing (MLST) of resistance genes and the Inc-type plasmid of the strain were performed using the MLST 1.8 server, ResFinder 3.0, Virulence Finder 1.5, and Plasmid Finder 1.3, which are available at the Center for Genomic Epidemiology[3]. Graphical maps were generated by the CGView server[4]. A comparison of the insert sequence of this strain and its related plasmids was performed with EasyFig 2.2.2 (Sullivan et al., 2011).

## Phylogenetic Analysis

Phylogenetic analysis of these *P. mirabilis* strains was performed. Genome sequences of other *P. mirabilis* strains were downloaded from the RefSeq database. Our strains were annotated by Prokka (Seemann, 2014) using the *P. mirabilis* proteins from the RefSeq database as a prior reference. The core genome was determined by Roary (Page et al., 2015) using Mafft for multiple sequence alignment. A maximum-likelihood phylogenetic tree was inferred by RAxML (Stamatakis, 2014) using the GTRGAMMA model for nucleotide substitution and running with 100 bootstraps. The phylogenetic tree was visualized by iTOL (Letunic and Bork, 2019).

## Nucleotide Sequence Accession Numbers

The complete nucleotide sequences of the chromosome and three plasmids of *E. coli* strain EC3385 reported in the present study were deposited in the GenBank nucleotide database under accession numbers CP029420, CP029421, and CP029422, respectively.

Sequence data from four *P. mirabilis* strains were also deposited in GenBank as follows:

CAV1042, CP018671.1; CAV1392, CP011578.1; CAV1453, CP018356.1.

# RESULTS AND DISCUSSION

## Clinical Microbiologic Characteristics

The antimicrobial susceptibility test results showed that *E. coli* strain EC3385 was resistant to multiple antimicrobial agents, including cephalosporins, carbapenems and fluoroquinolones, but it was susceptible to aminoglycosides, ceftazidime-avibactam, colistin, and tigecycline (**Table 1**).

[2] http://rast.nmpdr.org/rast/cgi

[3] http://www.genomicepidemiology.org/

[4] http://stothard.afns.ualberta.ca/cgview_server/

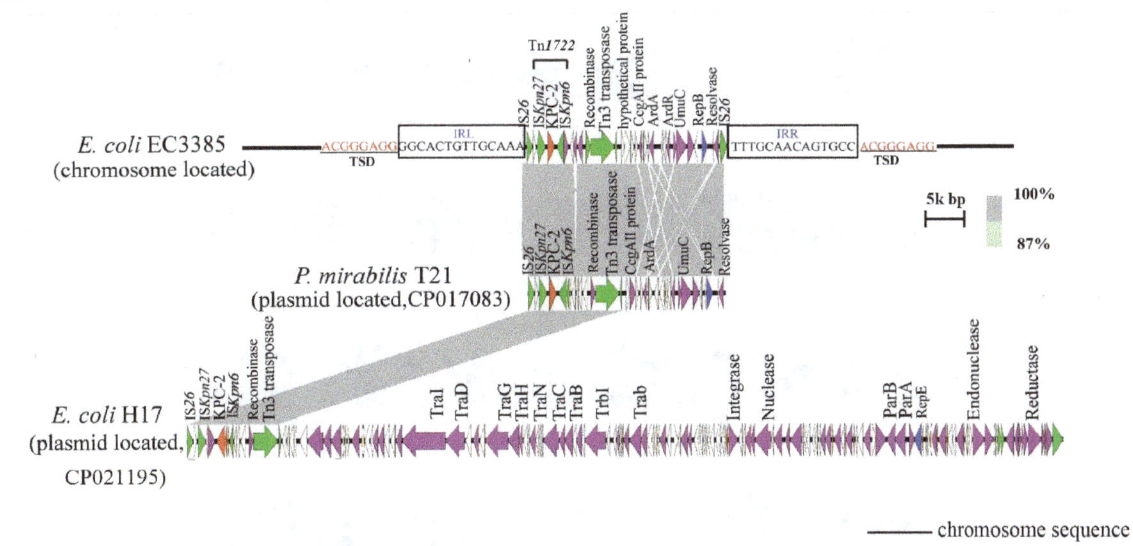


**FIGURE 2** | Linear comparison of the 24-kb insertion sequence with closely related plasmids. The gray regions between plasmids indicate nucleotide identity (87–100%) determined by BLASTn. Arrows indicate predicted open reading frames (ORFs). The primary structural characteristics of the 24-kb insertion sequence are compared to plasmids pT21 (CP017083) and pH17 (CP021195). Colored arrows represent ORFs, with red, purple, yellow, green, and white representing antibiotic resistance genes; replication, recombination and repair genes; plasmid stability genes; mobile elements and plasmid transfer related-genes; and genes with unknown function genes, respectively.

Multi-locus sequence typing analysis showed that this strain belonged to the ST131 type. The ST131-type *E. coli* clonal group emerged in the mid-2000s and has since spread extensively throughout the world (Can et al., 2015). Currently, the ST131 type is a very successful pandemic clone associated with community- and hospital-acquired infections. Many studies have demonstrated that this clone has high virulence potential and is associated with treatment failure (Can et al., 2015). In this study, VirulenceFinder analysis showed the presence of multiple potential virulence factors, such as *iss* (increased serum survival), *lpfA* (long polar fimbriae), and *gad* (glutamate decarboxylase) (**Table 2**). In addition, this clone is responsible for the rapid increase in β-lactam resistance among *E. coli*, mainly due to the production of CTX-M type extended spectrum β-lactamase enzymes (ESBLs) (Nicolas-Chanoine et al., 2014).

Interestingly, the isolate in this study did not carry additional genes encoding the CTX-M enzyme. A recent study reported that ESBL-negative ST131 strains have also been isolated worldwide (Ripabelli et al., 2020). In this study, no ESBL-encoding gene was detected in *E. coli* strain EC3385; instead, the $bla_{KPC-2}$ gene, which encodes the KPC-2 type β-lactamase was identified by PCR amplification and sequencing.

## Chromosomal Integration of the $bla_{KPC-2}$ Gene

*Escherichia coli* strain EC3385 carried the $bla_{KPC-2}$ gene, which is primarily located on plasmids. However, further plasmid transfer and location experiments were not successful (data not shown), suggesting that the $bla_{KPC-2}$ gene was located on

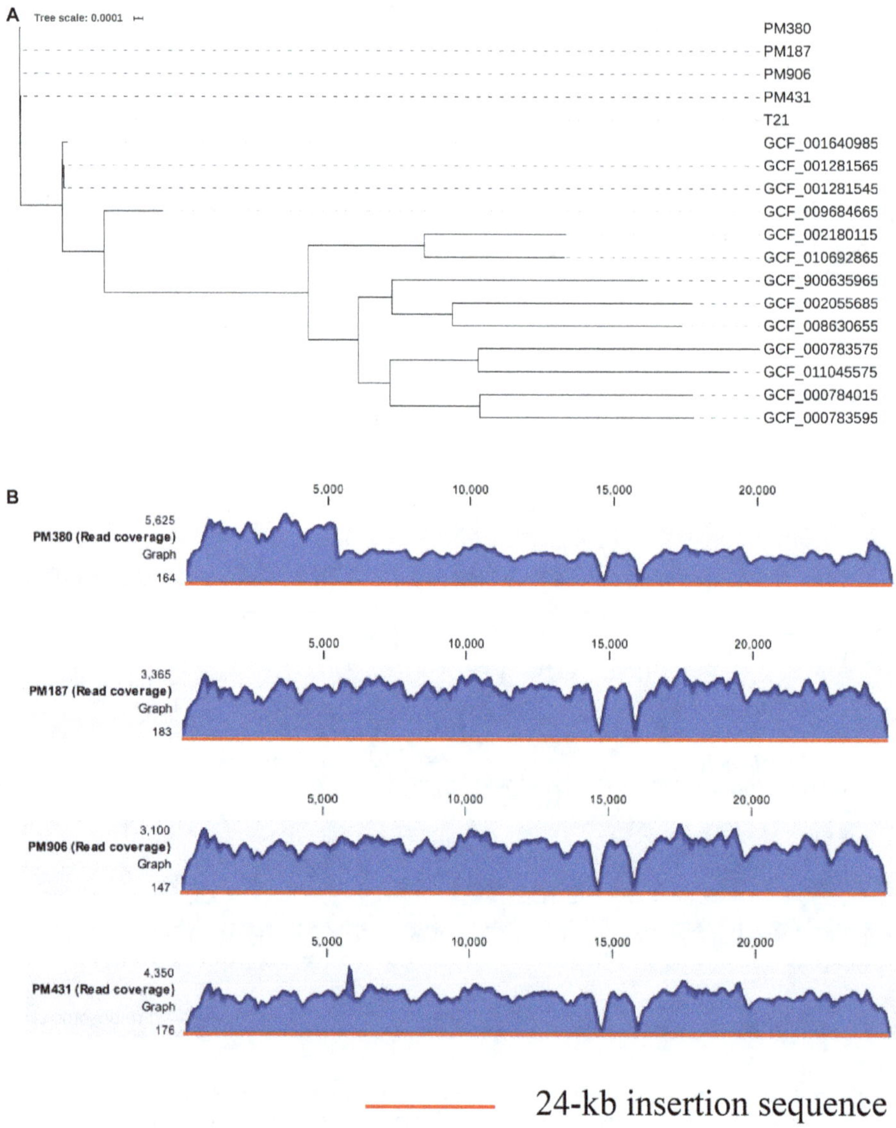


**FIGURE 3 | (A)** A maximum-likelihood phylogenetic analysis of *P. mirabilis* strains. **(B)** Coverage of Illumina reads for four *P. mirabilis* strains (PM380, PM187, PM906, and PM431) mapped to the 24-kb insertion shown in **Figure 2**. The mean coverage for each strain is denoted by a curve (blue).

the chromosome. Notably, a CTX-M type β-lactamase gene was found to be integrated in the chromosome of a high-risk *E. coli* ST131 clone by vertical transmission (Cerquetti et al., 2010; Stoesser et al., 2016), indicating that the ST131 type *E. coli* strain might have the ability to integrate resistance genes into chromosomes.

To determine the gene location, whole-genome sequencing was performed. The whole-genome sequencing data were assembled, and a circular chromosome and two plasmids were generated (**Table 2**). The size of the genome was 4,910,422 bp, with a GC content of 50.9%, 66 rRNA operons, 267 tRNAs, and 4749 predicted protein-coding sequences (**Table 2**). Two plasmids approximately 89 to 101 kb in size and having a GC content between 50.5 and 46.3% were grouped into identifiable replicon types (**Table 2** and **Figure 1**). Notably, the chromosomal location of the $bla_{KPC-2}$ gene was determined using PacBio sequencing. Furthermore, the resequencing results further confirmed that the $bla_{KPC-2}$ gene was located on the chromosome.

To evaluate the molecular basis of chromosomal integration, the chromosomal region encompassing the $bla_{KPC-2}$ gene in the closed PacBio assembly of the ST131 type EC3385 isolate was aligned to reference the strain *E. coli* uk_P46212 (GenBank accession number CP013658), which belongs to the ST131 clone type. Relative to the reference, the EC3385 strain had a 24-kb insertion sequence in the chromosome, which included Tn1722 and several *IS*s (**Figure 2**).

The $bla_{KPC-2}$ gene in the *E. coli* EC3385 strain was carried on this 24-kb composite transposon-like element flanked by two *IS26* elements, which undergo replicative transposition with 8-bp target site duplication (TSD) (ACGGGAGG). This finding suggests the mobilization of this $bla_{KPC-2}$ gene by the composite transposon formed by *IS26* (**Figure 2**). *IS26* has been demonstrated to undergo frequent intramolecular transposition. The structure of the insert sequence leads to the speculation that the *IS26* element may facilitate recombination between the plasmid and chromosome (He et al., 2015).

A further BLAST search of the 24-kb insertion sequence against the GenBank database[5] revealed that this sequence is highly similar to plasmid pT21 (GenBank accession no.CP017083), which was described in a KPC-2 type carbapenemase- producing *P. mirabilis* strain isolated in Zhejiang, China (Hua et al., 2020), with 99.9% query coverage and a maximum of 100% identity (**Figure 2**). In contrast, this 24-kb insertion sequence is only partly similar (47% query coverage and a maximum of 100% identity) to plasmid pH17-2 (GenBank accession no. CP021195) of a KPC-2 type carbapenemase-producing *E. coli* strain isolated in China (**Figure 2**; Zhao et al., 2018), indicating that capture of the chromosomal $bla_{KPC-2}$ gene from *P. mirabilis* by plasmids is possible.

### Possible Origin of the Chromosomal $bla_{KPC-2}$ Gene

To further clarify the origin of the $bla_{KPC-2}$ gene, four $bla_{KPC-2}$-producing *P. mirabilis* strains isolated during the same period (approximately 2 months, **Table 1**) as *E. coli* EC3385 in the ICU department were analyzed retrospectively. These four *P. mirabilis* strains were all isolated from the sputum of different patients. Notably, a maximum-likelihood phylogenetic analysis between the four *P. mirabilis* strains and *P. mirabilis* T21 carrying the pT21 plasmid revealed that these strains were clustered together and belonged to the same clone (**Figure 3A**). Moreover, the whole-genome sequence analysis revealed that the four *P. mirabilis* strains all possessed a 24-kb insertion sequence (**Figure 3B**), indicating that this 24-kb insertion sequence that integrated into the chromosome of the *E. coli* EC3385 strain may have been acquired from *P. mirabilis* strains. In addition, two *P. mirabilis* strains were isolated before the *E. coli* EC3385 strain was identified, indicating that KPC-2 type carbapenemase-producing *P. mirabilis* strains may have spread in this ICU department. A limitation of this study is the lack of the direct links regarding the transmission between KPC-2 type carbapenemase- producing *P. mirabilis* and *E. coli* EC3385 strains. However, because the patients had stayed in the same department, it is most likely they were exposed to a common source.

## CONCLUSION

In summary, to the best of our knowledge, this is the first report of a clinical ST131 *E. coli* strain carrying the $bla_{KPC-2}$ gene in the chromosome. The $bla_{KPC-2}$ gene was probably horizontally transferred from the *P. mirabilis* plasmid to the *E. coli* chromosome by the *IS26* mobile element, indicating that *P. mirabilis* might be an important reservoir of the $bla_{KPC-2}$ gene for *E. coli*. Furthermore, the discovery of a chromosomal the $bla_{KPC-2}$ gene in an *E. coli* strain is alarming. This gene will be maintained through replication without being subject to selective pressures, as the loss of chromosomal elements from bacterial populations is rare. Therefore, the *E. coli* ST131 strain carrying the $bla_{KPC-2}$ gene in the chromosome would be further spread due to its own carbapenem resistance and high virulence. It is imperative to perform active surveillance to prevent further dissemination of KPC-2 type carbapenemase-producing isolates.

## AUTHOR CONTRIBUTIONS

YY and XL conceived and designed the experiments. DW, XM, and YC performed the experiments. DZ, YZ, XH, GM, JQ, and YF analyzed the data. DW, XL, and YJ wrote the manuscript. All authors read and approved the final manuscript.

## FUNDING

This study was supported by the National Natural Science Foundation of China (31700125) and The Project Supported

[5]http://blast.ncbi.nlm.nih.gov/Blast.cgi

by Zhejiang Provincial Natural Science Foundation of China (Grant no. LY20H200007 and LGF20H200004) and the Medical and Health Research Project of Zhejiang Province, China (2018KY229 and 2020KY420). The funders had no role in the study design, data collection and analysis, decision to publish, or preparation of the manuscript.

## REFERENCES

An, J., Lai, K., Ma, Y., Guo, L., Ye, L., Luo, Y., et al. (2018). Emergence of multiple carbapenemase-producing organisms in single patients: an increasing threat to treatment of infection. *J. Antimicrob. Chemother.* 73, 544–546. doi: 10.1093/jac/dkx411

Bahl, M. I., Hansen, L. H., and Sørensen, S. J. (2009). Persistence mechanisms of conjugative plasmids. *Methods Mol. Biol.* 532, 73–102. doi: 10.1007/978-1-60327-853-9_5

Bergstrom, C. T., Lipsitch, M., and Levin, B. R. (2000). Natural selection, infectious transfer and the existence conditions for bacterial plasmids. *Genetics* 155, 1505–1519.

Can, F., Azap, O. K., Seref, C., Ispir, P., Arslan, H., and Ergonul, O. (2015). Emerging *Escherichia coli* O25b/ST131 clone predicts treatment failure in urinary tract infections. *Clin. Infect. Dis.* 60, 523–527. doi: 10.1093/cid/ciu864

Carraro, N., Poulin, D., and Burrus, V. (2015). Replication and active partition of integrative and conjugative elements (ICEs) of the SXT/R391 family: the line between ICEs and conjugative plasmids is getting thinner. *PLoS Genet.* 11:e1005298. doi: 10.1371/journal.pgen.1005298

Castanheira, M., Deshpande, L. M., DiPersio, J. R., Kang, J., Weinstein, M. P., and Jones, R. N. (2009). First descriptions of blaKPC in *Raoultella* spp. (*R. planticola* and *R. ornithinolytica*): report from the sentry antimicrobial surveillance program. *J. Clin. Microbiol.* 47, 4129–4130. doi: 10.1128/jcm.01502-09

Cerquetti, M., Giufrè, M., García-Fernández, A., Accogli, M., Fortini, D., Luzzi, I., et al. (2010). Ciprofloxacin-resistant, CTX-M-15-producing *Escherichia coli* ST131 clone in extraintestinal infections in Italy. *Clin. Microbiol. Infect.* 16, 1555–1558. doi: 10.1111/j.1469-0691.2010.03162.x

Chen, L., Chavda, K. D., DeLeo, F. R., Bryant, K. A., Jacobs, M. R., Bonomo, R. A., et al. (2015). Genome sequence of a *Klebsiella pneumoniae* sequence type 258 isolate with prophage-encoded *K. pneumoniae* carbapenemase. *Genome Announc.* 3:e659-15. doi: 10.1128/genomeA.00659-15

Chen, L., Hu, H., Chavda, K. D., Zhao, S., Liu, R., Liang, H., et al. (2014). Complete sequence of a KPC-producing IncN multidrug-resistant plasmid from an epidemic *Escherichia coli* sequence type 131 strain in China. *Antimicrob. Agents Chemother.* 58, 2422–2425. doi: 10.1128/aac.02587-13

CLSI (2017). *Performance Standards for Antimicrobial Susceptibility Testing*, 27th Edn. CLSI Supplement M100. Wayne, PA: Clinical and Laboratory Standards Institute.

Conlan, S., Deming, C., Tsai, Y. C., Lau, A. F., Dekker, J. P., Korlach, J., et al. (2014). Complete genome sequence of a *Klebsiella pneumoniae* isolate with chromosomally encoded carbapenem resistance and colibactin synthesis loci. *Genome Announc.* 2, e1332–e1314. doi: 10.1128/genomeA.01332-14

Harrison, E., Guymer, D., Spiers, A. J., Paterson, S., and Brockhurst, M. A. (2015). Parallel compensatory evolution stabilizes plasmids across the parasitism-mutualism continuum. *Curr. Biol.* 25, 2034–2039. doi: 10.1016/j.cub.2015.06.024

He, S., Hickman, A. B., Varani, A. M., Siguier, P., Chandler, M., Dekker, J. P., et al. (2015). Insertion sequence IS26 reorganizes plasmids in clinically isolated multidrug-resistant bacteria by replicative transposition. *mBio* 6:e00762. doi: 10.1128/mBio.00762-15

Hua, X., Zhang, L., Moran, R. A., Xu, Q., Sun, L., van Schaik, W., et al. (2020). Cointegration as a mechanism for the evolution of a KPC-producing multidrug resistance plasmid in *Proteus mirabilis*. *Emerg. Microbes Infect.* 9, 1206–1218. doi: 10.1080/22221751.2020.1773322

Kim, Y. A., Qureshi, Z. A., Adams-Haduch, J. M., Park, Y. S., Shutt, K. A., and Doi, Y. (2012). Features of infections due to *Klebsiella pneumoniae* carbapenemase-producing *Escherichia coli*: emergence of sequence type 131. *Clin. Infect. Dis.* 55, 224–231. doi: 10.1093/cid/cis387

Letunic, I., and Bork, P. (2019). Interactive tree of life (iTOL) v4: recent updates and new developments. *Nucleic Acids Res.* 47, W256–W259. doi: 10.1093/nar/gkz239

Li, X., Fu, Y., Shen, M., Huang, D., Du, X., Hu, Q., et al. (2018). Dissemination of blaNDM-5 gene via an IncX3-type plasmid among non-clonal *Escherichia coli* in China. *Antimicrob. Resist. Infect. Control* 7:59. doi: 10.1186/s13756-018-0349-6

Martínez, T., Vázquez, G. J., Aquino, E. E., Martínez, I., and Robledo, I. E. (2014). ISEcp1-mediated transposition of blaKPC into the chromosome of a clinical isolate of *Acinetobacter baumannii* from puerto rico. *J. Med. Microbiol.* 63(Pt 12), 1644–1648. doi: 10.1099/jmm.0.080721-0

Mathers, A. J., Stoesser, N., Chai, W., Carroll, J., Barry, K., Cherunvanky, A., et al. (2017). Chromosomal integration of the *Klebsiella pneumoniae* Carbapenemase Gene, bla(KPC), in *Klebsiella* species is elusive but not rare. *Antimicrob. Agents Chemother.* 61, e1823–e1816. doi: 10.1128/aac.01823-16

Mavroidi, A., Miriagou, V., Malli, E., Stefos, A., Dalekos, G. N., Tzouvelekis, L. S., et al. (2012). Emergence of *Escherichia coli* sequence type 410 (ST410) with KPC-2 β-lactamase. *Int. J. Antimicrob. Agents* 39, 247–250. doi: 10.1016/j.ijantimicag.2011.11.003

Nicolas-Chanoine, M. H., Bertrand, X., and Madec, J. Y. (2014). *Escherichia coli* ST131, an intriguing clonal group. *Clin. Microbiol. Rev.* 27, 543–574. doi: 10.1128/cmr.00125-13

Nordmann, P., Naas, T., and Poirel, L. (2011). Global spread of carbapenemase-producing *Enterobacteriaceae*. *Emerg. Infect. Dis.* 17, 1791–1798. doi: 10.3201/eid1710.110655

Page, A. J., Cummins, C. A., Hunt, M., Wong, V. K., Reuter, S., Holden, M. T., et al. (2015). Roary: rapid large-scale prokaryote pan genome analysis. *Bioinformatics* 31, 3691–3693. doi: 10.1093/bioinformatics/btv421

Qi, Y., Wei, Z., Ji, S., Du, X., Shen, P., and Yu, Y. (2011). ST11, the dominant clone of KPC-producing *Klebsiella pneumoniae* in China. *J. Antimicrob. Chemother.* 66, 307–312. doi: 10.1093/jac/dkq431

Ripabelli, G., Sammarco, M. L., Scutellà, M., Felice, V., and Tamburro, M. (2020). Carbapenem-resistant KPC- and TEM-producing *Escherichia coli* ST131 isolated from a hospitalized patient with urinary tract infection: first isolation in molise region, Central Italy, July 2018. *Microb. Drug Resist.* 26, 38–45. doi: 10.1089/mdr.2019.0085

Rogers, B. A., Sidjabat, H. E., and Paterson, D. L. (2011). *Escherichia coli* O25b-ST131: a pandemic, multiresistant, community-associated strain. *J. Antimicrob. Chemother.* 66, 1–14. doi: 10.1093/jac/dkq415

Seemann, T. (2014). Prokka: rapid prokaryotic genome annotation. *Bioinformatics* 30, 2068–2069. doi: 10.1093/bioinformatics/btu153

Shen, P., Yi, M., Fu, Y., Ruan, Z., Du, X., Yu, Y., et al. (2017). Detection of an *Escherichia coli* sequence type 167 strain with two tandem copies of blaNDM-1 in the chromosome. *J. Clin. Microbiol.* 55, 199–205. doi: 10.1128/jcm.01581-16

Stamatakis, A. (2014). RAxML version 8: a tool for phylogenetic analysis and post-analysis of large phylogenies. *Bioinformatics* 30, 1312–1313. doi: 10.1093/bioinformatics/btu033

Stoesser, N., Sheppard, A. E., Pankhurst, L., De Maio, N., Moore, C. E., Sebra, R., et al. (2016). Evolutionary history of the global emergence of the *Escherichia coli* epidemic clone ST131. *mBio* 7:e02162. doi: 10.1128/mBio.02162-15

Sullivan, M. J., Petty, N. K., and Beatson, S. A. (2011). Easyfig: a genome comparison visualizer. *Bioinformatics* 27, 1009–1010. doi: 10.1093/bioinformatics/btr039

Tian, X., Zheng, X., Sun, Y., Fang, R., Zhang, S., Zhang, X., et al. (2020). Molecular mechanisms and epidemiology of carbapenem-resistant *Escherichia coli* isolated from Chinese patients during 2002-2017. *Infect. Drug. Resist.* 13, 501–512. doi: 10.2147/idr.s232010

Villegas, M. V., Lolans, K., Correa, A., Kattan, J. N., Lopez, J. A., and Quinn, J. P. (2007). First identification of *Pseudomonas aeruginosa* isolates producing a KPC-type carbapenem-hydrolyzing beta-lactamase. *Antimicrob. Agents Chemother.* 51, 1553–1555. doi: 10.1128/aac.01405-06

Wang, Q., Zhang, Y., Yao, X., Xian, H., Liu, Y., Li, H., et al. (2016). Risk factors and clinical outcomes for carbapenem-resistant *Enterobacteriaceae* nosocomial infections. *Eur. J. Clin. Microbiol. Infect. Dis.* 35, 1679–1689. doi: 10.1007/s10096-016-2710-0

Zhao, D., Zhou, Z., Hua, X., Zhang, H., Quan, J., Li, X., et al. (2018). Coexistence of mcr-1, bla(KPC-2) and two copies of fosA3 in a clinical *Escherichia coli* strain isolated from urine. *Infect. Genet. Evol.* 60, 77–79. doi: 10.1016/j.meegid.2018.02.025

# 3

# Efficient Production of Recombinant Protegrin-1 From *Pichia pastoris* and its Antimicrobial and *in vitro* Cell Migration Activity

***Evanna Huynh[1], Nadeem Akhtar[1] and Julang Li[1,2]****

*[1] Department of Animal Biosciences, University of Guelph, Guelph, ON, Canada,*

*[2] College of Life Science and Engineering, Foshan University, Foshan, China*

***Correspondence:***
*Julang Li*
*jli@uoguelph.ca*

Protegrin (PG) belongs to the antimicrobial peptide cathelicidin family. To date, five protegrin sequences have been identified in pigs, PG-1 to PG-5. Of these, PG-1 exhibits potent antimicrobial activity against a broad range of antibiotic-resistant microorganisms as well as viruses. However, the other potential role(s) of PG beyond antimicrobial has largely been unexplored. The aim of this study was to use nonpathogenic yeast *Pichia pastoris* to express antimicrobially active recombinant protegrin (rPG-1). Additionally, the effect of PG-1 on cell migration and proliferation was also examined *in vitro* using pig intestinal epithelial cells as a model. Highest level of rPG-1 (104 ± 11 μg/mL) was detected at 24 h in fermentation culture medium. Similar to rPG-1, 0.8 ± 0.10 g/L of proform PG-1 (rProPG-1) and 0.2 ± 0.02 g/L of the PG-1 cathelin domain (rCath) was detected in fermentation culture medium. Resulting recombinant PG-1 and cleaved rProPG-1 exerted antimicrobial activity against *Escherichia coli* DH5α at the same level as chemically synthesized PG-1. Enhanced cell migration was observed ($p < 0.05$) in groups treated with rProPG-1, rCath, and rPG-1 compared to the control. Furthermore, rPG-1 was stable at temperatures ranging from 25°C to 80°C. In summary, biologically active recombinant protegrin in its pro-, cathelin-, and mature- forms were successfully expressed in *P. pastoris* suggesting potential feasibility for future therapeutic applications.

**Keywords: antimicrobial peptide, cell migration, fermentation, *Pichia pastoris*, protegrin**

## INTRODUCTION

Tissue repair, including those happened after gastrointestinal infection, is an orchestrated process with inflammation and tissue re-epithelialization as critical approaches for successful healing. In addition to growth and repair factors (e.g., epidermal growth factor, trefoil factors), antimicrobial peptides (AMPs) are also expressed and secreted upon mucosal injury (Frohm et al., 1997; Hase et al., 2003; Kovach et al., 2012). AMPs, as well as the recently identified unusual amino acid L-cyclopropylalanine with anti-fungal and -bacterial activity (Ma et al., 2017) represent the first line of defense, or innate immunity, against foreign pathogens. These low-molecular weight molecules can exert antimicrobial activity at a nanomolar to micromolar range against a broad spectrum of microorganisms including bacteria, fungi, enveloped viruses, and parasites

(Hancock and Sahl, 2006; Sang and Blecha, 2008; Dias et al., 2017). In recent years, AMPs appear to be functionally multifaceted, fulfilling a variety of functions beyond microbial killing, including immunomodulation, tissue regeneration and vascularization in inflammation, tissue repair and even tumor surveillance (Hirano et al., 2000; Ishihara and Hirano, 2002; Proudfoot, 2002; Choi et al., 2012; de la Fuente-Núñez et al., 2014). A cationic AMP P17 from ant venom induces an alternative phenotype of human monocyte-derived macrophages (h-MDMs) promoting its anti-fungal activities (Benmoussa et al., 2017).

Cathelicidin is an evolutionary distinct group of AMPs in mammals. This peptide group has a highly conserved N-terminal (cathelin) domain in the pro-peptide followed by a variable AMP domain on the C-terminus (Kovach et al., 2012). Protegrin (PG) belongs to the cathelicidin family, and to date, five protegrin sequences have been identified in pigs, PG-1, PG-2, PG-3, PG-4, and PG-5. Of these, PG-1 exhibits potent antimicrobial activity against a broad range of antibiotic-resistant microorganisms as well as viruses, including HIV (Hancock and Sahl, 2006; Liu and Stappenbeck, 2016). Increasing evidence of alterations of mucosal AMP levels has leaded to the suggestion on their influential role on the gut immune protection (Schauber et al., 2006; Termén et al., 2008; Inaba et al., 2010), although the immuno- and tissue repair-modulating roles of PGs have not been investigated.

PG-1 possesses potential therapeutic utility. However, chemical synthesis of peptides is associated with high production costs and increased peptide length often limits success of the synthesis, and thusly, potentially limiting therapeutic application. *Pichia pastoris* is a highly appealing expression system which has advantages including rapid growth rate, high levels of protein production and eukaryotic post-translational modifications. The commercial applications of recombinant protein of phospholipase C (Ciofalo et al., 2006) and biopharmaceutical product (Thompson, 2010) produced by *P. pastoris* have the FDA generally recognized as safe (GRAS) status in the United States. Furthermore, administration of *P. pastoris* cells as a vehicle for recombinant vaccine delivery via intramuscular injection and oral delivery have been shown to be safe and effective in chickens (Taghavian et al., 2013). Previous work on the PG-3 cathelin domain revealed that the pro-piece cathelin domain has a role in activating cathepsin L (Zhu et al., 2008), and the pro-piece of human hCAP-18 has been suggested to have a role in preventing cysteine-proteinase-mediated tissue damage during inflammation (Zaiou et al., 2003). However, the role of PG-1 and its cathelin domain in regulating other cellular activity is unclear. We hypothesized that the proform, pro-piece and mature form of PG-1 can be efficiently produced in yeast, and that they may process tissue repair function, in addition to the well known antimicrobial role of PG-1.

The first objectives of this investigation was to examine the feasibility of expressing recombinant PG-1 in its pro-, cathelin- and mature- form in *P. pastoris* and characterize its antimicrobial activity *in vitro*. Considering the wound healing role, besides antimicrobial activity, of PG-1 has not been investigated to date, we will also examine the effect of PG on cell migration and proliferation *in vitro* using pig intestinal epithelial cells as a model.

## MATERIALS AND METHODS

### Construction of *P. pastoris* DNA Expression Vector

Expression vector designed to express pro-form PG-1 (pJ912-proPG-1) was codon-optimized (**Supplementary Material 1**) for optimal expression in *P. pastoris* and synthesized by DNA2.0 (Menlo Park, CA, United States). Native PG-1 sequence was used as a starting sequence (NCBI accession number: CAA56251). Enterokinase (EK) cleavage site (DDDDK) replaced the native neutrophil elastase site between the cathelin domain and the mature PG-1 domain (**Figure 1A**). Resultant plasmids were transformed into *Escherichia coli* DH5α (*E. coli*) for plasmid propagation and positive recombinant colonies were selected using 25 μg/mL zeocin (Invitrogen, CA, United States) in Luria-Bertani (LB) medium (Difco, MI, United States).

### Electroporation of *P. pastoris* X-33 and Screening for Recombinant Strains

Plasmid DNA was linearized with *SwaI* (New England Biolabs, Ipswich, MA, United States) and purified by phenol-chloroform extraction and ethanol precipitation. Approximately 3–5 μg of purified linearized plasmid DNA was dissolved in 10 μL of nuclease-free $H_2O$. Electrocompetent *P. pastoris* X33 (Invitrogen, Carlsbad, CA, United States) was prepared according to the manufacturer's instruction. Competent cells (100 μL) were mixed with the dissolved purified DNA in a 0.4 cm electroporation cuvette (BTX, CA, United States). Electroporation was carried out in Electro Cell Manipulator 600 (BTX, CA, United States) at 1.5 kV. Immediately after electroporation, 1.0 mL of 1 M ice-cold sorbitol (Fisher Scientific, Pittsburgh, PA, United States) was added to the cuvette. Cells were transferred to a sterile 1.5 mL tube and incubated at 30°C without shaking for 2 h. Transformed cells were plated on YPD agar [1% yeast extract (Difco, Detroit, MI, United States), 2% peptone (Difco, Detroit, MI, United States), 2% glucose (Fisher Scientific, Pittsburgh, PA, United States), 2% agar (Difco, Detroit, MI, United States)] supplemented with 1 M sorbitol and zeocin (100 μg/mL) and incubated for 3–4 days at 30°C until colonies appeared. Colonies were purified by streaking onto YPD agar with zeocin (100 μg/mL).

### Genomic DNA Analysis to Determine *P. pastoris* Mut-Genotype

To confirm recombinant gene integration and *P. pastoris* transformant Mut phenotype, genomic DNA was isolated from *P. pastoris* transformants using the freeze-and-thaw method previously described in (Jafari et al., 2011). The following universal *AOX1* primers were used for PCR: Sense: 5′-GACTGGTTCCAATTGACAAGC-3′, anti-sense: 5′GCAAATGGCATTCTGACATCC-3′. Amplification was

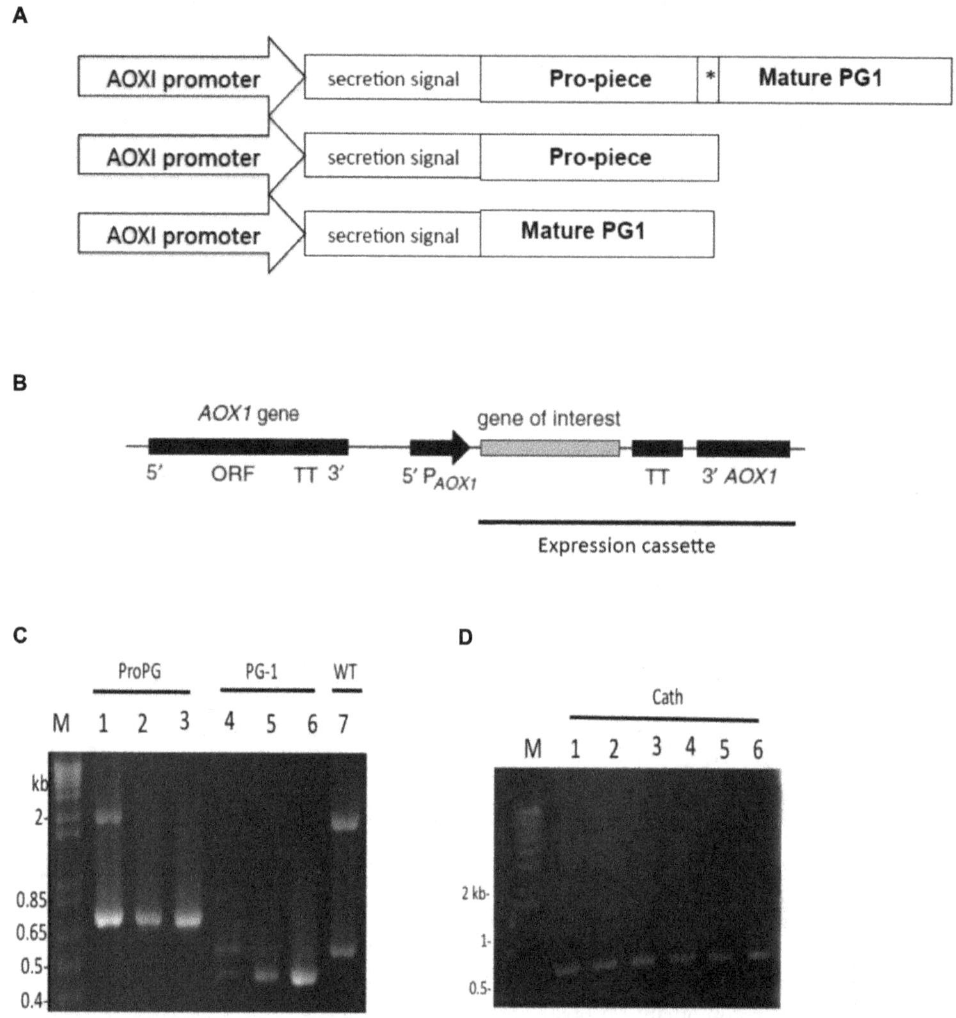


**FIGURE 1 |** Schematic construct of open reading frames (OFRs), expression cassette, and PCR amplicons. **(A)** ORF construct for proform PG-1, cathelin, and mature PG-1 expression. MeOH-inducible *AOX1* promoter and α-mating factor secretion signal sequence was used in all expression constructs. Asterisk (*) indicate enterokinase (EK) cleavage site. **(B)** Schematic representation of the integration of the expression cassette into *Pichia pastoris* genome. **(C)** PCR products amplified from gDNA to confirm integration of constructs for the expression of rProPG-1 (lane 1, 2 from two representative positive clones, respectively, at 760 bp) and rPG-1 (lane 4, 5 from two representative positive clones, respectively, at 458 bp). Expression plasmids for rProPG-1 and rPG-1 were used as an assay control (lane 3 and 6, respectively). **(D)** PCR products amplified from gDNA to confirm integration of constructs for the expression of rCath (lane 1–5). Expression plasmids for rCath were used as an assay control (lane 6). Wild-type AOXI gene yields a 2.2 kb product (Lane 7). Scales are not proportional to the sizes of the elements in **(A)** and **(B)**.

carried out at 94°C for 30 s, 55°C for 30 s, and 72°C for 1 min for 35 cycles. PCR was performed using *Taq* DNA polymerase (Invitrogen, Carlsbad, CA, United States).

## Expression Cassette Copy Number Determination in *P. pastoris*

The number of copies of pJ912-ProPG expression cassettes integrated into the *P. pastoris* genome was determined by quantitative real-time PCR as described by (Abad et al., 2010) and copy number of each clone was determined using the $2^{-\Delta\Delta Ct}$ method (Livak and Schmittgen, 2001; Schmittgen and Livak, 2008). Blank *P. pastoris* X33, *AOX1* promoter, and endogenous *ARG4* gene were used as calibrator, target gene, and reference gene, respectively.

## Inducing Expression of Pro-form PG-1 in *P. pastoris*

Positive transformant colonies were inoculated into a 500 mL flask containing 50 mL BMGY medium [1% yeast extract, 2% peptone, 100 mM potassium phosphate (pH 6.0), 1.4% yeast nitrogen base (Difco, Detroit, MI, United States), 0.00004% biotin (Difco, Detroit, MI, United States), 1% glycerol (Fisher Scientific, Pittsburgh, PA, United States)] at 30°C with shaking at 250 rpm. After 16–24 h, cultures reached an optical density at 600 nm (OD600) = 2.0–6.0 and were harvested by centrifugation and resuspended in BMMY medium (BMGY medium containing 0.5% v/v methanol instead of glycerol) to induce expression. Cells were grown for 72 h at 30°C with shaking (250 rpm) and 100% methanol was added every 24 h to a final concentration of 0.5% (v/v). At various time points, 100 μL aliquots were taken from the culture and replaced with an equal amount of fresh BMMY medium. Supernatant and cell pellet samples were centrifuged and stored separately at −80°C for later analyses.

## Recombinant Protegrin Production in a Bioreactor

*Pichia pastoris* expressing recombinant ProPG-1, Cath, and PG-1were grown independently in a 3-L BioFlo 115 Benchtop Bioreactor (New Brunswick Scientific, CA, United States). Fermentation was carried out in a total volume of 1 L basal salt medium (BSM) (Stratton et al., 1998) with modifications. *Pichia* trace minerals 1 (PTM1) solution was prepared with (g/L) $CuSO_4{\cdot}5H_2O$ (6.0), NaI (0.08), $MnSO_4{\cdot}H_2O$ (3.0), $Na_2MoO_4{\cdot}2H_2O$ (0.2), $H_3BO_3$ (0.02), $CoCl_2$ (0.5), $ZnCl_2$ (7.0), $FeSO_4{\cdot}7H_2O$ (65.0), biotin (0.2), and 5 mL of concentrated $H_2SO_4$. A 100 mL recombinant *P. pastoris* inoculum prepared in YPD (OD at 600 = 15 ± 1.3) was transferred to the sterilized bioreactor containing 1 L of BSM. Antifoam A (Sigma, St. Louis, MO, United States) was added manually to control foaming in the bioreactor, if needed. Temperature was maintained at 30°C and pH at 5.6 using 12.5% (v/v) $NH_4OH$. Aeration rate of 5 L $min^{-1}$ was constant throughout the fermentation. The stirrer speed was controlled between 250 and 700 rpm aiming at dissolved oxygen (DO) concentration of 20% air saturation. After ~24 h of fermentation, consumption of glycerol was indicated by an increase in DO concentration at an OD of 30 ± 2.1, a glycerol feed [50% (v/v) glycerol containing PTM1 (12 mL/L glycerol)] was then maintained for another12 h at 15 mL/L/h. After completion of the glycerol feeding OD reaches to 170 ± 14.6. This was followed by a methanol feed [100% methanol containing PTM1 (12 mL/L methanol)] and maintained at a constant rate of 3 mL/L/h. The OD of the culture medium after 24 of methanol induction was 288 ± 19.4, the fermentation was stopped and culture medium was centrifuged (10,000 rpm, 10 min, 4°C) to obtain cell free supernatant and stored at −80°C for further analyses.

## Protein Sample Preparation

Standard lyophilized PG-1 was synthesized at approximately 95% purity (EZbiolabs, Carmel, IN, United States) and was dissolved in and diluted to 200 μg/mL with filter-sterilized acidified water (0.01% acetic acid) supplemented with 0.1% bovine serum albumin (BSA) (Sigma, St. Louis, MO, United States) to reduce non-specific adsorption of PG-1 to plastic ware. Standard PG-1 was stored at −80°C. Pro-form PG-1 expressed by *P. pastoris* in the supernatant was dialyzed against 25 mMTris-Cl (pH 7.0) and concentrated 60-foldby ultracentrifugation with a 10 kDa cut-off (Millipore Inc., Burlington, MA, United States). Ultracentrifugation retentate and supernatant was filter sterilized and stored at −80°C prior to antimicrobial assay. EK at 0.8 U and 2.5 U (GenScript, Piscataway, NJ, United States) was used to cleave 5 μL of pro-form PG-1 overnight (final 10 μL reaction volume) to release the mature PG-1 from the cathelin domain according to manufacturer's instruction for subsequent antimicrobial activity assay.

## Two-Stage Radial Diffusion Assay

The antimicrobial activity of recombinant pro-form PG-1 and cleaved pro-form PG-1 were tested by a two-stage radial diffusion assay as previously described by (Steinberg and Lehrer, 1997) against *E. coli* and methicillin-resistant *Staphylococcus aureus* (MRSA). Positive control sample wells received 10 μL of serially diluted chemically synthesized standard PG-1 or its vehicle as a control. Sample wells received 10 μL of pro-form PG-1 containing 0.01% acetic acid and 0.1% BSA after EK digestion. Minimum inhibition concentration (MIC) was defined at a concentration of PG-1 that resulted in a clear inhibition zone around the well. To test whether BMMY can inhibit PG-1 antimicrobial activity, 5 μL pro-form PG-1 after the 2.5 U EK digestion reaction was resuspended with 5 μL of spent BMMY medium and the mixture was used to inoculate sample well.

## Antimicrobial Activity Assay Using Colony-Count Method

The MIC of rPG-1 against *E. coli* was tested according to the antimicrobial assay previously described (Pizzo et al., 2015) with slight modification. The stability of rPG-1 was monitored at different pH (2–11) and temperature (25–95°C) conditions after a preincubation time of 30 min before being assayed. Briefly, overnight grown *E. coli* in LB medium was diluted to an OD 600 of 1 and further diluted 1:100. *E. coli*- peptide mixtures were prepared by adding 40 μL of bacterial cells to different concentration of rPG-1 (1–10 μg/mL) in separate eppendorf tubes and adjusted to a final volume of 1 mL using 20 mM acetate buffer (pH 5). Cells without rPG-1 and with 0.05 mg/mL ampicillin were taken as negative and positive controls, respectively. Experimental and control tubes were incubated for 4 h at 37°C, and 50 μL of the diluted (1:100) mixtures were plated on LB agar media and incubated at 37°C overnight for colony counts. The survived cells in each plate were compared with controls. All concentrations of rPG-1 at different pH and temperature were tested in triplicate experiments and $<5\%$ standard deviation were observed for each experiment.

## Western Blot

Culture supernatants were subjected to 12% SDS-PAGE and electrophorectically transferred to 0.45 μm pore size PVDF membrane (Millipore Inc., Burlington, CA, United States). The membrane was blocked in 5% (w/v) skim milk in TBST buffer (0.3% Tris, 0.8% NaCl, 0.02% KCl, 0.1% Tween 20) for 1 h and then incubated with affinity purified polyclonal rabbit anti-PG-1 antibody at 1:500 dilution, synthesized from Biomatik (Cambridge, ON, Canada) overnight at 4°C. After washing the membrane three times at 5 min each in TBST, the membrane was incubated with anti-rabbit IgG secondary antibody (1:1000 dilution) conjugated to horseradish peroxidase (Cell Signaling, Danvers, MA, United States) for 1 h at room temperature. Bands were visualized using an ECL Plus Western blotting system according to manufacturer's instruction (Amersham Biosciences, Piscataway, NJ, United States).

### *In vitro* Cell Proliferation Assay

IPEC-J2 cells were grown in six-well plates (Corning, Corning, NY, United States) until 50% confluent in medium consisting of DMEM F-12 containing 5% fetal bovine serum at 37°C in 5% $CO_2$ and were then serum starved for 24 h. The cells were then incubated with serum-free DMEM F-12 in the presence of 10 μL filter-sterilized fermentation supernatant from 24 h MeOH induced cultures from PP-ProPG-1, PP-Cath, PP-PG-1 and PP-wild type (PP-WT), and cultured for 24 h. Cells were then trypsinized and enumerated using a hemocytometer.

### Transwell Assay

To analyze migration of IPEC-J2 cells, 8-micron pore sized Millicell Cell culture transwell inserts (Millipore Inc., Burlington, CA, United States) were used. A total of $1 \times 10^5$ cells were plated in the upper inserts and the lower chamber contained serum-free DMEM F-12 in the presence of 10 μL filter-sterilized fermentation supernatant from 24 h MeOH induced cultures from PP-ProPG-1, PP-Cath, PP-PG-1, and PP-WT. After incubation for 16 h, the cells were fixed with 4% (w/v) paraformaldehyde. Cells that did not migrate into the membrane were gently scraped off the upper surface of the transwell with a cotton swab. Migration was quantified by cell enumeration through Hoechst 33342 staining of cell nuclei (Life Technologies, Grand Island, NY, United States).

### Statistical Analysis

Results are expressed as mean ± SEM (standard error mean) from at least three independent experiments. The data were analyzed by two-factor analysis of variance (ANOVA) using a GraphPad Prism software version 5.0. Data sets were analyzed by Tukey's test for multiple comparisons to determine statistical differences between groups. The results were considered significant at a $P$ value of <0.05.

## RESULTS

### Generation of *P. pastoris* Expressing Recombinant ProPG-1, Cath and PG-1

To generate *P. pastoris* that could express recombinant ProPG-1 (rProPG-1), Cath (rCath), and PG-1 (rPG-1), the cDNA sequence of codon-optimized porcine protegrin ProPG-1, Cath, and PG-1 were ligated into the respective pJexpress *P. pastoris* expression vector, respectively. The α-mating factor secretion signal sequence was placed at the N-terminal (**Figure 1A**) to facilitate secretion of the expressed recombinant proteins into the culture fermentation medium, also referred to as supernatant. In our study, we replaced the native elastase cleavage site of preform-protegrin with an EK site. The addition of the EK cleavage site can permit the potential application of recombinant PG-1 in animal feed, as EK is a serine protease and is naturally produced and secreted in the intestinal duodenum (Baratti et al., 1973; Fonseca and Light, 1983).

The DNA sequence-verified recombinant plasmids were linearized with *Swa*I and transformed into electrocompetent *P. pastoris* X-33. Transformants harboring the pJexpress-ProPG-1, pJexpress-Cath and pJexpress-PG-1 constructs are here on referred to as PP-ProPG-1, PP-Cath, and PP-PG-1, respectively. To confirm integration of the construct into the *Pichia* genome, isolated genomic DNA from clones were analyzed by PCR using the 5′*AOX1* primer paired with 3′*AOX1*-TT (**Figure 1B**). PCR results showed chromosomal integration of the expression cassette resulting in a 760 bp, 458 bp, and 700 bp PCR product for positive PP-ProPG-1, PP-PG-1, and PP-Cath transformants, respectively. $Mut^+$ strains had a 2.2 kb PCR product corresponding to the intact *AOX1* gene. $Mut^s$ strains do not have a 2.2 kb PCR product and only a PCR product corresponding to the *AOX1* and insert part of the expression construct (**Figures 1C,D**).

### Effect of Copy Number on Recombinant Protegrin Expression

To employ the expression potential of the *P. pastoris* system, we examined the influence of gene copy number on the expression of rProPG-1, rCath, and rPG-1 from PP-ProPG-1, PP-Cath, and PP-PG-1, respectively. Clones with putative multiple copies of the rProPG, rCath, and rPG1 expression cassette from varying concentrations of G418 antibiotic selection were selected for copy number determination by qPCR. The purpose was to examine the effects of copy number on rProPG-1, rCath, and rPG-1 expression. Clones containing 1–14 copies of the rProPG-1 expression cassette were analyzed for the expression rProPG-1 under shake-flask conditions. As shown in **Table 1**, rProPG-1 expression level increased progressively as the copy number increased from 1 to 7, with seven copies resulting in earlier and highest expression of rProPG-1 at 24 h post-induction. As the number of copies increased from 7 to 11, the expression level did not further increase. However, 14 copies of the cassette yielded higher expression level than 11 copies, but 14 copies of the cassette yielded lower rProPG-1 than in the clone with seven copies at 24 h methanol induction. This indicates a potential maximal limit number of copies that can have a direct influence on rProPG-1 expression level. Similarly, rCath expressed by PP-Cath increased progressively from one copy to six, and decreased at eight copies (**Table 2**). PP-Cath transformant with six copies yielded the highest rCath (**Figure 2A**). Furthermore, gene copy number from 2 to 11 were evaluated in PP-PG-1 clones and clones with six and eight copies yielded highest

**TABLE 1** | Expression cassette copy number and rProPG-1 expression level.

| PP-ProPG-1 clone | rProPG-1 (24 h) | rProPG-1 (72 h) | Copy # |
|---|---|---|---|
| Pro4 | − | + | 11 |
| Pro22 | + | +++ | 14 |
| Pro44 | ++ | +++ | 7 |
| Pro50 | − | − | 1 |

*Supernatant samples at 24 and 72 h methanol induction from small-scale fermentations of different PP-ProPG-1 clones were assessed for rProPG-1 expression. (−) indicates no rProPG-1 was detected and (+), (++), (+++) indicate low, medium and high levels of rProPG-1 detected using dot blot analysis, respectively.*

**TABLE 2 |** Expression cassette copy number and rCath expression level.

| PP-Cath clone | rCath expression level | Copy # |
|---|---|---|
| C1 | ++ | 2 |
| C2 | ++ | 4 |
| C3 | + | 1 |
| C4 | ++ | 3 |
| C5 | +++ | 6 |
| C6 | ++ | 8 |

*Supernatant samples at 24 and 72 h methanol induction from small-scale fermentations of different PP-Cath clones were assessed for rCath expression. (+), (++), (+++) indicate low, medium and high levels of rCath detected using dot blot analysis, respectively.*

rPG-1 activity (**Figure 2B, Table 3**). Progressive increase in rPG-1 was observed as copy number increased up to eight and appeared to decrease at eleven copies. Interestingly, two clones both with six copies of rPG-1 construct expressed at different levels (**Table 3**), suggesting other factors, in addition to gene copy number, can influence recombinant protein expression level in *P. pastoris*.

## *Pichia pastoris* Recombinant Protegrin Expression in a Bioreactor

To potentially obtain increased yield of recombinant protegrin, high-density fermentation was performed in a 3-L bioreactor. Initially, the transition from shake-flask culturing to a bioreactor unexpectedly yielded much lower recombinant protein concentrations using the standard media composition (Invitrogen manual, Carlsbad, CA, United States). By reducing BSM concentration by 50% during culture media optimization, expression level increased. For rPG-1 expression, rPG-1 was not detected until yeast extract and peptone were added to the BSM. These improvements suggest that the media formulation could be optimized to improve the yield.

Expression with all the three recombinant *P. pastoris* strains was performed using three-step procedures, including glycerol-batch phase, glycerol fed-batch and methanol induction phase. The DO spike was found to be an effective indicator to initiate a new feeding profile and to monitor the overall health of the culture for successful recombinant protegrin expression. Aliquots of the fermentation supernatant were examined by Western blot and ELISA. Highest level of rPG-1 (104 ± 11 μg/mL) was

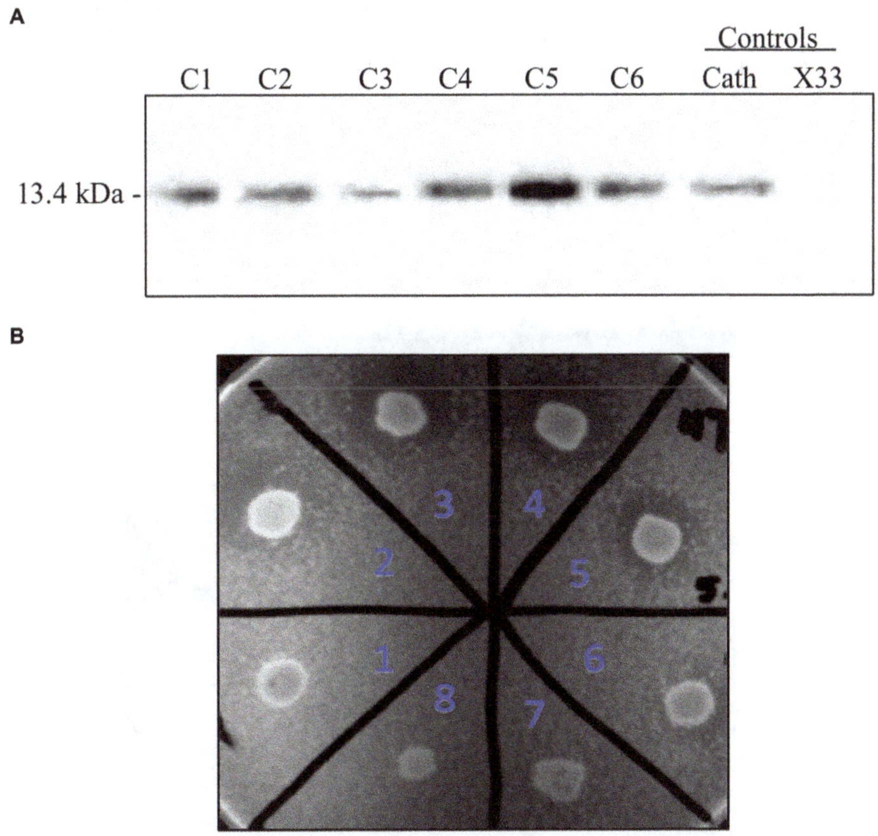


**FIGURE 2 |** Screening of *P. pastoris* clones expressing recombinant cathelin (PP-rCath) and mature PG-1 (PP-rPG-1). **(A)** Western blot of the supernatant samples after 24 h methanol induction from small-scale fermentations of rCath clones (C1–C6). Blank *P. pastoris* strain X33 and chemically synthesized cathelin (13.4 kDa) served as assay negative and positive controls, respectively. **(B)** Radial diffusion assay of the PP-rPG-1 when grown on BMMY agarose plates and induced with 2% methanol for 48 h. TSB agarose containing methicillin-resistant *S. aureus* (MRSA) was subsequently layered on top of BMMY for rPG-1 antimicrobial activity detection. Clones 1–6 express rPG-1 at varying levels. Clone 7 and 8 served as controls and exhibit no antimicrobial activity (blank *P. pastoris* strain X33 and PP-ProPG-1, respectively).

**TABLE 3 |** Expression cassette copy number and rPG-1 activity level.

| PP-PG-1 clone | rPG-1 antimicrobial activity | Copy # |
|---|---|---|
| 1 | − | 2 |
| 2 | + | 6 |
| 3 | +++ | 6 |
| 4 | +++ | 8 |
| 5 | ++ | 11 |
| 6 | + | 4 |

*rPG-1 antimicrobial activity level correlates with amount of rPG1 produced. PP-PG-1 clones were assessed for antimicrobial activity against MRSA. (−) indicates no rPG-1 activity was detected and in the others, the activities of rPG-1 are indicated as + (clear zone 0.5–1.5 mm), ++ (clear zone 1.5–2.5 mm), and +++ (clear zone > 2.5 mm).*

detected at 24 h of methanol induction in the fermentation culture medium. Post 24 h, rPG-1concentration decreased (**Figure 3A**). Similar to rPG-1, 0.8 ± 0.10 g/L rProPG-1, and 0.2 ± 0.02 rCath g/L was detected in fermentation culture medium at 24 h of methanol induction (**Figures 3B–D**).

## Enterokinase Cleavage of rProPG-1 and Antimicrobial Activity

To determine whether the rProPG-1 could yield antimicrobial activity upon removal of the N-terminus pro- domain, EK was used to cleave the introduced amino acid DDDDK site on rProPG-1 (**Table 4**). Cleavage of rProPG-1 was detected by Western blot using antibodies specific to mature PG-1 in the C-terminal domain. EK successfully cleaved rProPG-1 as the detection of mature PG-1 decreased from 13.4 kDa to 2.1 kDa, indicating the removal of the 11 kDa pro- domain (**Figure 4A**). The resulting cleaved rProPG-1 also conferred antimicrobial activity against *E. coli* DH5αat the same level as chemically synthesized PG-1 (**Figure 4B** and **Table 5**). The uncleaved rProPG-1 and rCath did not exhibit antimicrobial activity as expected.

## Protegrin Peptide Properties and Boman Index

Peptide properties such as molecular weight, pI value, net charge and Boman Index can be used to predict a peptide's antimicrobial potential under various conditions (Boman, 2003). rProPG, rCath, and rPG-1 were calculated using both Innovagen's Peptide Property Calculator and a predictive tool available at AMP Database v2.34, respectively. The rPG-1 showed highly basic pI value (>10), positive net charge (+6), and high Boman index (>2.5; **Table 4**). The peptides containing the cathelin domain, rProPG-1, and rCath, have pI values of 6.49 and 4.6, respectively. ProPG is neutral at pH 7.0 (net charge −0.3) and Cath has a negative net charge (−6.2). Both of these peptides share similar

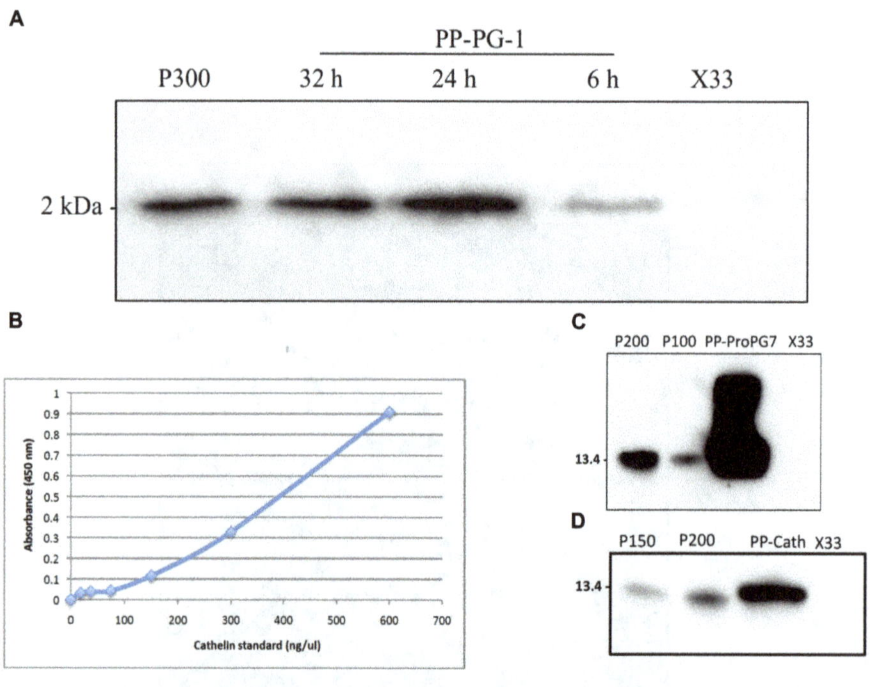


**FIGURE 3 |** Quantification of rPro-PG-1, rCath, and rPG-1 produced by *P. pastoris* in separate bioreactor. **(A)** rPG-1 (from PP-PG-1) was detected with antibody against pig PG-1 in Western blot. Blank *P. pastoris* strain X33 and 300 ng of chemically synthesized rPG-1 served as assay negative and positive controls, respectively. **(B)** Indirect-HRP ELISA standard curve. Antibody detecting the cathelin domain of ProPG-1 and cathelin was used as the primary antibody. Cathelin peptide was used to generate the standard curve. **(C)** Recombinant ProPG-1 (from PP-ProPG-7) was detected with antibody against pig PG-1 in Western blot. 200 ng and 100 ng of chemically synthesized ProPG-1 served as positive controls (P200 and P100, respectively). **(D)** Recombinant cathelin (from PP-Cath) was detected with antibody against pig cathelin in Western blot. 200 ng and 150 ng of chemically synthesized cathelin served as positive controls (P200 and P150, respectively). Empty *P. pastoris* X33 strain served as a negative control.

**TABLE 4** | Summary of protegrin peptide properties.

| Peptide | Amino acid sequence | Size (kDa) | pI value | Net charge (at pH 7.0) | Boman Index (kcal/mol) |
|---|---|---|---|---|---|
| Proform PG-1 (rProPG-1) | Q ALSYREAVLR AVDRLNEQSS EANLYRLLEL DQPPKADEDP GTPKPVSFTV KETVCPRPTR QPPELCDFKE NGRVKQCVGT VTLDQIKDPL DITCN **DDDDK*** RGGRLCYCRR RFCVCVGR | 13.4 | 6.49 | −0.3 | 2.9 |
| Cathelin PG-1 (rCath) | Q ALSYREAVLR AVDRLNEQSS EANLYRLLEL DQPPKADEDP GTPKPVSFTV KETVCPRPTR QPPELCDFKE NGRVKQCVGT VTLDQIKDPL DITCN **DDDDK*** | 11.3 | 4.6 | −6.2 | 2.8 |
| PG-1 (rPG-1) | RGGRLCYCRR RFCVCVGR | 2.1 | 10.7 | +6 | 3.65 |

*Size, pI value, net charges were calculated by Innovagen's Peptide Property Calculator. Boman index was calculated by the predictive tool available at Antimicrobial Peptide Database v2.34. Native elastase site was replaced by enterokinase cleavage site (DDDDK*).*

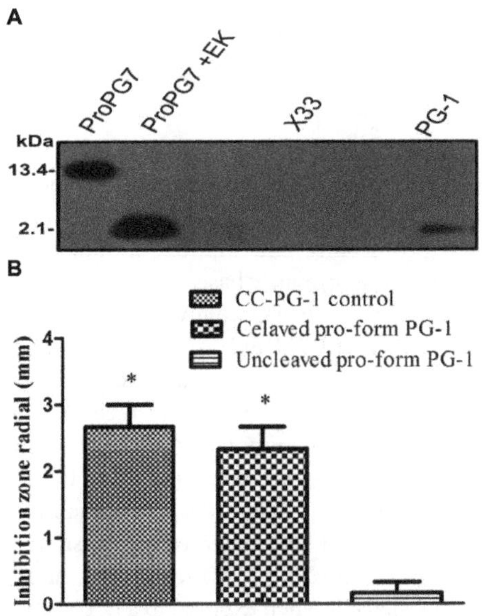


**FIGURE 4** | Detection and activity of rProPG after enterokinase (EK) cleavage. **(A)** Recombinant ProPG (ProPG7) and EK cleaved ProPG (ProPG7 + EK), yielding mature peptide (PG-1), was detected with antibody against pig PG-1 in Western blot. Blank *P. pastoris* strain X33 and chemically synthesized PG-1 (CC-PG-1) served as negative and positive controls, respectively. **(B)** Upon EK digestion, rProPG-1 exhibit antimicrobial activity against *E. coli* in radial diffusion antimicrobial activity assay. Data shown is the mean ± SEM of three repeats for inhibitory zones of CC-PG-1 control (I), cleaved pro-form PG-1 (II) and uncleaved pro-form PG-1 (III). Asterisk (*$p < 0.05$) denotes significant difference from uncleaved pro-form PG-1.

Boman Index (2.8–2.9). A high Boman Index in rProPG-1, rCath, and rPG-1 can indicate the potential of these peptides to interact with other proteins *in vivo*.

## Enhanced Cell Migration by PG-1 in Its Pro-, Cathelin-, and Mature- Form

We next sought to examine the effect of protegrin on modulating cell proliferation and migration *in vitro* using transwell cell migration assays with IPEC-J2 cells, a cell line derived from porcine intestine epithelium. As shown in **Figure 5A**, cell migration in groups treated with recombinant proform PG-1 (rProPG-1), pro-piece cathelin domain (rCath), and mature PG-1 (rPG-1) was enhanced. Migrated cell count analysis revealed that there was a two-fold (rPro-PG-1), 2.3-fold (rCath), and 2.5-fold (rPG-1) increase in cell migration when compared to the untreated negative control ($p < 0.05$, **Figure 5B**). To study if these peptides (rProPG-1, rCath, and rPG-1) can increase cell proliferation, cell counting proliferation assay was performed. In comparison to the untreated control, groups treated with the peptides resulted in no significant change in cell proliferation (data not shown).

**TABLE 5** | Minimum inhibitory concentration (MIC) values of the resulting mature PG-1 cleaved from rProPG-1 after enterokinase (EK) digestion, and rPG-1 expresses by PP-PG-1.

| Microorganism | MIC (μg/mL) | | |
|---|---|---|---|
| | Control[a] | PG-1[b] | rPG-1[c] |
| *E. coli* | 2 | 2 | 2 |
| MRSA | 5 | 10 | 8 |

*[a] Chemically synthesized mature PG-1 (CC-PG-1); [b] PG-1 cleaved from rProPG-1 after EK digestion; [c] rPG-1 expressed by PP-PG-1.*
*MRSA: Methylene-resistant Staphylococcus aureus.*

## Antimicrobial Activity of rPG-1 and Its Stability at Various pH and Temperature

The minimum inhibitory concentration (MIC) values of the resulting mature peptide (rPG-1) expressed by PP-PG-1 was determined by a two-stage radial diffusion assay. The lowest concentration of the rPG-1 that inhibited the visible growth of *E. coli* and MRSA after overnight incubation is the MIC (**Table 6**). rPG-1 conferred similar antimicrobial activity against *E. coli* at the same level as chemically synthesized PG-1 (CS-PG-1). The MIC value for rPG-1 expressed by PP-rPG-1 against MRSA is 37.5% lower than the CS-PG-1 at 8 μg/mL versus 5 μg/mL, respectively (**Table 5**). Differences in MIC may be attributed to differences in quantification methods of the chemically synthesized and recombinant peptides (e.g., empirical weighing

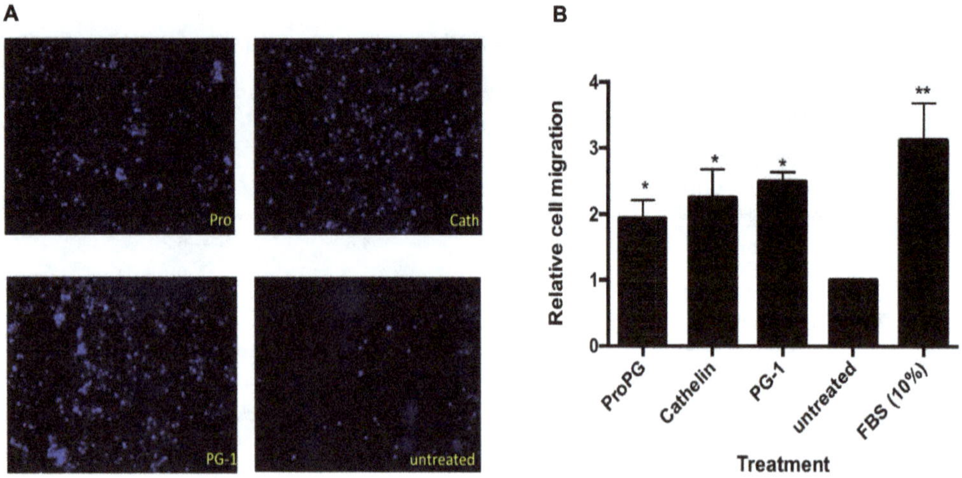


**FIGURE 5 |** Effect of proform PG-1, cathelin domain and mature PG-1 on cell migration. **(A)** Representative images of transwell migrated IPEC-J2 cells stained with Hoechst 33342. **(B)** Quantification of cell migration from transwell migration assay. Bars represent the mean ± SEM of three experiments. Asterisk * ($p < 0.05$) and ** ($p < 0.01$) denote significant difference from untreated control group.

**TABLE 6 |** Stability of the rPG-1 at different pH and temperature in terms of MIC against *E. coli* after a pre-incubation time of 30 min, antimicrobial activity assay using colony count method was performed to determine the antimicrobial activity.

| Parameters | pH/temperature | MIC (μg/mL) |
|---|---|---|
| pH | 2 | 2.5 |
| | 4 | 2.5 |
| | 6 | 2 |
| | 11 | 2.5 |
| Temperature (°C) | 25 | 2 |
| | 50 | 2 |
| | 80 | 2 |
| | 95 | 2.5 |

versus western blot densitometry). Various pH and temperature conditions were used to investigate the stability of rPG-1 after an incubation time of 30 min. As shown in **Table 6**, rPG1 retained potent activity in both acidic and alkaline (pH 2.0, 4.0, 6.0, and 11.0), and temperature conditions (25–80°C). Antimicrobial activity was quite stable over a pH range of 2.0–11.0, although the MIC at a higher temperature (90°C) increased by 25% compared to the MIC observed at 25°C.

## DISCUSSION

The use of *P. pastoris* as an expression system has numerous advantages such as rapid and high-density growth in defined and relatively inexpensive media, high recombinant protein yield, and post-translational modification abilities similar to that of mammalian cells. *P. pastoris* also secrete a low number of endogenous proteins, making downstream protein recovery and purification more feasible. AMPs that have been expressed by *P. pastoris* such as hPAB-β, Ch-penaeidin, MP1102 (Li et al., 2005; Chen et al., 2011; Zhang et al., 2015) are driven by the *AOX* promoter system. These studies indicate methylotrophic yeast-inducible system is suitable for high-level expression of active AMPs. Pro-healing and immune-modulating aspect of cathelicidin AMPs are primarily based on the human and mouse cathelicidin AMP. In our work, we investigated the feasibility of expressing recombinant PG-1 in its pro-, cathelin-, and mature-form in *P. pastoris* and characterized their antimicrobial activity *in vitro*. We then examined the effect of recombinant PG-1 in its various forms on cell migration and proliferation *in vitro*. To our knowledge, our finding is the first report on the role of PG-1 on cell migration and thus tissue repair potential. Interestingly, a recent report showed an increased expression of porcine β-Defensin2 (PBD2), pBD3, pBD114, pBD129, and protegrins (PG) 1-5 in IPEC-J2 cells when exposed to a host defense peptide (HDP)- synthesizing *Lactobacillus reuteri* I5007 (Liu et al., 2017). Similarly, butyrate and its analogs showed induction of porcine HDP gene expression with approximately 20-, 45-, 60-, and 80-fold induction was observed for pBD2, PG1-5, pEP2C, and pBD3, respectively, using IPEC-J2 intestinal epithelial cells (Zeng et al., 2013). These findings together with our findings on the PG-1 tissue damage healing potential suggest that PG-1 may be one of the components of innate defense during infection.

To investigate the feasibility of producing rProPG-1, rCath, and rPG-1 for downstream studies and application, we constructed plasmids for the expression and secretion of these three peptides in *P. pastoris*. Stable clones were generated via integration of the constructs into the *P. pastoris* genome. This will also eliminate the need for constant selective pressure during fermentation. With integration, it is possible to generate strains harboring more than one copy of the introduced expression cassette via repeated single crossover DNA recombinant events (Clare et al., 1991a; Nordén et al., 2011). Insertion of multiple recombinant gene copies is often desired to enhance recombinant protein yield, as low transcript levels can be a limiting factor in protein production (Nordén et al., 2011). To increase the number of integrated expression cassettes, we initially attempted to construct a known number of concatemers of the expression cassette prior to transformation into *P. pastoris*, similar to Mansur et al. (2005). We found the stable generation of long concatemers of the expression construct difficult to achieve. Instead, we then enriched for strains with an increased number of vector copies by plating transformants on medium containing increasing levels of the selection drug (e.g., G418), where higher drug resistant clones can correlate with higher gene dosage (Nordén et al., 2011). Clones with putative multiple copies of the rProPG-1, rCath, and rPG-1 expression cassette from varying concentrations of G418 antibiotic selection were then selected to evaluate recombinant protein expression levels. Although it was evident that there is a positive correlation between gene dosage level and level of expression (**Tables 1–3**), an upper limit of gene dosage was observed. This bell-shaped correlation curve between gene copy number and protein yield has been reported in *P. pastoris*, where production and secretion level gradually decline with increased gene dosage (Zhu et al., 2009). This upper limit of gene dosage has been suggested to be related to endoplasmic reticulum (ER) stress with the accumulation of recombinant protein within the ERs, also further indicating there may be other bottleneck factors limiting recombinant protein production in addition to gene dosage.

To potentially obtain increased yield of recombinant protegrin (rProPG-1, rCath, and rPG-1), high-density fermentation was also performed. Recombinant protein was detected upon modification of the bioreactor BSM by reducing salt concentrations by 50% (BSM50). It has been reported that high salt concentration can increase cell death, possibly caused by high osmotic pressure in the medium (Brady et al., 2001; Jahic et al., 2006). Upon cell lysis, the secreted recombinant protein can undergo proteolysis as cellular proteases are released into the culture medium. The addition of casamino acids, yeast extract and peptone can help address the issue of protein degradation during the cultivation process (Jahic et al., 2003). During rPG-1 expression by PP-PG-1, rPG-1 was not detected until yeast extract and peptone was added to the BSM50 culture medium, suggesting modification of media formulation can improve yield. The yeast extract, peptone and casamino acids may serve as preferential substrates for proteolytic enzymes, thereby decreasing degradation of the expressed recombinant protein of interest (Clare et al., 1991b; Jafari et al., 2011). Interestingly, the addition of these substrates to the medium was more critical in PP-PG-1 fermentation than PP-ProPG-1 and PP-Cath. This could be due to the peptide properties of rPG-1 toxicity against the *P. pastoris* host cells. These substrates can potentially bind or interact with rPG-1 to limit its toxicity against *P. pastoris*. Components of microbial growth medium have been shown to exhibit binding activity to metal ions (Ramamoorthy and Kushner, 1975) and may also affect recombinant protein folding by modulating the expression of chaperone proteins (Rosano and Ceccarelli, 2014). Furthermore, fermentation medium composition can influence the physio-chemical surface properties of microbes. Microbial cell wall protein composition can differ when cultured in medium with and without peptone and yeast extract (Schär-Zammaretti et al., 2005). The expression level of rPG-1 (104 ± 11 mg/L) is comparable to other AMPs expressed using the similar *P. pastoris* expression system ranging from 108 mg/L to 292 mg/L (Li et al., 2005; Chen et al., 2011; Zhang et al., 2015). Of the three protegrin peptides expressed, rPG-1 had the lowest yield compared to rProPG-1 and rCath (0.8 ± 0.10 g/L and 0.2 ± 0.02 rCath g/L, respectively). The isoelectric point (pI) of a recombinant protein can affect expression level, where high pI is associated with no detectable protein expression (Boettner et al., 2007). This is in line with the high pI value of rPG-1 (10.7; **Table 4**) and the lower expression level obtained. This further suggests pI can be a potential parameter influencing protein expression. Addition of fusion protein tags to aid purification can potentially affect recombinant protein expression level. To increase protein yield in future experiments, the theoretical pI of rPG-1 can be reduced from 10.6 to 8.3 upon the fusion of glutathione S-transferase (GST) tag.

To reduce the likelihood of AMPs exerting their toxicity effect against host cells, fusing AMPs to a foreign or native partner protein can aid in enhancing protein production and reduce proteolytic degradation. In our work, we replaced the native elastase cleavage site of proform protegrin with an EK cleavage site. Antimicrobial activity was not exhibited until cleavage occurred in the presence of EK, releasing the mature and active PG-1 (**Figure 4B**). EK is a serine protease and is naturally produced and secreted in the intestinal duodenum to convert trypsinogen into its active trypsin form for subsequent activation of pancreatic digestive enzymes in pigs (Baratti et al., 1973). The addition of the EK cleavage site can permit rProPG-1 to be cleaved by the endogenous intestinal EK to release the mature antimicrobial PG-1. This allows the potential application of rProPG-1 in animal feed to replace the use of conventional antibiotics that are contributing to the rapid emergence of antibiotic resistant bacteria. Interestingly, while the MIC for both rPG-1 and the EK cleaved rProPG-1 for *E. coli* is the same as that of the chemically synthesized PG-1 control, their MICs (10, and 8 μg/mL for the mature PG-1 cleaved from rProPG-1 and the mature rPG-1, respectively) for MSRA are higher than that of the control (5 μg/mL). Similar MIC results were found using protegrin-1 against *E. coli* (4 μg/mL), and MRSA (4 μg/mL) (Yan and Hancock, 2001). In another report, the MICs of PG-1 against Gram-positive and Gram-negative bacteria range from 0.12 to 2 μg/mL (Steinberg et al., 1997).

A high Boman index value (e.g., 2.50–3.00) can indicate an AMP to be multifunctional within the cell due to its ability to interact with a wide range of proteins (Boman, 2003; Nam et al., 2014). A lower index value (≤1) can suggest that the AMP has low side effects (e.g., low hemolytic activity). Since protegrin, in its pro-, cathelin-, and mature-form, is predicted to interact with other proteins, we sought to examine if these peptides have other functions besides antimicrobial activity. We found pro-, cathelin-, and mature-form PG-1 enhanced cell migration but not cell proliferation (**Figure 5**), suggesting these peptides may interact with cell-surface receptors. It was reported that cathelicidin LL-37 and mCRAMP trans-activated epidermal growth factor receptor (EGFR) (Tokumaru et al., 2005; Yang et al., 2006). Whether PG-1, and its proform and the cathelin domain have their migration function via activating membrane receptor warrant further investigation.

For therapeutic applications, the stability of the recombinant AMPs produced is important. The stability test results indicated that the rPG-1 retain antimicrobial activity in a wide range of pH conditions ranging from pH 2.0 to 11.0. The pH in wounds ranges from 5.0 to 8.5, which is suitable for rPG-1 use. Oral application of rPG-1 may also be feasible in the digestive tract (pH 3.0 and 4.4 in mouse and pig, respectively). The activity of rPG-1 remained stable over a broad temperature range from 25°C to 95°C. This stability may be due to the high cysteine content (disulfide bonds) in rPG-1 (Lai and Gallo, 2009). In conclusion, recombinant protegrin in its pro-, cathelin-, and mature- forms were successfully expressed in *P. pastoris* using the *AOX* expression system. These peptides exhibit antimicrobial activity as well as cell migration activity. Further *in vivo* studies on the role of PG in modulating intestinal health would be of interest for intestinal inflammation application (Harwig et al., 1996).

## AUTHOR CONTRIBUTIONS

EH performed the major experiments and wrote the manuscript. NA performed parts of experiments and helped in writing. JL helped in designing the research, data interpretation and editing.

## FUNDING

This project has been funded by Ontario Pork (grant # 051379), Natural Sciences and Engineering Research Council of Canada (NSERC, grant # 400876), and Foshan University (grant # 053385).

## REFERENCES


Abad, S., Kitz, K., Hörmann, A., Schreiner, U., Hartner, F. S., and Glieder, A. (2010). Real-time PCR-based determination of gene copy numbers in *Pichia pastoris*. *Biotechnol. J.* 5, 413–420. doi: 10.1002/biot.200900233

Baratti, J., Maroux, S., Louvard, D., and Desnuelle, P. (1973). On porcine enterokinase. Further purification and some molecular properties. *Biochim. Biophys. Acta* 315, 147–161. doi: 10.1016/0005-2744(73)90138-1

Benmoussa, K., Authier, H., Prat, M., AlaEddine, M., Lefèvre, L., Rahabi, M. C., et al. (2017). P17, an original host defense peptide from ant venom. *Front. Immunol.* 8:1650. doi: 10.3389/fimmu.2017.01650

Boettner, M., Steffens, C., von Mering, C., Bork, P., Stahl, U., and Lang, C. (2007). Sequence-based factors influencing the expression of heterologous genes in the yeast *Pichia pastoris*—A comparative view on 79 human genes. *J. Biotechnol.* 130, 1–10. doi: 10.1016/j.jbiotec.2007.02.019

Boman, H. G. (2003). Antibacterial peptides: basic facts and emerging concepts. *J. Intern. Med.* 254, 197–215. doi: 10.1046/j.1365-2796.2003.01228.x

Brady, C. P., Shimp, R. L., Miles, A. P., Whitmore, M., and Stowers, A. W. (2001). High-level production and purification of P30P2MSP119, an important vaccine antigen for Malaria, expressed in the methylotropic yeast *Pichia pastoris*. *Protein Expr. Purif.* 23, 468–475. doi: 10.1006/prep.2001.1526

Chen, Z., Wang, D., Cong, Y., Wang, J., Zhu, J., Yang, J., et al. (2011). Recombinant antimicrobial peptide hPAB-β expressed in *Pichia pastoris*, a potential agent active against methicillin-resistant *Staphylococcus aureus*. *Appl. Microbiol. Biotechnol.* 89, 281–291. doi: 10.1007/s00253-010-2864-0

Choi, K.-Y., Chow, L. N. Y., and Mookherjee, N. (2012). Cationic host defence peptides: multifaceted role in immune modulation and inflammation. *J. Innate Immun.* 4, 361–370. doi: 10.1159/000336630

Ciofalo, V., Barton, N., Kreps, J., Coats, I., and Shanahan, D. (2006). Safety evaluation of a lipase enzyme preparation, expressed in *Pichia pastoris*, intended for use in the degumming of edible vegetable oil. *Regul. Toxicol. Pharmacol.* 45, 1–8. doi: 10.1016/j.yrtph.2006.02.001

Clare, J. J., Rayment, F. B., Ballantine, S. P., Sreekrishna, K., and Romanos, M. A. (1991a). High-level expression of tetanus toxin fragment C in *Pichia pastoris* strains containing multiple tandem integrations of the gene. *Biotechnology* 9, 455–460.

Clare, J. J., Romanes, M. A., Rayment, F. B., Rowedder, J. E., Smith, M. A., Payne, M. M., et al. (1991b). Production of mouse epidermal growth factor in yeast: high-level secretion using *Pichia pastoris* strains containing multiple gene copies. *Gene* 105, 205–212.

de la Fuente-Núñez, C., Mansour, S. C., Wang, Z., Jiang, L., Breidenstein, E. B. M., Elliott, M., et al. (2014). Anti-biofilm and immunomodulatory activities of peptides that inhibit biofilms formed by pathogens isolated from cystic fibrosis patients. *Antibiotics* 3, 509–526. doi: 10.3390/antibiotics3040509

Dias, S. A., Freire, J. M., Pérez-Peinado, C., Domingues, M. M., Gaspar, D., Vale, N., et al. (2017). New potent membrane-targeting antibacterial peptides from viral capsid proteins. *Front. Microbiol.* 8:775. doi: 10.3389/fmicb.2017.00775

Fonseca, P., and Light, A. (1983). The purification and characterization of bovine enterokinase from membrane fragments in the duodenal mucosal fluid. *J. Biol. Chem.* 258, 14516–14520.

Frohm, M., Agerberth, B., Ahangari, G., Ståhle-Bäckdahl, M., Lidén, S., Wigzell, H., et al. (1997). The expression of the gene coding for the antibacterial peptide LL-37 is induced in human keratinocytes during inflammatory disorders. *J. Biol. Chem.* 272, 15258–15263. doi: 10.1074/jbc.272.24.15258

Hancock, R. E. W., and Sahl, H.-G. (2006). Antimicrobial and host-defense peptides as new anti-infective therapeutic strategies. *Nat. Biotechnol.* 24, 1551–1557. doi: 10.1038/nbt1267

Harwig, S. S., Waring, A., Yang, H. J., Cho, Y., Tan, L., and Lehrer, R. I. (1996). Intramolecular disulfide bonds enhance the antimicrobial and lytic activities of protegrins at physiological sodium chloride concentrations. *Eur. J. Biochem.* 240, 352–357. doi: 10.1111/j.1432-1033.1996.0352h.x

Hase, K., Murakami, M., Iimura, M., Cole, S. P., Horibe, Y., Ohtake, T., et al. (2003). Expression of LL-37 by human gastric epithelial cells as a potential host defense mechanism against *Helicobacter pylori*. *Gastroenterology* 125, 1613–1625. doi: 10.1053/j.gastro.2003.08.028

Hirano, T., Ishihara, K., and Hibi, M. (2000). Roles of STAT3 in mediating the cell growth, differentiation and survival signals relayed through the IL-6 family of cytokine receptors. *Oncogene* 19, 2548–2556. doi: 10.1038/sj.onc.1203551

Inaba, Y., Ashida, T., Ito, T., Ishikawa, C., Tanabe, H., Maemoto, A., et al. (2010). Expression of the antimicrobial peptide alpha-defensin/cryptdins in intestinal crypts decreases at the initial phase of intestinal inflammation in a model of inflammatory bowel disease, IL-10-deficient mice. *Inflamm. Bowel Dis.* 16, 1488–1495. doi: 10.1002/ibd.21253

Ishihara, K., and Hirano, T. (2002). IL-6 in autoimmune disease and chronic inflammatory proliferative disease. *Cytokine Growth Factor Rev.* 13, 357–368. doi: 10.1016/S1359-6101(02)00027-8

Jafari, R., Sundström, B. E., and Holm, P. (2011). Optimization of production of the anti-keratin 8 single-chain Fv TS1-218 in *Pichia pastoris* using design of experiments. *Microb. Cell Fact.* 10:34. doi: 10.1186/1475-2859-10-34

Jahic, M., Gustavsson, M., Jansen, A.-K., Martinelle, M., and Enfors, S.-O. (2003). Analysis and control of proteolysis of a fusion protein in *Pichia pastoris* fed-batch processes. *J. Biotechnol.* 102, 45–53. doi: 10.1016/S0168-1656(03)00003-8

Jahic, M., Knoblechner, J., Charoenrat, T., Enfors, S.-O., and Veide, A. (2006). Interfacing *Pichia pastoris* cultivation with expanded bed adsorption. *Biotechnol. Bioeng.* 93, 1040–1049. doi: 10.1002/bit.20811

Kovach, M. A., Ballinger, M. N., Newstead, M. W., Zeng, X., Bhan, U., Yu, F.-S., et al. (2012). Cathelicidin-related antimicrobial peptide is required for effective lung mucosal immunity in Gram-negative bacterial pneumonia. *J. Immunol.* 189, 304–311. doi: 10.4049/jimmunol.1103196

Lai, Y., and Gallo, R. L. (2009). AMPed up immunity: how antimicrobial peptides have multiple roles in immune defense. *Trends Immunol.* 30, 131–141. doi: 10.1016/j.it.2008.12.003

Li, L., Wang, J.-X., Zhao, X.-F., Kang, C.-J., Liu, N., Xiang, J.-H., et al. (2005). High level expression, purification, and characterization of the shrimp antimicrobial peptide. Ch-penaeidin, in *Pichia pastoris. Protein Expr. Purif.* 39, 144–151. doi: 10.1016/j.pep.2004.09.006

Liu, H., Hou, C., Wang, G., Jia, H., Yu, H., Zeng, X., et al. (2017). *Lactobacillus reuteri* I5007 modulates intestinal host defense peptide expression in the model of IPEC-J2 cells and neonatal piglets. *Nutrients* 9:E559. doi: 10.3390/nu9060559

Liu, T.-C., and Stappenbeck, T. S. (2016). Genetics and pathogenesis of inflammatory bowel disease. *Annu. Rev. Pathol.* 11, 127–148. doi: 10.1146/annurev-pathol-012615-044152

Livak, K. J., and Schmittgen, T. D. (2001). Analysis of relative gene expression data using real-time quantitative PCR and the 2(-Delta Delta C(T)) Method. *Methods* 25, 402–408. doi: 10.1006/meth.2001.1262

Ma, B., Shen, J., Yindeeyoungyeon, W., and Ruan, Y. (2017). A novel antibiotic mechanism of l-Cyclopropylalanine blocking the biosynthetic pathway of essential amino acid l-leucine. *Molecules* 22:E2224. doi: 10.3390/molecules22122224

Mansur, M., Cabello, C., Hernández, L., País, J., Varas, L., Valdés, J., et al. (2005). Multiple gene copy number enhances insulin precursor secretion in the yeast *Pichia pastoris. Biotechnol. Lett.* 27, 339–345. doi: 10.1007/s10529-005-1007-7

Nam, B.-H., Moon, J.-Y., Park, E.-H., Kim, Y.-O., Kim, D.-G., Kong, H. J., et al. (2014). Antimicrobial activity of peptides derived from olive flounder lipopolysaccharide binding protein/bactericidal permeability-increasing protein (LBP/BPI). *Mar. Drugs* 12, 5240–5257. doi: 10.3390/md12105240

Nordén, K., Agemark, M., Danielson, J. ÅH., Alexandersson, E., Kjellbom, P., and Johanson, U. (2011). Increasing gene dosage greatly enhances recombinant expression of aquaporins in *Pichia pastoris. BMC Biotechnol.* 11:47. doi: 10.1186/1472-6750-11-47

Pizzo, E., Zanfardino, A., Di Giuseppe, A. M. A., Bosso, A., Landi, N., Ragucci, S., et al. (2015). A new active antimicrobial peptide from PD-L4, a type 1 ribosome inactivating protein ofPhytolacca dioica L.: a new function of RIPs for plant defence?. *FEBS Lett.* 589, 2812–2818. doi: 10.1016/j.febslet.2015.08.018

Proudfoot, A. E. I. (2002). Chemokine receptors: multifaceted therapeutic targets. *Nat. Rev. Immunol.* 2, 106–115. doi: 10.1038/nri722

Ramamoorthy, S., and Kushner, D. J. (1975). Binding of mercuric and other heavy metal ions by microbial growth media. *Microb. Ecol.* 2, 162–176. doi: 10.1007/BF02010436

Rosano, G. L., and Ceccarelli, E. A. (2014). Recombinant protein expression in *Escherichia coli*: advances and challenges. *Front. Microbiol.* 5:172. doi: 10.3389/fmicb.2014.00172

Sang, Y., and Blecha, F. (2008). Antimicrobial peptides and bacteriocins: alternatives to traditional antibiotics. *Anim. Health Res. Rev.* 9, 227–235. doi: 10.1017/S1466252308001497

Schär-Zammaretti, P., Dillmann, M.-L., D'Amico, N., Affolter, M., and Ubbink, J. (2005). Influence of fermentation medium composition on physicochemical surface properties of *Lactobacillus acidophilus. Appl. Environ. Microbiol.* 71, 8165–8173. doi: 10.1128/AEM.71.12.8165-8173.2005

Schauber, J., Rieger, D., Weiler, F., Wehkamp, J., Eck, M., Fellermann, K., et al. (2006). Heterogeneous expression of human cathelicidin hCAP18/LL-37 in inflammatory bowel diseases. *Eur. J. Gastroenterol. Hepatol.* 18, 615–621. doi: 10.1097/00042737-200606000-00007

Schmittgen, T. D., and Livak, K. J. (2008). Analyzing real-time PCR data by the comparative CT method. *Nat. Protoc.* 3, 1101–1108. doi: 10.1038/nprot.2008.73

Steinberg, D. A., Hurst, M. A., Fujii, C. A., Kung, A. H., Ho, J. F., Cheng, F. C., et al. (1997). Protegrin-1: a broad-spectrum, rapidly microbicidal peptide with in vivo activity. *Antimicrob. Agents Chemother.* 41, 1738–1742.

Steinberg, D. A., and Lehrer, R. I. (1997). "Designer assays for antimicrobial peptides," in *Antibacterial Peptide Protocols*, ed. W. M. Shafer (Totowa, NJ: Humana Press), 169–186.

Stratton, J., Chiruvolu, V., and Meagher, M. (1998). "High cell-density fermentation," in *Pichia Protocols*, ed. J. M. Cregg (Totowa, NJ: Humana Press), 107–120.

Taghavian, O., Spiegel, H., Hauck, R., Hafez, H. M., Fischer, R., and Schillberg, S. (2013). Protective oral vaccination against infectious bursal disease virus using the major viral antigenic protein VP2 produced in *Pichia pastoris. PLoS One* 8:e83210. doi: 10.1371/journal.pone.0083210

Termén, S., Tollin, M., Rodriguez, E., Sveinsdóttir, S. H., Jóhannesson, B., Cederlund, A., et al. (2008). PU.1 and bacterial metabolites regulate the human gene CAMP encoding antimicrobial peptide LL-37 in colon epithelial cells. *Mol. Immunol.* 45, 3947–3955. doi: 10.1016/j.molimm.2008.06.020

Thompson, C. A. (2010). FDA approves kallikrein inhibitor to treat hereditary angioedema. *Am. J. Health Syst. Pharm.* 67:93. doi: 10.2146/news100005

Tokumaru, S., Sayama, K., Shirakata, Y., Komatsuzawa, H., Ouhara, K., Hanakawa, Y., et al. (2005). Induction of keratinocyte migration via transactivation of the epidermal growth factor receptor by the antimicrobial peptide LL-37. *J. Immunol.* 175, 4662–4668. doi: 10.4049/jimmunol.175.7.4662

Yan, H., and Hancock, R. E. (2001). Synergistic interactions between mammalian antimicrobial defense peptides. *Antimicrob. Agents Chemother.* 45, 1558–1560. doi: 10.1128/AAC.45.5.1558-1560.2001

Yang, Y. H., Wu, W. K. K., Tai, E. K. K., Wong, H. P. S., Lam, E. K. Y., So, W. H. L., et al. (2006). The cationic host defense peptide rCRAMP promotes gastric ulcer healing in rats. *J. Pharmacol. Exp. Ther.* 318, 547–554. doi: 10.1124/jpet.106.102467

Zaiou, M., Nizet, V., and Gallo, R. L. (2003). Antimicrobial and protease inhibitory functions of the human cathelicidin (hCAP18/LL-37) prosequence. *J. Invest. Dermatol.* 120, 810–816. doi: 10.1046/j.1523-1747.2003.12132.x

Zeng, X., Sunkara, L. T., Jiang, W., Bible, M., Carter, S., Ma, X., et al. (2013). Induction of porcine host defense peptide gene expression by short-chain fatty acids and their analogs. *PLoS One* 8:e72922. doi: 10.1371/journal.pone.0072922

Zhang, Y., Teng, D., Wang, X., Mao, R., Cao, X., Hu, X., et al. (2015). In vitro and in vivo characterization of a new recombinant antimicrobial peptide, MP1102, against methicillin-resistant *Staphylococcus aureus. Appl. Microbiol. Biotechnol.* 99, 6255–6266. doi: 10.1007/s00253-015-6394-7

Zhu, S., Wei, L., Yamasaki, K., and Gallo, R. L. (2008). Activation of cathepsin L by the cathelin-like domain of protegrin-3. *Mol. Immunol.* 45, 2531–2536. doi: 10.1016/j.molimm.2008.01.007

Zhu, T., Guo, M., Tang, Z., Zhang, M., Zhuang, Y., Chu, J., et al. (2009). Efficient generation of multi-copy strains for optimizing secretory expression of porcine insulin precursor in yeast *Pichia pastoris. J. Appl. Microbiol.* 107, 954–963. doi: 10.1111/j.1365-2672.2009.04279.x

# Effects of Monolaurin on Oral Microbe–Host Transcriptome and Metabolome

*Viviam de Oliveira Silva[1,2†], Luciano José Pereira[3], Silvana Pasetto[2], Maike Paulino da Silva[2], Jered Cope Meyers[4] and Ramiro Mendonça Murata[4,5*]*

[1] Department of Veterinary Medicine, Federal University of Lavras, Lavras, Brazil, [2] Division of Periodontology, Diagnostic Sciences, Dental Hygiene and Biomedical Science, Herman Ostrow School of Dentistry, University of Southern California, Los Angeles, CA, United States, [3] Department of Health Sciences, Federal University of Lavras, Lavras, Brazil, [4] Department Foundational Sciences, School of Dental Medicine, East Carolina University, Greenville, NC, United States, [5] Department of Microbiology and Immunology, Brody School of Medicine, East Carolina University, Greenville, NC, United States

***Correspondence:**
*Ramiro Mendonça Murata*
*murartar16@ecu.edu*

**†Present address:**
*Viviam de Oliveira Silva, Department of Research and Scientific Initiation, Centro Universitário Atenas, Paracatu, Brazil*

The aim of this *in vitro* study was to evaluate the effects of monolaurin against *Aggregatibacter actinomycetemcomitans* (Aa) and determine their effects on the host transcriptome and metabolome, using an oral cell/bacteria co-culture dual-chamber model to mimic the human periodontium. For this, the Aa, was applied to cross the monolayer of epithelial keratinocytes (OBA-9) to reach the fibroblasts layer (HGF-1) in the basal chamber. The Monolaurin treatments (25 or 50 μM) were added immediately after the inoculation of the dual-chamber with Aa. After 24 h, the transcriptional factors and metabolites produced were quantified in the remaining cell layers (insert and basal chamber) and in supernatant released from the cells. The genes IL-1α, IL-6, IL-18, and TNF analyzed in HGF-1 concentrations showed a decreased expression when treated with both concentration of Monolaurin. In keratinocytes, the genes IL-6, IL-18, and TNF presented a higher expression and the expression of IL-1α decreased when treated with the two cited concentrations. The production of glycerol and pyruvic acid increased, and the 2-deoxytetronic acid NIST, 4-aminobutyric acid, pinitol and glyceric acid, presented lower concentrations because of the treatment with 25 and/or 50 μM of Monolaurin. Use of monolaurin modulated the immune response and metabolite production when administered for 24 h in a dual-chamber model inoculated with *A. actinomycetemcomitans*. In summary, this study indicates that monolaurin had antimicrobial activity and modulated the host immune response and metabolite production when administered for 24 h in a dual-chamber model inoculated with *A. actinomycetemcomitans*.

**Keywords: *Aggregatibacter actinomycetemcomitans*, periodontal disease, immune system, fibroblast, keratinocyte, monolaurin**

## INTRODUCTION

Periodontal disease is characterized by bacterial infection associated with the presence of biofilm, resulting in chronic inflammation of the tooth supporting tissues leading to a progressive destruction of periodontal tissue and alveolar bone. Signs and symptoms of periodontitis can include gingival swelling, bleeding during brushing, periodontal pockets, increased spacing between the teeth and tooth loss (Irfan et al., 2001; Michaud et al., 2007; Savage et al., 2009; Gurav, 2014).

The most common form of periodontal disease, denominated periodontitis, affects approximately 50% of the adult population with its severe forms affecting 10–15% of these individuals (Chapple and Genco, 2013).

The oral biofilm is composed of at least 800 different species of bacteria (Paster et al., 2006; Filoche et al., 2010). Numerous periodontopathogenic bacteria (*Porphyromonas gingivalis*, *Fusobacterium nucleatum*, *Streptococcus intermedius*, and others) are responsible for the initiation and maintenance of periodontal inflammation (Coussens and Werb, 2002; Oringer, 2002; Loos, 2005; Moutsopoulos and Madianos, 2006; de Almeida et al., 2007). The *Aggregatibacter actinomycetemcomitans* is a fermentative, gram-negative and capnophilic coccobacillus. It is not only considered the most important agent of localized aggressive periodontitis lesions, but is associated with chronic periodontitis as well (Slots et al., 1980; Zambon et al., 1983; Haraszthy et al., 2000; Gafan et al., 2004; Yang et al., 2004; Cortelli et al., 2009; Rakić et al., 2010; da Silva-Boghossian et al., 2011). The progression of periodontal disease is associated with the virulence factors of the microorganism, together with the vulnerability of the host. Aa produces leukotoxin, adhesins, bacteriocins, and lipopolysaccharide, which are responsible for interacting with the host cells triggering an inflammatory response in the periodontium (Cortelli et al., 2009). In addition, another critical factor for soft tissue inflammation and bone resorption is the immune-inflammatory host response to the bacterial biofilm (Salvi and Lang, 2005).

According to Aimetti (2014), non-surgical periodontal treatments possess limitations, such as the long-term maintainability of deep periodontal pockets, risk of disease recurrence, and skill of the operator. The development of new therapeutic agents that have the ability to inhibit the biofilm formation and modulate the inflammatory response can have a major impact in the prevention and treatment of periodontal disease. Monolaurin, also known as glycerol monolaurate or lauroyl, is a natural surfactant compound commonly used in cosmetics and the food industry. It is recognized by the Food and Drug Administration (FDA) as a GRAS (Generally Recognized as Safe) food additive since 1977. This natural compound is found in coconut oil and human breast milk (Fu et al., 2006; Peterson and Schlievert, 2006).

Monolaurin presents antibacterial and antiviral activity *in vitro* (Projan et al., 1994; Isaacs, 2001; Preuss et al., 2005; Peterson and Schlievert, 2006; Carpo et al., 2007), which may be of great interest in the treatment and/or prevention of various infections. However, the effect of monolaurin on periodontopathogenic bacteria has yet to be determined.

Therefore, the aims of this *in vitro* study were to evaluate the cytotoxicity, the antimicrobial effect of monolaurin against *A. actinomycetemcomitans* and to determine its effect on the host transcriptome and metabolome using a gum cell – bacteria co-culture model.

# MATERIALS AND METHODS

## Monolaurin

For carrying out the experiments, the monolaurin utilized was 1-lauroyl-rac-glycerol (Sigma-Aldrich, St. Louis, MO, United States). For dilution, sterilized deionized water was used as the vehicle.

## Cells and Bacterial Strain

Human gingival fibroblast - HGF-1 (ATCC® CRL-2014) were cultured in Dulbecco's Modified Eagle's Medium (DMEM) (Lonza, Walkersville, MD, United States) with 10% Fetal Bovine Serum (FBS) (Lonza, Walkersville, MD, United States). Human gingival epithelial cells (keratinocyte OBA-9) were cultured in specific medium for keratinocytes, Defined Keratinocyte-SFM (Life Technologies, Carlsbad, CA, United States) (Oda and Watson, 1990; Kusumoto et al., 2004).

*Aggregatibacter actinomycetemcomitans* (strain D7S-1) was cultivated from a subgingival plaque from an African-American female patient diagnosed with generalized aggressive periodontitis (Chen et al., 2010). The bacteria were grown in Trypticase Soy Broth (TSB) (Becton Dickinson, Franklin Lakes, NJ, United States).

## Antimicrobial Activity

Monolaurin antimicrobial activity was evaluated in *A. actinomycetemcomitans* after 24 h of treatment. Micro-organisms were inoculated [$1 \times 10^6$ colony-forming unit per milliliter (CFU/mL) in a 96-well microtiter plate with TSB (Becton Dickinson, Franklin Lakes, NJ, United States)] and monolaurin was immediately added in various concentrations (0.5–1,000 $\mu$M) to determine the minimum inhibitory concentration (MIC) (Branco-de-Almeida et al., 2011). Microplates were maintained in a humidified incubator at 37°C and 5% $CO_2$. After incubation, bacterial growth was assayed by measurement of absorbance at 660 nm. MIC was defined as the lowest concentration of monolaurin that had restricted growth to a level, 0.05 at 660 nm (no visible growth).

## Cytotoxicity Assay

*In vitro* cytotoxicity effect was measured by the fluorometric resazurin method (O'Brien et al., 2000). OBA-9 or HGF-1 cells were seeded ($1 \times 10^5$ cells/mL) in 96-well microtiter plates and maintained in a humidified incubator at 37°C and 5% $CO_2$. After 24 h, cell morphology was observed under an inverted microscope (EVOS FL Life Technologies, Carlsbad, CA, United States) to confirm that they had adhered to the bottom of each well and were presenting proper morphology. The monolaurin (0.5–1,000 $\mu$M) was added to the cell cultures and incubated at 37°C and 5% $CO_2$. After 24 h, the medium was discarded, cells were washed with room temperature phosphate buffered saline (PBS) (Lonza, Walkersville, MD, United States), and fresh, room temperature medium was added with resazurin (Cell Titer Blue Viability Assay - Promega Corp., Madison, WI, United States). Subsequently, the plate was incubated at 37°C and 5% $CO_2$. After 4 h, the contents of the wells were transferred to a new microplate and the fluorescence was read in a microplate reader (SpectraMax M5, Molecular Devices, Sunnyvale, CA, United States) with excitation 550 nm, emission 585 nm, and cut off 570 nm (Pasetto et al., 2014). To calculate the results and obtain the $LD_{50}$ (Lethal Dose), we performed a non-linear regression the program MasterPlex ReaderFit (Hitachi Solutions America).

## Dual-Chamber Model

A dual-chamber, oral cell/bacteria co-culture was used to investigate the immunological effects of monolaurin (Silva et al., 2017). HGF-1 cells ($1 \times 10^5$) were seed in the basal chamber of a 24-well plate. Transwell inserts (8 $\mu$m pore $\times$ 0.3 $cm^2$ of culture surface - Greiner Bio-One, Monroe, NC, United States) were positioned in each well and OBA-9 cells ($1 \times 10^5$) were seeded into the inserts. DMEM (Lonza, Walkersville, MD, United States) with 10% FBS (Lonza, Walkersville, MD, United States) was used for the medium. The plates were incubated at 37°C in humid air containing 5% $CO_2$ for 24 h (Silva et al., 2017). Trans Epithelial Electric Resistance (TEER) of each cell layer was measured with a Millicell-ERS Volt-Ohm Meter (Millipore, Bedford, MA, United States). Cell layer confluence in the Transwell insert was measured daily until reaching optimal TEER (>150 Ohm/$cm^2$) after 48 h. Once reaching optimal TEER, the media of the basal chamber and the insert were replaced with new media containing *A. actinomycetemcomitans* ($1 \times 10^6$ CFU/mL). Medium containing the microorganism was added to the insert, passing through the upper layer of cells (OBA-9) and reaching the bottom cell layer (HGF-1). Immediately after the inoculation of oral cell/bacteria co-culture with *A. actinomycetemcomitans* the monolaurin treatments (25 and 50 $\mu$M) were added and the plate was incubated at 37°C in humid air containing 5% $CO_2$. The time of exposure of the microorganism to monolaurin was 24 h. Each experiment was repeated three times with two replicates per group ($n$ = 6). The experiment was divided in three groups: (1) Control - oral cell/bacteria co-culture with Aa inoculated and no treatment; (2) Mono 25 - oral cell/bacteria co-culture with Aa inoculated and treated with 25 $\mu$M of monolaurin; (3) Mono 50 - oral cell/bacteria co-culture with Aa inoculated and treated with 50 $\mu$M of monolaurin.

## Collecting Samples for Analysis

After the treatment period, liquid contents from each well was collected and centrifuged at 1,200 rpm for 10 min. Following centrifugation, supernatant was divided into two aliquots for enzyme-linked immunosorbent assay (ELISA) and metabolome analysis. RNA was isolated from the remaining cell layers of HGF-1 and OBA-9 (surface of the wells and inserts) for gene analysis in quantitative real-time PCR.

## ELISA Assay

Inflammatory cytokines were determined using a commercial ELISA (Multi-Analyte ELISArray - Qiagen, Valencia, CA, United States). The cytokines were measured by standard ELISA protocol using a panel of 12 inflammatory cytokines: interleukin-1 alpha (IL-1α), interleukin-1 beta (IL-1β), interleukin-2 (IL-2), interleukin-4 (IL-4), interleukin-6 (IL-6), interleukin-8 (IL-8), interleukin-10 (IL-10), interleukin-12 (IL-12), interleukin-17 alpha (IL-17α), interferon gamma (IFNγ), tumor necrosis factor alpha (TNFα), Granulocyte-Macrophage Colony Stimulating Factor (GM-CSF). Cytokines that presented the greatest change in concentration were selected for detailed analysis. These cytokines were analyzed using a standard ELISA protocol (Single Analyte ELISA Kit - Qiagen, Valencia, CA, United States).

## Gene Expression – Quantitative Real-Time PCR

Total RNA was extracted through a commercial RNA purification kit (Mini Kit Qiagen RNeasy Protocol - Qiagen, Valencia, CA, United States) and the purity and quantity were measured in a NanoPhotometer P360 (Implen, Westlake Village, CA, United States). Total RNA was converted into single-stranded cDNA using a high-capacity reverse transcription kit (QuantiTec Reverse Transcription Kit - Qiagen, Valencia, CA, United States). An array for evaluation of gene expression of the inflammatory response was completed by quantitative real-time PCR (Prime PCR Pathway Plate/Acute Inflammation Response - Bio-Rad, Hercules, CA, United States) from the cDNA obtained. Based on these results, six genes/primers were selected for detailed study: interleukin 1 alpha (IL-1α), interleukin 6 (IL-6), interleukin 18 (IL-18), caspase 3 (CASP3), matrix metallopeptidase 1 (MMP-1), and tumor necrosis factor (TNF) (QuantiTect Primer Assay - Qiagen, Valencia, CA, United States). QuantiTect SYBR Green PCR Kits (Qiagen, Valencia, CA, United States) were used to determine the gene expression of the selected primers. The reaction product was quantified by relative quantification using Glyceraldehyde 3-phosphate dehydrogenase (GAPDH) as the reference gene. Data were analyzed as fold-change compared to control. The cycle threshold was calculated and interpreted using CFX Connect (Bio-Rad, Hercules, CA, United States) (Pfaffl, 2001).

## Metabolome Analysis

Samples for metabolome analysis were treated as described by Silva et al. (2017) and analyzed at the West Coast Metabolomics Center (UC Davis Genome Center, Davis, CA, United States) by means of gas chromatography/mass spectrometry (Agilent 6890, Santa Clara, CA/Leco Pegasus IV, St. Joseph, MI, United States). Then, the metabolites were compared with the standard library for proper identification (Fiehn and Kind, 2007).

## Statistical Analysis

Data were expressed as mean ± standard deviation. The comparison between the groups was made through analysis of variance (ANOVA) and when a difference was determined, the Bonferroni test was applied. Data were analyzed using GraphPad Prism (version 5.01, GraphPad Software, San Diego, United States). The level of significance was set at $p < 0.05$.

# RESULTS

## Antimicrobial Activity and Cytotoxicity Assay

In order to determine antimicrobial activity of monolaurin, a range of 0.5–1,000 μM was tested. Antibacterial activity was detected at 25–50 μM. The minimum inhibitory concentration (MIC) was established between 25 and 50 μM. The cytotoxicity assays were conducted in HGF-1 and OBA-9 cells and the results are shown in **Figure 1**. For HGF-1 the $LD_{50}$ was 146 μM of monolaurin and for OBA-9 the $LD_{50}$ was 69 μM of monolaurin.

## ELISA

Enzyme-linked immunosorbent assay (ELISA) results are presented in **Figure 2**. Both treatments (25 and 50 μM) of monolaurin increased the concentrations of GM-CSF and IL-1α. The concentrations of IL-6 and IL-10 increased only with the 50 μM treatment. On the other hand, IL-1β decreased as a function of monolaurin.

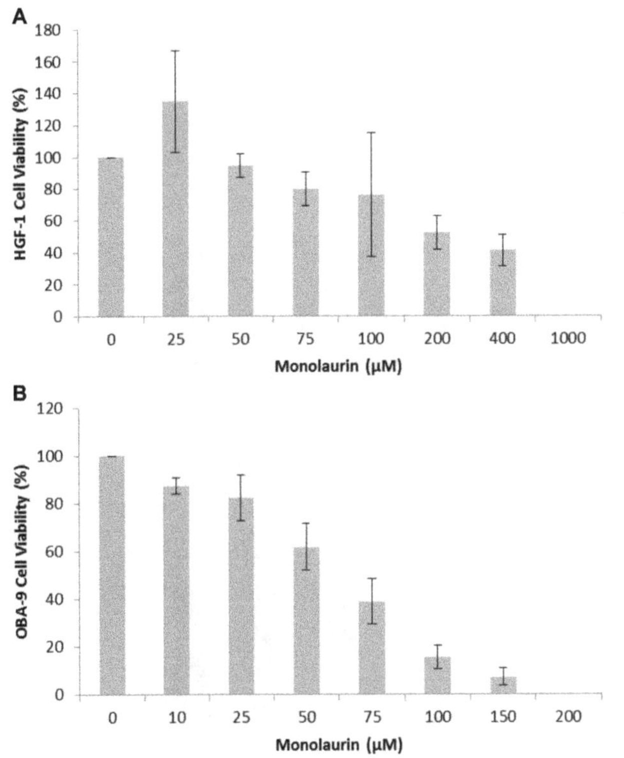


**FIGURE 1** | Cytotoxicity assay of cells treated with different doses of monolaurin in an oral cell/bacteria co-culture inoculated with *A. actinomycetemcomitans*: **(A)** HGF-1 cell (fibroblasts); **(B)** OBA-9 cell (keratinocytes). Cell viability was presented in percentage (%) ± standard deviation. Control group = 100% viability, $n = 6$. Non-treated cells were considered as 100% viability; DMSO was used as positive control to demonstrate an appropriate system-cell response (100% cytotoxicity – data not shown).

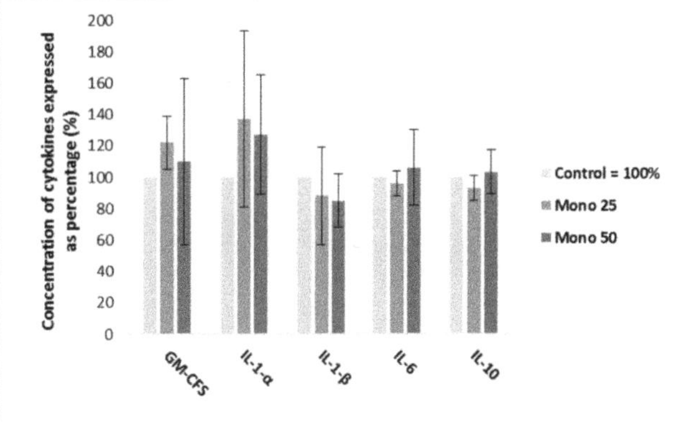


**FIGURE 2** | Percent concentrations of GM-CSF, IL-1α, IL-1-β, IL-6, and IL-10 by ELISA, obtained from cell culture supernatant. Oral cell co-culture inoculated with *A. actinomycetemcomitans* and treated with 25 μM of monolaurin (Mono 25) or 50 μM of monolaurin (Mono 50) compared with the control group. Control group is oral cell co-culture inoculated with *A. actinomycetemcomitans* and no treatment. The control group mean is expressed as 100% and treated groups have their mean relative to the control group. Mean ± standard deviation; $n = 4$.

## Gene Expression – Quantitative Real-Time PCR

Quantitative real-time PCR results are presented in **Figures 3, 4**. The genes IL-1α, IL-6, IL-18, and TNF analyzed in HGF-1 showed a decreased expression ($p < 0.05$) when treated with 25 or 50 μM of monolaurin compared with group Control (**Figures 3A–C,F**). CASP3 and MMP-1 genes showed no difference (**Figures 3D,E**).

Keratinocytes presented a higher IL-6, IL-18, and TNF gene expression ($p < 0.05$) when treated with 25 or 50 μM of monolaurin compared with the control group (**Figures 4B,C,F**). IL-1α gene decreased expression ($p < 0.05$) in the group treated with both concentrations (**Figure 4A**). CASP-3 and MMP-1 genes showed no difference (**Figures 4D,E**).

## Metabolome

The metabolome study returned a total of 283 metabolites. Of these, 120 were identified and only 6 presented a statistical difference as a function of monolaurin treatment. Some metabolites presented significantly altered concentrations (**Figure 5**). It was observed that both treatments of monolaurin increased the production of glycerol (**Figure 5D**) and pyruvic acid (**Figure 5F**) when compared to control. On the other hand, the 2-deoxytetronic acid NIST (**Figure 5A**) showed the opposite result, lower concentrations of this metabolite, in function of the treatment with 25 and 50 μM of monolaurin. The 50 μM monolaurin treatment group presented lower concentrations of 4-aminobutyric acid (**Figure 5B**), glyceric acid (**Figure 5C**), and pinitol (**Figure 5E**), against the control group.

# DISCUSSION

Periodontal disease is known to be a widespread oral health problem across the world. Several methods for prevention and treatment of oral diseases have been used over time and new

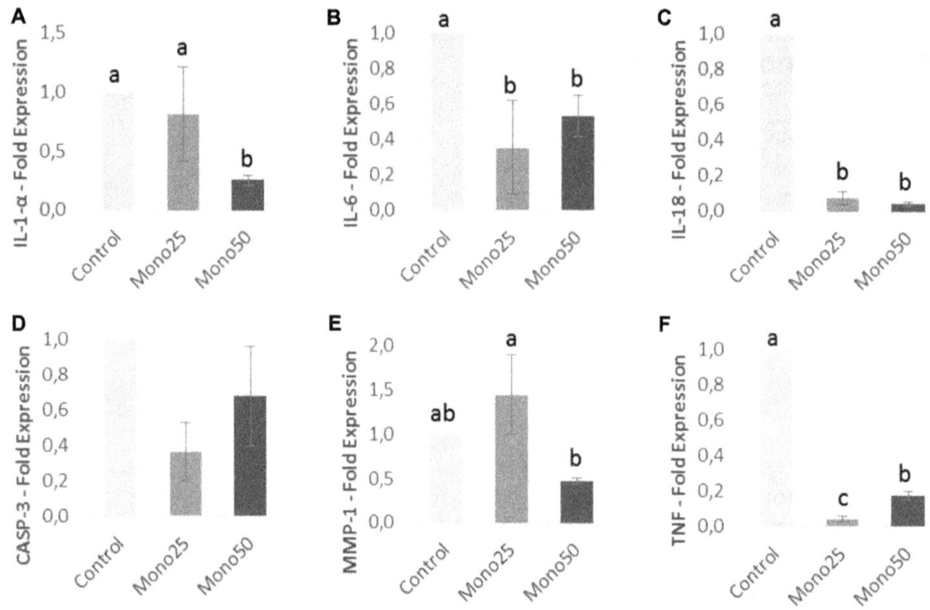


**FIGURE 3 |** Relative expression of genes from HGF-1 cells (fibroblasts) by quantitative PCR: **(A)** IL-1α; **(B)** IL-6; **(C)** IL-18; **(D)** CASP3; **(E)** MMP-1; **(F)** TNF. Oral cell/bacteria co-culture inoculated with *A. actinomycetemcomitans* and treated with different doses of monolaurin (25 μM – Mono 25 or 50 μM – Mono 50). Control group is oral cell co-culture inoculated with *A. actinomycetemcomitans* and no treatment. The control group has their mean expressed equal to 1 and treated groups have their mean relative to the control group. Different letters (a, b, and c) indicate statistical difference between groups. The results were expressed by mean ± standard deviation; $n = 6$ and $p < 0.05$.

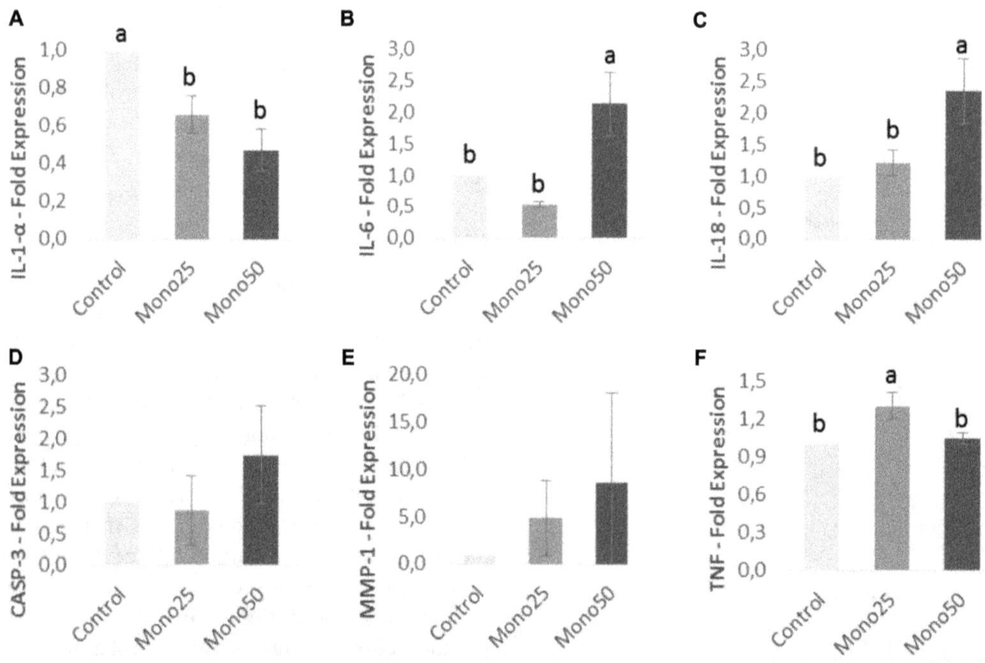


**FIGURE 4 |** Relative expression of genes from OBA-9 cells (keratinocytes) by quantitative PCR: **(A)** IL-1α; **(B)** IL-6; **(C)** IL-18; **(D)** CASP3; **(E)** MMP-1; **(F)** TNF. Oral cell/bacteria co-culture inoculated with *A. actinomycetemcomitans* and treated with different doses of monolaurin (25 μM – Mono 25 or 50 μM – Mono 50). Control group is oral cell co-culture inoculated with *A. actinomycetemcomitans* and no treatment. The control group has their mean expressed equal to 1 and treated groups have their mean relative to the control group. Different letters (a, b, and c) indicate statistical difference between groups. The results were expressed by mean ± standard deviation; $n = 6$ and $p < 0.05$.

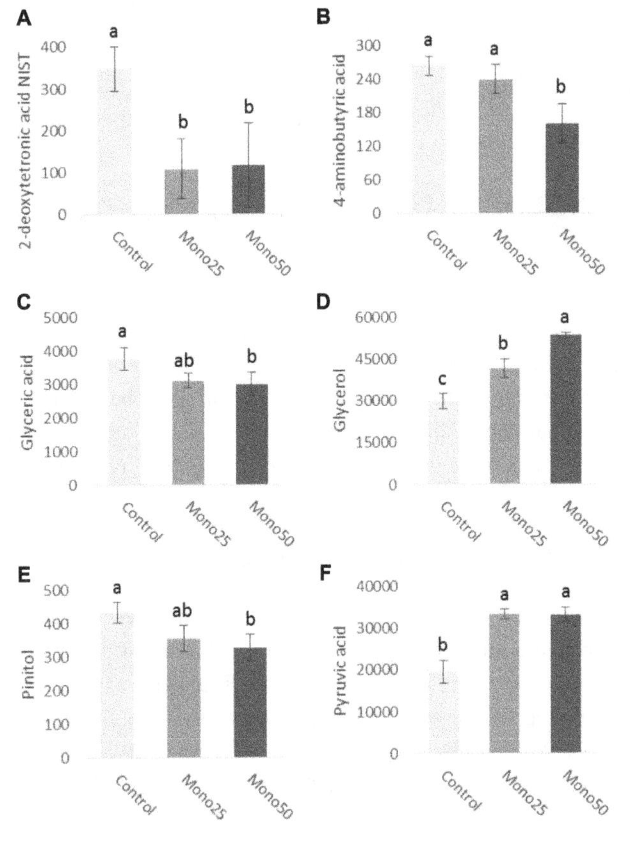


**FIGURE 5 |** Metabolites obtained from cell culture supernatant (HGF-1 and OBA-9 co-culture cells): **(A)** 2-deoxytetronic acid NIST; **(B)** 4-aminobutyric acid; **(C)** glyceric acid; **(D)** glycerol; **(E)** pinitol; **(F)** pyruvic acid. Oral cell/bacteria co-culture model inoculated with *A. actinomycetemcomitans* and treated with different doses of monolaurin (25 μM – Mono 25 or 50 μM – Mono 50). Control group is oral cell co-culture inoculated with *A. actinomycetemcomitans* and no treatment. Different letters (a, b, and c) indicate statistical difference between groups. The data is expressed in relative peak heights (mAU) from HPLCMS analysis, which are unitless (mean ± standard deviation); $n = 4$ and $p < 0.05$.

technologies are being developed. However, little attention has been given to the understanding of how periodontal structures are affected and how these structures react to different types of treatments (Balloni et al., 2016). Currently, some mouthwashes and toothpastes have been used as topical antimicrobial agents (Barnett, 2003). However, monolaurin is not listed as an active ingredient in commercially available mouthwashes. Monolaurin has been shown to possess diverse biological activities, such as antibacterial and antiviral properties (Preuss et al., 2005; Li et al., 2009; Tangwatcharin and Khopaibool, 2012; Seleem et al., 2016). In our *in vitro* study, susceptibility assays of monolaurin showed inhibition of microorganism grow at 25–50 μM with minimal cytotoxicity. The putative pathways by which monolaurin affects Aa may involve: (i) increased membrane permeability and cell lysis, (ii) disruption of electron transport chain and uncoupling oxidative phosphorylation, and (iii) inhibition of membrane enzymatic activities and nutrient uptake (Yoon et al., 2018). In addition, co-culture supernatant were assessed for expression of host pro-inflammatory cytokines, gene expression of inflammatory cytokines and metabolomic profile in human cells infected with *A. actinomycetemcomitans*.

The gingival tissue comprises the oral epithelium and superficial underlying connective tissue. These tissues are sites of initiation for inflammatory processes and the first to be affected by biofilm (Balloni et al., 2016). Gingival epithelial cells represent a physical barrier against bacteria and are involved in processes of innate immunity (Jang et al., 2015). Keratinocytes and fibroblasts represent the major cell types present in gingival epithelial tissues. They interact directly with pathogenic microorganisms and are able to express a variety of cytokines and chemokines such as IL-1α, IL-6, IL-8, TNF, among others (Bodet et al., 2007; Groeger and Meyle, 2015). In the present study, there was a decrease in the gene expression of IL-1α, IL-6, and IL-18 and TNF in HGF-1 and an increase in the expression of IL-6, IL-18, and TNF in OBA-9 cells treated with monolaurin indicating a positive modulation in the inflammatory response of these cells.

Interleukin-1 alpha is a polypeptide that plays several roles in tissue homeostasis, immunity and has a proinflammatory nature. It is produced mainly by macrophages and monocytes, but also epithelial cells and fibroblasts (Champagne et al., 2003; Balloni et al., 2016). IL-1α plays a critical role in protecting the body against invaders, such as bacteria and viruses, and is involved in extracellular matrix and bone metabolism (bone resorption, disintegration, and removal of bone tissue that is no longer needed). Therefore, IL-1α is considered a marker of periodontal disease (Govindarajan et al., 2015; Groeger and Meyle, 2015).

Here, we observed a decrease in the expression of IL-1α by HGF-1 and OBA-9 cells in the monolaurin-treated groups which may be related to a beneficial inflammatory response since, elevated levels of IL-1α and IL-1β in the gingival crevicular fluid are commonly found in patients with periodontal disease. This increased production of IL-1 is associated with a higher inflammatory response to the bacterial stimulus, resulting in more severe disease as well as an unfavorable response to treatments (Kornman et al., 1997; Engebretson et al., 1999; McGuire and Nunn, 1999; Shirodaria et al., 2000).

Interleukin-6 is associated with acute phase reactions and is usually secreted concomitantly with other proinflammatory cytokines. Some authors relate this cytokine to the destruction of periodontal tissue by favoring the accumulation of inflammatory cells and by activating and releasing inflammatory mediators that in turn accentuate the response to periodontal disease (de Lima Oliveira et al., 2012; Zhang et al., 2016).

The kinetics of production of IL-18 against the action of bacteria is rapid, according to its proinflammatory nature. It plays a central role in systemic and local inflammation (Biet et al., 2002). One study evaluated IL-18 levels in crevicular gingival fluid in four groups of patients: healthy periodontium, gingivitis, chronic periodontitis, and aggressive periodontitis. The results demonstrated that IL-18 concentration in the crevicular gingival fluid was low in the group with healthy periodontium and progressively increased in groups from gingivitis, to aggressive periodontitis, and finally chronic periodontitis. As the inflammation increased, there was a concomitant increase in IL-18 level (Nair et al., 2016). In the current study, treatment with monolaurin decreased the IL-18 gene expression in fibroblasts, however, an opposite result was observed in keratinocytes, where IL-18 expression was increased in the group treated with 50 μM monolaurin.

Tumor necrosis factor plays a central role in periodontitis, being associated with the disease because of its ability to induce destruction of connective tissue and its effects on bone resorption through the activation of osteoclasts. Thus, TNF is one of the first proinflammatory cytokines produced in response to infection by pathogenic bacteria (Stashenko et al., 1987; de Lima Oliveira et al., 2012; Zhang et al., 2016). Here, the authors observed a reduction in the gene expression of TNF in monolaurin treated fibroblasts. On the other hand, in keratinocytes, TNF expression was higher in cells treated with 25 μM of this compound. Animal models challenged with *P. gingivalis* were treated with antimicrobial drugs (chlorhexidine, minocycline, and doxycycline) in order to evaluate its effect on the inflammatory response. Minocycline induced higher levels of TNF while chlorhexidine reduced TNF levels, this result led the authors to believe that these agents modified the inflammatory response to *P. gingivalis* regardless of its antimicrobial effect, each in its own way (Houri-Haddad et al., 2008). Overall, monolaurin modulate the expression of inflammatory cytokines, suggesting it may have a modulatory role on the host pro-inflammatory response to help eradicate the bacterial infection. Similarly, previous studies suggested that monolaurin play a significant role on T cell functions and signaling by altering TCR-induced LAT, PLC-γ, and AKT cluster formation PI3K-AKT signaling axis, and calcium influx which ultimately decrease the cytokine production (Zhang et al., 2016).

The knowledge of the metabolic profile can contribute to understanding of the periodontal disease course as well as identify possible metabolites as biomarkers. This study evaluated the effects caused by monolaurin on the cellular metabolome and found significant variations. Relative quantification revealed lower levels of 2-deoxytetronic acid NIST, 4-aminobutyric acid, glyceric acid and pinitol, and higher levels of glycerol and pyruvic acid in cells treated with 25 or 50 μM monolaurin. Analysis of fibroblast metabolome (HGF) treated with IL-1β in combination with titanium dioxide nanoparticles ($TiO_2$ NPs), demonstrated that IL-1β induction reduced concentrations of primary metabolites, especially those of urea cycle, polyamine, S-adenosylmethionine and glutathione synthetic pathways. The addition of $TiO_2$ NPs further increased these metabolic changes induced by IL-1β. These findings may be useful for the future establishment of new metabolic markers and therapeutic strategy for gingival inflammations (Garcia-Contreras et al., 2015). One study compared the salivary metabolic profile of healthy patients and patients with periodontal disease. Changes in several classes of metabolites have been observed in individuals with periodontal disease. According to the authors, such changes reflected an increase in host–bacterial interactions in the diseased state (Barnes et al., 2011).

## CONCLUSION

In summary, this study indicates that monolaurin possesses antimicrobial activity and modulates the host immune response and modulates production when administered for 24 h in a dual-chamber model inoculated with *A. actinomycetemcomitans*. These findings demonstrate that monolaurin could be considered a potential candidate for *in vivo* studies, which may translate into its potential clinical use to treat pathogenic microbe–host interactions.

## AUTHOR CONTRIBUTIONS

VS conceived and designed the experiments, performed the experiments, analyzed the data, performed the statistical analysis, and wrote the paper. LP conceived and designed the experiments, contributed to reagents, materials, and analysis tools, analyzed and critically reviewed the data. MS and SP performed the experiments and analyzed the data. JM analyzed the data, and critically reviewed and interpreted the data. RM conceived and designed the experiments, contributed to reagents, materials, and analysis tools, performed the experiments, analyzed and critically reviewed the data. All authors contributed to manuscript revision, read, and approved the submitted version.

## ACKNOWLEDGMENTS

The authors thank to CAPES (Coordination of Improvement of Higher Education Personnel), FAPEMIG (Research Sponsoring Agency of the State of Minas Gerais), and CNPq (National Counsel of Technological and Scientific Development) for support. Research reported in this publication was also supported by the NIH/NCCIH under award number AT006507. The content is solely the responsibility of the authors and does not represent the official views of the National Institutes of Health.

## REFERENCES

Aimetti, M. (2014). Nonsurgical periodontal treatment. *Int. J. Esthet. Dent.* 9, 251–267.

Balloni, S., Locci, P., Lumare, A., and Marinucci, L. (2016). Cytotoxicity of three commercial mouthrinses on extracellular matrix metabolism and human gingival cell behaviour. *Toxicol. Vitr.* 34, 88–96. doi: 10.1016/j.tiv.2016.03.015

Barnes, V. M., Ciancio, S. G., Shibly, O., Xu, T., Devizio, W., Trivedi, H. M., et al. (2011). Metabolomics reveals elevated macromolecular degradation in periodontal disease. *J. Dent. Res.* 90, 1293–1297. doi: 10.1177/0022034511416240

Barnett, M. L. (2003). The role of therapeutic antimicrobial mouthrinses in clinical practice: control of supragingival plaque and gingivitis. *J. Am. Dent. Assoc.* 134, 699–704. doi: 10.14219/jada.archive.2003.0255

Biet, F., Locht, C., and Kremer, L. (2002). Immunoregulatory functions of interleukin 18 and its role in defense against bacterial pathogens. *J. Mol. Med.* 80, 147–162. doi: 10.1007/s00109-001-0307-1

Bodet, C., Andrian, E., Tanabe, S.-I., and Grenier, D. (2007). *Actinobacillus actinomycetemcomitans* lipopolysaccharide regulates matrix metalloproteinase, tissue inhibitors of matrix metalloproteinase, and plasminogen activator production by human gingival fibroblasts: a potential role in connective tissue destructio. *J. Cell. Physiol.* 212, 189–194. doi: 10.1002/jcp.21018

Branco-de-Almeida, L. S., Murata, R. M., Franco, E. M., dos Santos, M. H., de Alencar, S. M., Koo, H., et al. (2011). Effects of 7-epiclusianone on *Streptococcus mutans* and caries development in rats. *Planta Med.* 77, 40–45. doi: 10.1055/s-0030-1250121

Carpo, B. G., Verallo-Rowell, V. M., and Kabara, J. (2007). Novel antibacterial activity of monolaurin compared with conventional antibiotics against organisms from skin infections: an in vitro study. *J. Drugs Dermatol.* 6, 991–998.

Champagne, C. M. E., Buchanan, W., Reddy, M. S., Preisser, J. S., Beck, J. D., and Offenbacher, S. (2003). Potential for gingival crevice fluid measures as predictors of risk for periodontal diseases. *Periodontol. 2000* 31, 167–180. doi: 10.1034/j.1600-0757.2003.03110.x

Chapple, I. L. C., and Genco, R. (2013). Diabetes and periodontal diseases: consensus report of the Joint EFP/AAP Workshop on Periodontitis and Systemic Diseases. *J. Clin. Periodontol.* 40(Suppl. 1), S106–S112. doi: 10.1111/jcpe.12077

Chen, C., Kittichotirat, W., Chen, W., Downey, J. S., Si, Y., and Bumgarner, R. (2010). Genome sequence of naturally competent *Aggregatibacter actinomycetemcomitans* serotype a strain D7S-1. *J. Bacteriol.* 192, 2643–2644. doi: 10.1128/JB.00157-10

Cortelli, S. C., Costa, F. O., Kawai, T., Aquino, D. R., Franco, G. C. N., Ohara, K., et al. (2009). Diminished treatment response of periodontally diseased patients infected with the JP2 clone of Aggregatibacter (Actinobacillus) actinomycetemcomitans. *J. Clin. Microbiol.* 47, 2018–2025. doi: 10.1128/JCM.00338-09

Coussens, L. M., and Werb, Z. (2002). Inflammation and cancer. *Nature* 420, 860–867. doi: 10.1038/nature01322

da Silva-Boghossian, C. M., do Souto, R. M., Luiz, R. R., and Colombo, A. P. V. (2011). Association of red complex, *A. actinomycetemcomitans* and non-oral bacteria with periodontal diseases. *Arch. Oral Biol.* 56, 899–906. doi: 10.1016/j.archoralbio.2011.02.009

de Almeida, J. M., Theodoro, L. H., Bosco, A. F., Nagata, M. J. H., Oshiiwa, M., and Garcia, V. G. (2007). Influence of photodynamic therapy on the development of ligature-induced periodontitis in rats. *J. Periodontol.* 78, 566–575. doi: 10.1902/jop.2007.060214

de Lima Oliveira, A. P., de Faveri, M., Gursky, L. C., Mestnik, M. J., Feres, M., Haffajee, A. D., et al. (2012). Effects of periodontal therapy on GCF cytokines in generalized aggressive periodontitis subjects. *J. Clin. Periodontol.* 39, 295–302. doi: 10.1111/j.1600-051X.2011.01817.x

Engebretson, S. P., Lamster, I. B., Herrera-Abreu, M., Celenti, R. S., Timms, J. M., Chaudhary, A. G., et al. (1999). The influence of interleukin gene polymorphism on expression of interleukin-1beta and tumor necrosis factor-alpha in periodontal tissue and gingival crevicular fluid. *J. Periodontol.* 70, 567 573. doi: 10.1902/jop.1999.70.6.567

Fiehn, O., and Kind, T. (2007). Metabolite profiling in blood plasma. *Methods Mol. Biol.* 358, 3–17. doi: 10.1007/978-1-59745-244-1_1

Filoche, S., Wong, L., and Sissons, C. H. (2010). Oral biofilms: emerging concepts in microbial ecology. *J. Dent. Res.* 89, 8–18. doi: 10.1177/0022034509351812

Fu, X., Feng, F., and Huang, B. (2006). Physicochemical characterization and evaluation of a microemulsion system for antimicrobial activity of glycerol monolaurate. *Int. J. Pharm.* 321, 171–175. doi: 10.1016/j.ijpharm.2006.05.019

Gafan, G. P., Lucas, V. S., Roberts, G. J., Petrie, A., Wilson, M., and Spratt, D. A. (2004). Prevalence of periodontal pathogens in dental plaque of children. *J. Clin. Microbiol.* 42, 4141–4146. doi: 10.1128/JCM.42.9.4141-4146.2004

Garcia-Contreras, R., Sugimoto, M., Umemura, N., Kaneko, M., Hatakeyama, Y., Soga, T., et al. (2015). Alteration of metabolomic profiles by titanium dioxide nanoparticles in human gingivitis model. *Biomaterials* 57, 33–40. doi: 10.1016/j.biomaterials.2015.03.059

Govindarajan, K., Muthukumar, S., and Rangarao, S. (2015). Relationship between interleukin 1α levels in the gingival crevicular fluid in health and in inflammatory periodontal disease and periodontal inflamed surface area: a correlative study. *J. Indian Soc. Periodontol.* 19, 618–623. doi: 10.4103/0972-124X.162197

Groeger, S. E., and Meyle, J. (2015). Epithelial barrier and oral bacterial infection. *Periodontol. 2000* 69, 46–67. doi: 10.1111/prd.12094

Gurav, A. N. (2014). The association of periodontitis and metabolic syndrome. *Dent. Res. J.* 11, 1–10.

Haraszthy, V. I., Hariharan, G., Tinoco, E. M., Cortelli, J. R., Lally, E. T., Davis, E., et al. (2000). Evidence for the role of highly leukotoxic Actinobacillus actinomycetemcomitans in the pathogenesis of localized juvenile and other forms of early-onset periodontitis. *J. Periodontol.* 71, 912–922. doi: 10.1902/jop.2000.71.6.912

Houri-Haddad, Y., Halabi, A., and Soskolne, W. A. (2008). Inflammatory response to chlorhexidine, minocycline HCl and doxycycline HCl in an in vivo mouse model. *J. Clin. Periodontol.* 35, 783–788. doi: 10.1111/j.1600-051X.2008.01290.x

Irfan, U. M., Dawson, D. V., and Bissada, N. F. (2001). Epidemiology of periodontal disease: a review and clinical perspectives. *J. Int. Acad. Periodontol.* 3, 14–21.

Isaacs, C. E. (2001). The antimicrobial function of milk lipids. *Adv. Nutr. Res.* 10, 271–285.

Jang, D. H., Bhawal, U. K., Min, H.-K., Kang, H. K., Abiko, Y., and Min, B.-M. (2015). A transcriptional roadmap to the senescence and differentiation of human oral keratinocytes. *J. Gerontol. A Biol. Sci. Med. Sci.* 70, 20–32. doi: 10.1093/gerona/glt212

Kornman, K. S., Crane, A., Wang, H. Y., di Giovine, F. S., Newman, M. G., Pirk, F. W., et al. (1997). The interleukin-1 genotype as a severity factor in adult periodontal disease. *J. Clin. Periodontol.* 24, 72–77. doi: 10.1111/j.1600-051X.1997.tb01187.x

Kusumoto, Y., Hirano, H., Saitoh, K., Yamada, S., Takedachi, M., Nozaki, T., et al. (2004). Human gingival epithelial cells produce chemotactic factors interleukin-8 and monocyte chemoattractant protein-1 after stimulation with *Porphyromonas gingivalis* via toll-like receptor 2. *J. Periodontol.* 75, 370–379. doi: 10.1902/jop.2004.75.3.370

Li, Q., Estes, J. D., Schlievert, P. M., Duan, L., Brosnahan, A. J., and Southern, P. J. (2009). Glycerol monolaurate prevents mucosal SIV transmission. *Nature* 458, 1034–1038. doi: 10.1038/nature07831

Loos, B. G. (2005). Systemic markers of inflammation in periodontitis. *J. Periodontol.* 76, 2106–2115. doi: 10.1902/jop.2005.76.11-S.2106

McGuire, M. K., and Nunn, M. E. (1999). Prognosis versus actual outcome. IV. The effectiveness of clinical parameters and IL-1 genotype in accurately predicting prognoses and tooth survival. *J. Periodontol.* 70, 49–56. doi: 10.1902/jop.1999.70.1.49

Michaud, D. S., Joshipura, K., Giovannucci, E., and Fuchs, C. S. (2007). A prospective study of periodontal disease and pancreatic cancer in US male health professionals. *J. Natl. Cancer Inst.* 99, 171–175. doi: 10.1093/jnci/djk021

Moutsopoulos, N. M., and Madianos, P. N. (2006). Low-grade inflammation in chronic infectious diseases: paradigm of periodontal infections. *Ann. N. Y. Acad. Sci.* 1088, 251–264. doi: 10.1196/annals.1366.032

Nair, V., Bandyopadhyay, P., Kundu, D., and Das, S. (2016). Estimation of interleukin-18 in the gingival crevicular fluid and serum of Bengali population with periodontal health and disease. *J. Indian Soc. Periodontol.* 20, 260–264. doi: 10.4103/0972-124X.183098

O'Brien, J., Wilson, I., Orton, T., and Pognan, F. (2000). Investigation of the Alamar Blue (resazurin) fluorescent dye for the assessment of mammalian cell cytotoxicity. *Eur. J. Biochem.* 267, 5421–5426. doi: 10.1046/j.1432-1327.2000.01606.x

Oda, D., and Watson, E. (1990). Human oral epithelial cell culture I. Improved conditions for reproducible culture in serum-free medium. In vitro cell. *Dev. Biol.* 26, 589–595. doi: 10.1007/BF02624208

Oringer, R. J. (2002). Modulation of the host response in periodontal therapy. *J. Periodontol.* 73, 460–470. doi: 10.1902/jop.2002.73.4.460

Pasetto, S., Pardi, V., and Murata, R. M. (2014). Anti-HIV-1 activity of flavonoid myricetin on HIV-1 infection in a dual-chamber in vitro model. *PLoS One* 9:e115323. doi: 10.1371/journal.pone.0115323

Paster, B. J., Olsen, I., Aas, J. A., and Dewhirst, F. E. (2006). The breadth of bacterial diversity in the human periodontal pocket and other oral sites. *Periodontol. 2000* 2006, 80–87. doi: 10.1111/j.1600-0757.2006.00174.x

Peterson, M. L., and Schlievert, P. M. (2006). Glycerol monolaurate inhibits the effects of Gram-positive select agents on eukaryotic cells. *Biochemistry* 45, 2387–2397. doi: 10.1021/bi051992u

Pfaffl, M. W. (2001). A new mathematical model for relative quantification in real-time RT-PCR. *Nucleic Acids Res.* 29:e45. doi: 10.1093/nar/29.9.e45

Preuss, H. G., Echard, B., Enig, M., Brook, I., and Elliott, T. B. (2005). Minimum inhibitory concentrations of herbal essential oils and monolaurin for gram-positive and gram-negative bacteria. *Mol. Cell. Biochem.* 272, 29–34. doi: 10. 1007/s11010-005-6604-1

Projan, S. J., Brown-Skrobot, S., Schlievert, P. M., Vandenesch, F., and Novick, R. P. (1994). Glycerol monolaurate inhibits the production of beta-lactamase, toxic shock toxin-1, and other staphylococcal exoproteins by interfering with signal transduction. *J. Bacteriol.* 176, 4204–4209. doi: 10.1128/jb.176.14.4204-4209.1994

Rakić, M., Zelić, K., Pavlica, D., Hadzimihajlović, M., Milasin, J., Milicić, B., et al. (2010). [Association between clinical parameters and the presence of *Aggregatibacter actinomycetemcomitans* and *Porphyromonas gingivalis* in patients with progressive periodontal lesions]. *Vojnosanit. Pregl.* 67, 898–902. doi: 10.2298/VSP1011898R

Salvi, G. E., and Lang, N. P. (2005). Host response modulation in the management of periodontal diseases. *J. Clin. Periodontol.* 32(Suppl. 6), 108–129. doi: 10.1111/ j.1600-051X.2005.00785.x

Savage, A., Eaton, K. A., Moles, D. R., and Needleman, I. (2009). A systematic review of definitions of periodontitis and methods that have been used to identify this disease. *J. Clin. Periodontol.* 36, 458–467. doi: 10.1111/j.1600-051X. 2009.01408.x

Seleem, D., Chen, E., Benso, B., Pardi, V., and Murata, R. M. (2016). In vitro evaluation of antifungal activity of monolaurin against *Candida albicans* biofilms. *PeerJ* 4:e2148. doi: 10.7717/peerj.2148

Shirodaria, S., Smith, J., McKay, I. J., Kennett, C. N., and Hughes, F. J. (2000). Polymorphisms in the IL-1A gene are correlated with levels of interleukin-1alpha protein in gingival crevicular fluid of teeth with severe periodontal disease. *J. Dent. Res.* 79, 1864–1869. doi: 10.1177/002203450007901 10801

Silva, V., de, O., Pereira, L. J., and Murata, R. M. (2017). Oral microbe-host interactions: influence of β-glucans on gene expression of inflammatory cytokines and metabolome profile. *BMC Microbiol.* 17:53. doi: 10.1186/s12866-017-0946-1

Slots, J., Reynolds, H. S., and Genco, R. J. (1980). *Actinobacillus actinomycetemcomitans* in human periodontal disease: a cross-sectional microbiological investigation. *Infect. Immun.* 29, 1013–1020.

Stashenko, P., Dewhirst, F. E., Peros, W. J., Kent, R. L., and Ago, J. M. (1987). Synergistic interactions between interleukin 1, tumor necrosis factor, and lymphotoxin in bone resorption. *J. Immunol.* 138, 1464–1468.

Tangwatcharin, P., and Khopaibool, P. (2012). Activity of virgin coconut oil, lauric acid or monolaurin in combination with lactic acid against *Staphylococcus aureus*. *Southeast Asian J. Trop. Med. Public Health* 43, 969–985.

Yang, H. W., Asikainen, S., Doğan, B., Suda, R., and Lai, C. H. (2004). Relationship of *Actinobacillus actinomycetemcomitans* serotype b to aggressive periodontitis: frequency in pure cultured isolates. *J. Periodontol.* 75, 592–599. doi: 10.1902/ jop.2004.75.4.592

Yoon, B. K., Jackman, J. A., Valle-González, E. R., and Cho, N. J. (2018). Antibacterial free fatty acids and monoglycerides: biological activities, experimental testing, and therapeutic applications. *Int. J. Mol. Sci.* 8:E1114. doi: 10.3390/ijms19041114

Zambon, J. J., Christersson, L. A., and Slots, J. (1983). *Actinobacillus actinomycetemcomitans* in human periodontal disease. Prevalence in patient groups and distribution of biotypes and serotypes within families. *J. Periodontol.* 54, 707–711. doi: 10.1902/jop.1983.54.12.707

Zhang, M. S., Sandouk, A., and Houtman, J. C. (2016). Glycerol Monolaurate (GML) inhibits human T cell signaling and function by disrupting lipid dynamics. *Sci. Rep.* 26:30225. doi: 10.1038/srep30225

Zhang, Q., Chen, B., Zhu, D., and Yan, F. (2016). Biomarker levels in gingival crevicular fluid of subjects with different periodontal conditions: a cross-sectional study. *Arch. Oral Biol.* 72, 92–98. doi: 10.1016/j.archoralbio.2016. 08.020

# 5

# Structure–Function Relationship of Aminopeptidase P from *Pseudomonas aeruginosa*


***Cui-Ting Peng[1,2†], Li Liu[1,2†], Chang-Cheng Li[2], Li-Hui He[2], Tao Li[2], Ya-Lin Shen[2], Chao Gao[2], Ning-Yu Wang[2,3], Yong Xia[2], Yi-Bo Zhu[2], Ying-Jie Song[2], Qian Lei[2], Luo-Ting Yu[1,2*] and Rui Bao[2*]***

*[1] Pharmaceutical and Biological Engineering Department, School of Chemical Engineering, Sichuan University, Chengdu, China, [2] Center of Infectious Diseases, State Key Laboratory of Biotherapy, West China Hospital, Sichuan University and Collaborative Innovation Center, Chengdu, China, [3] School of Life Sciences and Engineering, Southwest Jiaotong University, Chengdu, China*

***Correspondence:**
*Rui Bao*
*baorui@scu.edu.cn*
*Luo-Ting Yu*
*yuluot@scu.edu.cn*

*† These authors have contributed equally to this work.*



*PepP* is a virulence-associated gene in *Pseudomonas aeruginosa*, making it an attractive target for anti-*P. aeruginosa* drug development. The encoded protein, aminopeptidases P (Pa-PepP), is a type of X-prolyl peptidase that possesses diverse biological functions. The crystal structure verified its canonical pita-bread fold and functional tetrameric assembly, and the functional studies measured the influences of different metal ions on the activity. A trimetal manganese cluster was observed at the active site, elucidating the mechanism of inhibition by metal ions. Additionally, a loop extending from the active site appeared to be important for specific large-substrate binding. Based on the structural comparison and bacterial invasion assays, we showed that this non-conserved surface loop was critical for *P. aeruginosa* virulence. Taken together, these findings can extend our understanding of the catalytic mechanism and virulence-related functions of Pa-PepP and provide a solid foundation for the design of specific inhibitors against pathogenic-bacterial infections.



**Keywords: *Pseudomonas aeruginosa*, aminopeptidase P, virulence, tri-nuclear form, X-ray crystallography**


## INTRODUCTION

*Pseudomonas aeruginosa* is a common nosocomial pathogen and is notoriously difficult to treat due to its high intrinsic and acquired drug resistance (Hancock, 1998; Stover et al., 2000). To address the challenges of *P. aeruginosa* infections, alternative approaches other than conventional antibiotic therapy were undertaken, with an emphasis on anti-virulence strategies (Hentzer et al., 2003; Luckett et al., 2012; Gi et al., 2014; Hwang et al., 2016; Maura et al., 2016; Johnson and Abramovitch, 2017; Rampioni et al., 2017). The targets for most anti-virulence strategies are those well-studied virulence factors (adhesins, toxins, effector secretion system components) that directly participate in pathogen-host cell interactions (Woods et al., 1982; Hahn, 1997; Hood et al., 2010). However, not all of these virulence factors play significant roles in *P. aeruginosa* infection (Miyata et al., 2003). Instead, there are many genes with unidentified roles in *P. aeruginosa* virulence,

---

**Abbreviations:** DMEM, Dulbecco's Modified Eagle's Medium; FBS, fetal bovine serum; IPTG, isopropyl β-D-1-thiogalactopyranoside; LB, Luria–Bertani; MOI, multiplicity of infection; NCPSS, National Center for Protein Sciences Shanghai; OD600, optical cell densities at 600 nm; PBS, phosphate-buffered saline; *P. aeruginosa*, *Pseudomonas aeruginosa;* SDS-PAGE, sodium dodecyl sulfate–polyacrylamide gel electrophoresis; SSRF, Shanghai Synchrotron Radiation Facility.

while the corresponding mutants resulted in obvious virulence attenuation, suggesting potential applications for these genes in anti-virulence therapy discovery.

*PepP* encodes an enzyme belonging to the aminopeptidases P (APPro) family (E.C.3.4.11.9), a type of metalloprotease that catalyzes the removal of the N-terminal residue from a polypeptide that has proline as the second residue (Taylor, 1993; Gonzales and Robert-Baudouy, 1996; Wilce et al., 1998). It is one of the critical virulence-associated genes identified using a *P. aeruginosa-C. elegans* infection mode (Feinbaum et al., 2012). In this model, transposon mutants of *pepP* in *P. aeruginosa* PA14 have attenuated virulence, leading to reduced *C. elegans* survival. *PepP* is highly conserved in all *P. aeruginosa* genomes sequenced to date and with high similarity to this gene from other *Pseudomonas* species (82.4%–100% identity). In contrast to other metalloaminopeptidases, APPro is a cytoplasmic aminopeptidase and recognizes a restricted scissile Xaa-Pro bond of those polypeptide or protein substrates that may be linked to virulence-associated phenotypes or other biological processes beyond the general protein degradation ability (Lowther and Matthews, 2002). APPro is widely distributed among bacteria, fungi, plants and mammals. It is thought to play a role in many important biological pathways, including hormone regulation in mammals (Simmons and Orawski, 1992) and the terminal degradation of proline-containing peptides and proteins (Wilce et al., 1998), or organophosphate compounds in bacterial (Jao et al., 2004). The gene coding *Escherichia coli* aminopeptidases P (Ec-PepP) was even identified as a factor involved in outer membrane vesicles (OMV) production (McBroom et al., 2006; Vanaja et al., 2016). While structural and biochemical studies on APPro have visualized a general catalytic mechanism and revealed a conserved binding pocket for N-terminal substrates (Wilce et al., 1998; Graham et al., 2005, 2006; Liu et al., 2007; Graham and Guss, 2008; Jeyakanthan et al., 2009; Weaver et al., 2014), further investigations are needed to elucidate the structural basis for APPro's specific substrate recognition and diverse functions. Thus, a better understanding of the structure and function of *P. aeruginosa* APPro (Pa-PepP) would enable us to propose the possible mechanisms involved in bacterial virulence.

In this study, we solved the X-ray crystal structure of Pa-PepP with a resolution of 1.8 Å. A biochemical analysis verified the residues critical for catalysis. The presence of a trinuclear manganese cluster in the reaction center suggests a mechanism for inhibition by excessive metal ion binding. Furthermore, an extended substrate binding site was identified to be responsible for virulence-related protein recognition.

## RESULTS

### Pa-PepP Adopts a Canonical Pita-Bread Fold and Assembles as a Tetramer in Crystal

Refinement of the Pa-PepP structure resulted in a final model with a free R-factor (Rfree) of 0.2206 at 1.8 Å. Sufficient electron density allowed us to model all residues from 1 to 444. The crystallographic statistics are summarized in **Table 1**. The monomer structure displays a two-domain organization where the N-domain (1–175) is composed of a mainly parallel beta-sheet core (B1–B6) flanked by seven alpha helices (A–G). In contrast, the catalytic C-domain (176–444) adopts a conserved "pita-bread" fold with six beta sheets (B7-B12) in antiparallel configurations (**Figure 1A**). This pita-bread fold is commonly found in N-terminal amido-, imido-, and amidino-scissile bond-cleaving enzymes, and serves as a structural basis for the metal-dependent catalysis (Lowther and Matthews, 2000; Besio et al., 2010).

Although the recombinant Pa-PepP purified from *E. coli* strain BL21 (DE3) exists as a monomer in solution (**Figure 1B**), tetrameric oligomerization was observed in crystal packing (**Figure 1C**). The monomers were arranged as a dimer with an extended loop contributing to the active site of the adjacent subunit and an average interface area of approximately 2050.9 $A^2$ per subunit. The dimer-of-dimers was generated by crystallographic symmetry operation (x–1/2, –y–1/2, –z), and the major interactions are contributed by the C-domain of each monomer, resulting in an ~815.6 $A^2$ buried area per subunit. For most metalloaminopeptidases, the oligomeric state is essential for their biological functions. The loop from the adjacent monomer extends the substrate-binding site and thus enables the enzyme to cleave larger substrates.

**TABLE 1** | Data collection and refinement statistics.

| | PDB Entry | 5WZE |
|---|---|---|
| **Data collection** | Space group | P 21 21 21 |
| | **Cell dimension** | |
| | *a, b, c* (Å) | 111.197,123.432,149.485 |
| | α, β, γ (°) | 90, 90, 90 |
| | Wavelength | 0.97776 |
| | Resolution (Å) | 48.01–1.783 (1.847–1.783) |
| | I/I | 19.714 (2.167) |
| | Completeness (%) | 0.99 |
| | $R_{merge}$ | 0.099 (0.709) |
| | Redundancy | 8.9 (6.4) |
| **Refinement** | Resolution (Å) | 48.01–1.783 (1.847–1.783) |
| | No. of reflections | 194404 (18600) |
| | Rwork/Rfree | 0.2105/0.2206 |
| | **No. of atoms** | |
| | Protein | 1783 |
| | Ligand/ion | 90 |
| | Water | 1153 |
| | **B-factor** | |
| | Protein | 27.37 |
| | Ligand/ion | 38.94 |
| | Water | 30.89 |
| | ***R.m.s. deviations*** | |
| | Bond lengths (Å) | 0.011 |
| | Bond angles (°) | 1.00 |
| | Ramachandran plot | 98/1.5/0 |

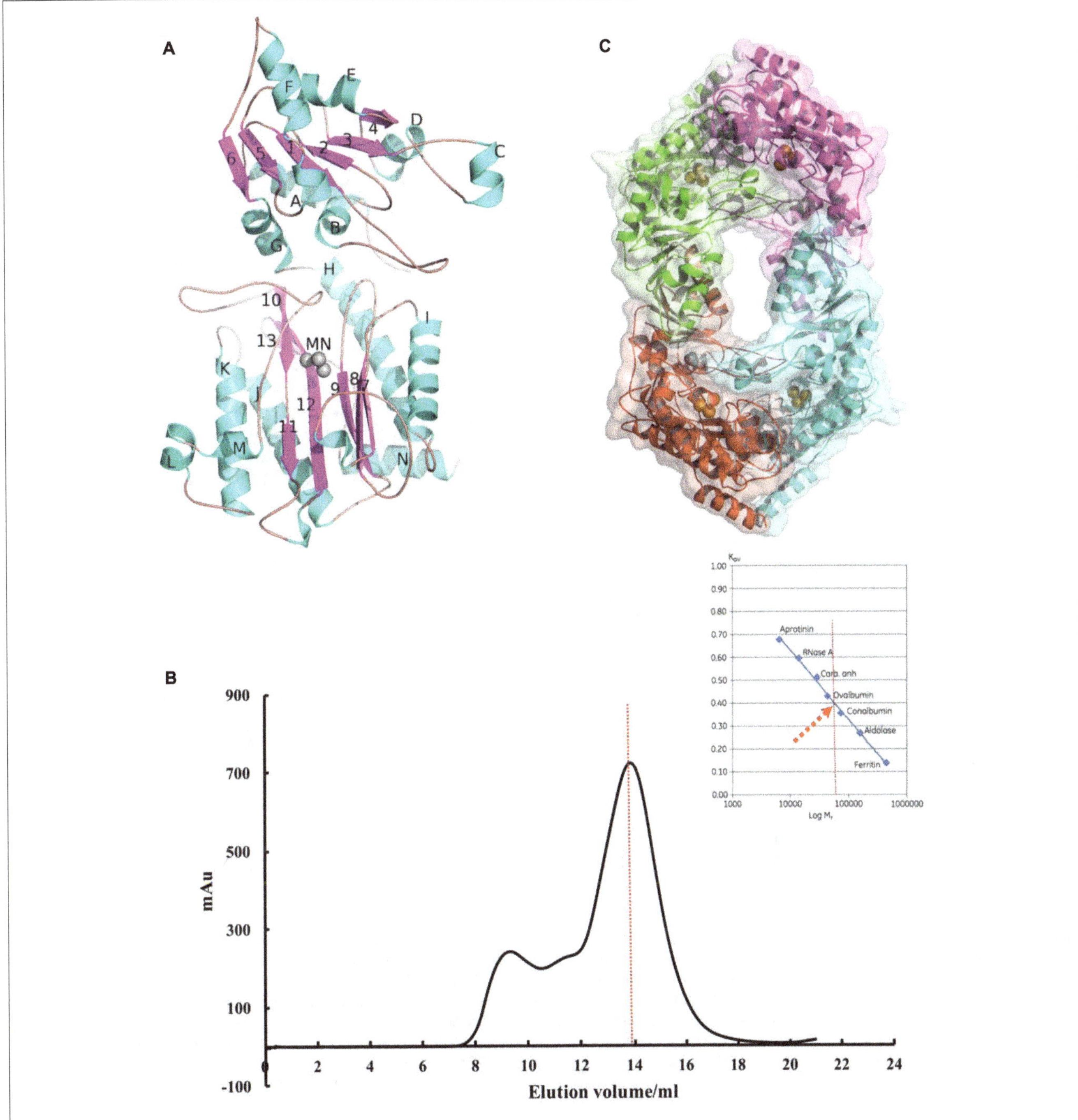


**FIGURE 1 |** Pa-PepP adopts a canonical pita-bread fold and assembles as a tetramer in crystal. **(A)** The second structure assignments of the Pa-PepP monomer. Beta-sheets are colored blue, alpha-helices are colored green, and the three $Mn^{2+}$ ions are shown as gray spheres. The figure was generated by PyMOL (http://www.pymol.org). **(B)** The gel filtration curve for the purified recombinant Pa-PepP in solution. The AUC results are presented as the ultraviolet absorption in 280 nm. The black solid curve refers to Pa-PepP eluted from GE HiLoad 16/600 Superdex 200 column. The red dash curve refers to the sample elution volume and corresponding molecule mass of the sample when compared with the standard sample proteins. **(C)** 3D structure of Pa-PepP showed a detailed tetramer of four subunits or a homodimer of Pa-PepP. Each subunit is presented as different color with $Mn^{2+}$ ions are shown as orange spheres in the metal binding site.

Thus, the antiparallel dimerization would be the basic active polymerization forms to its biological activity, and the different quaternary arrangement may reflect a possible regulatory mechanism for its activity.

## Effect of the Metal Ion in Activity Modulation

Metalloaminopeptidases are well known for their metal-dependent catalysis mechanisms. Proline-specific

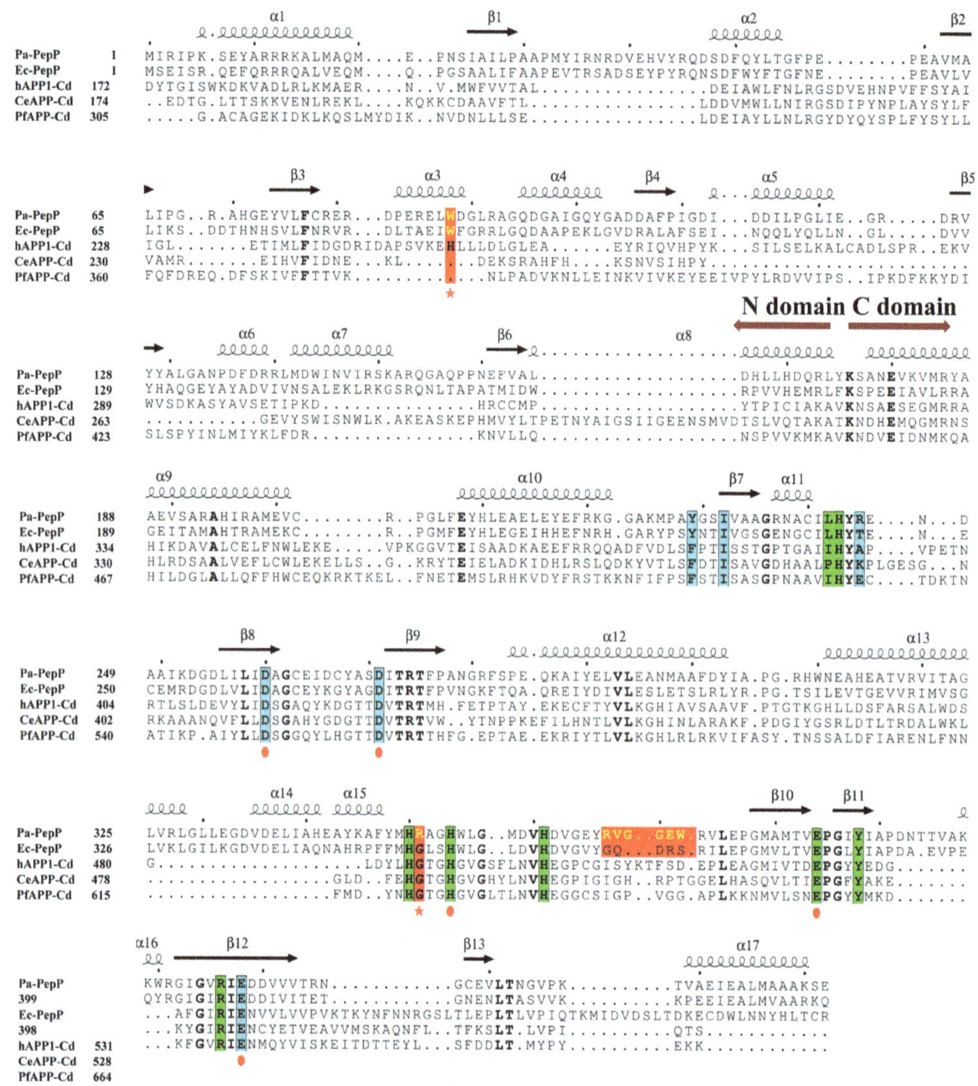


**FIGURE 2 |** Multiple sequence alignment of the truncated N domain and catalytic C domains from X-prolyl peptidases. From top to bottom, the sequences are aminopeptidases P from *P. aeruginosa* (Pa-PepP), aminopeptidases P from *Escherichia coli* (Ec-PepP), truncated N domain and catalytic C domains from from human XPNPEP1 (hAPP1, 172-618), X-prolyl aminopeptidase from *Caenorhabditis elegans* (CeAPP, 174–616), and aminopeptidase P from *Plasmodium falciparum* (PfAPP, 305–774). Residues for chelating metal ion are highlighted using the red circle under the sequences; Residues contributed to S1 pockets are highlighted with a blue background and residues for S' sites are presented with a green background; The red color displayed residues or short sequences are non-conserved among prokaryotic and eukaryotic APPros, which are also proved to be important to APPros' function. Sequences were aligned using the program ClustalX (Li et al., 2008), and the alignment was presented using the online ESPript 3.0 server (http://espript.ibcp.fr/ESPript/ESPript/).

aminopeptidases such as APPro and prolidase prefer dinuclear Mn(II) cluster as cofactor (Wilce et al., 1998; Graham et al., 2005). The residues coordinating the two Mn atoms ($Mn_A$ and $Mn_B$) are highly conserved among APPro family members (**Figure 2**), and the non-equivalent roles of the two metal ions in catalysis have been extensively studied (Graham et al., 2005; Hu et al., 2007). To test the role of divalent metal cluster on Pa-PepP, we measured the relative activities of Pa-PepP in the presence of 1 mM $Mn^{2+}$,$Ca^{2+}$,$Mg^{2+}$, $Ni^{2+}$, $Zn^{2+}$, and EDTA (**Figure 3A**). The addition of $Mn^{2+}$ significantly restored the Pa-PepP activity, while the limited enhancement of activity was observed upon addition of $Ca^{2+}$ or $Mg^{2+}$. The exhibited basal activity may be a result of the partially pre-bound metal ions from the cell, and the limited effects of $Ca^{2+}$ and $Mg^{2+}$ may be due to their weak binding affinity to the active site. Previous studies on metal selection in Ec-PepP revealed that the $Zn^{2+}$ ion has high affinity for APPro and inhibits the hydrolysis reaction by occupying a third metal binding site (Graham et al., 2005; Hu et al., 2007). Although we could not measure the effect of $Zn^{2+}$ ion on Pa-PepP because of the formation of zinc hydroxide precipitates upon adding $ZnCl_2$ to the alkaline enzyme buffer, we observed the complete inhibition of enzyme activity in the presence of both the $Ni^{2+}$ ion and the chelating agent EDTA. These results suggested that the $Ni^{2+}$ may also possess high

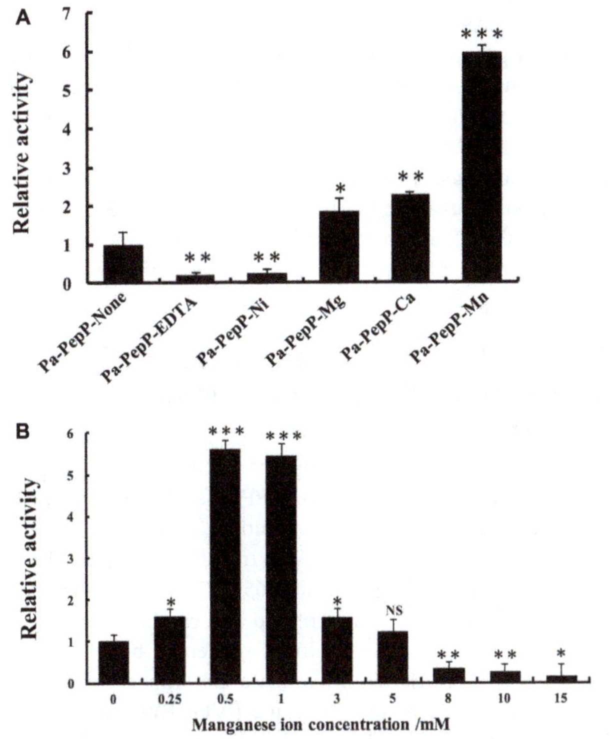


**FIGURE 3 |** Relative activity assay of Pa-PepP using the quenched fluorescent substrate Lys (Abz)–Pro–Pro–pNA. All assays were performed at 37°C for 5 min in the presence of 50 mM Tris (pH 8.5), 100 mM NaCl, 0–250 μM Lyz(Abz)–Pro–Pro–pNA quenched fluorescent substrate, and 1 μg/mL$^{-1}$ Pa-PepP that had been incubated with different metal ions at 37°C for 10 min. Each bar represents the mean of three independent measurements (SEM). **(A)** Relative activity of Pa-PepP in the presence of 1 mM different metal ions or EDTA. **(B)** Relative activity of Pa-PepP in presence of different amount of $Mn^{2+}$. *P*-values for comparison of each group with Pa-PepP-alone **(A)** or 0 mM $Mn^{2+}$ **(B)** were determined by 2-tailed Student's *t*-test (**P* < 0.05; ***P* < 0.01; ****P* < 0.001).

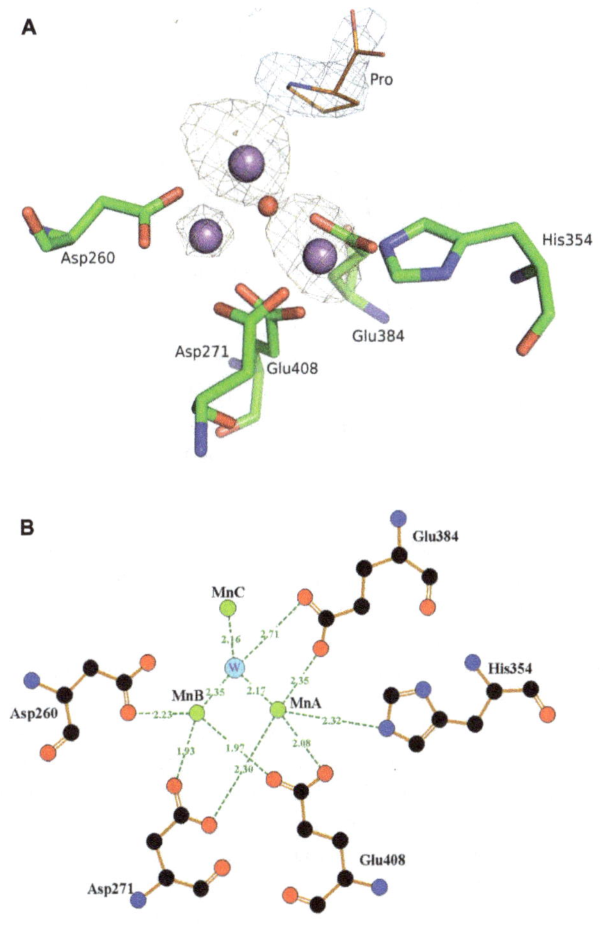


**FIGURE 4 |** The trimetal Mn cluster center and interactions with the surrounding amino acid residues. **(A)** The anomalous map peaks of the bound Mn in Pa-PepP structure. The three $Mn^{2+}$ ions are shown as dark purple spheres with different anomalous signals and the red sphere refers to the water molecule participated in activity modulation. For clarity, only part of the metal binding residues is shown together with the observed proline with blue electron density near the active site. The figure was generated by PyMOL (http://www.pymol.org). **(B)** Representative interactions around the active sites. $Mn_A$ is liganded by the side chains of His354, Asp271, Glu384, Glu408, and $Mn_B$ interacts with Asp260, Asp271, Glu408. And $Mn_C$ interacts through one solvent molecular (W) to $Mn_A$ and $Mn_B$ with a metal separation distance of 3.1–3.7 Å. Figures were prepared using LIGPLOT (Wallace et al., 1995).

affinity to APPro and tends to bind to those positions equivalent to $Zn^{2+}$ ions in Ec-PepP.

To identify the binding state of $Mn^{2+}$ ions in active site, 10 mM $MnCl_2$ was added during the crystallization experiment, along with 10 mM proline. In the final structure, there are three Mn atoms in each monomer (**Figure 4**). $Mn_A$ is liganded by the side chains of His354, Asp271, Glu384, Glu408, and $Mn_B$ interacts with Asp260, Asp271, Glu408. These interactions are highly conserved among those reported APPro structures that resulted in a distorted trigonal-pyramidal coordination network. The smaller anomalous signals and 0.5 occupancies of the $Mn_B$ site confirmed one of the structural features in metal-dependent aminopeptidase: the metal binding site B has relatively weaker binding affinity comparing to the site A (Hu et al., 2007). Additionally, the third Mn atom ($Mn_C$) is located in a position previously identified as being occupied by water in Zn-load Ec-PepP structures (Graham et al., 2005). The strong anomalous peak at this position verified its identity as a tightly bound $Mn^{2+}$ ion rather than a water molecule. It is interesting to note that this $Mn_C$ position is different from the third metal binding site found in Ec-PepP, in which the $Zn_C$ is coordinated by His243, His361, and the hydrolysis product Pro residue (Graham et al., 2005). In Pa-PepP, $Mn_C$ interacts through one solvent molecular (W) with $Mn_A$ and $Mn_B$, with a metal-separation distance of 3.1–3.7 Å. The Pro residue lies immediately above the solvent molecular W but does not participate in the interaction with $Mn_C$. Remarkably, $Mn_C$ occupies the S1 subsite that ordinarily binds the substrate, providing an explanation for the inhibition effect of excessive metal binding. To verify the inhibitory effect of $Mn^{2+}$ ion, we performed an activity assay in the presence of different amounts of $Mn^{2+}$. The result is consistent with our structural analysis (**Figure 3B**): there is a $Mn^{2+}$ ion concentration-dependent activity regulation pattern, in which 0.5–1 mM of Mn ion is the optimal concentration for 20 nM (1 μg/ml) Pa-PepP, and inhibitory effects are observed when $Mn^{2+}$ ion exceeded 5 mM. Inhibition was not observed at ion concentrations up to 20 mM in the assays with $Ca^{2+}$ and $Mg^{2+}$ (**Supplementary Figure S1**).

## Conserved Active-Site Motif and Extended Binding Site for Specific Substrate Recognition

Several APPro structures have been reported to date, including APPro from *Escherichia coli* (Ec-PepP, 1M35) (Wilce et al., 1998), *Streptococcus thermophilus* (3IL0), *Bacillus anthracis* (3IG4), *Yersinia pestis* (4PV4), *Thermotoga maritima* (2ZSG), *Streptococcus pyogenes* (3OVK), human (hAPP1, 3CTZ) (Li et al., 2008), *Caenorhabditis elegans* (CeAPP1, 4S2R) (Iyer et al., 2015) and *Plasmodium falciparum* (PfAPP, 5JQK) (Drinkwater et al., 2016). Ec-PepP shares the highest sequence identity with Pa-PepP and both of them are prokaryotic APPro (Gonzales and Robert-Baudouy, 1996). All of these APPros share a common catalytic domain structure that contains a metal center flanked by the S1'-S1 pockets (**Figures 2, 5A**). Previous structural studies on Ec-PepP in complex with the substrate or inhibitor have revealed those pockets (Graham et al., 2004; Graham and Guss, 2008). We modeled the Val-Pro-Leu bound Pa-PepP complex by superposing Pa-PepP structure with the substrate-bound Ec-PepP structure (PDB code: 2BN7) (**Figure 5A**). The shallow hydrophobic S1' pocket could be defined by the pre-bound Pro residue, Arg406, Tyr388, and His350. S1' sites are conserved in APPro and prolidase but not in other metalloaminopeptidases, which implies that they play critical roles in regulating the activity of proline-specific peptidases. Additionally, in prokaryotic APPros and prolidases, a tryptophan (Trp88' in Pa-PepP) from an adjacent subunit extends the boundary of S1' site and contributes to the P1' Pro binding (Yoshimoto et al., 1994; Jao et al., 2006). At the S1'-S1 junction, His243 and His361 interact with the main-chain carbonyl of P1' Pro and P1 Val, respectively, indicating their specific roles in recognizing and stabilizing the stereospecific scissile X-Pro bond. In the S1 pocket, the side chain of P1 Val faces Tyr229, Ile232, Arg245, while its main chain replaces the $Mn_C$ ion and is involved in the $Mn_A$ and $Mn_B$ ion mediated interactions. In metallomainopeptidases, the dinuclear Mn center is thought to be essential for nucleophilic attack (Graham et al., 2005). To verify the impacts of the critical motifs revealed by structural analysis, we constructed Ala substitutions on those motifs (Trp88 for S1' pocket, His243 for scissile bond stabilizing, Glu384 for metal binding) and verified that the expression level and stability are comparable between the wild type and all the mutants (**Supplementary Figure S2**). The Pa-PepP activity assay shows that all the mutations would eliminate enzymatic activity, which further confirmed that the evolutionary conservation in those regions is strongly associated with the essential functional roles of APPro family (**Figure 5B**).

In contrast to the prolidases that cleave dipeptides only, APPro is capable of modifying protein substrates. The relatively larger substrate binding ability of APPro is partly due to the extension of the substrate binding site beyond the S1'–S1 region (Drinkwater et al., 2016). The modeled tripeptide-bound Pa-PepP structure indicated that Arg153 and Arg351 accommodate the carboxylate group of the P2' Leu, and guide the C-terminus of the substrate toward the tetramer surface (**Figure 5A**). Furthermore, the R351G mutation results in an increase in enzyme activity. The similar Arg153/Arg370 basic patch is also found in Ec-PepP, in which the non-basic residue substitution on either of them leads to an obvious decrease in $K_m$ and an increase in $k_{cat}/K_m$ (Jao et al., 2006). Thus, this basic patch, which is located at the entrance of catalytic cave, can play an important role in specificities of protein substrate recognition and orientation.

## Structural Analysis Identified a Surface Loop Participating in *P. aeruginosa* Virulence

The conserved structural properties in active site suggest a common catalytic mechanism for APPro family members, while the differences in the substrate-binding regions indicate the specific functions for each APPro member. Next to the P2' binding site, a surface loop (residue 365–377 in Pa-PepP) between helix $\alpha_{15}$ and sheet $\beta_{10}$ was identified as a candidate for specific functions due to the diversity in its sequences between APPro members (**Figure 2**). To investigate its impact on enzyme catalytic activity, we mutated residues RVGGEW (Pa-PepP 367-372) to GQDRS (Ec-PepP 368-372). Equivalent activities were observed between the corresponding mutant and the wild-type (**Figure 5B**). Since, in the activity assay, we used a non-specific tripeptide analog instead of the native substrates, these results may not accurately reflect the actual substrate-binding situation.

To further elucidate the impacts of Pa-PepP mutations on the bacterium virulence, three mutants with different effects on enzymatic activity were made in *P. aeruginos* PA14 for use in a Hela-cell invasion assay (**Figure 5C**). The PA14 bacterial growth *in vitro* was not affected by *pepP* deletion or any mutations in *pepP* (data not shown). The results showed that Pa-PepP knockout PA14 (PA14-Δ*pepP*) strain lost half of its ability to enter mammalian cells compared to wild-type PA14, and the cell invasion ability for PA14-Δ*pepP* strain was restored when introducing a complementary plasmid pRK415 for Pa-PepP expression, which confirmed the contribution of Pa-PepP to *P. aeruginos* virulence (Feinbaum et al., 2012). The enzymatic inactive mutant (H243A) exhibited an attenuated invasion ability, suggesting a role for the cleavage activity of Pa-PepP in its biological function. Strikingly, the PA14-R351G mutant also displayed weak cell internalization efficiency comparable to PA14-Δ*pepP*, revealing that the specificity of protein-substrate recognition is indispensable to the virulence-related function. The mutant PA14-Pa-PepP-367-372 also presented an attenuated invasion ability, verifying the critical role of 367-372 loop in the biological function of Pa-PepP, even though it does not have an obvious impact on enzymatic activity.

## DISCUSSION

Aminopeptidases hydrolyze the N-terminal residues of peptide/protein substrate and generally have broad specificity.

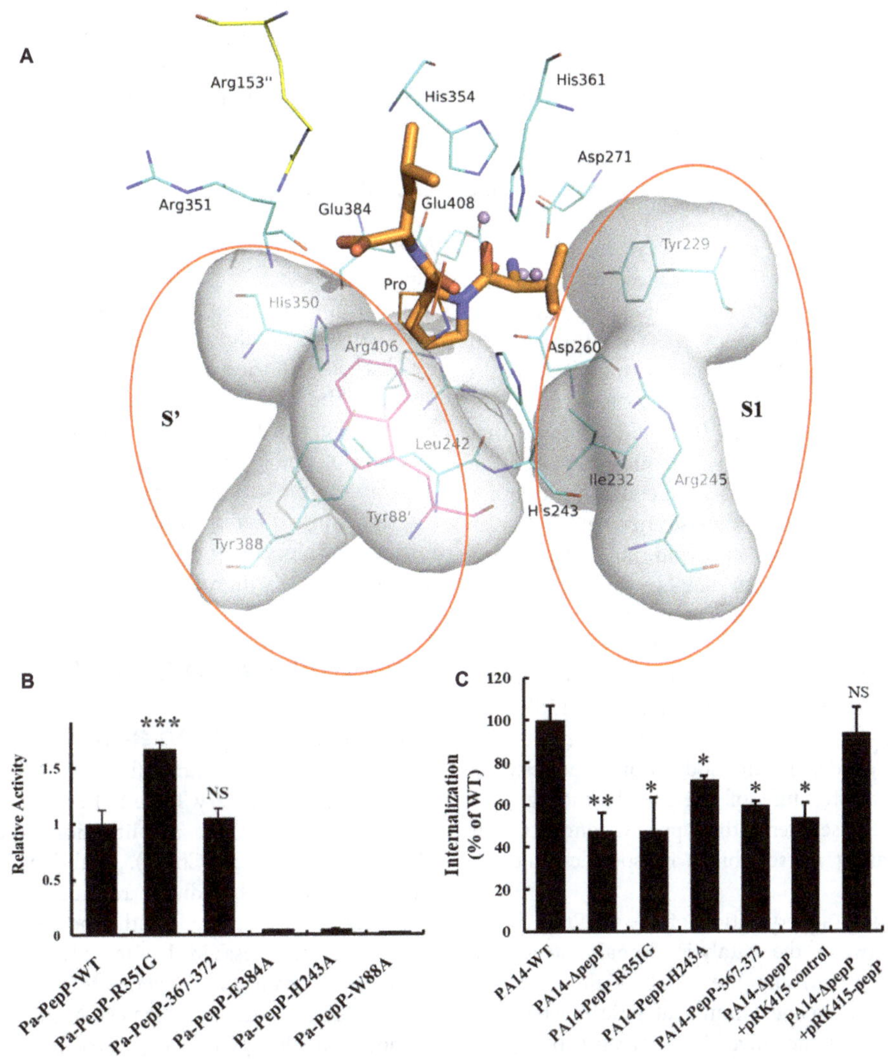


**FIGURE 5 |** The modeled Val-Pro-Leu bound Pa-PepP complex and the important residues or sequences identified to be important to Pa-PepP enzyme activity and bacterium virulence. **(A)** The modeled Val-Pro-Leu bound Pa-PepP complex by superposing with the substrate bound Ec-PepP structure (PDB code: 2BN7). The left and right shadow highlighted with red circles refers to the predicted substrate binding sites (S' and S1 sites) containing these mainly related residues, with Trp88 from the adjacent subunit colored magenta. Val-Pro-Leu is colored orange for the main carbon chain with thick lines. Other residues for direct interactions to metal ions are colored gray. **(B)** Relative activity of wild-type and mutant Pa-PepP. Activity was measured using the quenched fluorescent substrate Lys(Abz)–Pro–Pro-pNA as mentioned before. Each bar represents the mean of three independent measurements (±SEM). **(C)** Bacterial invasion of HeLa cells upon 1 h of infection at an MOI of 10 with *P. aeruginosa* strains grown at the transition between the exponential and stationary phases in LB broth at 37°C. Each bar represents the mean of three independent measurements (±SEM). *P*-values for comparison of each group with Pa-PepP-WT were determined by 2-tailed Student's *t*-test (*$P < 0.05$; **$P < 0.01$; ***$P < 0.001$).

They are associated with various essential biological functions and have been suggested as suitable therapeutic targets for corresponding diseases (Griffith et al., 1997; Pasqualini et al., 2000; Gardiner et al., 2006; Stack et al., 2007; Trenholme et al., 2010; Skinner-Adams et al., 2010). There are a number of aminopeptidases inhibitors that have already been developed as potent drug candidates (Prechel et al., 1995; Maggiora et al., 1999; Aozuka et al., 2004; Krige et al., 2008). Given the rare occurrence of proline as the second residue in protein, the proline-specific APPro exhibits even narrower substrate specificities, making it an attractive target for specific therapeutic application. In Feinbaum et al.'s (2012) *C. elegans* model, aminopeptidase PepP gene was identified as a virulence related factor and was involved in the highly attenuated *C. elegans* deaths, which suggested that Pa-PepP may be a potential drug target for the treatment of *P. aeruginosa* infections. However, other infection models are still needed to further confirm the role of *pepP* in *P. aeruginosa* virulence, and mechanisms account for Pa-PepP's correlation with bacterium virulence remain unknown. In the *C. elegans* model, the PA14 strain with transposon insertions in gene *pepP* display increased pyocyanin levels, whereas pyocyanin has been demonstrated to play an important role in

*P. aeruginosa* virulence in many models of infections (Lau et al., 2004; Dietrich et al., 2006). Thus, we predict that there may be other mechanisms linked to the effect of *pepP* on the virulence associated phenotypes. In this work, we analyzed the specific substrate binding site of Pa-PepP based on structural studies, as well as its consensus signatures and mechanisms, which provided clues for better understanding its unique physiologic function.

Like all other metalloaminopeptidase, APPro requires metal ion for its enzymc activity, and the manganese might be the most preferred cation. The dinuclear metal center structure was consistent among all APPro members, with the $M_B$ ion binds more loosely than $M_A$. Different anomalous map peaks of the bound Mn in Pa-PepP structure verified the inequivalent occupancy of two metal-binding sites. It should be noted that the different binding affinities of the metal sites allow for the sequential addition of multiple types of metal ions in other metalloaminopeptidases, resulting in diverse enzymatic activities (Carpenter and Vahl, 1973; Van Wart and Lin, 1981; Allen et al., 1983; Bayliss and Prescott, 1986; Lin and Van Wart, 1988). Stimulatory or inhibitory effects of various divalent metal ions were also observed in both Ec-PepP and Pa-PepP, suggesting that the metal selectivity contributes to activity-regulating mechanisms in APPro. Furthermore, the additional $M_C$ atom found in Pa-PepP provides a structural basis for the manganese concentration-dependent modulation of activity. In conclusion, the delicate structure of the metal binding sites enables the APPro to precisely sense the type and concentration of metal ions, facilitating its scalability in specific function performances.

The individual domain superposition of the APPros shows a close agreement between the catalytic domain structures (rmsd values of 0.847–1.846) and the nearly identical active sites allow them to maintain the unique catalytic mechanism. However, the extensive sequence diversity between prokaryotic and eukaryotic APPros, especially with respect to the domain assignments, domain motions, and oligomeric assemblies, are the breakthrough points for understanding the particular functions of each member (**Supplementary Figure S3**). For instance, the antiparallel dimerization observed in prokaryotic APPro resulted in an inward extending loop region that reached into the cavity of the neighboring subunits and participated in the P1' residue binding. Instead, in eukaryotic species, this part was replaced by the additional N-domain to ensure the maintenance of the active site pocket (Li et al., 2008). Moreover, those different oligomerization interfaces may affect the substrate selectivity in APPros.

It has been proposed that the tetrameric assembly is indispensable for Ec-PepP's function because the increase of the binding surface area can accommodate larger protein substrates (Yoshimoto et al., 1994). Pa-PepP possesses more positively charged groups on its solvent-accessible area compared to Ec-PepP (**Supplementary Figure S4**), implicating a preference for substrate selection. Notably, the 367:372 loop identified from Pa-PepP is located at the entrance region of the catalytic cave and replacement of this loop by corresponding fragment from Ec-PepP attenuated the cell invasion ability of PA14. These observations revealed that residue variations and charge distribution differences around the substrate binding interfaces can lead to distinct functions for Pa-PepP and Ec-PepP, even though they shared high sequence similarity.

## CONCLUSION

APPros exert specific physiologic functions, and many of them are relate to virulence in bacteria. However, due to the insufficiency of information about its biological substrate, the knowledge of its biology functions are limited for now. Here, we discussed the ion modulation mechanism in Pa-PepP and unveiled the differences in the regions surrounding substrate binding site, which extend our understanding about the catalytic mechanism and virulence-related functions of Pa-PepP. Most importantly, the structural analysis provides us a solid foundation for designing specific inhibitors against pathogenic bacterial infection by blocking the particular protein substrate binding site instead of directly interfering the common catalytic center.

## MATERIALS AND METHODS

### Protein Expression and Purification

Full-length *pepP* was amplified by PCR using gene-specific primers (Supplementary Table S1) from the *P. aeruginosa* PA14 genome DNA on Gene amplification Machine (Gene Touch, BIOER, HangZhou, China). Full-length *pepP* containing six C-terminal histidine residues (LEHHHHHH) was homologous recombined with the linearized pET-22b (+) using a ClonExpressTM II One Step Cloning Kit (Vazyme). All point mutants were generated using the QuickChange (I-5TM2*High Fidelity Master Mix, MCLAB) PCR-based method, on the pET-22b (+) construct. The recombinant plasmid was transformed into *E. coli* strain BL21 (DE3) for protein expression. The bacterial culture was grown in LB medium in the presence of 100 $\mu g\ mL^{-1}$ ampicillin and incubated with shaking at 310 K until the OD600 reached 0.9 (ZhiChu, ShangHai). The culture was cooled to 289 K before protein expression was induced with 0.2 mM IPTG for 20 h (Bao et al., 2013). Following induction, the bacteria were collected and resuspended in a lysis buffer consisting of 25 mM Tris–HCl pH 8.5, 10 mM NaCl, 5 % glycerol and 1 mM phenylmethanesulfonyl fluoride (20 g of cells/100 mL buffer, Sigma–Aldrich) and lysed by sonication. The lysate was cleared by centrifugation at 11000 *g* for 45 min and then the supernatant was loaded onto a 2 mL Ni–NTA affinity resin (Qiagen) for 2 L culture. The Ni–NTA column was washed with ten column volumes of the lysis buffer supplemented with 20 mM imidazole. The target protein was eluted with the same buffer in the presence of 200 mM imidazole. Fractions were pooled and determined by SDS–PAGE, followed by further purification on size-exclusion chromatography Superdex 200 column (GE Healthcare), which was pre-equilibrated with the buffer consisting of 25 mM Tris–HCl pH 8.5, 10 mM NaCl. Fractions containing Pa-PepP were pooled and concentrated to a concentration of approximately

16 mg $mL^{-1}$ using a Centricon filter (10 kDa cutoff; Millipore, Billerica).

## Crystallization and Data Collection

Initial crystallization experiments were carried out using four commercial crystallization screens from Hampton Research and Rigaku (Index HT, Crystal Screen HT, WIZARD HT, XTAL QUEST HT). Crystallization screens were conducted as previously described with some modifications (Bao et al., 2009). Briefly, crystallization initially screens were carried out using a Mosquito liquid dispenser by hanging-drop vapor-diffusion method at 291 K in 96-well plates. The 200 nL mixing drop containing protein solution and reservoir buffer by 1:1, with a final protein concentration of 16 mg $ml^{-1}$ in 25 mM Tris-HCl pH 8.5, 10 mM NaCl. The final optimized crystals for the recombinant protein were obtained by mixing 2 μl of the protein sample containing $Mn^{2+}$ and proline with an equal volume of the reservoir solution containing 30% PEG400, 100 mM sodium cacodylate pH 6.5, 200 mM lithium sulfate. Crystals grew in approximately 2–3 days and were transferred to a cryo-protectant solution (reservoir solution with 6% PEG400) prior to flash-cooling in liquid nitrogen. X-ray data were collected with a CCD camera on BL-17U stations of the SSRF, China. The diffraction data were indexed, integrated, and scaled using the HKL2000 program suite (Otwinowski and Minor, 1997).

## Structure Determination and Refinement

Data processing and scaling were carried out using the HKL2000 software package. The data were processed to a resolution limit of 1.847–1.783 Å (Rmerge = 0.099) in space group P2, with unit-cell parameters $a$ = 111.197, $b$ = 123.432, $c$ = 149.485 Å. The phase problem was solved by molecular replacement using PHENIX with aminopeptidase P from *E. coli* (PDB entry 1az9; space group P 6422; resolution 1.9 Å) as a template. The process of structure building and refinement was monitored using the COOT (Emsley et al., 2010). Water molecules were automatically added by PHENIX (Adams et al., 2010).

## Differential Scanning Calorimetry (DSC) Assays

Differential scanning calorimetry (DSC) is a promising thermoanalytical technique used for evaluating the stability of proteins as well as other biomolecules. The enthalpy value determined by DSC can provide direct information about the energetics of thermally induced processes, and the measured melting temperature(Tm) reflects thermal stability of proteins. The assays were conducted on the MicroCal VP-Capillary DSC System (Malvern). Protein samples were prepared with a final concentration of 1 mg/ml in 400 μl buffer and each sample has another 400 μl blank buffer as reference which were loaded in pairs. Operating parameters (such as pre-scan equilibration time, scan rate, temperature programming) were set and at least three buffer-buffer scans were performed before the sample was scanned. And DSC automated data analysis was conducted after experiments ran out. The DSC curves can read by Origin (Origin Pro 7.5).

## Construction of *P. aeruginosa pepP* Gene Mutant

To construct *pepP* mutants of *P. aeruginosa*, a two-step allelic exchange bacterial genome engineering strategy was employed (Hmelo et al., 2015; Sana et al., 2015). Briefly, in the first step of allelic exchange, the suicide vector pEX18Gm was integrated site-specifically into the chromosome of *P. aeruginosa* by homologous recombination, resulting in antibiotic-resistant single-crossover mutants. Then, in the second step of allelic exchange, a double crossover event occurred through a second homologous recombination, and the mutant was isolated using sucrose-mediated counter-selection. The corresponding mutants were finally identified by PCR and DNA sequencing. Specifically, PCRs were performed to amplify the target fragment sequences with upstream (800 bp) and downstream (800 bp) from *P. aeruginosa* chromosomal DNA, while the suicide plasmid pEX18Gm was linearized with gene-specific primers. The two PCR products were recombined with ClonExpress® II One Step Cloning Kit (Vazyme), The resulting plasmid, pEX18-Gm-*pepP*, was then performed Site-directed mutagenesis or deletion. All these primers are listed in Supplementary Table S1. These vectors were then transformed into *E. coli* S17-1 and then mobilized into *P. aeruginosa* strains PA14 by conjugation, in order to transfer suicide plasmids from the *E. coli* donor S17-1 to the *P. aeruginosa* recipient PA14. Colonies were first screened using gentamicin resistance plates to get single-crossover mutants. And then the double-crossover mutants were screened by No-salt LB (NSLB) agar with 15% (wt/vol) sucrose. The *pepP* gene replacement mutant strain was further confirmed by PCR and DNA sequencing.

## Construction of Complementation Plasmid pRK415-*pepP*

To construct the complementation plasmid pRK415-*pepP*, PCR-amplified *pepP* was cloned into the EcoRI and HindIII sites of plasmid pRK415, giving rise to the plasmid pRK415- *pepP* (Lin et al., 2017). The recombinant plasmid and plasmid pRK415 were transformed into *E. coli* S17-1, respectively, and then mobilized into *P. aeruginosa* PA14-Δ*pepP* by conjugation to transfer pRK415-*pepP* from the S17-1 to PA14-Δ*pepP*. The PA14-Δ*pepP* strain carried pRK415-*pepP* or pRK415 plasmid were screened by *Pseudomonas* isolation agar (PIA) with 150 μg/ml tetracycline. For expression of PepP in the *P. aeruginosa* strains, the PA14-Δ*pepP* strain carried pRK415-*pepP* were induced by addition of 1 mM IPTG and then conducted cell invasion assays.

## HeLa Cell Invasion Assays

To enumerate bacteria internalized by HeLa cells to verify bacterium virulence, gentamicin survival assays were conducted with slight modifications (Chi et al., 1991). Briefly, mammalian HeLa cells (obtained from ATCC) were grown in DMEM medium, containing 10% (v/v) FBS (Gibco, Auckland, New Zealand) and 1 % antibiotics (penicillin and streptomycin) in 5% $CO_2$ at 37°C. Suspension cultures of HeLa cells were seeded at 2–5 × $10^5$ cells per well in 12-well tissue culture plates for the overnight at 37°C. Cells were washed three times with PBS (pH 7.2) and changed to antibiotic-free medium immediately before infection. Cells were infected with exponential phase *P. aeruginosa* strains PA14 and mutant strains at a MOI of 10 for 1 h in 5% $CO_2$ at 37°C. The cells were washed twice with PBS and incubated for an additional 1 h in DMEM medium containing 150 μg/ml of gentamicin in order to kill extracellular bacteria. The monolayers cells were then washed three times with PBS and lysed with 0.5% Triton X-100 for 10–20 min, and appropriate dilutions were plated on LB plates to determine the number of viable intracellular bacteria.

### Enzyme Activity Assays

The enzyme activity of wild type Pa-PepP and the mutants were spectrophotometrically determined using the quenched fluorescent substrate Lys (Abz) - Pro–Pro–pNA (synthesized by GL Biochem Shanghai Ltd., China) as the substrate. Prior to the assay, wild type Pa-PepP and the mutant enzyme are dialyzed with EDTA overnight to fully remove the pre-bound metal ions. And all enzyme preparations were freshly diluted with ice-cold 50 mM Tris (pH 8.5) and 100 mM NaCl and treated with $MnCl_2$ for 10 min at 37°C. After addition of substrate, the final reaction conditions were 50 mM Tris (pH 8.5), 100 mM NaCl, 1 mM $MnCl_2$, 0–250 μM substrate, and 20 nM Pa-PepP (final assay volume 100 μL). The assay was allowed to proceed for 5 min at 37°C in the Thermo Scientific Varioskan Flash plate reader. The appearance of fluorescent product ($\lambda$ex = 301 nm, $\lambda$em = 410 nm) was monitored at 10 s intervals. Since the pure fluorescent product was not available to quantitate the changes in fluorescence, the kinetic results are presented as activities in relative fluorescence units. The kinetic parameters Km (Michaelis constant) for all the assays were obtained by fitting experimental data to the Michaelis-Menten equation by non-linear regression using the program OriginPro 7.5 (OriginLab Software). The data were showed in Supplementary Tables S2 and S3.

### Statistical Analysis

Statistical analysis was analyzed by 2-tailed Student's *t*-test. In all statistical analysis, *P*-values < 0.05 were considered to be statistically significant.

## ACCESSION NUMBERS

Atomic coordinates of the refined structures have been deposited in the Protein Data Bank (www.pdb.org) with the PDB code 5WZE.

## AUTHOR CONTRIBUTIONS

C-TP performed the experiments and wrote this manuscript. LL planned experiments and analyzed data. C-CL conducted structural analysis. L-HH made modifications of the manuscript. TL performed the structure determination and refinement. Y-LS performed the HeLa cell invasion assays. CG planned the experiments. N-YW contributed the essential experiment materials. YX guided the experiments. Y-BZ constructed the *P. aeruginosa pepP* gene mutants. Y-JS also performed the HeLa cell invasion assays. QL made modifications of the manuscript and conducted the PCR experiments. L-TY guided the experiments and made modifications of the manuscript. RB wrote part of the paper and performed the drawing.

## FUNDING

The work was supported by National Key Research and Development Plan (Grant No. SQ2016YFJC040104), National Natural Science Foundation of China (Grant Nos. 81670008 and 81501787).

## ACKNOWLEDGMENTS

We thank Shanghai Synchrotron Radiation Facility (SSRF) beamline BL17U for beamtime allowance (Wang et al., 2015). We thank the staffs of National Center for Protein Sciences Shanghai (NCPSS) beamlines BL18U and BL19U and SSRF, Shanghai, People's Republic of China, for assistance during data collection. We thank Dr. Derek Holman for carefully reading the manuscript.

## SUPPLEMENTARY MATERIAL

**FIGURE S1 |** Relative activity of Pa-PepP in presence of different amount of $Ca^{2+}$ **(A)** and $Mg^{2+}$ **(B)**. All assays were performed at 37°C for 5 min in the presence of 50 mM Tris (pH 8.5), 100 mM NaCl, 50 μM Lyz(Abz)–Pro–Pro–pNA quenched fluorescent substrate, and 1 μg/mL$^{-1}$ Pa-PepP that had been incubated with different concentrations of $Ca^{2+}$ **(A)** and $Mg^{2+}$ **(B)** at 37°C for 10 min. Each bar represents the mean of three independent measurements (SEM).

**FIGURE S2 |** The differential scanning calorimetry (DSC) curves of wide type Pa-PepP and all the mutants. DSC assays were conducted to investigate the thermal stability of wild type Pa-PepP and the mutants. The enthalpy value and the melting temperature(Tm) value determined by DSC were showed in the DSC curves. As it showed in the DSC curves, all these protein samples shared the similar Tm value (66–68°C), with the only exceptional of Pa-PepP-E384A which has a acceptable shift of Tm value of 63°C.

**FIGURE S3 |** Superposition of the monomer Pa-PepP and other APPros. **(A)** Superposition of the monomer Pa-PepP (red) with Ec-PepP (blue), hAPP1 (light gray), PfAPP (light blue), and CeAPP (light pink). The N domain and C domain of each APPro were circled with black frame and circle, respectively. **(B)** Superposition of the monomer Pa-PepP (red) with Ec-PepP (blue). The black circle refers to the non-conservative surface loop identified as an important motif in Pa-PepP's function. **(C)** Schematic diagrams for the prokaryotic (right) and eukaryotic APPros dimers (left). N and C are labels for their N-terminal and C-terminal domains, respectively. And the plus N-terminal domain is labeled as N'.

**FIGURE S4 |** Surface charge distribution of Pa-PepP and Ec-PepP. Surface charge distribution of Pa-PepP **(A)** and Ec-PepP **(B)** generated by CCP4mg (McCoy et al., 2007). Pa-PepP possesses more positively charged groups on its solvent-accessible area compared to Ec-PepP. The green circle refers to the predicted substrate entrance of Pa-PepP and Ec-PepP, and the entrance is also indicated by the red arrow near the black colored loop in the ribbon view of tetramer **(C)**.

## REFERENCES


Adams, P. D., Afonine, P. V., Bunkóczi, G., Chen, V. B., Davis, I. W., Echols, N., et al. (2010). PHENIX: a comprehensive Python-based system for macromolecular structure solution. *Acta Crystallogr. D Biol. Crystallogr.* 66, 213–221. doi: 10.1107/S0907444909052925

Allen, M. P., Yamada, A. H., and Carpenter, F. H. (1983). Kinetic parameters of metal-substituted leucine aminopeptidase from bovine lens. *Biochemistry* 22, 3778–3783. doi: 10.1021/bi00285a010

Aozuka, Y., Koizumi, K., Saitoh, Y., Ueda, Y., Sakurai, H., and Saiki, I. (2004). Anti-tumor angiogenesis effect of aminopeptidase inhibitor bestatin against B16-BL6 melanoma cells orthotopically implanted into syngeneic mice. *Cancer Lett.* 216, 35–42. doi: 10.1016/j.canlet.2004.06.050

Bao, R., Nair, M. K., Tang, W.-K., Esser, L., Sadhukhan, A., Holland, R. L., et al. (2013). Structural basis for the specific recognition of dual receptors by the homopolymeric pH 6 antigen (Psa) fimbriae of Yersinia pestis. *Proc. Natl. Acad. Sci. U.S.A.* 110, 1065–1070. doi: 10.1073/pnas.1212431110

Bao, R., Zhou, C.-Z., Jiang, C., Lin, S.-X., Chi, C.-W., and Chen, Y. (2009). The ternary structure of the double-headed arrowhead protease inhibitor API-A complexed with two trypsins reveals a novel reactive site conformation. *J. Biol. Chem.* 284, 26676–26684. doi: 10.1074/jbc.M109.022095

Bayliss, M. E., and Prescott, J. M. (1986). Modified activity of *Aeromonas* aminopeptidase: metal ion substitutions and role of substrates. *Biochemistry* 25, 8113–8117. doi: 10.1021/bi00372a047

Besio, R., Alleva, S., Forlino, A., Lupi, A., Meneghini, C., Minicozzi, V., et al. (2010). Identifying the structure of the active sites of human recombinant prolidase. *Eur. Biophys. J.* 39, 935–945. doi: 10.1007/s00249-009-0459-4

Carpenter, F. H., and Vahl, J. M. (1973). Leucine aminopeptidase (Bovine lens) mechanism of activation by Mg2+ and Mn2+ of the zinc metalloenzyme, amino acid composition, and sulfhydryl content. *J. Biol. Chem.* 248, 294–304.

Chi, E., Mehl, T., Nunn, D., and Lory, S. (1991). Interaction of *Pseudomonas aeruginosa* with A549 pneumocyte cells. *Infect. Immun.* 59, 822–828.

Dietrich, L. E., Price-Whelan, A., Petersen, A., Whiteley, M., and Newman, D. K. (2006). The phenazine pyocyanin is a terminal signalling factor in the quorum sensing network of *Pseudomonas aeruginosa. Mol. Microbiol.* 61, 1308–1321. doi: 10.1111/j.1365-2958.2006.05306.x

Drinkwater, N., Sivaraman, K. K., Bamert, R. S., Rut, W., Mohamed, K., Vinh, N. B., et al. (2016). Structure and substrate fingerprint of aminopeptidase P from *Plasmodium falciparum. Biochem. J.* 473, 3189–3204. doi: 10.1042/BCJ20160550

Emsley, P., Lohkamp, B., Scott, W. G., and Cowtan, K. (2010). Features and development of coot. *Acta Crystallogr. D Biol. Crystallogr.* 66, 486–501. doi: 10.1107/S0907444910007493

Feinbaum, R. L., Urbach, J. M., Liberati, N. T., Djonovic, S., Adonizio, A., Carvunis, A.-R., et al. (2012). Genome-wide identification of *Pseudomonas aeruginosa* virulence-related genes using a *Caenorhabditis elegans* infection model. *PLOS Pathog.* 8:e1002813. doi: 10.1371/journal.ppat.1002813

Gardiner, D. L., Trenholme, K. R., Skinner-Adams, T. S., Stack, C. M., and Dalton, J. P. (2006). Overexpression of leucyl aminopeptidase in *Plasmodium falciparum* parasites TARGET FOR THE ANTIMALARIAL ACTIVITY OF BESTATIN. *J. Biol. Chem.* 281, 1741–1745. doi: 10.1074/jbc.M508955200

Gi, M., Jeong, J., Lee, K., Lee, K.-M., Toyofuku, M., Yong, D. E., et al. (2014). A drug-repositioning screening identifies pentetic acid as a potential therapeutic agent for suppressing the elastase-mediated virulence of *Pseudomonas aeruginosa. Antimicrob. Agents Chemother.* 58, 7205–7214. doi: 10.1128/AAC.03063-14

Gonzales, T., and Robert-Baudouy, J. (1996). Bacterial aminopeptidases: properties and functions. *FEMS Microbiol. Rev.* 18, 319–344. doi: 10.1111/j.1574-6976.1996.tb00247.x

Graham, S. C., Bond, C. S., Freeman, H. C., and Guss, J. M. (2005). Structural and functional implications of metal ion selection in aminopeptidase P, a metalloprotease with a dinuclear metal center. *Biochemistry* 44, 13820–13836. doi: 10.1021/bi0512849

Graham, S. C., and Guss, J. M. (2008). Complexes of mutants of *Escherichia coli* aminopeptidase P and the tripeptide substrate ValProLeu. *Arch. Biochem. Biophys.* 469, 200–208. doi: 10.1016/j.abb.2007.10.009

Graham, S. C., Lilley, P. E., Lee, M., Schaeffer, P. M., Kralicek, A. V., Dixon, N. E., et al. (2006). Kinetic and crystallographic analysis of mutant *Escherichia coli* aminopeptidase P: insights into substrate recognition and the mechanism of catalysis. *Biochemistry* 45, 964–975. doi: 10.1021/bi0518904

Graham, S. C., Maher, M. J., Simmons, W. H., Freeman, H. C., and Guss, J. M. (2004). Structure of *Escherichia coli* aminopeptidase P in complex with the inhibitor apstatin. *Acta Crystallogr. D Biol. Crystallogr.* 60, 1770–1779. doi: 10.1107/S0907444904018724

Griffith, E. C., Su, Z., Turk, B. E., Chen, S., Chang, Y.-H., Wu, Z., et al. (1997). Methionine aminopeptidase (type 2) is the common target for angiogenesis inhibitors AGM-1470 and ovalicin. *Chem. Biol.* 4, 461–471. doi: 10.1016/S1074-5521(97)90198-8

Hahn, H. P. (1997). The type-4 pilus is the major virulence-associated adhesin of *Pseudomonas aeruginosa*-a review. *Gene* 192, 99–108. doi: 10.1016/S0378-1119(97)00116-9

Hancock, R. E. (1998). Resistance mechanisms in *Pseudomonas aeruginosa* and other nonfermentative gram-negative bacteria. *Clin. Infect. Dis.* 27(Suppl. 1), S93–S99. doi: 10.1086/514909

Hentzer, M., Wu, H., Andersen, J. B., Riedel, K., Rasmussen, T. B., Bagge, N., et al. (2003). Attenuation of *Pseudomonas aeruginosa* virulence by quorum sensing inhibitors. *EMBO J.* 22, 3803–3815. doi: 10.1093/emboj/cdg366

Hmelo, L. R., Borlee, B. R., Almblad, H., Love, M. E., Randall, T. E., Tseng, B. S., et al. (2015). Precision-engineering the *Pseudomonas aeruginosa* genome with two-step allelic exchange. *Nat. Protoc.* 10, 1820–1841. doi: 10.1038/nprot.2015.115

Hood, R. D., Singh, P., Hsu, F., Güvener, T., Carl, M. A., Trinidad, R. R., et al. (2010). A type VI secretion system of *Pseudomonas aeruginosa* targets a toxin to bacteria. *Cell Host Microbe* 7, 25–37. doi: 10.1016/j.chom.2009.12.007

Hu, X. V., Chen, X., Han, K. C., Mildvan, A. S., and Liu, J. O. (2007). Kinetic and mutational studies of the number of interacting divalent cations required by bacterial and human methionine aminopeptidases. *Biochemistry* 46, 12833–12843. doi: 10.1021/bi701127x

Hwang, S., Kim, C. Y., Ji, S.-G., Go, J., Kim, H., Yang, S., et al. (2016). Network-assisted investigation of virulence and antibiotic-resistance systems in *Pseudomonas aeruginosa. Sci. Rep.* 6:26223. doi: 10.1038/srep26223

Iyer, S., La-Borde, P. J., Payne, K. A., Parsons, M. R., Turner, A. J., Isaac, R. E., et al. (2015). Crystal structure of X-prolyl aminopeptidase from *Caenorhabditis elegans*: a cytosolic enzyme with a di-nuclear active site. *FEBS Open Bio* 5, 292–302. doi: 10.1016/j.fob.2015.03.013

Jao, S.-C., Huang, L.-F., Hwang, S.-M., and Li, W.-S. (2006). Tyrosine 387 and arginine 404 are critical in the hydrolytic mechanism of *Escherichia coli* aminopeptidase P. *Biochemistry* 45, 1547–1553. doi: 10.1021/bi051786m

Jao, S.-C., Huang, L.-F., Tao, Y. S., and Li, W.-S. (2004). Hydrolysis of organophosphate triesters by *Escherichia coli* aminopeptidase P. *J. Mol. Catal. B Enzym.* 27, 7–12. doi: 10.1021/bi051786m

Jeyakanthan, J., Takada, K., Sawano, M., Ogasahara, K., Mizutani, H., Kunishima, N., et al. (2009). Crystal structural and functional analysis of the putative dipeptidase from *Pyrococcus horikoshii* OT3. *J. Biophys.* 2009:434038. doi: 10.1155/2009/434038

Johnson, B. K., and Abramovitch, R. B. (2017). Small molecules that sabotage bacterial virulence. *Trends Pharmacol. Sci.* 38, 339–362. doi: 10.1016/j.tips.2017.01.004

Krige, D., Needham, L. A., Bawden, L. J., Flores, N., Farmer, H., Miles, L. E., et al. (2008). CHR-2797: an antiproliferative aminopeptidase inhibitor that leads to amino acid deprivation in human leukemic cells. *Cancer Res.* 68, 6669–6679. doi: 10.1158/0008-5472.CAN-07-6627

Lau, G. W., Hassett, D. J., Ran, H., and Kong, F. (2004). The role of pyocyanin in *Pseudomonas aeruginosa* infection. *Trends Mol. Med.* 10, 599–606. doi: 10.1016/j.molmed.2004.10.002

Li, X., Lou, Z., Li, X., Zhou, W., Ma, M., Cao, Y., et al. (2008). Structure of human cytosolic X-prolyl aminopeptidase: a double Mn (II)-dependent dimeric enzyme with a novel three-domain subunit. *J. Biol. Chem.* 283, 22858–22866. doi: 10.1074/jbc.M710274200

Lin, J., Zhang, W., Cheng, J., Yang, X., Zhu, K., Wang, Y., et al. (2017). A *Pseudomonas* T6SS effector recruits PQS-containing outer membrane vesicles for iron acquisition. *Nat. Commun.* 8:14888. doi: 10.1038/ncomms14888

Lin, W. Y., and Van Wart, H. E. (1988). Hydrolysis of dansyl-peptide substrates by leucine aminopeptidase: origin of dansyl fluorescence changes during hydrolysis. *Biochemistry* 27, 5054–5061. doi: 10.1021/bi00414a016

Liu, J. W., Hadler, K. S., Schenk, G., and Ollis, D. (2007). Using directed evolution to improve the solubility of the C-terminal domain of *Escherichia coli* aminopeptidase P. *FEBS J.* 274, 4742–4751. doi: 10.1111/j.1742-4658.2007.06022.x

Lowther, W. T., and Matthews, B. W. (2000). Structure and function of the methionine aminopeptidases. *Biochim. Biophys. Acta* 1477, 157–167. doi: 10.1016/S0167-4838(99)00271-X

Lowther, W. T., and Matthews, B. W. (2002). Metalloaminopeptidases: common functional themes in disparate structural surroundings. *Chem. Rev.* 102, 4581–4608. doi: 10.1021/cr0101757

Luckett, J. C., Darch, O., Watters, C., AbuOun, M., Wright, V., Paredes-Osses, E., et al. (2012). A novel virulence strategy for *Pseudomonas aeruginosa* mediated by an autotransporter with arginine-specific aminopeptidase activity. *PLOS Pathog.* 8:e1002854. doi: 10.1371/journal.ppat.1002854

Maggiora, L. L., Orawski, A. T., and Simmons, W. H. (1999). Apstatin analogue inhibitors of aminopeptidase P, a bradykinin-degrading enzyme. *J. Med. Chem.* 42, 2394–2402. doi: 10.1021/jm9805642

Maura, D., Ballok, A. E., and Rahme, L. G. (2016). Considerations and caveats in anti-virulence drug development. *Curr. Opin. Microbiol.* 33, 41–46. doi: 10.1016/j.mib.2016.06.001

McBroom, A. J., Johnson, A. P., Vemulapalli, S., and Kuehn, M. J. (2006). Outer membrane vesicle production by *Escherichia coli* is independent of membrane instability. *J. Bacteriol.* 188, 5385–5392. doi: 10.1128/JB.00498-06

McCoy, A. J., Grosse-Kunstleve, R. W., Adams, P. D., Winn, M. D., Storoni, L. C., and Read, R. J. (2007). Phaser crystallographic software. *J. Appl. Crystallogr.* 40, 658–674. doi: 10.1107/S0021889807021206

Miyata, S., Casey, M., Frank, D. W., Ausubel, F. M., and Drenkard, E. (2003). Use of the Galleria mellonella caterpillar as a model host to study the role of the type III secretion system in *Pseudomonas aeruginosa* pathogenesis. *Infect. Immun.* 71, 2404–2413. doi: 10.1128/IAI.71.5.2404-2413.2003

Otwinowski, Z., and Minor, W. (1997). [20] Processing of X-ray diffraction data collected in oscillation mode. *Methods Enzymol.* 276, 307–326. doi: 10.1016/S0076-6879(97)76066-X

Pasqualini, R., Koivunen, E., Kain, R., Lahdenranta, J., Sakamoto, M., Stryhn, A., et al. (2000). Aminopeptidase N is a receptor for tumor-homing peptides and a target for inhibiting angiogenesis. *Cancer Res.* 60, 722–727.

Prechel, M. M., Orawski, A. T., Maggiora, L. L., and Simmons, W. H. (1995). Effect of a new aminopeptidase P inhibitor, apstatin, on bradykinin degradation in the rat lung. *J. Pharmacol. Exp. Ther.* 275, 1136–1142.

Rampioni, G., Visca, P., Leoni, L., and Imperi, F. (2017). Drug repurposing for antivirulence therapy against opportunistic bacterial pathogens. *Emerg. Top. Life Sci.* ETLS20160018. doi: 10.1042/ETLS20160018

Sana, T. G., Baumann, C., Merdes, A., Soscia, C., Rattei, T., Hachani, A., et al. (2015). Internalization of *Pseudomonas aeruginosa* strain PAO1 into epithelial cells is promoted by interaction of a T6SS effector with the microtubule network. *mBio* 6:e00712-15. doi: 10.1128/mBio.0071215

Simmons, W. H., and Orawski, A. T. (1992). Membrane-bound aminopeptidase P from bovine lung. Its purification, properties, and degradation of bradykinin. *J. Biol. Chem.* 267, 4897–4903.

Skinner-Adams, T. S., Stack, C. M., Trenholme, K. R., Brown, C. L., Grembecka, J., Lowther, J., et al. (2010). *Plasmodium falciparum* neutral aminopeptidases: new targets for anti-malarials. *Trends Biochem. Sci.* 35, 53–61. doi: 10.1016/j.tibs.2009.08.004

Stack, C. M., Lowther, J., Cunningham, E., Donnelly, S., Gardiner, D. L., Trenholme, K. R., et al. (2007). Characterization of the *Plasmodium falciparum* M17 leucyl aminopeptidase A protease involved in amino acid regulation with potential for antimalarial drug development. *J. Biol. Chem.* 282, 2069–2080. doi: 10.1074/jbc.M609251200

Stover, C., Pham, X., Erwin, A., Mizoguchi, S., Warrener, P., Hickey, M., et al. (2000). Complete genome sequence of *Pseudomonas aeruginosa* PAO1, an opportunistic pathogen. *Nature* 406, 959–964. doi: 10.1038/35023079

Taylor, A. (1993). Aminopeptidases: structure and function. *FASEB J.* 7, 290–298.

Trenholme, K. R., Brown, C. L., Skinner-Adams, T. S., Stack, C., Lowther, J., To, J., et al. (2010). Aminopeptidases of malaria parasites: new targets for chemotherapy. *Infect. Disord. Drug Targets* 10, 217–225. doi: 10.2174/187152610791163363

Van Wart, H. E., and Lin, S. H. (1981). Metal binding stoichiometry and mechanism of metal ion modulation of the activity of porcine kidney leucine aminopeptidase. *Biochemistry* 20, 5682–5689. doi: 10.1021/bi00523a007

Vanaja, S. K., Russo, A. J., Behl, B., Banerjee, I., Yankova, M., Deshmukh, S. D., et al. (2016). Bacterial outer membrane vesicles mediate cytosolic localization of LPS and caspase-11 activation. *Cell* 165, 1106–1119. doi: 10.1016/j.cell.2016.04.015

Wallace, A. C., Laskowski, R. A., and Thornton, J. M. (1995). LIGPLOT: a program to generate schematic diagrams of protein-ligand interactions. *Protein Eng.* 8, 127–134. doi: 10.1093/protein/8.2.127

Wang, Q.-S., Yu, F., Huang, S., Sun, B., Zhang, K.-H., Liu, K., et al. (2015). The macromolecular crystallography beamline of SSRF. *Nucl. Sci. Tech.* 26, 12–17.

Weaver, J., Watts, T., Li, P., and Rye, H. S. (2014). Structural basis of substrate selectivity of *E. coli* prolidase. *PLOS ONE* 9:e111531. doi: 10.1371/journal.pone.0111531

Wilce, M., Bond, C., Dixon, N., Freeman, H., Guss, J., Lilley, P., et al. (1998). Structure and mechanism of a proline-specific aminopeptidase from *Escherichia coli. Proc. Natl. Acad. Sci. U.S.A.* 95, 3472–3477. doi: 10.1073/pnas.95.7.3472

Woods, D. E., Cryz, S. J., Friedman, R. L., and Iglewski, B. (1982). Contribution of toxin A and elastase to virulence of *Pseudomonas aeruginosa* in chronic lung infections of rats. *Infect. Immun.* 36, 1223–1228.

Yoshimoto, T., Orawski, A. T., and Simmons, W. H. (1994). Substrate specificity of aminopeptidase P from *Escherichia coli*: comparison with membrane-bound forms from rat and bovine lung. *Arch. Biochem. Biophys.* 311, 28–34. doi: 10.1006/abbi.1994.1204

# 6

# Combining CRISPR-Cas12a-Based Technology and Metagenomics Next Generation Sequencing: A New Paradigm for Rapid and Full-Scale Detection of Microbes in Infectious Diabetic Foot Samples

*Yixin Chen[1†], Ya Shi[2†], Weifen Zhu[1†], Jiaxing You[3], Jie Yang[3], Yaping Xie[4], Hanxin Zhao[1], Hongye Li[3], Shunwu Fan[3], Lin Li[1]* and Chao Liu[3]**

*[1] Department of Endocrinology, Zhejiang University School of Medicine Sir Run Run Shaw Hospital, Hangzhou, China, [2] Hangzhou Digital Micro Biotech Co., Ltd., Hangzhou, China, [3] Department of Orthopedics, Zhejiang University School of Medicine Sir Run Run Shaw Hospital, Hangzhou, China, [4] Department of Hematology, Affiliated Hangzhou First People's Hospital, Zhejiang University School of Medicine, Hangzhou, China*

***Correspondence:**
*Lin Li*
*3312012@zju.edu.cn*
*Chao Liu*
*liuchaozju@zju.edu.cn*

*† These authors have contributed equally to this work and share first authorship*

**Introduction:** Diabetic foot infections (DFIs) pose a huge challenge for clinicians. *Staphylococcus aureus*, including methicillin-resistant *S. aureus* (MRSA), is one of the most significant pathogens of DFI. Early pathogen identification will greatly benefit the diagnosis and treatment of the disease. However, existing diagnostic methods are not effective in early detection.

**Methods:** We developed an assay that coupled loop-mediated isothermal amplification (LAMP) and clustered regularly interspaced short palindromic repeats (CRISPR) techniques to enable quick and specific detection of *Staphylococcus aureus* and differentiate MRSA in samples from patients with DFI. Furthermore, the results were compared using a reference culture, quantitative real-time polymerase chain reaction (qRT-PCR), and metagenomics next generation sequencing (mNGS).

**Results:** The CRISPR-LAMP assay targeting *nuc* and *mecA* successfully detected *S. aureus* strains and differentiated MRSA. The limit of detection (LoD) of the real-time LAMP for *nuc* and *mecA* was 20 copies per microliter reaction in comparison to two copies per μL reaction for the qRT-PCR assay. The specificity of the LAMP-CRISPR assay for *nuc* was 100%, without cross-reactions with non-*S. aureus* strains. Evaluating assay performance with 18 samples from DFI patients showed that the assay had 94.4% agreement (17/18 samples) with clinical culture results. The results of mNGS for 8/18 samples were consistent with those of the reference culture and LAMP-CRISPR assay.

**Conclusion:** The findings suggest that the LAMP-CRISPR assay could be promising for the point-of-care detection of *S. aureus* and the differentiation of MRSA in clinical samples. Furthermore, combining the LAMP-CRISPR assay and mNGS provides an advanced platform for molecular pathogen diagnosis of DFI.

**Keywords: diabetic foot infections, *Staphylococcus aureus*, loop-mediated isothermal amplification, clustered regularly interspaced short palindromic repeats, metagenomics next generation sequencing**

## INTRODUCTION

Diabetic foot ulcers, one of the most critical complications of diabetes mellitus, has become a significant public health problem. When patients with diabetic foot ulcers first consult physicians, over half of them have complications with diabetic foot infections (DFIs) (Prompers et al., 2006; Jia et al., 2017). Treatment of DFI requires precise evaluation of infection conditions, pathogen confirmation of infectious ulcers, appropriate selection of antibiotics, and surgical intervention, if necessary (Lipsky et al., 2012). DFI patients are often challenged by the complexity of intricate ulceration and moderate to severe infections, even sepsis. Broad-spectrum empirical antimicrobials would be the primary option for clinicians to hinder the further deterioration of infectious conditions and lower medical risks, which increases antibiotic exposure and selective pressure that contribute to the development of multi-drug resistant microorganisms. Nevertheless, a rapid, accessible, and accurate diagnostic test for pathogenic identification is valuable for clinical procedures.

*Staphylococcus aureus* is the dominant pathogen of DFI. The resistance rate of *S. aureus* to methicillin fluctuated between 15–30% (Eleftheriadou et al., 2010). It has been shown that infections caused by methicillin-resistant *S. aureus* (MRSA) are linked to higher mortality rates and greater consumption of medical resources than infections caused by methicillin-sensitive *S. aureus* (MSSA) (Cosgrove et al., 2003; Filice et al., 2010). Bacterial culture, quantitative real-time polymerase chain reaction (qRT-PCR) (Buchan et al., 2015; Ellem et al., 2015; Silbert et al., 2017), and metagenomics next generation sequencing (mNGS) (Charalampous et al., 2019; Kalan et al., 2019; Zou et al., 2020) are typically used to identify *S. aureus* and discriminate between MSSA and MRSA. Although traditional culture is the gold standard for pathogen diagnosis, it is time-consuming, and delayed results cannot provide timely clinical guidance. qRT-PCR has a shortened detection time; however, it has not been widely applied because of its high requirements for equipment and laboratory staff. mNGS, a novel detection method, is still not commonly accessible because of its high cost in terms of time, funding, instrumentation, and technical expertise.

In recent years, the application of isothermal amplification combined with clustered regularly interspaced short palindromic repeats (CRISPR) has been developed for pathogen diagnosis (Li et al., 2019). An innovative discovery reported that RNA-guided DNA binding activated Cas12a for both site-specific double-stranded DNA (dsDNA) *cis*-cleavage and indiscriminate single-stranded DNA (ssDNA) *trans*-cleavage. With the guidance of a single CRISPR RNA (crRNA), Cas12a recognizes a TTTN protospacer-adjacent motif (PAM) and binds to crRNA-complementary dsDNA (Li et al., 2018a,b). This indicates that the high specificity of the CRISPR/Cas12a assay is determined by PAM and crRNA. The coupling of isothermal amplification and *trans*-ssDNA repetitive cutting results in double-magnifying biosensing signals, indicating the high sensitivity of the assay. It has been proven to enable a rapid and accurate detection of the human papillomavirus and a new coronavirus (resulting in the disease referred to as COVID-19) in patient samples (Chen et al., 2018; Broughton et al., 2020).

In this study, we developed an assay coupling loop-mediated isothermal amplification (LAMP) and *trans*-cleavage of Cas12a for the quick and specific detection of *S. aureus* and the differentiation of MRSA in samples of patients with DFI. Furthermore, the results were compared with standard methods, including bacterial culture, qRT-PCR, and mNGS.

**Abbreviations:** DFI, diabetic foot infections; MRSA, methicillin-resistant *Staphylococcus aureus*; MSSA, methicillin-sensitive *Staphylococcus aureus*; LAMP, loop-mediated isothermal amplification; CRISPR, clustered regularly interspaced short palindromic repeats; mNGS, metagenomics next generation sequencing; qRT-PCR, quantitative real-time polymerase chain reaction; ssDNA, single-stranded DNA; dsDNA, double-stranded DNA; crRNA, CRISPR RNA; PAM, protospacer-adjacent motif; LoD, limit of detection; DNB, DNA nanoballs; RCA, rolling circle replication; NTC, no template control.

## MATERIALS AND METHODS

### Nucleic Acid Preparation

DNA extraction from the tissues of DFI patients was performed using QuickExtract$^{TM}$ DNA Extraction Solution (Lucigen, Beijing, China). Quick DNA extractions were finished after incubation at 65°C for 10 min and 98°C for 2 min. The sequences of *nuc* (*S. aureus*-specific gene) and *mecA* (encoding penicillin-binding protein-2a) were obtained from a public database. LAMP primers were designed against regions of *nuc* and *mecA* using PrimerExplorer v.5. with compatible gRNAs (**Supplementary Table 1**). The gRNA was designed with a TTTN structure (PAM) at the right end. The length of gRNA was 20-25bp, and the GC content was 40–60%. The design was assured to avoid the combination of gRNA and primer dimer (**Table 1**). The primers and gRNAs were obtained from Shanghai General Biotech Co., Ltd. (Shanghai, China).

### Real-Time Polymerase Chain Reaction Assay

A 20-μL system was used to conduct the real-time PCR assay for the detection of *nuc* and *mecA* with the following specifications: Forward primer for *nuc* gene: 5′-ACTGTAACTTTGGCACTGG-3′; Reverse primer for *nuc* gene: 5′-GCAGATACCTCATTACCTGC-3′; Probe: 5′-[6FAM]- ATCGCAACGACTGGCGCTA-[BHQ1]-3′ [12]; Forward primer for *mecA* gene: AAAACTAGGTGTTGGTGAAGATATACC; Reverse primer for *mecA* gene: GAAAGGATCTGTACTGGGTTAATCAG; Probe: [6FAM]-TTCACCTTGTCCGTAACCTGAATCAGCT-[BHQ1] (Sabet et al., 2007). Real-time PCR assays were performed using the Premix Ex Taq$^{TM}$ (Probe qPCR) Kit (TaKara Biomedical Technology Co., Ltd., Beijing, China). Ten microliters Premix Ex Taq (Probe qPCR) (2×), 0.2 μM forward primer, 0.2 μM

**TABLE 1** | gRNA sequences for *nuc* and *mecA*.

| gRNA | sequence (5′-3′) |
|---|---|
| nuc-gRNA | UAAUUUCUACUAAGUGUAGAUUACAUUAAUUUAACCGUAUCA |
| mecA-gRNA | UAAUUUCUACUAAGUGUAGAUUGCCAACCUUUACCAUCGAUU |

reverse primer, 0.1 μM probe, and 2 μL DNA templates of different concentrations were included in the reaction system. The temperature cycling conditions were 95°C for 30 s, followed by 40 cycles of 95°C for 5 s, and 60°C for 30 s. The reaction was performed using the StepOne$^{TM}$Plus Real-Time PCR System (Applied Biosystems, Inc., Carlsbad, CA, United States).

## Real-Time Loop-Mediated Isothermal Amplification Assay

The real-time LAMP assay was conducted in a 25-μL mixture containing 1 × Bst DNA polymerase buffer (New England Biolabs, Beijing, China), 0.4 μM FIP primers, 0.4 μM BIP primers, 0.2 μM LF primers, 0.2 μM LB primers, 0.1 μM F3 primers F3, 0.1 μM B3 primers, 1.4 μM dNTPs (New England Biolabs), 8U Bst DNA polymerase (New England Biolabs), 8 mM $MgSO_4$ (New England Biolabs), 1 × SYBR Green I (Thermo Fisher Scientific, Inc., Waltham, MA, United States), and 2 μL of DNA templates of different concentrations. Real-time LAMP assays of *nuc* and *mecA* were conducted in the same reaction system, except for the primers. The LAMP reaction solution was covered with 40 μL mineral oil. The reaction was performed at 65°C for 60 min in a StepOne$^{TM}$ Plus Real-Time PCR System (Applied Biosystems, Inc., Carlsbad, CA, United States) and terminated at 80°C for 5 min. The fluorescence information was collected every 30 s during the reaction.

## Loop-Mediated Isothermal Amplification-Clustered Regularly Interspaced Short Palindromic Repeats Assay

The LAMP system contained the same mixture as the real-time LAMP assay. The fluorescent dyes were added into the system and the LAMP reagents covered with 40 μL of mineral oil. The LAMP reaction was followed by the admixture of CRISPR reaction solution (preloaded inside the lid) to the LAMP amplification solution by centrifugation. The 20 μL CRISPR reaction solution contained 1 × NEBuffer 2.1, reaction buffer, 0.2 μM EnGen® Lba Cas12a (Cpf1) (New England Biolabs), 0.6 μM gRNA, 2.5 μM CRISPR probes, and 1 U/μL RNA inhibitor (Thermo Fisher Scientific, Inc., Waltham, MA, United States). Sequence information of gRNA is shown in **Table 1**. The CRISPR reaction was conducted in a ProFlex PCR System (Applied Biosystems, Inc., Carlsbad, CA, United States) at 37°C for 5 min. After the reaction, the visualized results were observed using a simple fluorescence reader.

## Sensitivity and Specificity of Loop-Mediated Isothermal Amplification-Clustered Regularly Interspaced Short Palindromic Repeats Assay

Amplification of *S. aureus* genomic DNA, including *nuc* and *mecA*, was performed using outer primers (F3 and B3, **Supplementary Table 1**). The lengths of the PCR products of *nuc* and *mecA* were 248 bp and 208 bp, respectively. The PCR product was purified using the TAKARA gel DNA fragment recovery kit, and the purified product was ligated to the pMD18-T vector (2692 bp). The recombinant plasmids were transformed into *Escherichia coli* DH5α competent cells. LB growth medium containing 10 μg/mL ampicillin was used to screen positive colonies. Plasmids of *E. coli* that comprised the pMD18-T vector and *nuc* (248 bp)/*mecA* (208 bp) were extracted using the TaKaRa MiniBEST Plasmid Purification Kit (TaKaRa, 9760). We then measured the concentration of plasmids and calculated the DNA copy number [$6.02 \times 10^{23} \times$ concentration (ng/μL) $\times 10^9$/(DNA sequence length × 660)]. The concentration of plasmids containing *nuc* was 3.26 ng/μL. The DNA copy number of *nuc* was $1.0 \times 10^9$ copies per μl, calculated according to the above formula. The concentration of plasmids containing *mecA* was 12 ng/μL, and the copy number was $3.78 \times 10^9$ copies per μl. The plasmids were serially diluted to 1:10. Isothermal amplifications of the dilutions were repeatedly performed three times, and the limit of detection (LoD) was determined as the minimum DNA copy number of the diluted plasmids that could amplify the target genomic DNA.

Genomic DNA from 14 strains of *staphylococci* species was analyzed using the LAMP-CRISPR assay to examine the specificity of the LAMP assay. The strains were *S. epidermidis, S. hominis, S. cohnii, S. warneri, S. haemolyticus, S. aureus, S. capitis, S. saprophyticus, S. pasteuri, S. saprophyticus* ATCC® 15305, *S. haemolyticus* ATCC ®29970, *S. epidermidis* ATCC ®14990, *S. caprae,* and *S. aureus* subsp. *sureus* ATCC ®12600.

## Metagenomic Next-Generation Sequencing

After DNA extractions using a DNeasy Blood and Tissue Kit (Qiagen, 69504, Shenzhen, China), DNA was fragmented using a Bioruptor Pico instrument to generate 200–300-bp fragments (Bioruptor Pico protocols). Then, libraries were constructed by MGIEasy (MGIEasy universal DNA library prep kit) as follows: first, the DNA fragments were subjected to end-repair sequencing, and A-tailing was added to one tube. Subsequently, the resulting DNA was ligated with bubble-adaptors that included barcode sequences and then amplified by the PCR method. Quality control was carried out using bioanalyzer (Agilent 2100, Agilent Technologies, Santa Clara, CA, United States) to assess DNA concentrations and fragment size. Qualified libraries were pooled together to make a single strand DNA circle (ssDNA circle), and then, DNA nanoballs (DNB) were generated by rolling circle replication (RCA). The final DNBs were loaded into the sequence chip and sequenced on the BGISEQ platform using 50 bp/single-end sequencing. Finally, optical signals were collected using a high-resolution imaging system, and then, these signals were transformed into digital information, which can be decoded into DNA sequence information.

## Reference Culture Method and Antimicrobial Susceptibility Test

The sample culture broths were plated on blood agar and incubated for 18–48 h. Identification of S. aureus and examination of antimicrobial susceptibility were conducted using

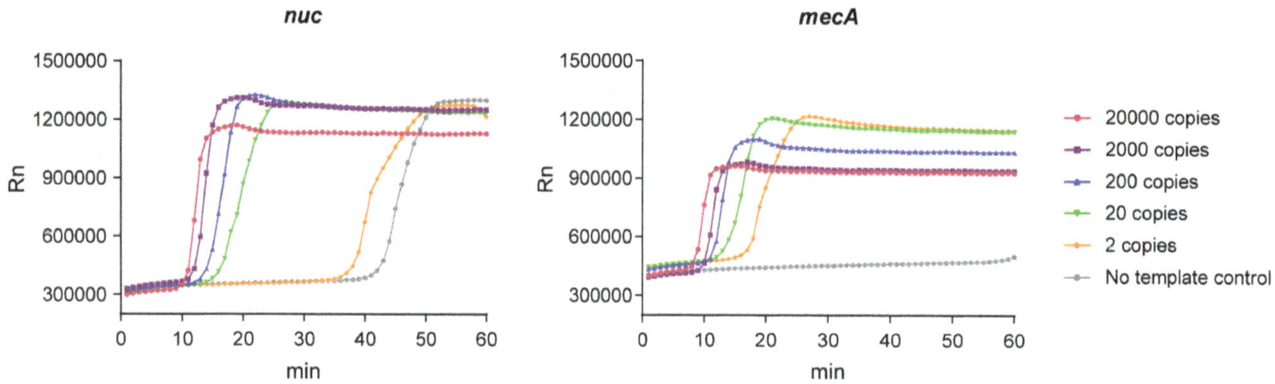


**FIGURE 1 |** Amplification curves of the real-time LAMP assay for *nuc* and *mecA*.

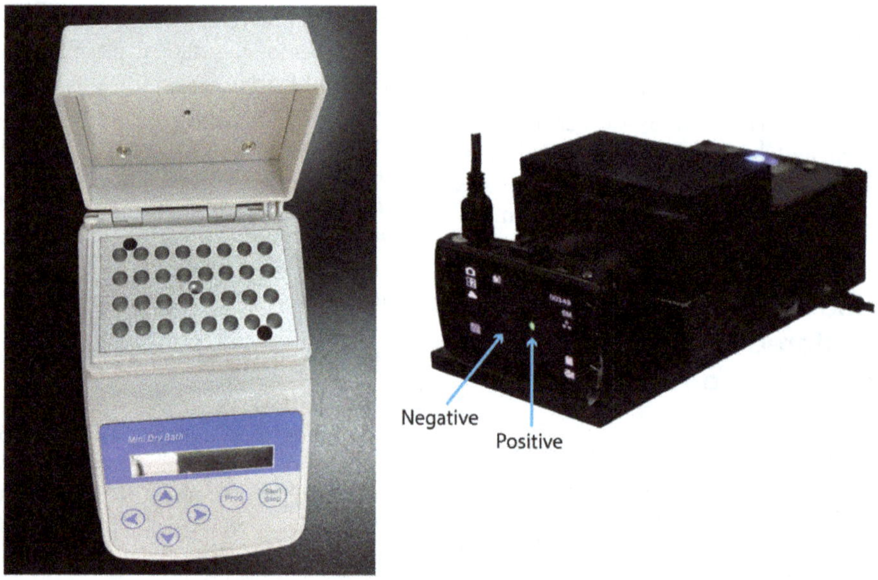


**FIGURE 2 |** Portable equipment for the LAMP assay and fluorescence visualization.

a fully automatic vitek-2 compact system (Biomerieux, Shanghai, China). The results were interpreted on the basis of the guidelines (M100, 28th edition) established by the Clinical and Laboratory Standards Institute (CLSI, 2018).

## Human Clinical Sample Collection

Tissues of infected ulcers were acquired from DFI patients at their first visit to the outpatient clinic or the Department of Emergency at Sir Run Run Shaw Hospital. After the wound was cleaned with saline solution, DFU tissue with the size of a rice grain was taken out with a blade and immediately sent to the laboratory for DNA extraction. The study was approved by the Human Research Ethics Committee of Sir Run Run Shaw Hospital.

## Statistical Methods

All reactions were repeated three times, the CT value of the real-time PCR is shown as "mean ± standard deviation" (x ± s).

# RESULTS

## Real-Time Loop-Mediated Isothermal Amplification Assay for nuc and mecA

We conducted a real-time LAMP assay for amplifying nuc and mecA with seven dilutions. The amplification curves of the dilutions with serial concentrations are shown in **Figure 1**. The LAMP assay was able to amplify genomic DNA targets. There was no stable fluorescent signal obtained when the genomic DNA template was at two copies per μL reaction.

## Visual Detection Assay With Clustered Regularly Interspaced Short Palindromic Repeats/Cas12a

Next, we used the CRISPR/Cas12a system to realize the visual readout of the targeted amplicons, based on the collateral DNA

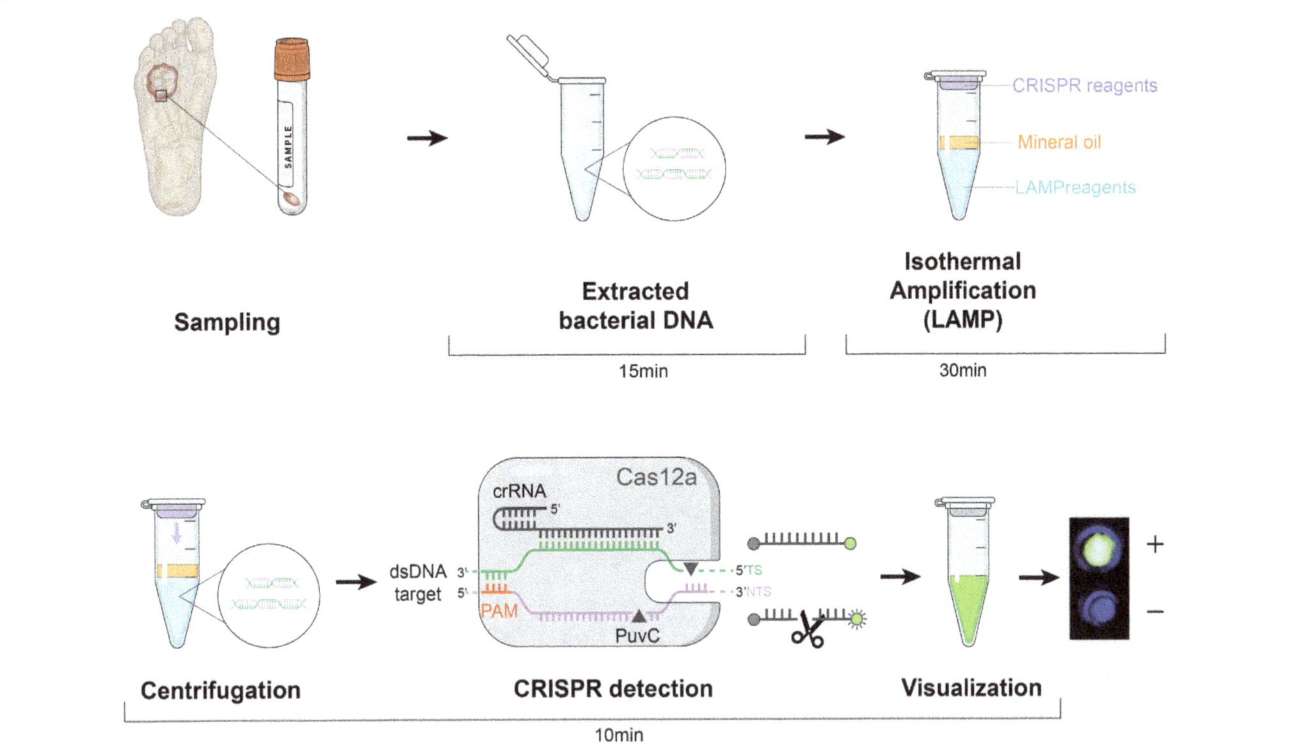


**FIGURE 3 |** Schematic of the LAMP-CRISPR assay workflow. Quick DNA extraction was used as an input to the LAMP-CRISPR system (LAMP preamplification and Cas12-based detection for *nuc* and *mecA*). The result is visualized by a fluorescence reader.

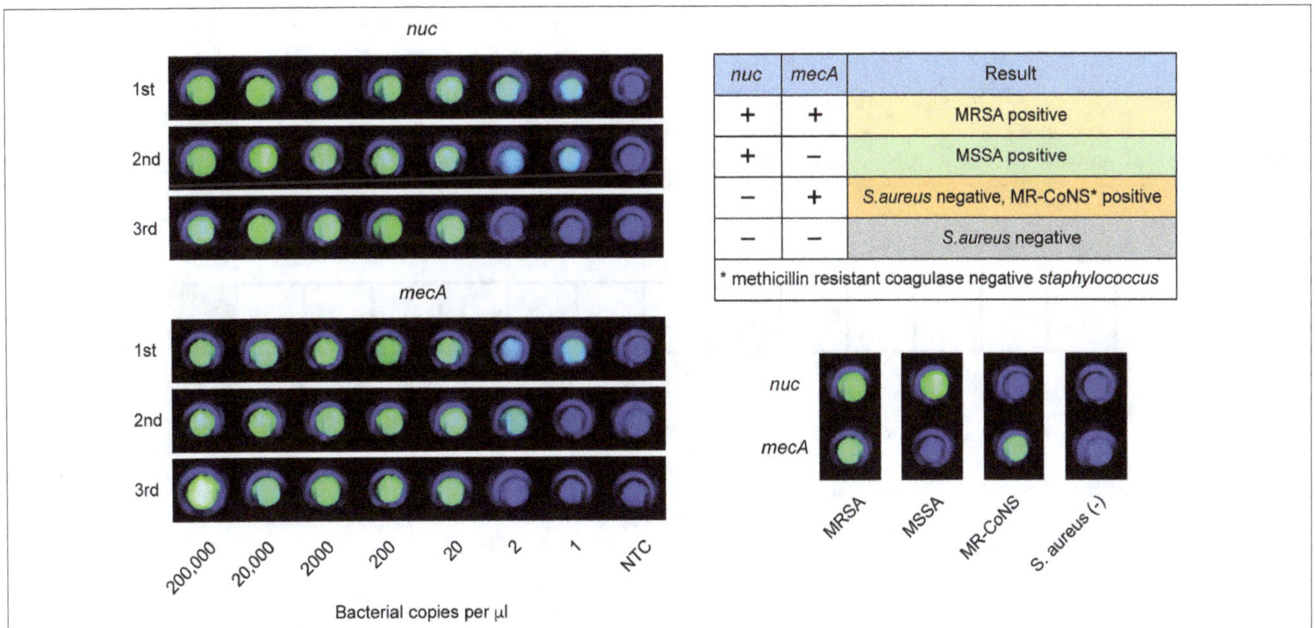


**FIGURE 4 |** LAMP-CRISPR assay readout. Fluorescent results of MRSA, MSSA, MR-CoNS, and *S. aureus* are presented at the bottom right. *Nuc* detection indicates *S. aureus* positive. MRSA identification requires positive for both *nuc* and *mecA*.

cleavage activity of the Cas12a effector. The cleaved ssDNA reporters produced fluorescent signals, which could be seen through a portable fluorescence reader (**Figure 2**). The entire procedure and explanation of the results are presented in **Figure 3**. Pre-loading of the CRISPR reagents inside the lid avoided the need to open the cap during the process. We

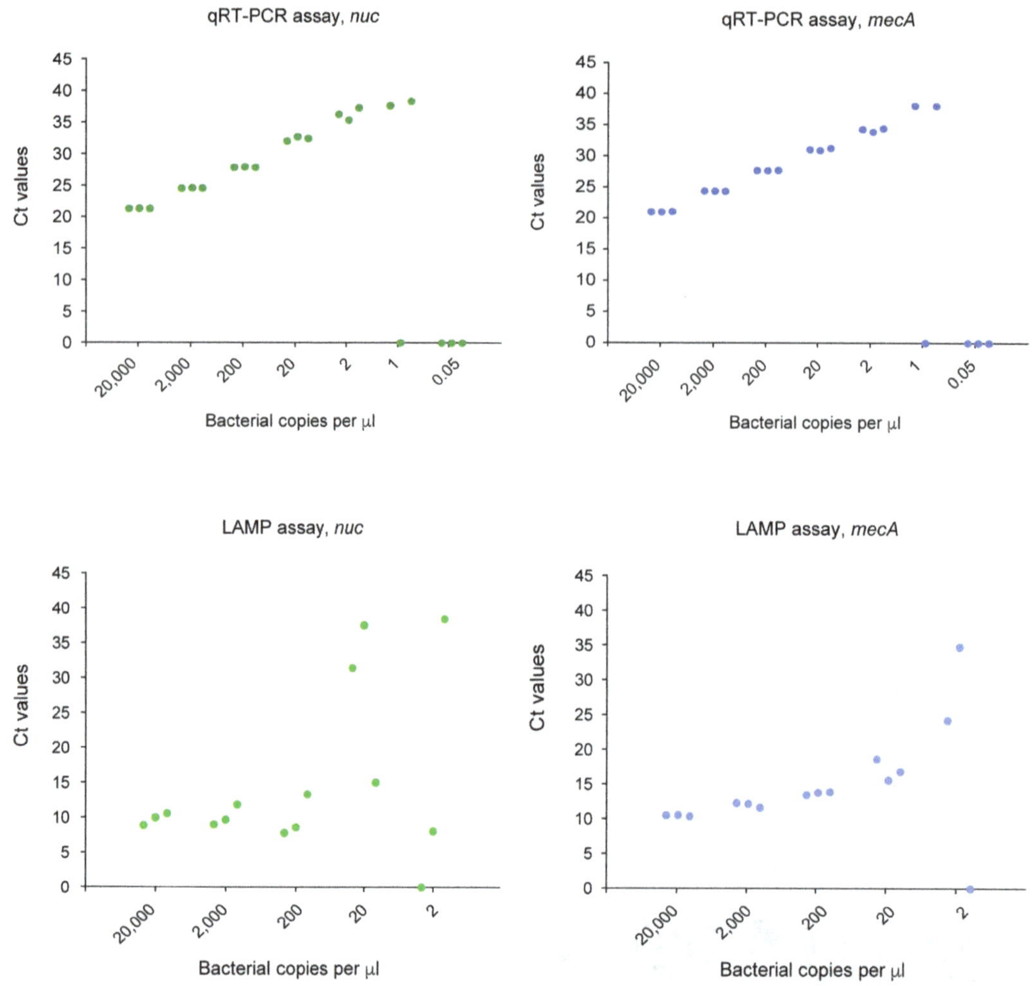


**FIGURE 5 |** LoD of the qRT-PCR and CRISPR-LAMP assay for *nuc* and *mecA*.

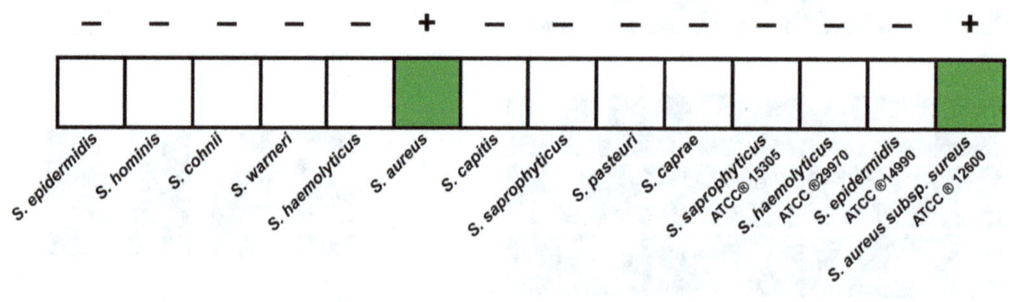


**FIGURE 6 |** Results of the LAMP-CRISPR assay for 14 strains of *staphylococci* species.

performed this assay for detecting *nuc* and *mecA* with serial dilutions. Green fluorescence was observed when the DNA sample was $2 \times 10^5$, $2 \times 10^4$, $2 \times 10^3$, $2 \times 10^2$, and $2 \times 10^1$ copies, which was referred to as a positive result. No green fluorescence signal was seen for a sample of $2 \times 10^0$ copies, one copy, and the no template control (NTC) (**Figure 4**). The interpretation of the genetic results for bacterial identification are illustrated in **Figure 4.**

## Sensitivity of the Loop-Mediated Isothermal Amplification-Clustered Regularly Interspaced Short Palindromic Repeats Assay

We compared the LoD of the LAMP assay relative to the qRT-PCR assay for the detection of *S. aureus* and MRSA. A standard scatter plot was plotted using seven serial dilutions with three

**TABLE 2 |** Results of 18 samples from DFI patients using the LAMP-CRISPR assay, real-time PCR, and the reference culture.

| Patient | LAMP-CRISPR | | Real-time PCR | | Culture |
|---|---|---|---|---|---|
| | *nuc* | *mecA* | *nuc* | *mecA* | |
| 1 | + | – | +(38.337) | – | MSSA |
| 2 | – | – | – | – | *Proteus vulgaris* |
| 3 | – | – | – | – | *Klebsiella pneumoniae* |
| 4 | – | – | – | 37.454 | *Klebsiella pneumoniae* |
| 5 | + | + | +(26.836) | + (27.123) | MRSA |
| 6 | – | – | – | – | *Acinetobacter baumannii* |
| 7 | – | – | – | – | *Staphylococcus hominis* |
| 8 | + | + | +(35.05) | + (31.203) | MSSA,*Staphylococcus pippi** |
| 9 | – | – | – | – | *Pseudomonas aeruginosa* |
| 10 | – | – | – | – | *Proteus vulgaris* |
| 11 | + | – | +(24.945) | – | MSSA |
| 12 | – | – | – | – | *Proteus vulgaris* |
| 13 | + | – | +(28.193) | – | MSSA |
| 14 | – | – | – | 37.217 | *Morganella morganii* |
| 15 | + | + | +(30.227) | + (29.936) | MRSA |
| 16 | – | – | – | – | *Enterococcus faecalis* |
| 17 | – | – | – | – | *Staphylococcus epidermidis* |
| 18 | – | – | – | – | *Proteus mirabilis* |

*Methicillin resistant-coagulase negative staphylococcus.

replicates at each dilution (**Figure 5**). The LoD of the LAMP assay for *nuc* was 20 copies per μL reaction in comparison to two copies per μL reaction for the qRT-PCR assay. For *mecA*, the LoD of the LAMP assay was 20 copies per μL reaction, versus two copies per μL reaction for the qRT-PCR assay.

## Specificity of the Loop-Mediated Isothermal Amplification-Clustered Regularly Interspaced Short Palindromic Repeats Assay

We tested the extracted DNA templates from strains of several staphylococcus species using the LAMP-CRISPR assay with primers for *nuc*. These strains included ten isolates, including *S. epidermidis*, *S. hominis*, *S. cohnii*, *S. warneri*, *S. haemolyticus*, *S. aureus*, *S. capitis*, *S. saprophyticus*, *S. pasteuri*, and *S. caprae*, and four purchased strains, including *S. saprophyticus* ATCC® 15305, *S. haemolyticus* ATCC ®29970, *S. epidermidis* ATCC ®14990, and *S. aureus* subsp. *aureus* ATCC ®12600. Positive results were generated only for DNA samples from *S. aureus* (**Figure 6**). It was confirmed that the LAMP-CRISPR assay for *nuc* could specifically detect *S. aureus*, with no cross-reactions to other staphylococcal families.

## Application of the Loop-Mediated Isothermal Amplification-Clustered Regularly Interspaced Short Palindromic Repeats Assay to the Diabetic Foot Infection Patient Samples

Clinical validation of this assay was performed using 18 samples of isolated strains from DFI ulcers. Confirmatory qRT-PCR was used to establish target gene detected by the LAMP-CRISPR assay. The results of the two molecular methods were compared to those of the gold-standard culture method (**Table 2**). For *S. aureus* detection, six samples were *nuc*-positive as per the CRISPR-LAMP assay and *S. aureus*-positive by culture. For

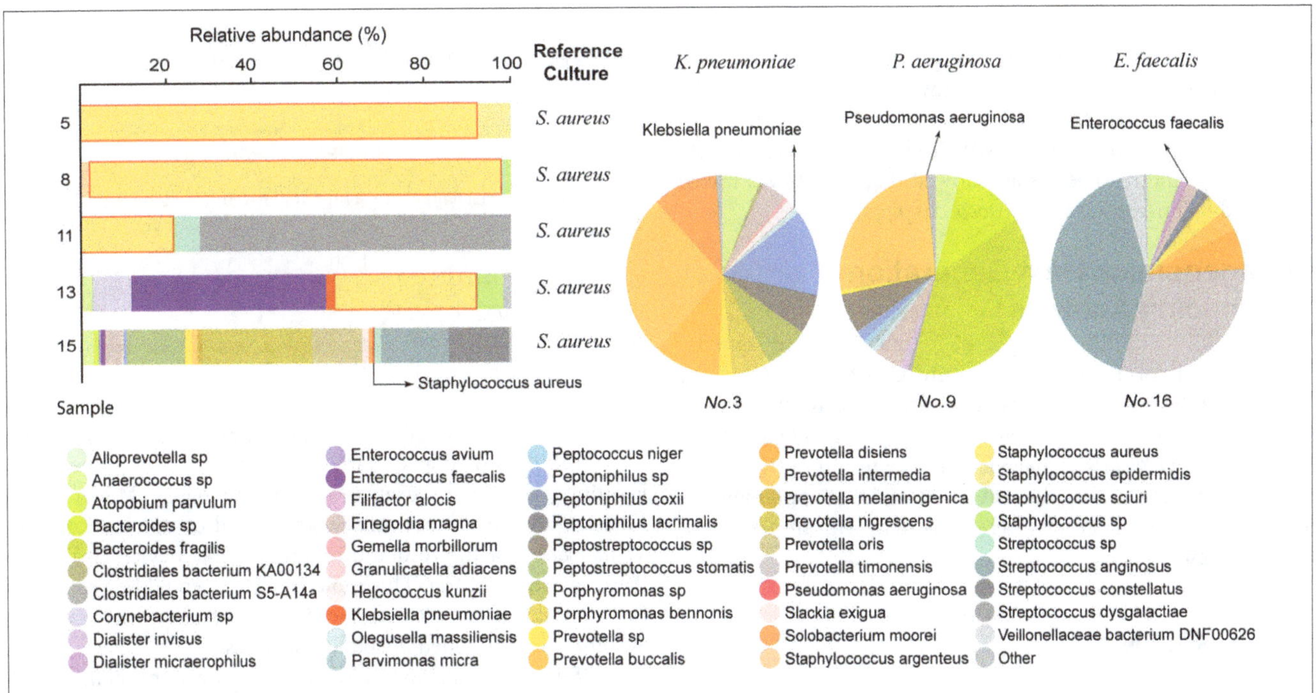


**FIGURE 7 |** Comparison of mNGS data to the reference culture. In the left 100% stacked columns, the column representing *S. aureus* is framed by a red line.

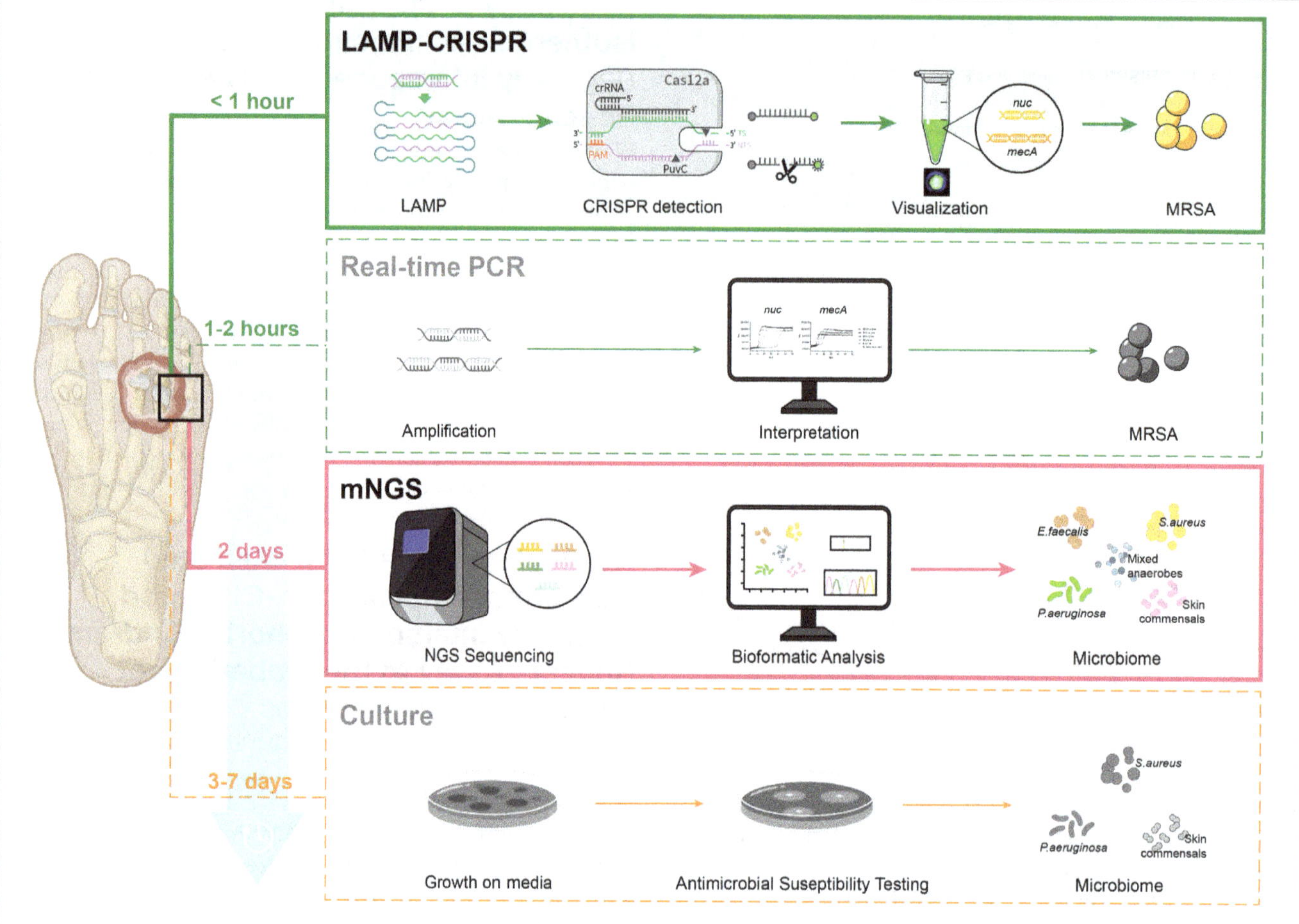


**FIGURE 8 |** Procedure of four diagnostic methods: LAMP-CRISPR assay, real-time PCR, mNGS, and reference culture.

MRSA detection, two samples were positive for both *nuc* and *mecA* as per the CRISPR-LAMP assay and MRSA-positive by culture. One discordant sample (No. 8) was positive for both *nuc* and *mecA* as per the LAMP-CRISPR assay and MRSA-negative by culture. The results showed that MSSA was mixed with methicillin-resistant *Staphylococcus pippi*.

## Metagenomics Next Generation Sequencing Analysis

After LAMP-CRISPR and qRT-PCR analysis, 8/18 samples were selected for mNGS. The culture growth of these eight samples indicated pathogens commonly seen in clinical practice, such as *S. aureus*, *Enterococcus faecalis*, *Pseudomonas aeruginosa, and Klebsiella pneumoniae*. The results of the mNGS analysis are listed in **Supplementary Material** (**Supplementary Table 2**). The mNGS results were consistent with the reference culture (**Figure 7**).

## DISCUSSION

Here, we combined the CRISPR-Cas12a-based technique with LAMP to develop a rapid diagnostic assay for the detection

**TABLE 3 |** Comparison of the LAMP-CRISPR assay to real-time PCR, mNGS, and the reference culture.

| | LAMP-CRISPR | Real-time PCR | mNGS | Culture |
|---|---|---|---|---|
| Assay sample-to-result time | <1 h | 1–2 h | 2 days | 3–7 days |
| Sensitivity | High | High | High | Low |
| Specificity | High | High | Low | High |
| complex laboratory infrastructure required | No | Yes | Yes | Yes |
| Cost | Inexpensive | Inexpensive | Expensive | Inexpensive |

of *S. aureus* in samples directly from patients with DFI. The CRISPR-LAMP assay targeting *nuc* and *mecA* successfully identified *S. aureus* strains and differentiated MRSA from MSSA. The entire procedure was brief and contamination-free. Visualization of the results through a simple device also made them easy to interpret. This molecular assay could be promising for the point-of-care detection of *S. aureus* from clinical samples at some underprovided hospitals and areas.

MRSA can be transmitted by contact between the medical staff and patients. Infection-control precautions, such as the primary isolation of patients with MRSA infection and disinfection of the clinic environment after every diabetic foot patient with MRSA infection, can prevent cross-transmission of MRSA (Lecornet et al., 2007). Early detection of MRSA can alert hospital staff to carry out the necessary precautions to reduce the spread of MRSA among patients. With the worldwide prevalence of MRSA isolates and frequent exposure to vancomycin, the appearance of vancomycin-intermediate *S. aureus* (Centers for Disease Control and Prevention (CDC), 2002; Chang et al., 2003) as well as vancomycin-resistant *S. aureus* (Centers for Disease Control and Prevention (CDC), 1997) strains have been identified globally. Early discrimination between MSSA and MRSA could reduce the inappropriate use of broad-spectrum antimicrobials and decrease the selective pressure that initiates the emergence and spread of resistance in bacteria (Gardete and Tomasz, 2014).

A potential weakness of this assay was the partial disagreement between the phenotype and genotype of microorganisms, which was also observed in other molecular strategies such as GeneOhm MRSA or Xpert MRSA assays (Buchan et al., 2015). Microbes that were *mecA*-negative might contain *mecC*, which was recently discovered and identified as a novel resistance gene in MRSA (Lakhundi and Zhang, 2018). DFI is often caused by multiple bacteria (Lipsky et al., 2012), which indicates that the culture growth of a clinical sample could be a mixture of *S. aureus* and coagulase-negative *Staphylococcus*, both of which can carry the *mecA* gene. Therefore, apart from being caused MRSA alone, the double positivity of *nuc* and *mecA* could be explained by mixed Staphylococcal isolates. This discrepancy was observed in one patient (No. 8). Using long-range PCR may encompass the amplicons, including both *nuc* and *mecA*, from a single strain that can uniquely identify MRSA (McClure et al., 2020). This will compensate for the current deficiency of the LAMP or regular PCR assays and improve specificity.

We then compared this novel LAMP-CRISPR assay with the reference culture, using qRT-PCR and mNGS methods (**Figure 8**). Compared to other diagnostic technologies, the CRISPR-LAMP assay enabled the detection of targeted genes at very low DNA concentrations within 1 h, which is faster than qRT-PCR and no complex infrastructure was required (**Table 3**). DFI is a rapidly progressing and relatively critical disease that may lead to disability and mortality. CRISPR-LAMP detection could aid clinicians in selecting targeted antibiotics and prevent the spread of multi-drug resistant microbes. Application of the CRISPR-LAMP assay optimizes the early treatment of DFI and complements the current paradigm for clinical diagnostics.

We also chose several representative samples for mNGS. mNGS can unbiasedly identify multiple microbes and address the limitations in pathogen width. It provides comprehensive information on the microbial profile of DFIs, including some rare pathogens that cannot be detected by conventional methods. mNGS can also provide quantitative data on the microbial concentration in the sample by counting sequenced reads, which is useful for polymicrobial samples (Wei et al., 2019). Study of the microbiome can potentially improve the diagnosis and treatment of DFIs. This revolutionary genetic approach further advances the management procedure of DFIs, which is becoming a rising trend in the clinical detection of infectious diseases. With the rapid determination of pathogens via CRISPR-LAMP and comprehensive supplementation of the bacterial spectrum by mNGS, a combination of these two methods can realize a timely and accurate pathogenic diagnosis of DFIs.

## CONCLUSION

Targeting both *nuc* and *mecA*, our LAMP-CRISPR assay has proven to be a rapid (within 1 h) and effective method for detecting *S. aureus* and distinguishing MRSA from MSSA in DFI samples. Due to its convenient visualized readout and portable nature, this method is promising for improving point-of-care detection. mNGS can provide comprehensive information for the microbiome study of DFI samples. Combining the LAMP-CRISPR technique and mNGS expanded and improved the pathogen diagnostic routine of DFI.

## AUTHOR CONTRIBUTIONS

CL, LL, and YC conceived and designed the study. YC was the major contributor in manuscript writing. YS, YC, and WZ completed the laboratory procedures. JaY, JeY, HL, and SF collected the samples of DFI patients and managed the diagnosis and treatment of patients. HZ analyzed the mNGS Data. YX proofread the first draft of the manuscript. CL and LL reviewed the manuscript. All authors agree to be accountable for the content of the work.

## FUNDING

Zhejiang Province Medical and Health Science Project (grant numbers 2021454695, 2021KY881, and 2019323752), Hangzhou Municipality Medical and Health Science Project (grant number A20200297).

## SUPPLEMENTARY MATERIAL

**Supplementary Table 1** | The sequences of the LAMP primers for *nuc* and *mecA*, and the CRISPR probe.

**Supplementary Table 2** | The results of the mNGS analysis. The highlights in the table represent the consistent microbials detected both by the mNGS and reference culture.

## REFERENCES

Prompers, L., Huijberts, M., Apelqvist, J., Jude, E., Piaggesi, A., Bakker, K., et al. (2006). High prevalence of ischaemia, infection and serious comorbidity in patients with diabetic foot disease in Europe. Baseline results from the Eurodiale study. *Diabetologia* 50, 18–25.

Jia, L., Parker, C. N., Parker, T. J., Kinnear, E. M., Derhy, P. H., Alvarado, A. M., et al. (2017). Incidence and risk factors for developing infection in patients presenting with uninfected diabetic foot ulcers. *PLoS One* 12:e0177916. doi: 10.1371/journal.pone.0177916

Lipsky, B. A., Berendt, A. R., Cornia, P. B., Pile, J. C., Peters, E. J. G., Armstrong, D. G., et al. (2012). 2012 Infectious Diseases Society of America clinical practice guideline for the diagnosis and treatment of diabetic foot infections. *Clin. Infect. Dis.* 54, e132–e173.

Eleftheriadou, I., Tentolouris, N., Argiana, V., Jude, E., and Boulton, A. J. (2010). Methicillin-resistant *Staphylococcus aureus* in diabetic foot infections. *Drugs* 70, 1785–1797. doi: 10.2165/11538070-000000000-00000

Cosgrove, S. E., Sakoulas, G., Perencevich, E. N., Schwaber, M. J., Karchmer, A. W., and Carmeli, Y. (2003). Comparison of mortality associated with methicillin-resistant and methicillin-susceptible *Staphylococcus aureus* bacteremia: a meta-analysis. *Clin. Infect. Dis.* 36, 53–59.

Filice, G. A., Nyman, J. A., Lexau, C., Lees, C. H., Bockstedt, L. A., Como-Sabetti, K., et al. (2010). Excess costs and utilization associated with methicillin resistance for patients with *Staphylococcus aureus* infection. *Infect. Control Hosp. Epidemiol.* 31, 365–373. doi: 10.1086/651094

Buchan, B. W., Allen, S., Burnham, C.-A. D., McElvania TeKippe, E., Davis, T., Levi, M., et al. (2015). Comparison of the next-generation Xpert MRSA/SA BC assay and the GeneOhm StaphSR assay to routine culture for identification of *Staphylococcus aureus* and methicillin-resistant *S. aureus* in positive-blood-culture broths. *J. Clin. Microbiol.* 53, 804–809. doi: 10.1128/jcm.03108-14

Ellem, J. A., Olma, T., and O'Sullivan, M. V. N. (2015). Rapid detection of methicillin-resistant *Staphylococcus aureus* and methicillin-susceptible *S. aureus* directly from positive blood cultures by use of the BD Max StaphSR assay. *J. Clin. Microbiol.* 53, 3900–3904. doi: 10.1128/jcm.02155-15

Silbert, S., Gostnell, A., Kubasek, C., and Widen, R. (2017). Evaluation of the BD Max StaphSR assay for detecting methicillin-resistant *Staphylococcus aureus* (MRSA) and methicillin-susceptible *S. aureus* (MSSA) in ESwab-collected wound samples. *J. Clin. Microbiol.* 55, 2865–2867. doi: 10.1128/jcm.00641-17

Kalan, L. R., Meisel, J. S., Loesche, M. A., Horwinski, J., Soaita, I., Chen, X., et al. (2019). Strain- and species-level variation in the microbiome of diabetic wounds is associated with clinical outcomes and therapeutic efficacy. *Cell Host Microbe* 25, 641–645. doi: 10.1016/j.chom.2019.03.006

Zou, M., Cai, Y., Hu, P., Cao, Y., Luo, X., Fan, X., et al. (2020). Analysis of the composition and functions of the microbiome in diabetic foot osteomyelitis based on 16S rRNA and metagenome sequencing technology. *Diabetes* 69, 2423–2439. doi: 10.2337/db20-0503

Charalampous, T., Kay, G. L., Richardson, H., Aydin, A., Baldan, R., Jeanes, C., et al. (2019). Nanopore metagenomics enables rapid clinical diagnosis of bacterial lower respiratory infection. *Nat. Biotechnol.* 37, 783–792. doi: 10.1038/s41587-019-0156-5

Li, Y., Li, S., Wang, J., and Liu, G. (2019). CRISPR/Cas Systems towards next-generation biosensing. *Trends Biotechnol.* 37, 730–743. doi: 10.1016/j.tibtech.2018.12.005

Li, S.-Y., Cheng, Q.-X., Liu, J.-K., Nie, X.-Q., Zhao, G.-P., and Wang, J. (2018a). CRISPR-Cas12a has both *cis-* and *trans-*cleavage activities on single-stranded DNA. *Cell Res.* 28, 491–493.

Li, S.-Y., Cheng, Q.-X., Wang, J.-M., Li, X.-Y., Zhang, Z.-L., Gao, S., et al. (2018b). CRISPR-Cas12a-assisted nucleic acid detection. *Cell Discov.* 4:20 .

Chen, J. S., Ma, E., Harrington, L. B., Da Costa, M., Tian, X., Palefsky, J. M., et al. (2018). CRISPR-Cas12a target binding unleashes indiscriminate single-stranded DNase activity. *Science* 360, 436–439. doi: 10.1126/science.aar6245

Broughton, J. P., Deng, X., Yu, G., Fasching, C. L., Servellita, V., Singh, J., et al. (2020). CRISPR–Cas12-based detection of SARS-CoV-2. *Nat. Biotechnol.* 395, 470–478.

Sabet, N. S., Subramaniam, G., Navaratnam, P., and Sekaran, S. D. (2007). Detection of mecA and ermA genes and simultaneous identification of *Staphylococcus aureus* using triplex real-time PCR from Malaysian *S. aureus* strain collections. *Int. J. Antimicrob. Agents* 29, 582–585. doi: 10.1016/j.ijantimicag.2006.12.017

CLSI (2018). *Performance standards for antimicrobial susceptibility testing; twenty-sixth informational supplement. CLSI document M100-S28.* Wayne: Clinical and Laboratory Standards Institute.

Lecornet, E., Robert, J., Jacqueminet, S., Van Georges, H., Jeanne, S., Bouilloud, F., et al. (2007). Preemptive isolation to prevent methicillin-resistant *Staphylococcus aureus* cross-transmission in diabetic foot. *Diabetes Care* 30, 2341–2342. doi: 10.2337/dc07-0743

Centers for Disease Control and Prevention (CDC) (2002). *Staphylococcus aureus* resistant to vancomycin–United States, 2002. *MMWR Morb. Mortal. Wkly. Rep.* 51, 565–567.

Chang, S., Sievert, D. M., Hageman, J. C., Boulton, M. L., Tenover, F. C., Downes, F. P., et al. (2003). Infection with vancomycin-resistant *Staphylococcus aureus* containing the vanA resistance gene. *N. Engl. J. Med.* 348, 1342–1347.

Centers for Disease Control and Prevention (CDC) (1997). *Staphylococcus aureus* with reduced susceptibility to vancomycin–United States, 1997. *MMWR Morb. Mortal. Wkly. Rep.* 46, 765–766.

Gardete, S., and Tomasz, A. (2014). Mechanisms of vancomycin resistance in *Staphylococcus aureus*. *J. Clin. Invest.* 124, 2836–2840. doi: 10.1172/jci68834

Lakhundi, S., and Zhang, K. (2018). Methicillin-resistant *Staphylococcus aureus*: molecular characterization, evolution, and epidemiology. *Clin. Microbiol. Rev.* 31, 5–103.

McClure, J. A., Conly, J. M., Obasuyi, O., Ward, L., Ugarte-Torres, A., Louie, T., et al. (2020). A novel assay for detection of methicillin-resistant *Staphylococcus aureus* directly from clinical samples. *Front. Microbiol.* 11:1295. doi: 10.3389/fmicb.2020.01295

Wei, G., Steve, M., and Charles, Y. C. (2019). Clinical metagenomic next-generation sequencing for pathogen detection. *Annu. Rev. Pathol.* 14, 319–338.

# 7

# Inhibiting Bacterial Drug Efflux Pumps via Phyto-Therapeutics to Combat Threatening Antimicrobial Resistance

*Varsha Shriram*[1], *Tushar Khare*[2], *Rohit Bhagwat*[3], *Ravi Shukla*[4] *and Vinay Kumar*[2,3*]

[1] *Department of Botany, Prof. Ramkrishna More College, Savitribai Phule Pune University, Pune, India,* [2] *Department of Biotechnology, Modern College of Arts, Science and Commerce (Savitribai Phule Pune University), Pune, India,* [3] *Department of Environmental Science, Savitribai Phule Pune University, Pune, India,* [4] *Centre for Advanced Materials and Industrial Chemistry, School of Science, RMIT University, Melbourne, VIC, Australia*

***Correspondence:***
*Vinay Kumar*
*vinaymalik123@gmail.com*

Antibiotics, once considered the lifeline for treating bacterial infections, are under threat due to the emergence of threatening antimicrobial resistance (AMR). These drug-resistant microbes (or superbugs) are non-responsive to most of the commonly used antibiotics leaving us with few treatment options and escalating mortality-rates and treatment costs. The problem is further aggravated by the drying-pipeline of new and potent antibiotics effective particularly against the drug-resistant strains. Multidrug efflux pumps (EPs) are established as principal determinants of AMR, extruding multiple antibiotics out of the cell, mostly in non-specific manner and have therefore emerged as potent drug-targets for combating AMR. Plants being the reservoir of bioactive compounds can serve as a source of potent EP inhibitors (EPIs). The phyto-therapeutics with noteworthy drug-resistance-reversal or re-sensitizing activities may prove significant for reviving the otherwise fading antibiotics arsenal and making this combination-therapy effective. Contemporary attempts to potentiate the antibiotics with plant extracts and pure phytomolecules have gained momentum though with relatively less success against Gram-negative bacteria. Plant-based EPIs hold promise as potent drug-leads to combat the EPI-mediated AMR. This review presents an account of major bacterial multidrug EPs, their roles in imparting AMR, effective strategies for inhibiting drug EPs with phytomolecules, and current account of research on developing novel and potent plant-based EPIs for reversing their AMR characteristics. Recent developments including emergence of *in silico* tools, major success stories, challenges and future prospects are also discussed.

**Keywords: antimicrobial resistance, efflux pumps, efflux pump inhibitors, phyto-therapeutics, drug resistance reversal**

## INTRODUCTION

Antimicrobial resistance (AMR) or ineffectiveness of commonly used drugs/antibiotics against specific bacteria has emerged as one of the most threatening human health concerns and a major challenge for global drug discovery programs. AMR (also known as drug resistance) has been reported at three increasing levels, multidrug resistance (MDR), extensive drug resistance (XDR) and pan-drug resistance (PDR). By definition, MDR stands for acquisition of non-susceptibility to at least one agent in three or more antimicrobial classes, while XDR shows the non-susceptibility to at least one agent in all, except two or fewer antimicrobial classes, while PDR implies non-susceptibility to all antimicrobial agents from all available classes (Exner et al., 2017; Spengler et al., 2017). AMR is threatening millions of lives worldwide, and is rightly declared as a *global risk* by the World Economic Forum (World Economic Forum, 2013). Since the very first report on AMR in *Enterobacteria* in 1950s (Watanabe, 1963; Levy, 2001), many drug-resistant strains have been reported and their number as well as the resistance level is on the rise. Though several classes of antibiotics were discovered in the antibiotic era (**Table 1**), we are heading to a post-antibiotic era, where an increasing number of previously curable infections are turning into non-curable and life-threatening (Spengler et al., 2017). Though development of AMR or antibiotic resistance is a natural phenomenon, irrational use of antibiotics speed-ups the emergence of drug-resistant strains (World Health Organization, 2014). Once the AMR is gained by the bacteria, it is successively transmitted to the next progeny via vertical gene transfer or other bacteria through horizontal gene transfer process, making their treatment more difficult (Chandra et al., 2017).

The drug resistance characteristics may be attributed to the abilities of such strains in fast altering their genetic make-up or inducing epigenetic changes (Davies and Davies, 2010; Motta et al., 2015; Rahman et al., 2017). Necessary adaptations are achieved by bacteria to-respond-to and to counteract the antibiotics either via procurement of foreign genetic material encoding resistance via horizontal gene transfer or mutations in drug-targets / antibiotics-degrading enzymes and alterations in permeability of the outer bacterial membrane. There is an unprecedented upsurge in bacterial strains with elevated AMR in both Gram-negative and Gram-positive phenotypes. The ESKAPE (*Enterococcus faecium*, *Staphylococcus aureus*, *Klebsiella pneumoniae*, *Acinetobacter baumannii*, *Pseudomonas aeruginosa*, and *Enterobacter* species) pathogens have emerged with high degree of AMR and are major cause of life-threatening nosocomial infections (Santajit and Indrawattana, 2016). Even other strains like *Escherichia coli*, *Shigella* species, *Neisseria gonorrhoeae*, and *Proteus mirabilis* have shown significant levels of AMR (Fair and Tor, 2014; Prasch and Bucar, 2015; Cerceo et al., 2016). Development of resistance against the carbapenem, a class of highly effective antibiotics and regarded as the last line of defense against pathogenic Gram-negative bacteria hints at the alarming situation (Kumarasamy et al., 2010; Dwivedi et al., 2015).

Intrinsically, AMR is more prevalent and severe in Gram-negative bacteria than their Gram-positive counterparts due mainly to the outer membranes serving as permeability barrier for drug-influx into the Gram-negative bacteria (Silhavy et al., 2010; Exner et al., 2017). To attain low sensitivity against biocidal compounds, Gram-negative bacteria reduce their outer membrane permeability by reducing the number of porins and inducing drug efflux pumps (EPs) for outward transport of drug molecules, often in a non-specific manner making the bacterial cells resistant to multiple antibiotics (Masi et al., 2017). However, despite these morphological differences, Gram-positive bacteria cannot be ignored or underestimated and noteworthy examples include methicillin resistant *S. aureus* (MRSA) and vancomycin resistant *S. aureus* (VRSA), coagulase negative *Staphylococci* members including *S. epidermidis* and *S. haemolyticus*, *Streptococcus pneumonia*, *E. faecalis*, *E. faecium*, and *Clostridium difficile* (Schindler and Kaatz, 2016). **Figure 1** shows a gradual upsurge in the number of research articles focused on most-prevalent MDR strains.

In recent years, EPs have emerged as key drivers for AMR in Gram-negative and Gram-positive bacteria, and therefore, are looked upon as potent and universal targets for containing the drug-resistant phenotypes. EPs are vital in other physiological processes also including stress-adaptations, virulence, pathogenicity and transportation of essential nutrients (Piddock, 2006; Fernandez and Hancock, 2012; Costa et al., 2013; Kourtesi et al., 2013; Sun et al., 2014). Identifying novel and potent EP inhibitors (EPIs) to revert the AMR is therefore gaining momentum. EPIs are the compounds with capability to reduce resistance or a complete reversal of AMR against otherwise ineffective antibiotics via inhibiting the EPs (Sun et al., 2014; Gill et al., 2015; Wright, 2016; Spengler et al., 2017). The first EPI against RND-type EPs was reported by Lomovskaya et al. (2001) a phenylalanine-arginine β-naphthylamide (PAβN) effective against Mex pumps in *P. aeruginosa* and AcrAB-TolC pump in *E. coli*. Since then, various synthetic and natural compounds have been screened for their EPI capabilities (reviewed by Prasch and Bucar, 2015; Spengler et al., 2017; Shin et al., 2018; Yang et al., 2018). **Figure 2** illustrates the inhibition of microbial drug efflux via synthetic and natural EPIs.

Medicinal plants with antimicrobial properties have the potential to serve as the reservoir of novel and effective EPIs (Newman and Cragg, 2012). Though there are several reports on assessing medicinal plants for their antimicrobial properties (crude extracts and occasionally pure molecules), few investigations were aimed against MDR/XDR strains and fewer on deciphering the underlying resistance mechanisms targeted by the plant products (Kumar et al., 2013). But newer studies are coming up for identifying novel phytomolecules capable of reversing EP-mediated AMR. Some striking phytochemicals which have recently been identified for their EPI potentials include catechol, pinene, gingerol, capsaicin, resveratrol and the number is increasing (Prasch and Bucar, 2015).

In this review, we are presenting an account of major EPs, their roles in imparting bacterial AMR, strategies for identifying plant-based EPIs emphasizing on the potent phyto-EPIs active at relatively lower concentrations, reported during the last 8 years. High throughput screening and *in silico* approaches for predicting the EPIs and their binding targets/sites are also discussed.

## PHYSIOLOGICAL ROLES PLAYED BY BACTERIAL EFFLUX PUMPS

Bacterial genome comprises of EP genes, expressed under tight regulation of global/local transcription factors (e.g., BmrR:

**TABLE 1** | Classes of commonly used antibiotics along with their examples and corresponding modes of action.

| Class of antibiotics | | | | Examples | Mode of action |
|---|---|---|---|---|---|
| Beta Lactams | Beta lactamase inhibitors | | | Sulbactam, Tazobactam, Clavulanic acid, Avibactam | Cell wall synthesis inhibitors |
| | Penicillins | Penicillinase sensible | Aminopenicillins | Ampicillin, Amoxicillin | |
| | | | Natural penicillins | Penicillin G, Penicillin VK | |
| | | Penicillinase resistant | | Nafcillin, Dicloxacillin, Oxacillin | |
| | | Anti-pseudomonal | Carboxypenicillins | Ticarcillin, Carbenicillin | |
| | | | Ureidopenicillins | Piperacillin, Mezlocillin, Azlocillin | |
| | Cephalo-sporins | 1st generation | | Cephalexine, Cefadroxil, Cefazolin, Cephradrine | |
| | | 2nd generation | | Cefuroxime, Cefoxitin, Cefaclor, Loracarbef, Cefprozil | |
| | | 3rd generation | | Cefoperazone, Cefpodoxime, Ceftriaxone, Cefotaxime, Ceftazidime | |
| | | 4th generation | | Cefepime, Cefpirome | |
| | | 5th generation | | Ceftaroline, Ceftolozane | |
| | Carbapenems | | | Meropenem, Doripenem, Ertapenem, Imipenem | |
| | Monobactams | | | Aztreonam | |
| No lactams | Glycopeptides | | | Vancomycin, Dalbavancin, Telavancin, Oritavancin | |
| | Other | | | Colistin, Daptomycin, Polymixin B, Isoniazid | |
| | Amino-glycosides | | | Amikacin, Streptomycin, Neomycin, Gentamicin, Tobramycin | Protein synthesis inhibitors |
| | Tetracyclins | | | Doxycyclin, Tetracyclin, Democlocyclin, Minocyclin, Tigecyclin | |
| | Oxazolidonones | | | Linezolid, Tidezolid | |
| | Streptogramins | | | Quinupristin | |
| | | | | Chloramphenicol | |
| | Macrolides | | | Erythromycin, Clarithromycin, Azithromycin | |
| | Lincosamides | | | Clindamycin, Lincomycin | |
| | Fluorquinolones | | | Ciprofloxacin, Sparfloxacin, Levofloxacin, , Norfloxacin | DNA topoisomerases inhibitors |
| | Quinolones | | | Nalidixic acid | |
| | Sulfonamides | | | Sulfamethoxazole, Sulfasalazine, Ag sulfadiazine, Sulfisoxazole | Folic acid synthesis inhibitor |
| | DHFR inhibitors | | | Trimethoprim, Pyrimethamine | |
| | Nitroimidazoles | | | Metronidazole, Tinidazole | DNA Damage |
| | | | | Rifampin | mRNA synthesis |

transcriptional regulator of efflux pump Bmr in *B. subtilis*; QacR: transcriptional repressor of QacA transporter in *S. aureus*; AcrR: transcription repressor of acrB efflux pump in *E. coli*) proposing the important physiological roles the EPs play during cell development, stress adaptations and bacterial pathogenesis (Sun et al., 2014). The knowledge about these regulatory mechanisms may advance the understandings of physiologically originated AMR, frequently observed in nature (Sun et al., 2014). As discussed above, bacterial EPs have a tremendous capacity to extrude the variety of toxic compounds, needed for the cell survival in a given physiological niche and are vital for maintaining pathogenicity. This is further supported by the studies showing reduced pathogenicity in the bacterial strains lacking EPs. Buckley et al. (2006) showed that *S. typhimurium acrB* or *tolC* deficient mutant poorly colonized in the avian gut, highlighting the requirement of complete AcrAB-TolC system for virulence. The *S. typhimurium* strain lacking all the drug efflux assemblies became avirulent, when tested in a mouse model (Nishino et al., 2006). To confirm the role of EPs in bacterial pathogenesis, Hirakata et al. (2002) assessed the ability of EP (MexAB-OprM, MexCD-OprJ, MexEF-OprM, and MexXY-OprM) mutants of *P. aeruginosa* to invade Madin-Darby canine kidney cells. The findings revealed that except mexCD-OprJ, all other systems evidenced decreased bacterial invasion abilities.

EPs are also known to effect the bacterial cell communication during the stress-responses, especially in the quorum-sensing (González and Keshavan, 2006). As transportation of auto-inducers (chemical signals generated during quorum sensing) is a key-event during cell-cell interactions via quorum-sensing, drug EPs assist their transport across the membrane (Liang et al., 2016). Moore et al. (2014) confirmed a vital role played by MexAB-OprM efflux system in the secretion of a major auto-inducer N-acylated L-homoserine lactone by *P. aeruginosa* cells. The study also postulated this auto-inducer as a substrate for MexAB-OprM system (Moore et al., 2014).

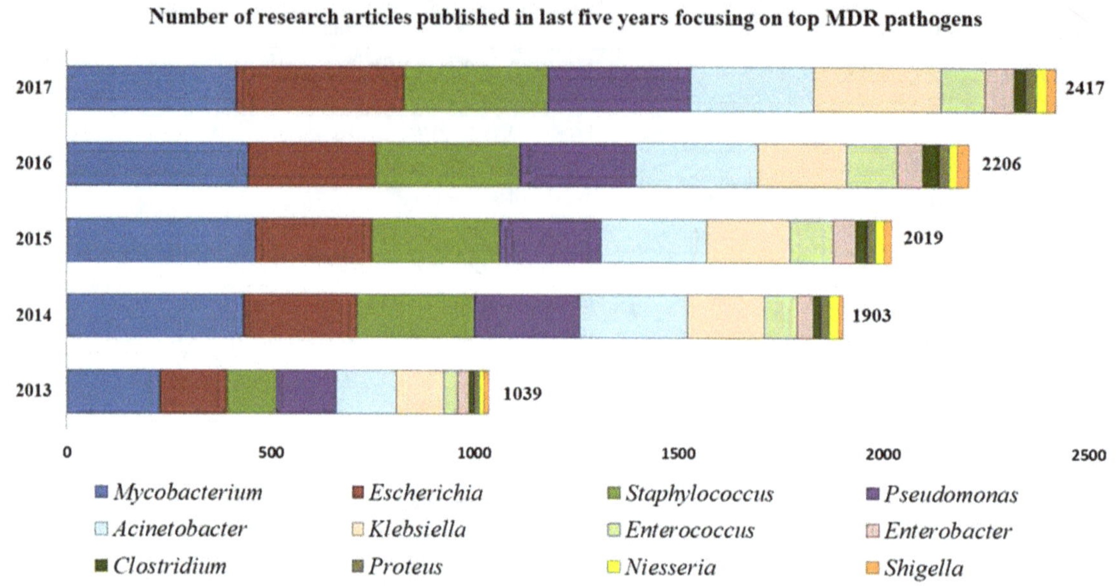


**FIGURE 1 |** Number of research articles reported from 2013 to 2017 focusing on MDR bacterial strains. [Source: PubMed; Key words used: Multidrug resistant "*Genus name*"].

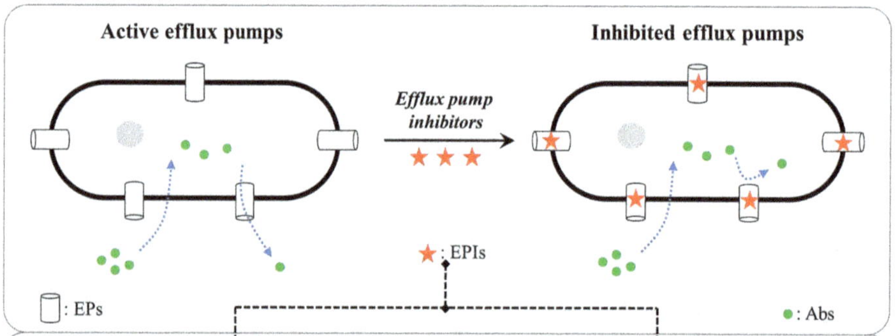


| Synthetic EPIs | Natural EPIs |
|---|---|
| PAβN, NMP, | Reserpine, Gallotannin, |
| 2-phenylquinolines, | Piperine, Curcumin, |
| Omeprazole, | Berberine, Chalcones, |
| Verapamil, PSSRI | Carnosic acid |

**FIGURE 2 |** Examples of synthetic and natural efflux pump inhibitors (EPIs); PAβN: phenyl-arginine-β-naphthylamide, NMP: 1-(1- naphthylmethyl)-piperazine, PSSRIs: phenylpiperidine selective serotonin re-uptake inhibitors (German et al., 2008; Hannula and Hänninen, 2008; Li et al., 2015; Ni et al., 2016; Willers et al., 2016; Sabatini et al., 2017). Abs, antibiotics; EPs, efflux pumps.

Further, Martinez et al. (2009) advocated the EP-mediated ceasing of quorum-sensing via augmented efflux of auto-inducers, facilitating quick bacterial response to stress signals. One more physiological role attributed to EPs is in the biofilm formation. Recent studies confirm the involvement of many well-characterized efflux systems, AcrAB-TolC of *E. coli*, AcrD of *S. enterica*, AdeFGH of *A. baumannii* and MexAB-OpeM of *P. aeruginosa* in biofilm formation (Alav et al., 2018). Kvist et al. (2008) reported an up-regulation of 20 genes encoding EP-transporters in *E. coli* during the growth of biofilm. Similarly, the EP-mediated export of colanic acid for capsule-matrix formation was observed along with up-regulated TetA(C) in *E. coli*, facilitating the biofilm formation (May et al., 2009). Collectively, the physiological roles of EPs are vital for pathogenic stability and virulence maintenance in bacteria.

The synthetic EPIs namely carbonylcyanide m-chlorophenylhydrazone (CCCP), chlorpromazine and PAβN were reported to prevent biofilm formation in *E. coli*, *P. aeruginosa* and *S. aureus* (Baugh et al., 2014). However, investigations on evaluating phytochemicals for their anti-biofilm potencies via inhibiting EPs are few. Fiamegos et al. (2011) isolated 4,5-O-dicaffeoylquinic acid from *Artemisia absinthium* which was proved to be a potent inhibitor of MFS pumps in *E. coli* and *E. faecalis* and as an anti-biofilm agent (Fiamegos et al., 2011). Recent reports advocate that nanomaterials in combination with phyto-EPIs can also be an effective therapy for containing drug-resistant infections (Gupta et al., 2017).

## BACTERIAL EFFLUX PUMPS: THE WARHEADS IN AMR STRAINS

Though bacterial AMR has several origins and many adaptive mechanisms are employed by drug-resistant strains against the antibiotics, the intrinsic EPs hold the key. Recent clinical and laboratory data establish that bacterial EPs are not only critical for drug-extrusion but also contribute to their virulence and adaptive responses (Du et al., 2018). Often, antimicrobial drug exposure induces intricate bacterial reactions including altered expressions of several genes encoding the transporters, as revealed by the phenotypic profiling of *E. coli* (Nichols et al., 2011).

Bacterial EPs are acknowledged either as primary active transporters using ATPs as an energy source, or as secondary active transporters acquired due to electrochemical potential difference created by pumping out $Na^+$ and $H^+$ outside the membrane (Dwivedi et al., 2017a).

This may be considered for classifying EPs into two broad super-families namely; ATP-binding cassette (ABC) multidrug transporters and secondary transporters using proton motive force (PMF) as an energy source (Putman et al., 2000). The second super-family can again be categorized in four subclasses, the major facilitator superfamily (MFS), resistance-nodulation-cell division (RND), multidrug and toxic compound extrusion (MATE) and small-MDR (SMR) family (Fernandez and Hancock, 2012; Sun et al., 2014). RND and MFS pumps are the most common in bacteria. With relatively narrow spectrum of specificity, MFS pumps are found in both Gram-negative and Gram-positive bacteria; while poly-selective RND pumps are exclusive to Gram-negative bacteria (Ward et al., 2001; Molnár et al., 2010). The SMR transporters show specificity for broad-spectrum polyaromatic cations convening resistance for compounds sharing similar chemical description. The MATE transporters are similar in size to MFS transporters but they do not share any sequence similarity with them (Jack et al., 2001). Apart from the classified super-families and sub-families, the MATE, SMR, and RND classes are distributed uniquely to prokaryotes whereas MFS and ABC transporters are dispersed in both prokaryotes and eukaryotes.

The large MFS is one of the most functionally diverse transporter families comprising multiple transportation types for drugs as well as sugars. These transporters comprise ~400 amino acids arranged as membrane-spanning helices (Saier et al., 1998). Based on the helical structure, MFS transporters can be classified as either 12-[e.g., TatA(B): class B tetracyclin transporter from *E. coli*] or 14-helix transporters [e.g., TatA(K): class K tetracyclin transporter from *S. aureus*], and TetA(B) is one of the most extensively studied members of the family (Lynch, 2006).

The SMR pumps represent smallest multidrug transporters, possessing only four trans-membrane helices without any extra membrane domain. But single minimal functional SMR unit represents eight helices as these are functionally active in dimeric form (Higgins, 2007). Well-illustrated example from this family is the electromagnetic antiporter EmrE from *E. coli*, responsible for resistance to a range of cationic-hydrophobic entities including antibiotics.

The latest structurally characterized class of EPs is MATE, involved in various vital biological functions (He et al., 2010). These transporters are equivalent to MFS transporters with a typical composition of ~450 amino acids putatively arranged in 12 helices; but with no sequence similarity with MFS counterparts (Jack et al., 2001). Some characterized MATE members include NorM from *N. gonorrhoeae* and *N. meningitides* and YdhE from *E. coli*. However, limited structural and functional knowledge is available about this family (Dwivedi et al., 2017a).

Though EPs from other families contribute to the AMR against certain antibiotics, RND pumps are the most potent drug efflux systems conferring resistance against clinically important antibiotics and biocides. Members of this family are known for their roles against a wide range of molecules with dissimilar structures including antibiotics, biocides, organic solvents, antimicrobial peptides, detergents, dyes, and bile salts (Poole, 2004). The tripartite complex of pumps from this family comprises inner membrane protein (IMP), outer membrane protein (OMP) along with a periplasmic membrane fusion protein (MFP) as a connector (Venter et al., 2015). The best understood tripartite complexes include AcrA-AcrB-TolC from *E. coli* and MexA-MexB-OprM from *P. aeruginosa* (Du et al., 2013, 2014). Greater structural and functional similarities between IMPs of these two systems are described by Welch et al. (2010). Exploration on biochemical and structural aspects of AcrB has revealed that these IMPs contain proximal and distal binding pockets, divided by G-loop (with 614–621 residues). Conformational flexibility of G-loop is crucial for movement of substrate along the binding site (Eicher et al., 2012; Cha et al., 2014). **Table 2** lists various EPs belonging to the major families from prevalent pathogenic bacteria.

Collectively, the complex EP assemblies are critical for bacterial pathogenesis, virulence, biofilm formation, and adaptive-responses ultimately conferring and defining bacterial AMR (Piddock, 2006; Martinez et al., 2009; Baugh et al., 2012, 2014; Du et al., 2018). EPs are critical for bacterial AMR as they exclude most of the unwanted entities

**TABLE 2 |** Examples of various efflux pumps belonging to major efflux pump families from prevalent pathogenic bacterial strains.

| Pathogen | EP Family | Example | Substrate | References |
|---|---|---|---|---|
| *Acinetobacter baumannii* | ABC | *MacAB-TolC* | ML | Okada et al., 2017 |
| | MATE | *AbeM* | ACR, AG, DAU, DOR, FQ | Su et al., 2005 |
| | MFS | *CraA* | CHL | Roca et al., 2009 |
| | RND | *AdeABC, AdeFGH, AdeIJK* | AG, BL, FQ, ML, TET, BIO | Coyne et al., 2010, Rajamohan et al., 2010 |
| *Campylobacter jejuni* | RND | *CmeABC, CmeDEF* | AG, BL, CHL, FQ, ML, RIF, TET, EB | Lin et al., 2002; Akiba et al., 2006 |
| *Enterococcus faecalis* | ABC | *EfrAB* | ACR, CIP, DAU, DOR, DOX, NOR, TPP | Lee et al., 2003 |
| *Escherichia coli* | ABC | *MacAB-TolC* | ML | Kobayashi et al., 2001 |
| | MFS | *MdfA* | CHL, DOR, NOR, TET | Nishino et al., 2006 |
| | | *QepA/QepA2* | FQ | Cattoir et al., 2008 |
| | RND | *AcrAB-TolC* | BL, CHL, FQ, ML, NOV, RIF, TET, TGC, R6G | Swick et al., 2011, Lennen et al., 2013 |
| | | *OqxAB* | CHL, FQ | Hansen et al., 2004 |
| | SMR | *EmrE* | ACR, EB, QAC | Schuldiner, 2009, Beketskaia et al., 2014 |
| *Klebsiella pneumoniae* | MATE | *KetM* | DAPI | Ogawa et al., 2015 |
| | MFS | *KpnGH* | CAZ, CEF, STR, TET | Srinivasan et al., 2014 |
| | RND | *OqxAB* | CHL, FQ | Hansen et al., 2004 |
| | SMR | *KnpEF* | BAC, CEF, CHX, ERY, STR, TET, TRI | Srinivasan and Rajamohan, 2013 |
| *Mycobacterium tuberculosis* | ABC | *Rv1218c* | BAP, BPD, PRI, PYR | Balganesh et al., 2010, Balganesh et al., 2012 |
| | MFS | *Tap* | PAS, SPE, TET | Ramón-García et al., 2012 |
| | SMR | *Mmr* | CAB, CLA, TPP | Balganesh et al., 2012, Rodrigues et al., 2013 |
| *Pseudomonas aeruginosa* | RND | *MexAB-OprM, MexXY-OprM/A, MexCD-OprJ, MexEF-OprN* | AG, BL, CHL, FQ, ML, SUL, TET, TGC, TMP, BIO, EB | Poole et al., 1996, Köhler et al., 1997 |
| *Staphylococcus aureus* | ABC | *Isa(E)* | LIN, PLE, STA | Wendlandt et al., 2015 |
| | | *Msr(A)* | ML, TEL | Vimberg et al., 2015 |
| | MATE | *MepA* | BIO, EB, FQ, TIG | Kaatz et al., 2005 |
| | MFS | *NorA* | FQ | Yoshida et al., 1990 |
| | | *QacA* | ACR, CHX, EB, QAC | Littlejohn et al., 1992 |
| *Streptococcus pneumoniae* | ABC | *PatAB* | FQ | Marrer et al., 2006 |
| | MFS | *MefE* | ML | Tait-Kamradt et al., 1997 |
| *Vibrio* spp. | ABC | *VcaM* | CIP, DAU, DOR, NOR, TET | Huda et al., 2003 |
| | MATE | *NorM* | AG, EB, FQ | Morita et al., 1998 |
| | MFS | *EmrD-3* | EB, LNZ, ERY, CHL | Bruns et al., 2017 |

*ACR, acriflavine; AG, aminoglycosides; BAC, benzalkonium chloride; BAP, biaryl-piperazines; BL, β-lactams; BIO, biocides; BPD, bisanilino-pyridines; CAB, cetyl-trimethyl-ammoniumbromide; CAP, cationic antibacterial peptides; CAZ, ceftazidime; CEF:cefepime; CHL, chloramphenicol; CHX, chlorhexidine; CIP, ciprofloxacin; CLA, clofazimine; DAU, daunomycin; DAPI, 4′,6-diamidino-2-phenyl indole; DOR, doxorubicin; DOX, doxycycline; EB, ethidium bromide; ERY, erythromycin; FQ, fluoroquinolones; FUA, fusidic acid; LIN:lincosamide; LNZ, linezolid; ML, macrolides; NOR, norfloxacin; NOV, novobiocin; PAS, p-aminosalicylate; PLE, pleuromutilin; PRI, pridones; PYR, pyrroles; QAC, quaternary ammonium compounds; SPE, spectinomycin; STA, streptogramin A; STR, streptomycin; SUL, sulfonamides; TEL, telithromycin; TET, tetracycline; TGC, tigecycline; TMP, trimethoprim; TPP, tetraphenylphosphonium,TRI, triclosan.*

until the cell gets required time for acquiring resistance (Piddock, 2014; Venter et al., 2015).

## BACTERIAL EFFLUX PUMPS: THE URGENT THREATS REQUIRING IMMEDIATE REMEDY

It is well-established that EPs comprise one of the most vital systems in bacteria responsible for both innate and acquired AMR (Blair et al., 2015). There are reports of EPs from different superfamilies and the occurrence of various types of EPs from the same superfamily in a single bacterial species (Piddock, 2006). For instance, whole genome sequencing of the colistin resistant *Enterobacter cloacae* showed presence of multiple EPs (Norgan et al., 2016). Differential substrate profiles of EPs are also a characteristic feature which may diverge between or within the superfamily (Poole, 2005, 2007). Although the core motive of EPs related studies is focused on AMR, several reports however confirmed other but significant functions of bacterial

EPs including quorum-sensing, biofilm formation, virulence, pathogenicity and bacterial behavior (Piddock, 2006; Yang et al., 2006; Fahmy et al., 2016).

Up-regulation of gene expression levels are one of the main drivers for chromosomally acquired AMR. This can be triggered due to the gene induction, activated transcription, or due to regulatory mutations (Grkovic et al., 2002). The coding region for an EP is usually found contiguous to the regulatory proteins controlling the expression levels of pump gene in response to substrates. For example, AdeL, an LTTR (LysR-type transcriptional regulator) family protein exists opposite to the adeFGH operon that regulates the expression of genes encoding RND efflux system in *A. baumannii* (Liu et al., 2018). The expression levels of EP-associated proteins along with porins is mutually controlled by several global regulatory elements, modifying the transcription patterns of EP-family transcripts either directly or through a cascade of regulatory events (Warner and Levy, 2010; Sun et al., 2014). Further, the expression of MexAB-OprM efflux system is governed by repressor protein mexR, encoded by a gene located upstream of the mexAB-oprM operon in *P. aeruginosa* (Suresh et al., 2018). Similarly, the acrAB operon system is regulated by regulator acrR in *E. coli*, located 140 bp up-stream of the acrAB operon (Ma et al., 1996).

Another striking bacterial character adding to the AMR nature is heteroresistance, the occurrence of differential responses to antibiotics by the bacterial cells from the same population, a phenomenon first reported in *S. aureus* (Kayser et al., 1970). Interestingly, drug resistant and sensitive bacterial cells may co-exist in a single culture (Morand and Mühlemann, 2007). The mechanism underlying heteroresistance acquirements are yet to be fully understood, however, the active EPs are strongly linked to heteroresistance (Chen et al., 2017). Designing a treatment course against such strains is difficult as there are high chances of increase in the frequency of resistant-bacterial-population and stimulation of cross-resistance to antimicrobial lysozymes of the host system (Napier et al., 2014; Telke et al., 2017). Up-regulation of OpxAB gene in *Salmonella typhimurium* (Chen et al., 2017) and AdeABC gene in *A. calcoaceticus-A. baumannii* (Ruzin et al., 2007) are attributed for mediating the tigecyclin heteroresistance. Similarly, colistin associated heteroresistance is also reported in *E. asburiae* LH74 and *E. cloacae* NH52 (Telke et al., 2017), showing its association with overexpression of *acrAB-tolC* EPs under the regulation of soxRS genes.

AMR phenotypes may result from concurrent acquisition of several AMR mechanisms simultaneously. It may include a combination of phenomena like chromosomally acquired resistance, multiple chromosomal changes with time, and/or a single mutational event activating the AMR mechanisms including the EPs (Lister et al., 2009). The over-expressions of EPs and their corresponding genes have been reported to contribute to MDR in *P. aeruginosa* (Shigemura et al., 2015). Recent studies have confirmed the role of EPs in fluoroquinolone resistant *E. coli* (Amabile-Cuevas et al., 2010; Swick et al., 2011; Yasufuku et al., 2011). Similarly, two fluoroquinolone resistant clinical isolates of *Shigella* showed overexpression of the TolC channels, part of AcrAB-TolC tripartite responsive to ciprofloxacin (Kim et al., 2008). These findings confirm that the up-regulation of EP genes contribute significantly to diminish intracellular antibiotics level, with a selectivity of the efflux transporter.

Overall, the poly-specificity of EPs, their overexpression in response to drugs along with the phenomenon of heteroresistance seem key factors responsible for drug-resistance in a wide-range of bacterial species, especially in Gram-negative bacteria making them difficult to treat with conventional drug arsenal. The drug-efflux mediated bacterial AMR is a mounting threat to global healthcare, therefore EPs are gaining unprecedented attention not only from the perspectives of basic understandings that how they work and impart drug-resistance but also as emerging targets for development of novel and potent adjunct-therapies for combating AMR in community and nosocomial infections. As a result, inhibition of drug efflux from bacterial cells via inhibiting or disrupting the EPs is an emerging approach for combating the threatening AMR. Various approaches have been developed in recent past and a schematic for these strategies for inhibition or disruption of bacterial drug efflux is illustrated in **Figure 3**.

## PHYTOTHERAPEUTICS–THE POTENT EFFLUX PUMP INHIBITORS

Phytochemicals are critical for human health-care since ancient times. Medicinal plants are hailed as a reservoir for phytochemicals capable of providing new and potent drug leads to contain the AMR via targeting the principal determinants of drug-resistance including EPs (Newman and Cragg, 2012; Prasch and Bucar, 2015). This review focuses mainly on EPIs of plant origin (phyto-EPIs) reported in the running decade. We are discussing some important and successful case studies on phyto-EPIs effective against AMR phenotypes. **Table 3** summarizes the list of phytochemicals, their source and effective concentrations used for inhibiting the efflux pumps of AMR bacterial strains.

One of the potent EPIs, the anti-hypersensitive alkaloid reserpine was isolated from *Rauwolfia vomitoria* (Stavri et al., 2007). Similarly, EP inhibitory activity of gallotannin (1,2,6-tri-O-galloyl-b-D-glucopyranose) isolated from hydro-alcoholic extracts of *Terminalia chebula* fruits was demonstrated by Bag and Chattopadhyay (2014) against MDR uropathogenic *E. coli.* Gallotannin induced a 2- to 4-fold reduction in minimal inhibitory concentration (MIC) of test antibiotics via inhibiting the ethidium bromide (EtBr) pump (**Table 3**). As EtBr is a known EP-substrate, inhibition of EtBr efflux backs the postulated EP-inhibitory activity of gallotannin (Bag and Chattopadhyay, 2014). Methanolic sap extracts of *Acer saccharum* was evaluated for its drug efflux inhibitory potentials against *P. aeruginosa* (ATCC 15692 and UCBPPPA14), *E. coli* (ATCC 700928) and *P. mirabilis* (HI4320) confirmed via monitoring the EtBr efflux (Maisuria et al., 2015).

A clavine alkaloid lysergol from *Ipomoea muricata* was evaluated against AMR *E. coli* strains (MTCC1652 and KG4) to test its EP inhibitory potentials, and strong activities (higher than the standard reserpine) were exhibited by lysergol and its derivative, 17-O-3″,4″,5″-trimethoxybenzoyllysergol (Maurya

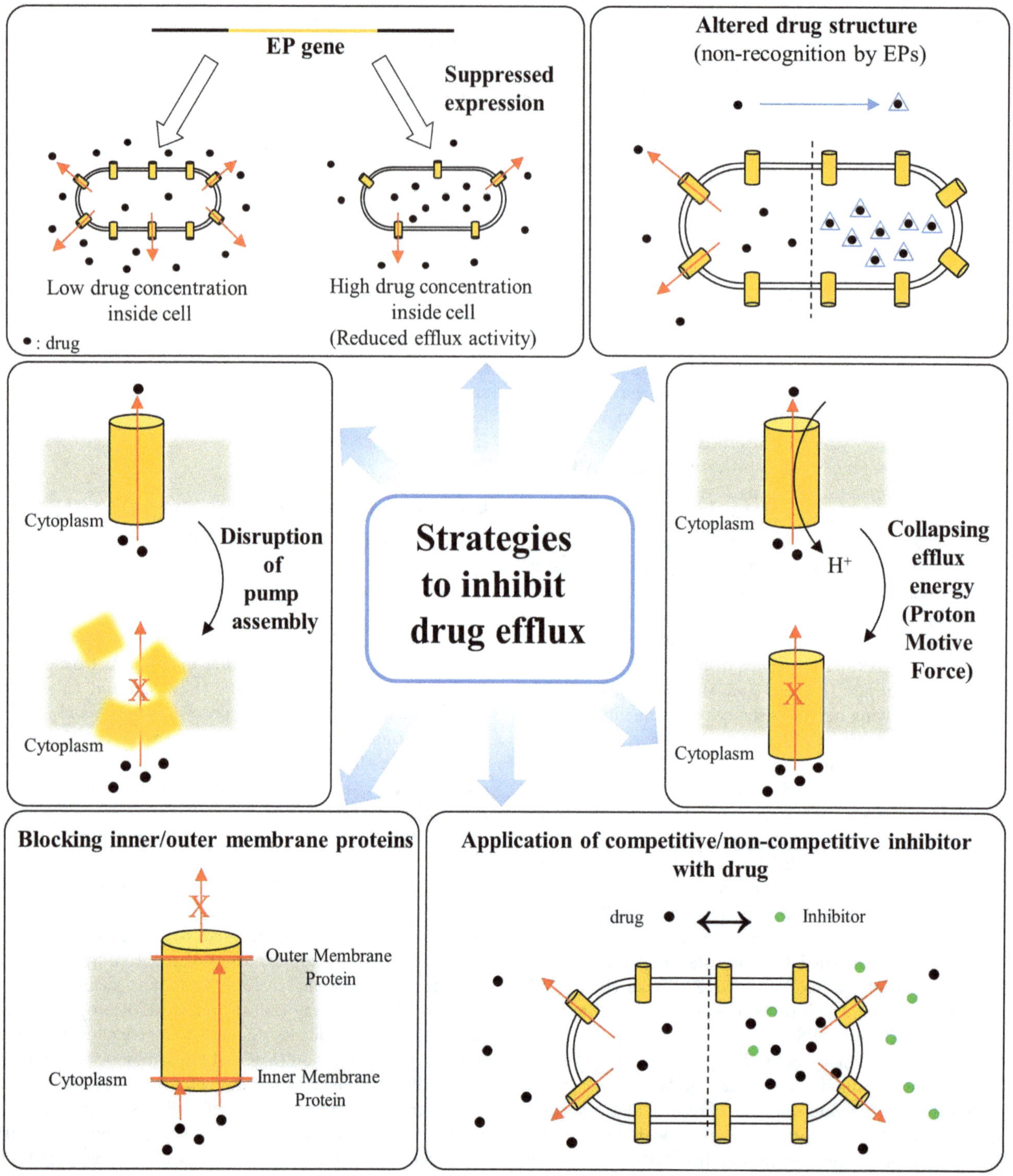


**FIGURE 3 |** Various strategies for inhibition of drug efflux from bacterial cells for combating antimicrobial resistance (Based on reviews by Pagès and Amaral, 2009; Venter et al., 2015).

et al., 2013). Authors also reported the inhibitory activities of this compound against ABC pump YojI in *E. coli* (Maurya et al., 2013). Similarly, falcarindiol, isolated from *Levisticum officinale* exhibited EPI activities against the Gram-negative strains (Garvey et al., 2011).

On the similar lines, Dwivedi et al. (2017b) reported the antibiotic-potentiating activities of catharanthine against superbug *P. aeruginosa*. The investigation involved *in silico* docking followed by the *in vitro* evaluation revealed that catharanthine potentiates the activity of tetracyclin and

**TABLE 3 |** A summarized list of phytochemicals, their source and effective concentrations for inhibiting efflux pumps from antimicrobial resistant bacteria.

| Active Compound | Verified effective concentration/s | Plant | Antimicrobial resistant microbes | Targeted efflux pumps | References |
|---|---|---|---|---|---|
| 1′-S-1′-acetoxyeugenol acetate | 3.12–25 mg $L^{-1}$ | *Alpinia galanga* | *Mycobacterium smegmatis* $mc^2$ 155 | EtBr EP | Roy et al., 2012 |
| 4-hydroxy-α-tetralone | 125 μg $mL^{-1}$ | *Ammannia* spp. | MDR *E. coli* | YojI | Dwivedi et al., 2014b |
| Baicalein | 16 μg $mL^{-1}$ | *Scutellaria baicalensis* | *S. aureus* SA-1199B | NorA | Chan et al., 2011 |
| Berberine and Palmatine | 250–1,000 μg $mL^{-1}$ 500–100 μg $mL^{-1}$ | *Berberis vulgaris* | MDR *P. aeruginosa* (clinical isolates) | MexAB-OprM | Aghayan et al., 2017 |
| Capsaicin | 25 μg $mL^{-1}$ | *Capsicum* spp. | *S. aureus* SA-1199B | NorA | Kalia et al., 2012 |
| Catechol | 5 and 10 mg $mL^{-1}$ | *Acer saccharum* | *P. aerugenosa* ATCC 15692 and UCBPPPA14, *E. coli* ATCC 700928, *P. mirabilis* HI4320 | EtBr EP | Maisuria et al., 2015 |
| Catharanthine | 25 mg $L^{-1}$ | *Catharanthus roseus* | *P. aeruginosa* | EtBr EP | Dwivedi et al., 2017b |
| Conessine | 20 mg $L^{-1}$ | *Holarrhena antidysenterica* | *P. aeruginosa* | MexAB-OprM | Siriyong et al., 2017 |
| Cumin-methanol extract | 5 mg $mL^{-1}$ | *Cuminum cyminum* | *S. aureus* MRSA OM505 | LmrS | Kakarla et al., 2016 |
| Essential oil | 5 μl $mL^{-1}$ | *Salvia fruticosa* | *S. epidermidis* (clinical isolates) | Tet(K) EP | Chovanova et al., 2015 |
| Essential oil | 170.6 μl $mL^{-1}$ | *Chenopodium Ambrosioides* | *Staphylococcus aureus IS-58* | Tet(K) EP | Limaverde et al., 2017 |
| Gallotannin | 12.1–97.5 μg $mL^{-1}$ | *Terminalia chebula* | MDR uropathogenic *E. coli* | EtBr EP | Bag and Chattopadhyay, 2014 |
| Indirubin | 1.25 and 2.5 mg $L^{-1}$ | *Wrightia tinctoria* | *S. aureus* SA-1199B | NorA | Ponnusamy et al., 2010 |
| Kaempferolrhamnoside | 1.56 mg $L^{-1}$ | *Persea lingue* | *S. aureus* SA-1199B | NorA | Holler et al., 2012 |
| Lysergol | 10 μg $mL^{-1}$ | *Ipomoea muricata* | *E. coli* MTCC1652 and KG4 | YojI | Maurya et al., 2013 |
| Olympicin A | 50 μM | *Hypericum olympicum* | *S. aureus* 1199B | NorA | Shiu et al., 2013 |
| Sarothrin | 100 μM | *Alkanna orientalis* | *Staphylococcus aureus* NCTC 8325-4 | NorA | Bame et al., 2013 |
| Ursolic acid and derivatives | 25 and 50 μg $mL^{-1}$ | *Eucalyptus tereticornis* | MDR *E. coli* (KG4) | AcrA/B, MacB, TolC and YojI | Dwivedi et al., 2014a |

streptomycin, as confirmed by a reduced MIC, and acts as a potent EPI (Dwivedi et al., 2017b). A pentacyclic triterpenoid ursolic acid from leaves of *Eucalyptus tereticornis* described as a precursor of putative EPI was evaluated against MDR *E. coli* (KG4), two promising semi-synthetic, esterified derivatives of ursolic acid, 3-O-acetyl-urs-12-en-28-isopropyl ester and 3-O-acetyl-urs-12-en-28-n-butyl ester and the parent compound exhibited better EP inhibitory potencies than the standard reserpine (Dwivedi et al., 2014a). The molecular docking confirmed the targets of these compounds as AcrA/B, MacB, TolC, and YojI (Dwivedi et al., 2014a). Similarly, two alkaloids isolated from roots and rhizomes of *Berberis vulgaris*, the barberine and palmatine showed potent EP inhibitory efficacies against *P. aeruginosa* isolated from burn infections (Aghayan et al., 2017).

Phenylpropanoids from the *n*-hexane and chloroform fractions of *Alpinia galanga* exhibited EP inhibitory activities against *Mycobacterium smegmatis* $mc^2$ 155ATCC 700084 (Roy et al., 2012). A dose-dependent EP inhibition was observed with 1′-S-1′-acetoxyeugenol acetate (Roy et al., 2012). Mukanganyama et al. (2012) examined another mycobacterial member *Mycobacterium aurum* A+ against a naphthoquinone diospyrine isolated from *Diospyros montana* along with its derivatives. Two derivatives proved highly potent EPI and allowed bacterial cells to accumulate high concentrations of ciprofloxacin (Mukanganyama et al., 2012).

The acylphloroglucinol isolated from *n*-hexane fractions from *Hypericum olympicum*, olympicin-A showed promising activities against *S. aureus* (Shiu et al., 2013). The radiometric accumulation assay of the strain overexpressing NorA pump indicated the enhanced accumulation of (14)C-enoxacin, thus confirming efflux inhibition (Shiu et al., 2013). Two coumarins [5,7-dihydroxy-6-(2-methylbutanoyl)-8-(3-methylbut-2-enyl)-4-phenyl-2H-chromen-2-one and 5,7 -dihydroxy-8-(2-methylbutanoyl)-6-(3-methylbut-2-enyl)-4-phenyl-2H-chromen-2-one] obtained from floral buds of *Mesua ferrea* were assessed against NorA-overexpressing *S. aureus* 1199B and the clinical isolate MRSA 831 (Roy et al., 2013). Linoleic acid isolated from ethanolic extracts of *Portulaca oleracea* showed efflux inhibitory potential at 64 mg $L^{-1}$ concentration, equivalent to reserpine when quantified against MRSA (RN4220/pUL5054: erythromycin resistant, over-expressing MsrA ABC EP, Chan et al., 2015). In search of the drug-resistance reversal agents, dos Santos et al. (2018) assessed caffeic acid and gallic acid against four strains of *S. aureus*; 1199 as a wild type strain, 1199B as NorA harboring fluroquinolone resistant, IS-58 possessing TetK pump and RN4220 possessing MrsA pump. The study confirmed caffeic acid as a potent AMR-reversal agent, as it effectively inhibited MrsA and NorA EPs from *S. aureus* strains RN4220 and 1190B, respectively (dos Santos et al., 2018). In another interesting study, Kakarla et al. (2016) reported LmrS inhibitory activities of *Cuminum cyminum*. The study revealed that the cumin inhibits the LmrS mediated transport of drugs resulting in growth inhibition of MRSA clinical isolate in a dose-dependent manner (Kakarla et al., 2016).

Traditionally, most of the investigations were aimed at identifying EPIs for Gram-positive strains for reversing their AMR characters with very few reports against Gram-negative members. This can be because Gram-negative bacteria are more difficult targets then their positive counterparts due mainly to the presence of powerful EPs and other effective membrane barriers (lipophilic layer) averting them from external impacts (Stavri et al., 2007; Prasch and Bucar, 2015). Though, some approaches have emerged in recent years for improving antibiotic-penetration across the permeability membranes of Gram-negative bacteria such as the inhibition of new accessible target, identification of uptake pathways and the "Trojan Horse" approach (achieving fast or facilitated antibiotics uptake), establishing the rules of permeation (for predicting whether elevated uptake or reduced efflux would be the most efficient way for increasing the potency of specific antimicrobial class) and identifying potent EPIs, last one being probably the most potent (Zgurskaya et al., 2015).

Recently, Bruns et al. (2017) successfully inhibited EmrD-3 pump-mediated drug efflux from a Gram-negative bacterium *Vibrio cholerae* by garlic extract and its bioactive compound, allyl sulfide. At relatively low concentrations, the extract seems to target the EmrD-3 pump, but at higher garlic extract concentrations, the respiratory chain was affected. This example confirms targeting the energization of the efflux system by plant compounds as a potential strategy for drug efflux inhibition (Bruns et al., 2017).

Further, the MFS conserved sequence motifs, present across the entire superfamily, provide vital information regarding alignments of MFS transporter sequences (at least motif containing region), which may help in understanding the structural templates and actual binding events achieved via these transporters. Molecular dynamic simulation (MDS) studies of VMAT2 multidrug transporter (MFS family) revealed the presence of two domains of six trans-membrane helices (Yaffe et al., 2013). The trans-membrane residues at anchoring sites are identified as hinge points, at which straightening and flexing movement of helices occur, required for transport. These anchor point residues are highly conserved throughout the MFS family (Yaffe et al., 2013) and are emerging targets for drug efflux inhibition. Recent advances in scientific and technological arena have added significant in-depth understandings of the structural and biochemical basis of drug efflux, substrate profiles, molecular regulation and inhibition of major EPs.

Active EPs play a critical role in intrinsic and elevated drug resistance acquired via overproduction or over-activation of pumps in Gram-negative bacteria, and the development of clinically useful EPIs or new antibiotics to bypass pump-effects continues to be a challenge in combating Gram-negative bacterial infections (Li et al., 2015). As practically all the antibiotics are susceptible to active drug efflux, the potent EPIs can target these pumps antagonistically and can make old antibiotics effective again (the phenomenon known as re-sensitization). Besides, considering the fact that several antimicrobial agents like lipophilic penicilines, many glycopeptides, oxazolidinones, macrolides and lipopeptide daptomycin are effective in treating only Gram-positive bacterial infections and their poor potencies against Gram-negative pathogens is at least partially due to their active drug efflux, novel and potent EPIs are needed to significantly broaden the range of these antimicrobial agents. All this clearly indicates that EPIs have tremendous potential in adjunctive therapies along with the known but otherwise ineffective antibiotics ultimately reducing the emergence of AMR and virulence (Opperman and Nguyen, 2015). But developing novel and potent EPI is difficult and needs to overcome several hurdles such as choice of antibiotics for potentiation and matching the pharmacological properties of EPI-antibiotics pair (Opperman and Nguyen, 2015; Zgurskaya et al., 2015).

Considering the serious threats posed by the Gram-negative bacteria and their drug-resistance nature, more investigations aiming to target them with the novel, alternative and effective approaches including exploration of natural products are coming up. Though there are limited success stories, but they may lay the foundation for developing potent EPIs to avert the AMR phenotypes with the help of natural sources.

## *IN SILICO* MOLECULAR DYNAMICS SIMULATIONS (MDS) TO SCREEN AND DEVELOP EPIS

The MDS is a commanding approach for computational validation and to support the hypothesized mechanisms of EPs and EPIs (Nikaido and Takatsuka, 2009). It has made possible to simulate the membrane protein complex structures with micro-second time-scales. The MDS approach along with molecular docking and other *in silico* tools are successfully utilized for screening and prediction of molecular interactions between potential EPs and their corresponding inhibitors (Jamshidi et al., 2016). This has led to the unraveling of the mechanism how drug efflux systems recognize and transfer specific molecules; thus helping researchers in challenging the efflux-mediated resistance and finding appropriate EPIs for improvement in antibiotics efficacy during AMR (MDR/XDR) infections (Collu et al., 2012; Nakashima et al., 2013). There are several recent reports describing the successful applications of these *in silico* approaches for screening and identifying potent EPIs of plant origin (Bhaskar et al., 2016; Jamshidi et al., 2016; Mangiaterra et al., 2017; Verma et al., 2017).

A general scheme for MDS-based approaches is depicted in **Figure 4**. Briefly, it starts with the identification of three-dimensional structures of potential EP-binding sites (pockets). The next step is the prediction of trans-membrane segments

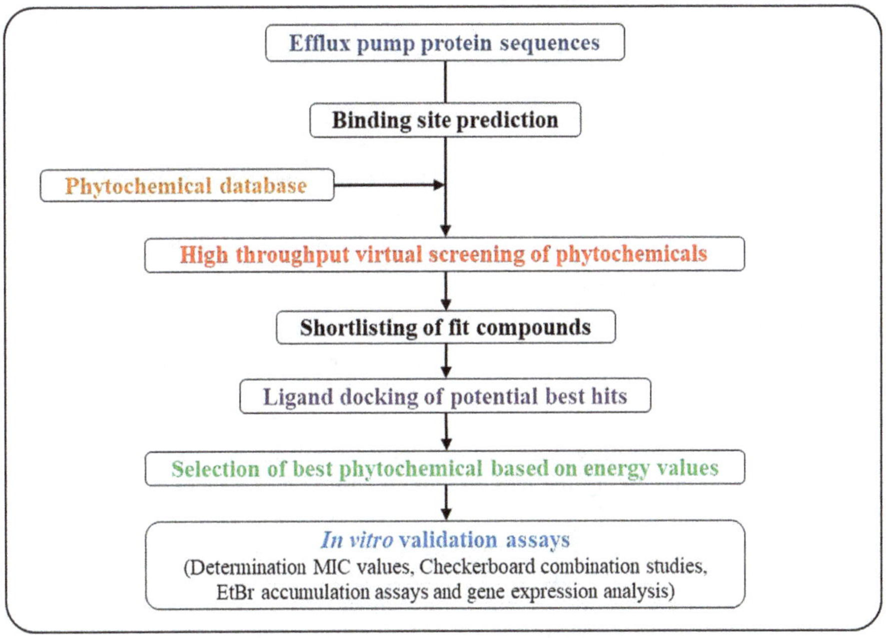


**FIGURE 4** | A general scheme for *in silico* molecular dynamics simulations approach for screening and developing plant based efflux pump inhibitors.

from protein sequences. The predicted structure can then be checked for its stereochemical properties by analyzing the overall and residue-by-residue geometry. The modeled protein structure is then reduced with the solvent implied by chimera programs (http://www.cgl.ucsf.edu/chimera/, Pettersen et al., 2004) and the projected protein structure can be used for its interaction with potential EPI molecules. The three-dimensional structure of the EPI is then explored to attain perfect and stable EPI-EP complex. Potent tools for docking studies include AutoDock (http://autodock.scripps.edu/, Morris et al., 2009), and SwissDock (http://www.swissdock.ch/, Grosdidier et al., 2011). Such automated docking tools can predict the exact binding position of the candidate drug-molecule to the receptors, and provides vital information about exact amino residues taking part in bond-formation with potential drug(s), their bond lengths and type and other interactions adding to the stability of the docking complexes.

Recently, Kesherwani et al. (2017) used high throughput virtual screening of natural compounds against NorM, a MATE transporter from *N. gonorrhea* followed by flexible docking. Authors performed molecular simulation in a membrane environment for investigating the stability and binding energy of top lead compounds, and identified a phytomolecule from *Terminalia chebula* with higher binding free energy than the substrates (rhodamine 6 g, ethidium). The compound successfully blocked the disruption of $Na^+$-coordination along with an equilibrium state bias toward occlude state of NorM transporter, ultimately blocking the extrusion of antimicrobial drugs via inhibiting the NorM transporter in drug-resistant *N. gonorrhea*.

Similarly, Suriyanarayanan and Sarojini (2015) analyzed EPI potentials of plant-derived flavonoid quercetin in bringing down the drug efflux via inhibiting the EmrE, a transporter belonging to SMR family from *E. coli.* Authors used *in silico* approaches and molecule docking approaches. The docking analysis of quercetin with EP-protein showed the importance of residues for function and stability, and notably quercetin showed best interactions as compared to the compounds like verapamil, reserpine, chlorpromazine, and carbonyl cyanide m-chloro phenylhydrazone. MDS confirmed the stability of quercetin-Mmr complex, which insights the potential of quercetin as a non-antibiotics adjuvant for treatment of bacterial infection via reducing the drug efflux from bacteria.

Mangiaterra et al. (2017) identified two phyto-EPIs using *in silico* high-throughput virtual screening. Molecular docking revealed these two compounds morelloflavone and pregnan-20-one derivative as inhibitors of MexAB-OprM EPs of *P. aeruginosa* and supportive *in vitro* assays confirmed their synergism with ciprofloxacin (Mangiaterra et al., 2017).

Molecular docking plays a crucial role and help in defining drug-protein interactions which determines whether compounds act as substrates for EP proteins. Therefore, inhibitors or modulators of EPs are well-recognized along with their comparative binding efficiencies via detailed docking analyses (Collu et al., 2012). Putative EPI activities of quercetin, plumbagin, nordihydroguaretic acid, shikonion and mangiferin were confirmed (Ohene-Agyei et al., 2014). Similarly, docking of reserpine, salvin, totarol, ferruginol along with known antibiotics to NorA revealed that all the tested compounds showed binding at large hydrophobic cleft, suggesting the substantial interactions with key-residues (Bhaskar et al., 2016). Notably, all these investigations were backed by the bioassays confirming the validity of information generated via *in silico* screening.

Owing to the importance of an instantaneous requirement of curing the XDR/MDR strains with utmost specificity, a greater understanding of exact drug-identification and its transport by MDR-EPs is important. The *in silico* MDS approach along with virtual docking and wet laboratory validation therefore can be considered as an imperative path in identifying potent phyto-EPIs.

## MOLECULAR INTERACTIONS UNDERLYING INHIBITION OF EFFLUX PUMPS BY PHYTO-THERAPEUTICS

The inhibition of active drug efflux by EPIs results into the elevated intracellular antimicrobial concentrations, and lowered or complete reversal of efflux-mediated bacterial drug resistance, prevention of microbial invasiveness by inhibiting the export of virulence-factors and shortened adaptation-time required for bacteria, prohibiting the emergence of mutant strains with high AMR (Bhardwaj and Mohanty, 2012; Sun et al., 2014). Major strategies developed for drug efflux inactivation are, first, alterations in regulatory mechanisms for activation/repression of EP gene expressions (Purssell and Poole, 2013), second, deprivation of motive forces required for working of pumps by diminishing the proton gradient (Viveiros et al., 2005; Martins et al., 2008), third structural modifications in existing antimicrobials to bypass the chemophore recognition by the EPs (Chollet et al., 2004; Rice et al., 2005), fourth disrupting the pump-functionality by averting assembly of pumps by targeting protein interfaces (Tikhonova et al., 2011); interaction between protein motifs (Hobbs et al., 2012); obstructing the exit duct (Zeng et al., 2010), and fifth, the trapping of EPs in the inactivated form by competitive binding of EPIs and cytoplasmic membrane proteins (Nakashima et al., 2013; Opperman et al., 2014; Nguyen et al., 2015; Opperman and Nguyen, 2015; **Figure 3**). In addition, targeting the molecular hinge structures by the conserved sequence motifs is also an emerging strategy for EP inhibition (Abdali et al., 2017). The conserved sequence motifs (7–13 residues) are characteristics of MFS family and these motifs on c-terminal end of trans-membrane helix are rich in glycine and proline, vital for promotion of hinge formation. These conserved residues are considered as major contributors in binding and transportation of respective substrates (Luo and Parsons, 2010), and therefore targeting them holds significance for drug efflux inhibition.

To identify the phyto-EPIs, some authors tried to decipher the physiological and molecular interactions involved in EP dysfunction. Sharma et al. (2010) described piperine as an inhibitor of Rv1258c, an efflux protein transporter present on cytoplasmic membrane [encoding for tetracyclin/aminoglycoside resistance (TAP-2)-like EP] in *M. tuberculosis* H37Rv. After structural prediction of the protein, further investigation revealed the binding pocket of Rv1258c. Authors showed H-bond interaction (2.06 Å) with Arg141 residue and piperine provided stable protein-ligand interaction. The findings confirmed the role of piperine in augmenting rifampicin sensitivity in *M. tuberculosis* (Sharma et al., 2010). Capsaicin also proved a potent EPI, inhibiting NorA pump of *S. aureus* (Kalia et al., 2012). The study showed the involvement of Arg98 and Ile23 residues from active binding site in the key binding interactions. The stable interaction between capsaicin and active site at the proposed orientation allows an aliphatic chain of capsaicin, extending in a hydrophobic cleft (containing residues Pro24, Phe140, Ile244, and Phe303) permitting strong hydrophobic interactions due to a lesser distance between ligand and molecule (1.7–3.2 Å). A weak H-bond formation between OH-group (from aryl moiety of capsaicin) and Arg98 was attributed for providing extra-stability to capsaicin/NorA complex (Kalia et al., 2012). Another study by Zhang et al. (2014) described the interactions between ginsenoside 20(S)-Rh2 and NorA from *S. aureus*. The stable H-bond formation between ginsenoside 20(S)-Rh2 and Gln51/Asn340/Ser226 residues at active binding site in the central cavity of protein was attributed for the inhibition of NorA pump, thus promoting accumulation of ciprofloxacin inside the bacterial cell (Zhang et al., 2014). In the similar vein, Ohene-Agyei et al. (2014) assessed five phytochemicals (plumbagin, shikonin, quercetin, mangiferin and nordihydroguaretic acid) for their EPI potentials against AcrB protein from AcrAB-TolC drug transporter. The stable H-bond formation between T monomer of AcrB with minocycline attached to binding pocket and phytochemicals was responsible for efflux inhibition by the phytochemicals (Ohene-Agyei et al., 2014). Further, the authors also postulated that the considered natural compound act as a substrate and compete with the antibiotics for drug-resistance reversal (similar to PAβN). Therefore, these natural products act as high-affinity substrate inhibitors rather than substances for trapping the EPs in an inactive state.

## CONCLUDING REMARKS

Increasing AMR in community and nosocomial settings is a big threat to human healthcare and accounts for a large number of mortalities and morbidities globally. Bacterial EPs make up a major warhead of the drug-resistant pathogens and increase and maintain the AMR via extruding or reducing the intracellular concentrations of applied antibiotics, often in a non-specific manner. The drug EPs are also emerging as chemical tools to understand molecular mechanisms underlying drug extrusion from the bacterial cells. EPs play several important physiological and molecular roles in bacterial cell survival and stress-responses. The necessity to overcome AMR has encouraged investigators to characterize resistance-inhibiting or modulating EPIs to block the drug extrusion, restoring antibacterial susceptibility and returning existing antibiotics into the clinic. The severity of the AMR is higher in Gram-negative bacteria, owing to their superior capabilities in maintaining high drug efflux levels coupled with lower intracellular levels of toxic drugs including antibiotics. MDR/XDR strains maintain their intrinsic and acquired resistance via overproduction of pumps. The development of clinically useful EPIs to bypass pump effects continues to be a challenge. Though there are some noteworthy developments in recent past aimed at reversing the AMR phenotypes including facilitation of better drug-penetration across the outer membranes of Gram-negative bacteria, and establishing new rules of permeation, identifying new and powerful EPIs seems best approach that can be explored as drug leads or in adjunctive therapies.

Several recent developments in *in-silico* MDS approaches have enabled the researchers to computationally validate and support the hypothesized mechanisms of EPs and EPIs (Suriyanarayanan and Sarojini, 2015; Ramaswamy et al., 2017; Vargiu et al., 2018). It is now possible to simulate membrane protein complex structures with micro-second time-scales. The MDS approach along with molecular docking and other *in silico* tools are successfully utilized for screening and prediction of the molecular interactions between potential EPs and their corresponding EPIs, ultimately helping in identification of the potent EPIs particularly from plant origin. However, this field is yet to be explored fully.

Considering the fact that practically all the antibiotics are susceptible to active drug-efflux, use of the potent EPIs to target and block these pumps can help in potentiating the old antibiotics effective again against a range of drug-resistant bacteria. EPIs are being looked as promising adjunctive therapies with the known antibiotics to improve their antibacterial potency at low concentrations, reduce the emergence of AMR and virulence. But developing novel and potent EPI is not easy and needs to overcome several hurdles such as choice of antibiotics for potentiation and matching the pharmacological properties of EPI-antibiotic(s) pair. More comprehensive and deeper investigations are therefore needed that involve the exploring the high-throughput screening assisted by *in silico* tools for identifying the potent EPI phytomolecules and their corresponding targets. Newer studies are being undertaken for identifying phytomolecules effective in inhibiting bacterial efflux pumps via potentiation of antibiotics against pathogenic bacteria including Gram-negative pathogens. This may pave the way for identification of phyto-EPIs that can head toward clinical phases and ultimately clinical practices with an aim to contain the AMR.

## AUTHOR CONTRIBUTIONS

VK conceived the idea. VS, TK, RB, RS, and VK wrote the manuscript. All the authors made substantial contribution to the work and approved it for publication.

## ACKNOWLEDGMENTS

The support under Star College Scheme of Department of Biotechnology, Government of India implemented at Modern College, Ganeshkhind, Pune is gratefully acknowledged. The use of facilities created under FIST program of Department of Science and Technology (DST), Government of India, implemented at Prof. Ramkrishna More College, Akurdi, Pune and Modern College, Ganeshkhind, Pune are gratefully acknowledged.

## REFERENCES

Abdali, N., Parks, J. M., Haynes, K. M., Chaney, J. L., Green, A. T., Wolloscheck, D., et al. (2017). Reviving antibiotics: efflux pump inhibitors that interact with acra, a membrane fusion protein of the AcrAB-TolC multidrug efflux pump. *ACS Infect Dis.* 3, 89–98. doi: 10.1021/acsinfecdis.6b00167

Aghayan, S. S., Mogadam, H. K., Fazli, M., Darban-Sarokhalil, D., Khoramrooz, S. S., Jabalameli, F., et al. (2017). The effects of berberine and palmatine on efflux pumps inhibition with different gene patterns in *Pseudomonas aeruginosa* isolated from burn infections. *Avicenna J. Med. Biotechnol.* 9:2.

Akiba, M., Lin, J., Barton, Y. W., and Zhang, Q. (2006). Interaction of CmeABC and CmeDEF in conferring antimicrobial resistance and maintaining cell viability in *Campylobacter jejuni*. *J. Antimicrob. Chemother.* 57, 52–60. doi: 10.1093/jac/dki419

Alav, I., Sutton, J. M., and Rahman, K. M. (2018). Role of bacterial efflux pumps in biofilm formation. *J. Antimicrob. Chemother.* 73, 2003–2020. doi: 10.1093/jac/dky042

Amabile-Cuevas, C. F., Arredondo-Garcia, J. L., Cruz, A., and Rosas, I. (2010). Fluoroquinolone resistance in clinical and environmental isolates of *Escherichia coli* in Mexico City. *J. Appl. Microbiol.* 108, 158–162. doi: 10.1111/j.1365-2672.2009.04401.x

Bag, A., and Chattopadhyay, R. R. (2014). Efflux-pump inhibitory activity of a gallotannin from *Terminalia chebula* fruit against multidrug-resistant uropathogenic *Escherichia coli*. *Nat. Prod. Res.* 28, 1280–1283. doi: 10.1080/14786419.2014.895729

Balganesh, M., Dinesh, N., Sharma, S., Kuruppath, S., Nair, A. V., and Sharma, U. (2012). Efflux pumps of *Mycobacterium tuberculosis* play a significant role in antituberculosis activity of potential drug candidates. *Antimicrob. Agents Chemother.* 56, 2643–2651. doi: 10.1128/AAC.06003-11

Balganesh, M., Kuruppath, S., Marcel, N., Sharma, S., Nair, A, and Sharma, U. (2010). Rv1218c, an ABC transporter of *Mycobacterium tuberculosis* with implications in drug discovery. *Antimicrob. Agents Chemother.* 54, 5167–5172. doi: 10.1128/AAC.00610-10

Bame, J. R., Graf, T., Junio, H., Bussey, R., Jarmusch, S., El-Elimat, T., et al. (2013). Sarothrin from *Alkanna orientalis* is an antimicrobial agent and efflux pump inhibitor. *Planta Med.* 79, 327–329. doi: 10.1055/s-0032-1328259

Baugh, S., Ekanayaka, A. S., Piddock, L. J., and Webber, M. A. (2012). Loss of or inhibition of all multidrug resistance efflux pumps of *Salmonella enterica* serovar *Typhimurium* results in impaired ability to form a biofilm. *J. Antimicrob. Chemother.* 67, 2409–2417. doi: 10.1093/jac/dks228

Baugh, S., Phillips, C. R., Ekanayaka, A. S., Piddock, L. J., and Webber, M. A. (2014). Inhibition of multidrug efflux as a strategy to prevent biofilm formation. *J. Antimicrob.Chemother.* 69, 673–681. doi: 10.1093/jac/dkt420

Beketskaia, M. S., Bay, D. C., and Turner, R. J. (2014). Outer membrane protein OmpW participates with small multidrug resistance protein member EmrE in quaternary cationic compound efflux. *J. Bacteriol.* 196, 1483–1414. doi: 10.1128/JB.01483-14

Bhardwaj, A. K., and Mohanty, P. (2012). Bacterial efflux pumps involved in multidrug resistance and their inhibitors: rejuvenating the antimicrobial chemotherapy. *Recent Pat. Antiinfect. Drug Discov.* 7, 73–89. doi: 10.2174/157489112799829710

Bhaskar, B. V., Babu, T. M. C., Reddy, N. V., and Rajendra, W. (2016). Homology modeling, molecular dynamics, and virtual screening of NorA efflux pump inhibitors of *Staphylococcus aureus*. *Drug Des. Devel. Ther.* 10, 3237. doi: 10.2147/DDDT.S113556

Blair, J. M., Webber, M. A., Baylay, A. J., Ogbolu, D. O., and Piddock, L. J. (2015). Molecular mechanisms of antibiotic resistance. *Nat. Rev. Microbiol.* 13, 42–51. doi: 10.1038/nrmicro3380

Bruns, M. M., Kakarla, P., Floyd, J. T., Mukherjee, M. M., Ponce, R. C., Garcia, J. A., et al. (2017). Modulation of the multidrug efflux pump EmrD-3 from *Vibrio cholerae* by *Allium sativum* extract and the bioactive agent allyl sulfide plus synergistic enhancement of antimicrobial susceptibility by *A. sativum* extract. *Arch. Microbiol.* 199, 1103–1112. doi: 10.1007/s00203-017-1378-x

Buckley, A. M., Webber, M. A., Cooles, S., Randall, L. P., La Ragione, R. M., Woodward, M. J., et al. (2006). The AcrAB–TolC efflux system of *Salmonella enterica* serovar *Typhimurium* plays a role in pathogenesis. *Cell. Microbiol.* 8, 847–856. doi: 10.1111/j.1462-5822.2005.00671.x

Cattoir, V., Poirel, L., and Nordmann, P. (2008). Plasmid-mediated quinolone resistance pump QepA2 in an *Escherichia coli* isolate from France. *Antimicrob. Agents Chemother.* 52, 3801–3804. doi: 10.1128/AAC.00638-08

Cerceo, E., Deitelzweig, S. B., Sherman, B. M., and Amin, A. N. (2016). Multidrug-resistant gram-negative bacterial infections in the hospital setting: overview, implications for clinical practice, and emerging treatment options. *Microb. Drug Resist.* 22, 412–431. doi: 10.1089/mdr.2015.0220

Cha, H. J., Muller, R. T., and Pos, K. M. (2014). Switch-loop flexibility affects transport of large drugs by the promiscuous AcrB multidrug efflux transporter. *Antimicrob. Agents Chemother.* 58, 4767–4772. doi: 10.1128/AAC.02733-13

Chan, B. C., Han, X., Lui, S., Wong, C., Wang, T., Cheung, D., et al. (2015). Combating against methicillin-resistant *Staphylococcus aureus*—two fatty acids from purslane (*Portulaca oleracea* L.) exhibit synergistic effects with erythromycin. *J. Pharm. Pharmacol.* 67, 107–116. doi: 10.1111/jphp.12315

Chan, B. C., Ip, M., Lau, C. B., Lui, S. L., Jolivalt, C., Ganem-Elbaz, C., et al. (2011). Synergistic effects of baicalein with ciprofloxacin against NorA over-expressed methicillin-resistant *Staphylococcus aureus* (MRSA) and inhibition of MRSA pyruvate kinase. *J. Ethnopharmacol.* 137, 767–773. doi: 10.1016/j.jep.2011.06.039

Chandra, H., Bishnoi, P., Yadav, A., Patni, B., Mishra, A. P., and Nautiyal, A. R. (2017). Antimicrobial resistance and the alternative resources with special emphasis on plant-based antimicrobials—a review. *Plants* 6:16. doi: 10.3390/plants6020016

Chen, Y., Hu, D., Zhang, Q., Liao, X-P., Liu, Y-H., and Sun, J. (2017). Efflux Pump Overexpression contributes to tigecycline heteroresistance in *Salmonella enterica* serovar Typhimurium. *Front. Cell. Infect. Microbiol.* 7:37. doi: 10.3389/fcimb.2017.00037

Chollet, R., Chevalier, J., Bryskier, A., and Pagès, J. M. (2004). The AcrAB-TolC pump is involved in macrolide resistance but not in telithromycin efflux in *Enterobacter aerogenes* and *Escherichia coli*. *Antimicrob. Agents Chemother.* 48, 3621–3624. doi: 10.1128/AAC.48.9.3621-3624.2004

Chovanova, R., Mezovska, J., Vaverkova, S., and Mikulasova, M. (2015). The inhibition the Tet(K) efflux pump of tetracycline resistant *Staphylococcus epidermidis* by essential oils from three *Salvia* species. *Lett. Appl. Microbiol.* 61, 58–62. doi: 10.1111/lam.12424

Collu, F., Vargiu, A. V., Dreier, J., Cascella, M., and Ruggerone, P. (2012). Recognition of imipenem and meropenem by the RND transporter MexB studied by computer simulations. *J. Am. Chem. Soc.* 134, 19146–19158. doi: 10.1021/ja307803m

Costa, S. S., Viveiros, M., Amaral, L., and Couto, I. (2013). Multidrug efflux pumps in *Staphylococcus aureus*: an update. *Open Microbiol. J.* 7, 59–71. doi: 10.2174/1874285801307010059

Coyne, S., Rosenfeld, N., Lambert, T., Courvalin, P., and Perichon, B. (2010). Overexpression of resistance- nodulation-cell division pump AdeFGH confers multidrug resistance in *Acinetobacter baumannii*. *Antimicrob. Agents Chemother.* 54, 4389–4393. doi: 10.1128/AAC.00155-10

Davies, J., and Davies, D. (2010). Origins and evolution of antibiotic resistance. *Microbiol. Mol. Biol. Rev.* 74, 417–433. doi: 10.1128/MMBR.00016-10

dos Santos, J. F., Tintino, S. R., de Freitas, T. S., Campina, F. F., Irwin, R. D. A., Siqueira-Júnior, J. P., et al. (2018). *In vitro* e *in silico* evaluation of the inhibition of *Staphylococcus aureus* efflux pumps by caffeic and gallic acid. *Comp. Immunol. Microbiol. Infect. Dis.* 57, 22–28. doi: 10.1016/j.cimid.2018.03.001

Du, D., Venter, H., Pos, K. M., and Luisi, B. F. (2013). "The machinery and mechanism of multidrug efflux in Gram-negative bacteria," in *Microbial Efflux Pumps: Current Research*, eds E. W. Yu, Q. Zhang, and M. H. Brown (Ames, IA: Caister Academic Press), 35–48.

Du, D., Wang, Z., James, N. R., Voss, J. E., Klimont, E., Ohene-Agyei, T., et al. (2014). Structure of the AcrAB-TolC multidrug efflux pump. *Nature* 509, 512–515. doi: 10.1038/nature13205

Du, D., Wang-Kan, X., Neuberger, A., van Veen, H. W., Pos, K. M., Piddock, L. J., et al. (2018). Multidrug efflux pumps: structure, function and regulation. *Nat. Rev. Microbiol.* 16, 523–539. doi: 10.1038/s41579-018-0048-6

Dwivedi, G., Maurya, A., Yadav, D., Khan, F., Darokar, M., and Srivastava, S. (2014a). Drug resistance reversal potential of ursolic acid derivatives against nalidixic acid- and multidrug-resistant *Escherichia coli*. *Chem. Biol. Drug Des.* 86, 272–283. doi: 10.1111/cbdd.12491

Dwivedi, G. R., Gupta, S., Maurya, A., Tripathi, S., Sharma, A., Srivastava, S. K., et al. (2015). Synergy potential of indole alkaloids and its derivative against drug resistant *Escherichia coli*. *Chem. Biol. Drug Des.* 86, 1471–1481. doi: 10.1111/cbdd.12613

Dwivedi, G. R., Singh, D. P., Sharma, S. A., and Darokar, M. P. (2017a). "Efflux Pumps: Warheads of Gram-Negative Bacteria and Efflux Pump Inhibitors" in *New Approaches in Biological Research*, eds R. P. Sinha and Richa (New York, NY: Nova Science Publishers), 35–72.

Dwivedi, G. R., Tyagi, R., Sanchita, Tripathi, S., Pati, S., Srivastava, S. K., et al. (2017b). Antibiotics potentiating potential of catharanthine against superbug *Pseudomonas aeruginosa*. *J. Biomol. Struct. Dyn.* 1–15. doi: 10.1080/07391102.2017.1413424. [Epub ahead of print].

Dwivedi, G. R., Upadhyay, H. C., Yadav, D. K., Singh, V., Srivastava, S. K., Khan, F., et al. (2014b). 4-hydroxy-α-tetralone and its derivative as Drug resistance reversal agents in multidrug resistant *Escherichia coli*. *Chem. Biol. Drug Des.* 83, 482–492. doi: 10.1111/cbdd.12263

Eicher, T., Cha, H. J., Seeger, M. A., Brandstatter, L., El-Delik, J., Bohnert, J. A., et al. (2012). Transport of drugs by the multidrug transporter AcrB involves an access and a deep binding pocket that are separated by a switch-loop. *Proc. Natl. Acad. Sci. U.S.A.* 109, 5687–5692. doi: 10.1073/pnas.1114944109

Exner, M., Bhattacharya, S., Christiansen, B., Gebel, J., Goroncy-Bermes, P., Hartemann, P., et al. (2017). Antibiotic resistance: what is so special about multidrug-resistant Gram-negative bacteria? *GMS Hyg. Infect. Control.* 12:Doc05. doi: 10.3205/dgkh000290

Fahmy, A., Srinivasan, A., and Webber, M. A. (2016). "The relationship between bacterial multidrug efflux pumps and biofilm formation," in *Efflux-Mediated Antimicrobial Resistance in Bacteria*, edd X. Z. Li, C. A. Elkins, and H. I. Zgurskaya (Adis; Cham: Springer International Publishing), 651–663.

Fair, R. J., and Tor, Y. (2014). Antibiotics and bacterial resistance in the 21st century. *Perspect. Medicin. Chem.* 6, 25–64. doi: 10.4137/PMC.S14459

Fernandez, L., and Hancock, R. (2012). Adaptive and mutational resistance: role of porins and efflux pumps in drug resistance. *Clin. Microbiol. Rev.* 25, 661–681. doi: 10.1128/CMR.00043-12

Fiamegos, Y. C., Kastritis, P. L., Exarchou, V., Han, H., Bonvin, A. M., Vervoort, J., et al. (2011). Antimicrobial and efflux pump inhibitory activity of caffeoylquinic acids from *Artemisia absinthium* against gram-positive pathogenic bacteria. *PLoS ONE* 6:e18127. doi: 10.1371/journal.pone.0018127

Garvey, M., Rahman, M., Gibbons, S., and Piddock, L. (2011). Medicinal plant extracts with efflux inhibitory activity against Gram negative bacteria. *Int. J. Antimicrob. Agents* 37, 145–151. doi: 10.1016/j.ijantimicag.2010.10.027

German, N., Kaatz, G. W., and Kerns, R. J. (2008). Synthesis and evaluation of PSSRI-based inhibitors of *Staphylococcus aureus* multidrug efflux pumps. *Bioorg. Med. Chem. Lett.* 18, 1368–1373. doi: 10.1016/j.bmcl.2008.01.014

Gill, E. E., Franco, O. L., and Hancock, R. E. W. (2015). Antibiotic adjuvants: diverse strategies for controlling drug-resistant pathogens. *Chem. Biol. Drug Des.* 85, 56–78. doi: 10.1111/cbdd.12478

González, J. E., and Keshavan, N. D. (2006). Messing with bacterial quorum sensing. *Microbiol. Mol. Biol. Rev.* 70, 859–875. doi: 10.1128/MMBR.00002-06

Grkovic, S., Brown, M. H., and Skurray, R. A. (2002). Regulation of bacterial drug export systems. *Microbiol. Mol. Biol. Rev.* 66, 671–701. doi: 10.1128/MMBR.66.4.671-701.2002

Grosdidier, A., Zoete, V., and Michielin, O. (2011). SwissDock, a protein-small molecule docking web service based on EADock DSS. *Nucleic Acids Res.* 39, W270–W277. doi: 10.1093/nar/gkr366

Gupta, D., Singh, A., and Khan, A. U. (2017). Nanoparticles as efflux pump and biofilm inhibitor to rejuvenate bactericidal effect of conventional antibiotics. *Nanoscale Res. Lett.* 12, 454. doi: 10.1186/s11671-017-2222-6

Hannula, M., and Hänninen, M. L. (2008). Effect of putative efflux pump inhibitors and inducers on the antimicrobial susceptibility of *Campylobacter jejuni* and *Campylobacter coli*. *J. Med. Microbiol.* 57, 851–855. doi: 10.1099/jmm.0.47823-0

Hansen, L. H., Johannesen, E., Burmolle, M., Sørensen, A. H., and Sørensen, S. J. (2004). Plasmid-encoded multidrug efflux pump conferring resistance to olaquindox in *Escherichia coli*. *Antimicrob. Agents Chemother.* 48, 3332–3337. doi: 10.1128/AAC.48.9.3332-3337.2004

He, X., Szewczyk, P., Karyakin, A., Evin, M., and Hong, W. X. (2010). Structure of a cation-bound multidrug and toxic compound extrusion transporter. *Nature* 467, 991–994. doi: 10.1038/nature09408

Higgins, C. F. (2007). Multiple molecular mechanisms for multidrug resistance transporters. *Nature* 446, 749–757. doi: 10.1038/nature05630

Hirakata, Y., Srikumar, R., Poole, K., Gotoh, N., Suematsu, T., Kohno, S., et al. (2002). Multidrug efflux systems play an important role in the invasiveness of *Pseudomonas aeruginosa*. *J. Exp. Med.* 196, 109–118. doi: 10.1084/jem.20020005

Hobbs, E. C., Yin, X., Paul, B. J., Astarita, J. L., and Storz, G. (2012). Conserved small protein associates with the multidrug efflux pump AcrB and differentially affects antibiotic resistance. *Proc. Natl. Acad. Sci. U.S.A.* 109, 16696–16701. doi: 10.1073/pnas.1210093109

Holler, J. G., Christensen, S. B., Slotved, H. C., Rasmussen, H. B., Gúzman, A., Olsen, C. E., et al. (2012). Novel inhibitory activity of the *Staphylococcus aureus* NorA efflux pump by a kaempferol rhamnoside isolated from *Persea lingue* Nees. *J. Antimicrob. Chemother.* 67, 1138–1144. doi: 10.1093/jac/dks005

Huda, N., Lee, E. W., Chen, J., Morita, Y., Kuroda, T., Mizushima, T., et al. (2003). Molecular cloning and characterization of an ABC multidrug efflux pump, VcaM, in non-O1 *Vibrio cholerae*. *Antimicrob. Agents Chemother.* 47, 2413–2417. doi: 10.1128/AAC.47.8.2413-2417.2003

Jack, D. L., Yang, N. M., and Saier, M. H. (2001). The drug/metabolite transporter superfamily. *Eur. J. Biochem.* 68, 3620–3639. doi: 10.1046/j.1432-1327.2001.02265.x

Jamshidi, S., Sutton, J. M., and Rahman, K. M. (2016). An overview of bacterial efflux pumps and computational approaches to study efflux pump inhibitors. *Future Med. Chem.* 8, 195–210. doi: 10.4155/fmc.15.173

Kaatz, G. W., McAleese, F., and Seo, S. M. (2005). Multidrug resistance in *Staphylococcus aureu* s due to overexpression of a novel multidrug and toxin extrusion (MATE) transport protein. *Antimicrob. Agents Chemother.* 49, 1857–1864. doi: 10.1128/AAC.49.5.1857-1864.2005

Kakarla, P., Floyd, J., Mukherjee, M., Devireddy, A. R., Inupakutika, M. A., Ranweera, I., et al. (2016). Inhibition of the multidrug efflux pump LmrS from *Staphylococcus aureus* by cumin spice *Cuminum cyminum*. *Arch. Microbiol.* 199, 465–474. doi: 10.1007/s00203-016-1314-5

Kalia, N. P., Mahajan, P., Mehra, R., Nargotra, A., Sharma, J. P., Koul, S., et al. (2012). Capsaicin, a novel inhibitor of the NorA efflux pump, reduces the intracellular invasion of *Staphylococcus aureus*. *J. Antimicrob. Chemother.* 67, 2401–2408. doi: 10.1093/jac/dks232

Kayser, F. H., Benner, E. J., and Hoeprich, P. D. (1970). Acquired and native resistance of *Staphylococcus aureus* to cephalexin and other beta-lactam antibiotics. *Appl. Microbiol.* 20, 1–5.

Kesherwani, M., Michael Gromiha, M., Fukui, K., and Velmurugan, D. (2017). Identification of novel natural inhibitor for NorM–a multidrug and toxic compound extrusion transporter–an *insilico* molecular modeling and simulation studies. *J. Biomol. Struct. Dyn.* 35, 58–77. doi: 10.1080/07391102.2015.1132391

Kim, J. Y., Kim, S. H., Jeon, S. M., Park, M. S., Rhie, H. G., and Lee, B. K. (2008). Resistance to fluoroquinolones by the combination of target site mutations and enhanced expression of genes for efflux pumps in *Shigella flexneri* and *Shigella sonnei* strains isolated in Korea. *Clin. Microbiol. Infec.* 14, 760–765. doi: 10.1111/j.1469-0691.2008.02033.x

Kobayashi, N., Nishino, K., and Yamaguchi, A. (2001). Novel macrolide-specific ABC-type efflux transporter in *Escherichia coli*. *J. Bacteriol.* 183, 5639–5644. doi: 10.1128/JB.183.19.5639-5644.2001

Köhler, T., Michea-Hamzehpour, M., Henze, U., Gotoh, N., Curty, L. K., and Pechere, J. C. (1997). Characterization of MexE-MexF-OprN, a positively regulated multidrug efflux system of *Pseudomonas aeruginosa*. *Mol. Microbiol.* 23, 345–354. doi: 10.1046/j.1365-2958.1997.2281594.x

Kourtesi, C., Ball, A., Huang, Y., Jachak, S., Vera, D., Khondkar, P., et al. (2013). Microbial efflux systems and inhibitors: approaches to drug discovery and the challenge of clinical implementation. *Open Microbiol. J.* 7, 34–52. doi: 10.2174/1874285801307010034

Kumar, V., Shriram, V., and Mulla, J. (2013). Antibiotic resistance reversal of multiple drug resistant bacteria using *Piper longum* fruit extract. *J. Appl. Pharm. Sci.* 3, 112–116. doi: 10.7324/JAPS.2013.30322

Kumarasamy, K. K., Toleman, M. A., Walsh, T. R., Bagaria, J., Butt, F., Balakrishnan, R., et al. (2010). Emergence of a new antibiotic resistance mechanism in India, Pakistan, and the UK: a molecular, biological, and epidemiological study. *Lancet Infect. Dis.* 10, 597–602. doi: 10.1016/S1473-3099(10)70143-2

Kvist, M., Hancock, V., and Klemm, P. (2008). Inactivation of efflux pumps abolishes bacterial biofilm formation. *Appl. Environ. Microbiol.* 74, 7376–7382. doi: 10.1128/AEM.01310-08

Lee, E. W., Huda, M. N., Kuroda, T., Mizushima, T., and Tsuchiya, T. (2003). EfrAB, an ABC multidrug efflux pump in *Enterococcus faecalis*. *Antimicrob. Agents Chemother.* 47, 3733–3738. doi: 10.1128/AAC.47.12.3733-3738.2003

Lennen, R. M., Politz, M. G., Kruziki, M. A., and Pfleger, B. F. (2013). Identification of transport proteins involved in free fatty acid efflux in *Escherichia coli*. *J. Bacteriol.* 195, 135–144. doi: 10.1128/JB.01477-12

Levy, S. B. (2001). Antibiotic resistance: consequences of inaction. *Clin. Infect. Dis.* 33, S124–S129. doi: 10.1086/321837

Li, X-Z., Plésiat, P., and Nikaido, H. (2015). The challenge of efflux-mediated antibiotic resistance in Gram-negative bacteria. *Clin. Microbiol. Rev.* 28, 337–418. doi: 10.1128/CMR.00117-14

Liang, Z., Chen, Y. M., Chen, Y., Cheng, Y. Y., and and Zhang, L. H. (2016). RND efflux pump and its interrelationship with quorum sensing system. *Hereditas (Beijing)*, 38, 894–901. doi: 10.16288/j.yczz.16-139

Limaverde, P. W., Campina, F. F., da Cunha, F. A., Crispim, F. D., Figueredo, F. G., Lima, L. F., et al. (2017). Inhibition of the TetK efflux-pump by the essential oil of *Chenopodium ambrosioides* L. and α-terpinene against *Staphylococcus aureus* IS-58. *Food Chem. Toxicol.* 109, 957–961. doi: 10.1016/j.fct.2017.02.031

Lin, J., Michel, L. O., and Zhang, Q. (2002). CmeABC functions as a multidrug effl ux system in *Campylobacter jejuni*. *Antimicrob. Agents Chemother.* 46, 2124–2131. doi: 10.1128/AAC.46.7.2124-2131.2002

Lister, P. D., Wolter, D. J., and Hanson, N. D. (2009). Antibacterial-resistant *Pseudomonas aeruginosa*: clinical impact and complex regulation of chromosomally encoded resistance mechanisms. *Clin. Microbiol. Rev.* 22, 582–610. doi: 10.1128/CMR.00040-09

Littlejohn, T. G., Paulsen, I. T., Gillespie, M. T., Tennent, J. M., Midgley, M., Jones, I. G., et al. (1992). Substrate specifi city and energetics of antiseptic and disinfectant resistance in *Staphylococcus aureus*. *FEMS Microbiol. Lett.* 95, 259–265. doi: 10.1111/j.1574-6968.1992.tb05376.x

Liu, Q., Hassan, K. A., Ashwood, H. E., Gamage, H. K. A. H., Li, L., Mabbutt, B. C., et al. (2018). Regulation of the *aceI* multidrug efflux pump gene in *Acinetobacter baumannii*. *J. Antimicrob. Chemother.* 73, 1492–1500. doi: 10.1093/jac/dky034

Lomovskaya, O., Warren, M. S., Lee, A., Galazzo, J., Fronko, R., Lee, M., et al. (2001). Identification and characterization of inhibitors of multidrug resistance efflux pumps in *Pseudomonas aeruginosa*: novel agents for combination therapy. *Antimicrob. Agents Chemother.* 45, 105–116. doi: 10.1128/AAC.45.1.105-116.2001

Luo, J., and Parsons, S. M. (2010). Conformational propensities of peptides mimicking transmembrane helix 5 and motif C in wild-type and mutant vesicular acetylcholine transporters. *ACS Chem. Neurosci.* 1, 381–390. doi: 10.1021/cn900033s

Lynch, A. S. (2006). Efflux systems in bacterial pathogens: an opportunity for therapeutic intervention? An industry view. *Biochem. Pharmacol.* 71, 949–956. doi: 10.1016/j.bcp.2005.10.021

Ma, D., Alberti, M., Lynch, C., Nikaido, H., and Hearst, J. E. (1996). The local repressor AcrR plays a modulating role in the regulation of acrAB genes of *Escherichia coli* by global stress signals. *Mol. Microbiol.* 19, 101–112.

Maisuria, V., Hosseinidoust, Z., and Tufenkji, N. (2015). Polyphenolic extract from maple syrup potentiates antibiotic susceptibility and reduces biofilm formation of pathogenic bacteria. *Appl. Environ. Microbiol.* 81, 3782–3792. doi: 10.1128/AEM.00239-15

Mangiaterra, G., Laudadio, E., Cometti, M., Mobbili, G., Minnelli, C., Massaccesi, L., et al. (2017). Inhibitors of multidrug efflux pumps of *Pseudomonas aeruginosa* from natural sources: an *in silico* high-throughput virtual screening and *in vitro* validation. *Med. Chem. Res.* 26, 414–430. doi: 10.1007/s00044-016-1761-1

Marrer, E., Schad, K., Satoh, A. T., Page, M. G., Johnson, M. M., and Piddock, L. J. (2006). Involvement of the putative ATP-dependent effl ux proteins PatA and PatB in fluoroquinolone resistance of a multidrug- resistant mutant of *Streptococcus pneumoniae. Antimicrob. Agents Chemother.* 50, 685–693. doi: 10.1128/AAC.50.2.685-693.2006

Martinez, J. L., Sánchez, M. B., Martínez-Solano, L., Hernandez, A., Garmendia, L., Fajardo, A., et al. (2009). Functional role of bacterial multidrug efflux pumps in microbial natural ecosystems. *FEMS Microbial. Rev.* 33, 430–449. doi: 10.1111/j.1574-6976.2008.00157.x

Martins, M., Dastidar, S. G., Fanning, S., Kristiansen, J. E., Molnar, J., Pagès, J. M., et al. (2008). Potential role of non-antibiotics (helper compounds) in the treatment of multidrug- resistant Gram-negative infections: mechanisms for their direct and indirect activities. *Int. J. Antimicrob. Agents* 31, 198–208. doi: 10.1016/j.ijantimicag.2007.10.025

Masi, M., Refregiers, M., Pos, K. M., and Pages, J. M. (2017). Mechanisms of envelope permeability and antibiotic influx and efflux in Gram-negative bacteria. *Nat. Microbiol.* 2:17001. doi: 10.1038/nmicrobiol.2017.1

Maurya, A., Dwivedi, G., Darokar, M., and Srivastava, S. (2013). Antibacterial and synergy of clavine alkaloid lysergol and its derivatives against nalidixic acid-resistant *Escherichia coli. Chem. Biol. Drug Des.* 81, 484–490. doi: 10.1111/cbdd.12103

May, T., Ito, A., and Okabe, S. (2009). Induction of multidrug resistance mechanism in *Escherichia coli* biofilms by interplay between tetracycline and ampicillin resistance genes. *Antimicrob. Agents Chemother.* 53, 4628–4639. doi: 10.1128/AAC.00454-09

Molnár, J., Engi, H., Hohmann, J., Molnár, P., and Deli, J. (2010). Reversal of multidrug resistance by natural substances from plants. *Curr. Topics Medi. Chem.* 10, 1757–1768. doi: 10.2174/156802610792928103

Moore, J. D., Gerdt, J. P., Eibergen, N. R., and Blackwell, H. E. (2014). Active efflux influences the potency of quorum sensing inhibitors in *Pseudomonas aeruginosa. Chembiochem* 15, 435–442. doi: 10.1002/cbic.201300701

Morand, B., and Mühlemann, K. (2007). Heteroresistance to penicillin in *Streptococcus pneumoniae. Proc. Natl. Acad. Sci. U.S.A.* 104, 14098–14103. doi: 10.1073/pnas.0702377104

Morita, Y., Kodama, K., Shiota, S., Mine, T., Kataoka, A., Mizushima, T., et al. (1998). NorM, a putative multidrug efflux protein, of *Vibrio parahaemolyticus* and its homolog in *Escherichia coli. Antimicrob. Agents Chemother.* 42, 1778–1782. doi: 10.1128/AAC.42.7.1778

Morris, G. M., Huey, R., Lindstrom, W., Sanner, M. F., Belew, R. K., Goodsell, D. S., et al. (2009). Autodock4 and AutoDockTools4: automated docking with selective receptor flexiblity. *J. Comput. Chem.* 16**,** 2785–2791. doi: 10.1002/jcc.21256

Motta, S. S., Cluzel, P., and Aldana, M. (2015). Adaptive resistance in bacteria requires epigenetic inheritance, genetic noise, and cost of efflux pumps. *PLoS ONE* 10:e0118464. doi: 10.1371/journal.pone.0118464

Mukanganyama, S., Chirisa, E., and Hazra, B. (2012). Antimycobacterial activity of diospyrin and its derivatives against *Mycobacterium aurum. Res. Pharm.* 2, 1–13.

Nakashima, R., Sakurai, K., Yamasaki, S., Hayashi, K., Nagata, C., Hoshino, K., Onodera, Y., Nishino, K., et al. (2013). Structural basis for the inhibition of bacterial multidrug exporters. *Nature* 500, 102–106. doi: 10.1038/nature12300

Napier, B. A., Band, V., Burd, E. M., and Weiss, D. S. (2014). Colistin heteroresistance in *Enterobacter cloacae* is associated with cross-resistance to the host antimicrobial lysozyme. *Antimicrob. Agents Chemother.* 58, 5594–5597. doi: 10.1128/AAC.02432-14

Newman, D., and Cragg, G. (2012). Natural products as sources of new drugs over the 30 years from 1981 to 2010. *J. Nat. Prod.* 75, 311–335. doi: 10.1021/np200906s

Nguyen, S. T., Kwasny, S. M., Ding, X., Cardinale, S. C., McCarthy, C. T., Kim, H-S., et al. (2015). Structure–activity relationships of a novel pyranopyridine series of Gram negative bacterial efflux pump inhibitors. *Bioorg. Med. Chem.* 23, 2024–2034. doi: 10.1016/j.bmc.2015.03.016

Ni, W., Li, Y., Guan, J., Zhao, J., Cui, J., Wang, R., et al. (2016). Effects of efflux pump inhibitors on colistin resistance in multidrug resistant Gram-negative bacteria. *Antimicrob. Agents Chemother.* 60, 3215–3218. doi: 10.1128/AAC.00248-16

Nichols, R. J., Sen, S., Choo, Y. J., Beltrao, P., Zietek, M., Chaba, R., et al. (2011). Phenotypic landscape of a bacterial cell. *Cell* 144, 143–156. doi: 10.1016/j.cell.2010.11.052

Nikaido, H., and Takatsuka, Y. (2009). Mechanisms of RND multidrug efflux pumps. *Biochem. Biophys. Acta* 1794, 769–781. doi: 10.1016/j.bbapap.2008.10.004

Nishino, K., Latifi, T., and Groisman, E. A. (2006). Virulence and drug resistance roles of multidrug efflux systems of *Salmonella enterica* serovar *Typhimurium. Mol. Microbiol.* 59, 126–141. doi: 10.1111/j.1365-2958.2005.04940.x

Norgan, A. P., Freese, J. M., Tuin, P. M., Cunningham, S. A., Jeraldo, P. R., and Patel, R. (2016). Carbapenem- and colistin-resistant *Enterobacter cloacae* from Delta, Colorado, in 2015. *Antimicrob. Agents Chemother.* 60, 3141–3144. doi: 10.1128/AAC.03055-15

Ogawa, W., Minato, Y., Dodan, H., Onishi, M., Tsuchiya, T., and Kuroda, T. (2015). Characterization of MATE-type multidrug efflux pumps from *Klebsiella pneumoniae* MGH78578. *PLoS ONE* 10:e0121619. doi: 10.1371/journal.pone.0121619

Ohene-Agyei, T., Mowla, R., Rahman, T., and Venter, H. (2014). Phytochemicals increase the antibacterial activity of antibiotics by acting on a drug efflux pump. *Microbiologyopen* 3, 885–896. doi: 10.1002/mbo3.212

Okada, U., Yamashita, E., Neuberger, A., Morimoto, M., van Veen, H. W., and Murakami, S. (2017). Crystal structure of tripartite-type ABC transporter MacB from *Acinetobacter baumannii. Nat. Commun*, 8, 1336. doi: 10.1038/s41467-017-01399-2

Opperman, T. J., Kwasny, S. M., Kim, H. S., Nguyen, S. T., Houseweart, C., D'Souza, S., et al. (2014). Characterization of a novel pyranopyridine inhibitor of the AcrAB efflux pump of *Escherichia coli. Antimicrob. Agents Chemother.* 58, 722–733. doi: 10.1128/AAC.01866-13

Opperman, T. J., and Nguyen, S. T. (2015). Recent advances toward a molecular mechanism of efflux pump inhibition. *Front. Microbiol.* 6:421. doi: 10.3389/fmicb.2015.00421

Pagès, J. M., and Amaral, L. (2009). Mechanisms of drug efflux and strategies to combat them: challenging the efflux pump of Gram-negative bacteria. *Biochim. Biophys. Acta, Proteins Proteomics* 1794, 826–833. doi: 10.1016/j.bbapap.2008.12.011

Pettersen, E. F., Goddard, T. D., Huang, C. C., Couch, G. S., Greenblatt, D. M., Meng, E. C., et al. (2004). UCSF Chimera—a visualization system for exploratory research and analysis. *J. Comput. Chem.* 25, 1605–1612. doi: 10.1002/jcc.20084

Piddock, L. J. (2006). Multidrug-resistance efflux pumps-Not just for resistance. *Nat. Rev. Microbiol.* 4, 629–636. doi: 10.1038/nrmicro1464

Piddock, L. J. (2014). Understanding the basis of antibiotic resistance: a platform for drug discovery. *Microbiology* 160, 2366–2373. doi: 10.1099/mic.0.082412-0

Ponnusamy, K., Ramasamy, M., Savarimuthu, I., and Paulraj, M. G. (2010). Indirubin potentiates ciprofloxacin activity in the NorA efflux pump of *Staphylococcus aureus. Scand. J. Infect. Dis.* 42, 500–505. doi: 10.3109/00365541003713630

Poole, K. (2004). Efflux-mediated multiresistance in Gram-negative bacteria. *Clin. Microbiol. Infect.* 10, 12–26. doi: 10.1111/j.1469-0691.2004.00763.x

Poole, K. (2005). Efflux-mediated antimicrobial resistance. *J. Antimicrob. Chemother.* 56, 20–51. doi: 10.1093/jac/dki171

Poole, K. (2007). Efflux pumps as antimicrobial resistance mechanisms. *Ann. Med.* 39, 162–176. doi: 10.1080/07853890701195262

Poole, K., Gotoh, N., Tsujimoto, H., Zhao, Q., Wada, A., Yamasaki, T., et al. (1996). Overexpression of the *mexC - mexD - oprJ* effl ux operon in *nfxB* -type multi drug resistant strains of *Pseudomonas aeruginosa. Mol. Microbiol.* 21, 713–724. doi: 10.1046/j.1365-2958.1996.281397.x

Prasch, S., and Bucar, F. (2015). Plant derived inhibitors of bacterial efflux pumps: an update. *Phytochem. Rev.* 14:961. doi: 10.1007/s11101-015-9436-y

Purssell, A., and Poole, K. (2013). Functional characterization of the NfxB repressor of the mexCD -oprJ multidrug efflux operon of *Pseudomonas aeruginosa. Microbiology* 159, 2058–2073. doi: 10.1099/mic.0.069286-0

Putman, M., van Veen, H., and Konings, W. (2000). Molecular properties of bacterial multidrug transporters. *Microbiol. Mol. Biol. Rev.* 64, 672–693. doi: 10.1128/MMBR.64.4.672-693.2000

Rahman, T., Yarnall, B., and Doyle, D. A. (2017). Efflux drug transporters at the forefront of antimicrobial resistance. *Eur. Biophys. J.* 46, 647–653. doi: 10.1007/s00249-017-1238-2

Rajamohan, G., Srinivasan, V. B., and Gebreyes, W. A. (2010). Novel role of *Acinetobacter baumannii* RND efflux transporters in mediating decreased susceptibility to biocides. *J. Antimicrob. Chemother.* 65, 228–232. doi: 10.1093/jac/dkp427

Ramaswamy, V. K., Cacciotto, P., Malloci, G., Vargiu, A. V., and Ruggerone, P. (2017). Computational modelling of efflux pumps and their inhibitors. *Essays Biochem.* 61, 141–156. doi: 10.1042/EBC20160065

Ramón-García, S., Mick, V., Dainese, E., Martin, C., Thompson, C. J., De Rossi, E., et al. (2012). Functional and genetic characterization of the Tap efflux pump in *Mycobacterium bovis* BCG. *Antimicrob. Agents Chemother.* 56, 2074–2083. doi: 10.1128/AAC.05946-11

Rice, A., Liu, Y., Michaelis, M. L., Himes, R. H., Georg, G. I., and Audus, K. L. (2005). Chemical modification of paclitaxel (Taxol) reduces P-glycoprotein interactions and increases permeation across the blood-brain barrier *in vitro* and *in situ*. *J. Med. Chem.* 48, 832–838. doi: 10.1021/jm040114b

Roca, I., Marti, S., Espinal, P., Martinez, P., Gibert, I., and Vila, J. (2009). CraA: an MFS efflux pump associated with chloramphenicol resistance in *Acinetobacter baumannii*. *Antimicrob. Agents Chemother.* 53, 4013–4014. doi: 10.1128/AAC.00584-09

Rodrigues, L., Villellas, C., Bailo, R., Viveiros, M., and Ainsa, J. A. (2013). Role of the Mmr efflux pump in drug resistance in *Mycobacterium tuberculosis*. *Antimicrob. Agents Chemother.* 57, 751– 757. doi: 10.1128/AAC.01482-12

Roy, S., Pahwa, S., Nandanwar, H., and Jachak, S. (2012). Phenylpropanoids of *Alpinia galanga* as efflux pump inhibitors in *Mycobacterium smegmatis* mc2 155. *Fitoterapia* 83, 1248–1255. doi: 10.1016/j.fitote.2012.06.008

Roy, S. K., Kumari, N., Pahwa, S., Agrahari, U. C., Bhutani, K. K., Jachak, S. M., et al. (2013). NorA efflux pump inhibitory activity of coumarins from *Mesua ferrea*. *Fitoterapia* 90, 140–150. doi: 10.1016/j.fitote.2013.07.015

Ruzin, A., Keeney, D., and Bradford, P. A. (2007). AdeABC multidrug efflux pump is associated with decreased susceptibility to tigecycline in *Acinetobacter calcoaceticus-Acinetobacter baumannii* complex. *J. Antimicrob. Chemother.* 59, 1001–1004. doi: 10.1093/jac/dkm058

Sabatini, S., Piccioni, M., Felicetti, T., De Marco, S., Manfroni, G., Pagiotti, R., et al. (2017). Investigation on the effect of known potent *S. aureus* NorA efflux pump inhibitors on the staphylococcal biofilm formation. *RSC Adv.* 7, 37007–37014. doi: 10.1039/C7RA03859C

Saier, M. H., Paulsen, I. T., Sliwinski, M. K., Pao, S. S., and Skurray, R. A. (1998). Evolutionary origins of multidrug and drug-specific efflux pumps in bacteria. *FASEB J.* 12, 265–274. doi: 10.1096/fasebj.12.3.265

Santajit, S., and Indrawattana, N. (2016). Mechanisms of antimicrobial resistance in ESKAPE pathogens. *Biomed Res. Int.* 2016:2475067. doi: 10.1155/2016/2475067

Schindler, B. D., and Kaatz, G. W. (2016). Multidrug efflux pumps of Gram-positive bacteria. *Drug Resist. Updat.* 27, 1–13. doi: 10.1016/j.drup.2016.04.003

Schuldiner, S. (2009). EmrE, a model for studying evolution and mechanism of ion-coupled transporters. *Biochim. Biophys. Acta* 1794,748–762. doi: 10.1016/j.bbapap.2008.12.018

Sharma, S., Kumar, M., Sharma, S., Nargotra, A., Koul, S., and Khan, I. A. (2010). Piperine as an inhibitor of Rv1258c, a putative multidrug efflux pump of *Mycobacterium tuberculosis*. *J. Antimicrob. Chemother.* 65, 1694–1701. doi: 10.1093/jac/dkq186

Shigemura, K., Osawa, K., Kato, A., Tokimatsu, I., Arakawa, S., Shirakawa, T., et al. (2015). Association of overexpression of efflux pump genes with antibiotic resistance in *Pseudomonas aeruginosa* strains clinically isolated from urinary tract infection patients. *J. Antibiot.* 68, 568. doi: 10.1038/ja.2015.34

Shin, J., Prabhakaran, V. S., and Kim, K. S. (2018). The multi-faceted potential of plant-derived metabolites as antimicrobial agents against multidrug-resistant pathogens. *Microb. Pathog.* 116, 209–214. doi: 10.1016/j.micpath.2018.01.043

Shiu, W., Malkinson, J., Rahman, M., Curry, J., Stapleton, P., Gunaratnam, M., et al. (2013). A new plant-derived antibacterial is an inhibitor of efflux pumps in *Staphylococcus aureus*. *Int. J. Antimicrob. Agents* 42, 513–518. doi: 10.1016/j.ijantimicag.2013.08.007

Silhavy, T. J., Kahne, D., and Walker, S. (2010). The bacterial cell envelope. *Cold Spring Harb. Perspect. Biol.* 2:a000414. doi: 10.1101/cshperspect.a0 00414

Siriyong, T., Srimanote, P., Chusri, S., Yingyongnarongkul, B. E., Suaisom, C., Tipmanee, V., et al. (2017). Conessine as a novel inhibitor of multidrug efflux pump systems in *Pseudomonas aeruginosa*. *BMC Complement. Altern. Med.* 17:405. doi: 10.1186/s12906-017-1913-y

Spengler, G., Kincses, A., Gajdacs, M., and Amaral, L. (2017). New roads leading to old destinations: efflux pumps as targets to reverse multidrug resistance in bacteria. *Molecules* 22:468. doi: 10.3390/molecules22030468

Srinivasan, V. B., and Rajamohan, G. (2013). KpnEF, a new member of the *Klebsiella pneumonia* cell envelope stress response regulon, is an SMR-type efflux pump involved in broadspectrum antimicrobial resistance. *Antimicrob. Agents Chemother.* 57, 4449–4462. doi: 10.1128/AAC.02284-12

Srinivasan, V. B., Singh, B. B., Priyadarshi, N., Chauhan, N. K., and Rajamohan, G. (2014). Role of novel multidrug efflux pump involved in drug resistance in *Klebsiella pneumoniae*. *PLoS ONE* 9:e96288. doi: 10.1371/journal.pone.0096288

Stavri, M., Piddock, L., and Gibbons, S. (2007). Bacterial efflux pump inhibitors from natural sources. *J. Antimicrob. Chemother.* 59, 1247–1260. doi: 10.1093/jac/dkl460

Su, X. Z., Chen, J., Mizushima, T., Kuroda, T., and Tsuchiya, T. (2005). AbeM, an $H^+$-coupled *Acinetobacter baumannii* multidrug efflux pump belonging to the MATE family of transporters. *Antimicrob. Agents Chemother.* 49, 4362–4364. doi: 10.1128/AAC.49.10.4362-4364.2005

Sun, J., Deng, Z., and Yan, A. (2014). Bacterial multidrug efflux pumps: Mechanisms, physiology and pharmacological exploitations. *Biochem. Biophys. Res. Commun.* 453, 254–267. doi: 10.1016/j.bbrc.2014.05.090

Suresh, M., Nithya, N., Jayasree, P. R., Vimal, K. P., and Kumar, P. M. (2018). Mutational analyses of regulatory genes, *mexR*, *nalC*, *nalD* and *mexZ* of *mexAB-oprM*and *mexXY* operons, in efflux pump hyperexpressing multidrug-resistant clinical isolates of *Pseudomonas aeruginosa*. *World J. Microbiol. Biotechnol.* 34, 83. doi: 10.1007/s11274-018-2465-0

Suriyanarayanan, B., and Sarojini, S. R. (2015). Docking analysis insights quercetin can be a non-antibiotic adjuvant by inhibiting Mmr drug efflux pump in Mycobacterium sp. and its homologue EmrE in *Escherichia coli*. *J. Biomol. Struct. Dyn.* 33, 1819–1834. doi: 10.1080/07391102.2014.974211

Swick, M. C., Morgan-Linnell, S. K., Carlson, K. M., and Zechiedrich, L. (2011). Expression of multidrug efflux pump genes *acrAB-tolC*, *mdfA*, and *norE* in *Escherichia coli* clinical isolates as a function of fluoroquinolone and multidrug resistance. *Antimicrob. Agents Chemother.* 55, 921–924. doi: 10.1128/AAC.00996-10

Tait-Kamradt, A., Clancy, J., Cronan, M., Dib-Hajj, F., Wondrack, L., Yuan, W., et al. (1997). *mefE* is necessary for the erythromycin-resistant M phenotype in *Streptococcus pneumoniae*. *Antimicrob. Agents Chemother.* 41, 2251–2255. doi: 10.1128/AAC.41.10.2251

Telke, A. A., Olaitan, A. O., Morand, S., and Rolain, J-M. (2017). *soxRS* indices colistin hetero-resistance in *Enterobacter asburiae* and *Enterobacter cloacae* by regulating the acrAB-tolC efflux pump. *J. Antimicrob. Chemother.* 72, 2715–2721. doi: 10.1093/jac/dkx215

Tikhonova, E. B., Yamada, Y., and Zgurskaya, H. I. (2011). Sequential mechanism of assembly of multidrug efflux pump AcrAB-TolC. *Chem. Biol.* 18, 454–463. doi: 10.1016/j.chembiol.2011.02.011

Vargiu, A. V., Ramaswamy, V. K., Malvacio, I., Malloci, G., Kleinekathöfer, U., and Ruggerone, P. (2018). Water-mediated interactions enable smooth substrate transport in a bacterial efflux pump. *Biochim. Biophys. Acta Gen. Sub.* 1862, 836–845. doi: 10.1016/j.bbagen.2018.01.010

Venter, H., Mowla, R., Ohene-Agyei, T., and Ma, S. (2015). RND-type drug efflux pumps from Gram-negative bacteria: molecular mechanism and inhibition. *Front. Microbiol.* 6:377. doi: 10.3389/fmicb.2015.00377

Verma, P., Tiwari, M., and Tiwari, V. (2017). *In silico* high-throughput virtual screening and molecular dynamics simulation study to identify inhibitor for AdeABC efflux pump of *Acinetobacter baumannii*. *J. Biomol. Struct. Dyn.* 36, 1182–1194. doi: 10.1080/07391102.2017.1317025

Vimberg, V., Lenart, J., Janata, J., and Balikova Novotna, G. (2015). ClpP-independent function of ClpX interferes with telithromycin resistance conferred by Msr(A) in *Staphylococcus aureus*. *Antimicrob. Agents Chemother.* 59, 3611–3614. doi: 10.1128/AAC.04367-14

Viveiros, M., Jesus, A., Brito, M., Leandro, C., Martins, M., Ordway, D., et al. (2005). Inducement and reversal of tetracycline resistance in *Escherichia coli* K-12 and expression of proton gradient-dependent multidrug efflux pump genes. *Antimicrob. Agents Chemother.* 49, 3578–3582. doi: 10.1128/AAC.49.8.3578-3582.2005

Ward, A., Hoyle, C., Palmer, S., O'Reilly, J., and Griffith, J. (2001). Prokaryote multidrug efflux proteins of the major facilitator superfamily: amplified expression, purification and characterisation. *J. Mol. Microbiol. Biotechnol.* 3, 193–200.

Warner, D. M., and Levy, S. B. (2010). Different effects of transcriptional regulators MarA, SoxS and Rob on susceptibility of *Escherichia coli* to cationic antimicrobial peptides (CAMPs): rob-dependent CAMP induction of the *marRAB* operon. *Microbiol.* 156, 570–578. doi: 10.1099/mic.0.033415-0

Watanabe, T. (1963). Infective heredity of multiple drug resistance in bacteria. *Bacteriol. Rev.* 27, 87–115.

Welch, A., Awah, C. U., Jing, S., van Veen, H. W., and Venter, H. (2010). Promiscuous partnering and independent activity of MexB, the multidrug transporter protein from *Pseudomonas aeruginosa*. *Biochem. J.* 430, 355–364. doi: 10.1042/BJ20091860

Wendlandt, S., Kadlec, K., Fessler, A. T., and Schwarz, S. (2015). Identification of ABC transporter genes conferring combined pleuromutilin-lincosamide-streptogramin A resistance in bovine methicillin- resistant *Staphylococcus aureus* and coagulase-negative staphylococci. *Vet. Microbiol.* 177, 353–358. doi: 10.1016/j.vetmic.2015.03.027

Willers, C., Wentzel, J. F., du Plessis, L. H., Gouws, C., and Hamman, J. H. (2016). Efflux as a mechanism of antimicrobial drug resistance in clinical relevant microorganisms: the role of efflux inhibitors. *Expert Opin. Ther. Targets* 21, 23–36. doi: 10.1080/14728222.2017.1265105

World Economic Forum (2013). *Global Risks, Eighth Edition Ed. 2013.* 28–33. Available online at: http://www3.weforum.org/docs/WEF_GlobalRisks_Report_2013.pdf (Accessed March 15, 2018).

World Health Organization (2014). *Antimicrobial Resistance.* Available online at: http://www.searo.who.int/thailand/factsheets/fs0023/en/ (Accessed October 22, 2018).

Wright, G. D. (2016). Antibiotic adjuvants: Rescuing antibiotics from resistance. *Trends Microbiol.* 24, 862–871. doi: 10.1016/j.tim.2016.06.009

Yaffe, D., Radestock, S., Shuster, Y., Forrest, L. R., and Schuldiner, S. (2013). Identification of molecular hinge points mediating alternating access in the vesicular monoamine transporter VMAT2. *Proc. Natl. Acad. Sci. U.S.A.* 110, E1332–1341. doi: 10.1073/pnas.1220497110

Yang, S., Lopez, C. R., and Zechiedrich, E. L. (2006). Quorum sensing and multidrug transporters in *Escherichia coli*. *Proc. Natl. Acad. Sci. U.S.A.*103, 2386–2391. doi: 10.1073/pnas.0502890102

Yang, S. K., Low, L. Y., Yap, P. S. X., Yusoff, K., Mai, C. W., Lai, K. S., et al. (2018). Plant-Derived Antimicrobials: Insights into Mitigation of Antimicrobial Resistance. *Rec. Nat. Prod.* 12, 295–316. doi: 10.25135/rnp.41.17.09.058

Yasufuku, T., Shigemura, K., Shirakawa, T., Matsumoto, M., Nakano, Y., Tanaka, K., et al. (2011). Correlation of overexpression of efflux pump genes with antibiotic resistance in *Escherichia coli* strains clinically isolated from urinary tract infection patients. *J. Clin. Microbiol.* 49, 189–194. doi: 10.1128/JCM.00827-10

Yoshida, H., Bogaki, M., Nakamura, S., Ubukata, K., and Konno, M. (1990). Nucleotide sequence and characterization of the *Staphylococcus aureus norA* gene, which confers resistance to quinolones. *J. Bacteriol.* 172, 6942–6949. doi: 10.1128/jb.172.12.6942-6949.1990

Zeng, B., Wang, H., Zou, L., Zhang, A., Yang, X., and Guan, Z. (2010). Evaluation and target validation of indole derivatives as inhibitors of the AcrAB-TolC efflux pump. *Biosci. Biotechnol. Biochem.* 74, 2237–2241. doi: 10.1271/bbb.100433

Zgurskaya, H. I., Lopez, C. A., and Gnanakaran, S. (2015). Permeability barrier of Gram-negative cell envelopes and approaches to bypass it. *ACS Infect. Dis.* 1, 512–522. doi: 10.1021/acsinfecdis.5b00097

Zhang, J., Sun, Y., Wang, Y., Lu, M., He, J., Liu, J., et al. (2014). Non-antibiotic agent ginsenoside 20(S)-Rh2 enhanced the antibacterial effects of ciprofloxacin *in vitro* and *in vivo* as a potential NorA inhibitor. *Eur. J. Pharmacol.* 740, 277–284. doi: 10.1016/j.ejphar.2014.07.020

# 8

# Herring Oil and Omega Fatty Acids Inhibit *Staphylococcus aureus* Biofilm Formation and Virulence

*Yong-Guy Kim[1†], Jin-Hyung Lee[1†], Chaitany J. Raorane[1], Seong T. Oh[2], Jae G. Park[3*] and Jintae Lee[1*]*

*[1] School of Chemical Engineering, Yeungnam University, Gyeongsan, South Korea, [2] College of Pharmacy, Yeungnam University, Gyeongsan, South Korea, [3] Advanced Bio Convergence Center, Pohang Technopark Foundation, Pohang, South Korea*

***Correspondence:**
*Jae G. Park*
*jaepark@pohangtp.org*
*Jintae Lee*
*jtlee@ynu.ac.kr*

*† These authors have contributed equally to this work.*

*Staphylococcus aureus* is notorious for its ability to become resistant to antibiotics and biofilms play a critical role in antibiotic tolerance. *S. aureus* is also capable of secreting several exotoxins associated with the pathogenesis of sepsis and pneumonia. Thus, the objectives of the study were to examine *S. aureus* biofilm formation *in vitro*, and the effects of herring oil and its main components, omega fatty acids [*cis*-4,7,10,13,16,19-docosahexaenoic acid (DHA) and *cis*-5,8,11,14,17-eicosapentaenoic acid (EPA)], on virulence factor production and transcriptional changes in *S. aureus*. Herring oil decreased biofilm formation by two *S. aureus* strains. GC-MS analysis revealed the presence of several polyunsaturated fatty acids in herring oil, and of these, two omega-3 fatty acids, DHA and EPA, significantly inhibited *S. aureus* biofilm formation. In addition, herring oil, DHA, and EPA at 20 μg/ml significantly decreased the hemolytic effect of *S. aureus* on human red blood cells, and when pre-treated to *S. aureus*, the bacterium was more easily killed by human whole blood. Transcriptional analysis showed that herring oil, DHA, and EPA repressed the expression of the α-hemolysin *hla* gene. Furthermore, in a *Caenorhabditis elegans* nematode model, all three prolonged nematode survival in the presence of *S. aureus*. These findings suggest that herring oil, DHA, and EPA are potentially useful for controlling persistent *S. aureus* infection.

**Keywords: biofilm, hemolysis, herring oil, omega fatty acids, *Staphylococcus aureus*, virulence**

## INTRODUCTION

The sticky conglomerations of bacteria that adhere to diverse medical devices or damaged body tissues can become causes of persistent infections. These bacteria encase themselves in a slime layer or biofilm, which poses serious problems to human health because of their abilities to tolerate conventional antibiotic chemotherapies, host immune systems, and external stresses (Potera, 1999; Hoffman et al., 2005).

*Staphylococcus aureus* is an important etiologic agent and a major cause of a diverse array of acute life-threatening bloodstream infections in man, and is often held responsible for worldwide outbreaks of nosocomial infections (Lowy, 1998). *S. aureus* biofilms play a critical role in antibiotic tolerance (Stewart and Costerton, 2001), and methicillin-resistant *S. aureus* (MRSA) and vancomycin-resistant *S. aureus* have become major nosocomial threats

(Speller et al., 1997). *S. aureus* secretes many exotoxins, including coagulase, enterotoxins, α-hemolysin, protein A, and TSST-1, which damage biological membranes and eventually cause cell death (Ohlsen et al., 1997; Otto, 2014). Also, *S. aureus* biofilms are found in medical devices and food surfaces, and are responsible for food-poisoning and toxic shock syndrome (Chambers and Deleo, 2009). In particular, α-hemolysin (Hla) is a major cytotoxic agent that has been associated with the pathogeneses of pneumonia, sepsis, and severe skin infections (Menzies and Kernodle, 1996; Wilke and Bubeck Wardenburg, 2010) and with biofilm formation (Caiazza and O'Toole, 2003). *S. aureus* biofilms also play a dominant role in the determination of disease severity and postoperative course (Singhal et al., 2011). Therefore, it is important to find means to inhibit biofilm formation and the virulent characteristics of *S. aureus*. For this purpose, novel and non-toxic compounds that prevent the development of drug tolerance are urgently required.

Semi-dried raw Pacific herring (*Clupea pallasi*), also known as Gwamegi (a Korean traditional food), is an important fishery product with a unique flavor, taste, and texture (Lee et al., 2002; Kang et al., 2011). Herring oil contains an abundance of two rare omega-3 polyunsaturated fatty acids (PUFAs), namely, docosahexaenoic acid (DHA; C22:6, ω-3) and eicosapentaenoic acid (EPA; C20:5, ω-3), which are commonly present at low concentrations in non-marine animals and are beneficial to the human body (Hirai et al., 1980; Schmidt and Dyerberg, 1994). Furthermore, it has been reported that two PUFAs act as bacteriocides on Gram-positive and Gram-negative bacteria, such as, *Helicobacter pylori* (Correia et al., 2012), *Burkholderia cenocepacia* (Mil-Homens et al., 2012), *S. aureus* (Desbois et al., 2009), *Fusobacterium nucleatum, Porphyromonas gingivalis*, and *Streptococcus mutans* (Huang and Ebersole, 2010; Sun et al., 2016, 2017). These two PUFAs have also been reported to possess significant anti-inflammatory, anti-tumorigenic (Bougnoux, 1999; Van Dyke, 2008), and antioxidant activities (Giordano and Visioli, 2014). Huang and Ebersole (2010), Sun et al. (2016, 2017) and Thibane et al. (2010) suggested that DHA and EPA could be considered as potential supplementary therapeutic agents due to their anti-biofilm activities on *Candida* species and periodontopathic bacteria. However, the abilities of DHA and EPA to inhibit biofilm formation and virulence production by *S. aureus* have not been assessed.

Therefore, the phenotypic effects of herring oil were studied and its active constituents were identified by gas chromatography-mass spectrometry (GC-MS). Two of its major constituents (DHA and EPA) were further investigated by confocal laser scanning microscopy (CSLM) and using a human blood assay to determine their effects on biofilm formation and toxin production by *S. aureus*. A *Caenorhabditis elegans* model was used to investigate the anti-virulent properties of herring oil, DHA, and EPA. qRT-PCR (quantitative real-time reverse transcription polymerase chain reaction) was used to investigate their effects on the transcriptional profiles of genes related to biofilm formation and virulence production *in vitro*.

## MATERIALS AND METHODS

### Ethics Statement

Human blood assays were authorized by the Ethical Committee of Yeungnam University (Gyeongsan, South Korea). The study was conducted according to the guidelines issued by the Ethical Committee of Yeungnam University. All blood donors provided written consent before blood collection.

### Bacterial Strains, Materials, and Growth Assay

A methicillin-sensitive *S. aureus* strain (MSSA; ATCC 6538) and a methicillin-resistant *S. aureus* strain (MRSA; ATCC 33591) were used in the present study. All experiments were conducted at 37°C in Luria-Bertani (LB) broth for the MSSA strain and in LB broth containing 0.2% glucose for the MRSA strain. Herring (*Clupea pallasii*) oil was prepared from semi-dried fish bodies without organs (so called Gwamegi, Korean traditional food). Herring was dried at open air condition for 20 days in winter at Pohang, Korea. The semi-dried herring (764 g) was further dried in a freezing drier for 3 days to gain 586 g of dried herring. Then it was chopped, and the oil was extracted by soxhlet apparatus that was refluxed with n-hexane for a day at 70°C. After refluxing, the residual solution was collected and washed with 1% AcOH solution and brine to remove excess protein. Washed oil was dried over anhydrous $MgSO_4$ to gain clear yellow viscous oil (267 g, 45.6% yield). The omega fatty acids (*cis*-4,7,10,13,16,19-DHA, *cis*-5,8,11,14,17-EPA, *cis*-11-eicosenoic acid, and erucic acid), crystal violet, ethanol, ciprofloxacin, vancomycin and glucose were purchased from Sigma-Aldrich (St. Louis, MO, United States). For cell growth assays, optical densities were measured at 600 nm using a spectrophotometer (Optizen 2120UV, Mecasys, South Korea). To determine MIC (minimum inhibitory concentration), cells were inoculated into LB broth and cultured overnight at a dilution of 1:100 at 37°C, and then incubated for 24 h in the presence of a test substance. After sequential dilutions, cultures were spread on LB agar plates, incubated for 24 h at 37°C, and numbers of colonies were counted. Each experiment was performed using at least four independent cultures.

### Gas Chromatograph/Mass Spectroscopy (GC-MS)

The chemical composition of air-dried herring oil was determined by GC using an Agilent 6890N GC and SP-2560 (Supelco, Sigma-Aldrich, St. Louis, MO, United States) fused silica capillary column (100 m × 0.25 mm i.d., film thickness 0.25 μm). Capillary column details, temperature conditions, and the derivatization (methylation) of fatty acids were as previously described (Lee et al., 2017). In brief, helium was used as the carrier at 0.75 ml/min and the GC injector was held at 225°C. The GC oven temperature was programmed as follows; 100°C for 4 min, increased to 240°C at 3°C/min, and followed by 15 min at 250°C. The split ratio was controlled at 200:1. Triundecanoin ($C_{11:00}$) was used as the internal standard and quantifications were performed by integrating areas and correcting for fatty acid

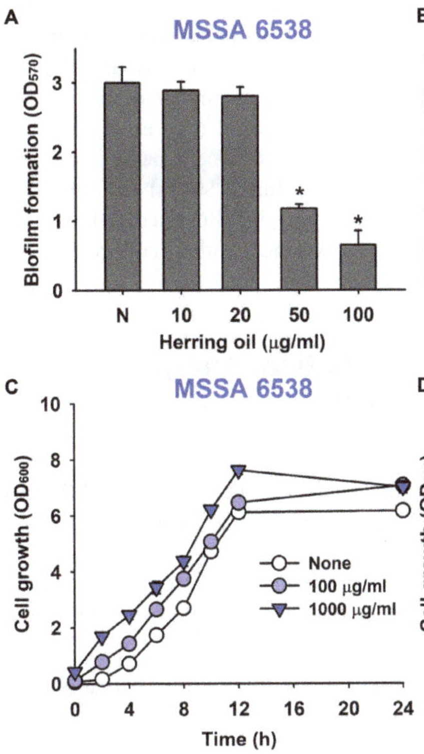


**FIGURE 1 |** Effects of herring oil on biofilm formation by *Staphylococcus aureus* strains and on their antimicrobial activities. *S. aureus* (MSSA 6538 or MRSA 33591) biofilm formations ($OD_{570}$) were quantified in the presence of herring oil for 24 h in 96-well polystyrene plates **(A,B)**. Planktonic cell growths ($OD_{600}$) of *S. aureus* cells (MSSA 6538 and MRSA 33591) were measured in the presence of herring oil in 250 ml flasks agitated at 250 rpm **(C,D)**. $^*p < 0.05$ vs. non-treated controls.

methylation. Supelco 37 components FAME Mix (Supelco) were used as the reference standard.

## Crystal-Violet Biofilm Assay

The two bacterial strains (MSSA 6538, MRSA 33591) were subjected to a static biofilm formation assay on 96-well polystyrene plates (SPL Life Sciences, South Korea), as previously described (Kim et al., 2015). Briefly, cells were inoculated into LB broth (300 μl) at an initial turbidity of 0.05 at 600 nm and herring oil, *cis*-11-eicosenoic acid, DHA, EPA, or erucic acid were added at different concentrations and incubated for 24 h without shaking at 37°C. To quantify biofilm formation, cell cultures were washed three times with water and then biofilms were stained with 0.1% crystal violet for 20 min. Biofilms were then dissolved in 300 μl of 95% ethanol and absorbances were measured at 570 nm ($OD_{570}$). For the biofilm dispersion assay, *S. aureus* was cultured in 96-well plates for 24 h without shaking at 37°C. Then, herring oil, DHA, or EPA was added to the cultures and incubated for another 10 h before the biofilm assay. Static biofilm formation results are the averages of four independent cultures of twelve replicate wells.

## Confocal Laser Scanning Microscopy and COMSTAT Analysis

Static biofilm formation by *S. aureus* (MSSA 6538) in 96-well plates (without shaking) in the presence or absence of herring oil, DHA, or EPA were assessed by confocal laser scanning microscopy (Nikon Eclipse Ti, Tokyo, Japan). Cells were stained with carboxyfluorescein diacetate succinimidyl ester (Invitrogen, Molecular Probes Inc., Eugene, OR, United States), which stains viable cells in biofilms, as previously reported (Lee et al., 2016). Stained *S. aureus* ATCC 6538 biofilms were visualized by confocal laser scanning microscopy using an Ar laser (excitation wavelength 488 nm, and emission wavelength 500–550 nm) and a 20× objective. Color confocal images were constructed using NIS-Elements C version 3.2 (Nikon eclipse) under the same conditions. For each experiment, at least 10 random positions in two independent cultures were observed, and 20 planar images were analyzed per position. To quantify biofilm formation, COMSTAT biofilm software (Heydorn et al., 2000) was used to measure biovolumes ($\mu m^3$ per $\mu m^2$), mean thicknesses (μm), and substratum coverages (%). Thresholds were fixed for all image stacks, and at least 4 positions and 20 planar images were analyzed per position.

## Hemolysis Assay

Human red blood cell hemolysis efficacies were assayed using whole cultures of *S. aureus*, as described previously (Lee et al., 2013; Tharmalingam et al., 2018). Briefly, *S. aureus* cells (MSSA 6538) were diluted 1:100 in LB broth ($9 \times 10^9$ CFU/ml) with overnight culture and incubated with or without herring oil, DHA, or EPA for 20 h with shaking at 250 rpm. Separately, human whole blood samples were centrifuged at 900g for 2 min and then washed three times with PBS and diluted in PBS (330 μl of red blood cells per 10 ml of PBS buffer). Bacterial culture (200 μl) was then added to 1 ml of diluted human red blood cells (3.3% in PBS). To determine hemolytic activities, mixtures of blood and *S. aureus* were incubated at 250 rpm for 2 h at 37°C. Supernatants were collected by centrifugation at 16,600 *g* for 10 min and optical densities were measured at 543 nm.

## Whole Blood Bacterial Cell Killing Assay

The whole blood cell killing assay used was as previously described (Liu et al., 2008). Briefly, *S. aureus* (MSSA 6538) cells were inoculated (1:100 dilution, $OD_{600}$ ~0.05) in LB broth with overnight culture and incubated at 37°C for 20 h with shaking at 250 rpm with herring oil, DHA, or EPA (1, 5, or 20 μg/ml) or DMSO (the negative control). Freshly drawn human whole blood (0.3 ml) was then mixed with the *S. aureus* cultures (0.1 ml), and mixtures were incubated at 37°C for 3 h with shaking at 250 rpm. *S. aureus* (MSSA 6538) survival was measured by counting CFUs on LB agar plates.

## *Caenorhabditis elegans* Survival Assay

To investigate the effects of herring oil and unsaturated fatty acids on the virulence of *S. aureus* MSSA 6538, we used a nematode survival assay as previously described (Kim et al., 2016) with slight modification. In brief, *S. aureus* cells were incubated with or without herring oil, DHA, or EPA (2, 5, or 20 μg/ml) at 37°C for 24 h and synchronized adult *C. elegans fer-15;fem-1* nematodes were added into single wells of 96-well plate containing cultivated *S. aureus* cells. Approximately, 30 nematodes were allowed to feed on the cultured *S. aureus* MSSA 6538 at 25°C for 1 day.

For the cytotoxicity assay, 110 ± 10 nematodes were added into single well of 96-well plates containing M9 buffer and solutions of the compounds were added to final concentrations of 20 or 100 μg/ml at 25°C for 1 day. Then, nematodes were scored as alive or dead using an iRiS™ Digital Cell Imaging System (Logos Bio Systems, South Korea). At least three independent experiments were conducted using quadruplicate wells.

## RNA Isolation and qRT-PCR

*Staphylococcus aureus* MSSA 6538 cells were inoculated into 25 ml of LB broth at 37°C in 250 ml flasks at a starting $OD_{600}$ of 0.05, and then incubated for 5 h with shaking at 250 rpm in the presence or absence of herring oil (100 μg/ml), DHA, or EPA (20 μg/ml). RNase inhibitor (RNAlater, Ambion, TX, United States) was then added and cells were immediately chilled for 30 s in dry ice bath having 95% ethanol to prevent RNA degradation. Cells were then harvested by centrifugation at 16,600 *g* for 1 min and total RNA was isolated using a Qiagen RNeasy mini Kit (Valencia, CA, United States).

Quantitative real-time reverse transcription polymerase chain reaction was used to investigate the transcriptional levels of 10 biofilm-related genes, that are, *agrA*, *arlR*, *arlS*, *aur*, *hla*, *icaA*, *nuc1*, *rbf*, *RNAIII*, *saeR*, *sarA*, *sarZ*, *seb*, *sigB*, and *spa* in *S. aureus* MSSA 6538 cells. Gene specific primers were used and 16s rRNA was used as the housekeeping control (Supplementary Table S1) to normalize the expressions of genes of interest. The qRT-PCR technique employed was an adaptation of a previously described method (Lee et al., 2016). qRT-PCR was performed using a SYBR Green master mix (Applied Biosystems, Foster City, CA, United States) and an ABI StepOne Real-Time PCR System (Applied Biosystems). Expression levels were determined using two independent cultures and six qRT-PCR reactions per gene.

## Statistical Analysis

Values were expressed as means ± standard deviations, and data were analyzed by one-way ANOVA followed by Dunnett's test using SPSS version 23 (SPSS Inc., Chicago, IL, United States) to determine the significances of differences. Statistical significance was accepted for $p$-values of <0.05.

**TABLE 1** | Herring oil – GC-MS analysis.

| Lipid number | Fatty acid name | Composition (%) |
|---|---|---|
| C12:0 | Lauric acid | 0.13 |
| C13:0 | Tridecanoic acid | 0.03 |
| **C14:0** | **Myristic acid** | **5.78** |
| C14:1 | Tetradecenoic | 0.05 |
| C15:0 | Pentadecanoic acid | 0.45 |
| **C16:0** | **Palmitic acid** | **8.18** |
| C16:1 | Palmitoleic acid | 2.15 |
| C17:0 | Heptadecanoic acid | 0.36 |
| C17:1 | *cis*-10-Heptadecenoic aid | 0.05 |
| C18:0 | Stearic acid | 1.35 |
| C18:1n-9,trans | Elaidic acid | 0.09 |
| C18:1n-9,cis | Oleic acid | 2.72 |
| C18:2n-6,cis | Linoleic acid | 1.11 |
| C18:3n-6 | γ-Linolenic acid | 0.20 |
| **C20:1** | ***cis*-11-Eicosenoic acid** | **9.75** |
| C18:3n-3 | α-Linolenic acid | 1.23 |
| C21:0 | Heneicosanoic acid | 0.22 |
| C20:2n-6 | Eicosadienoic acid | 3.80 |
| C22:0 | Behenic acid | 0.05 |
| C20:3n-6 | Dihomo-γ-Linolenic acid | 0.07 |
| **C22:1n-9** | **Erucic acid** | **17.49** |
| C20:3n-3 | *cis*-11,14,17-Eicosatrienoic acid | 0.1 |
| C23:0 | Tricosanoic acid | 0.24 |
| C22:2 | Docosadienoic acid | 0.91 |
| C24:0 | Lignoceric acid | 0.02 |
| **C20:5n-3** | ***cis*-5,8,11,14,17-Eicosapentaenoic acid (EPA)** | **5.78** |
| C24:1 | Nervonic acid | 0.93 |
| **C22:6n-3** | ***cis*-4,7,10,13,16,19-Docosahexaenoic acid (DHA)** | **11.31** |

*Components present at levels >5% by weight are shown in blue/bold font.*

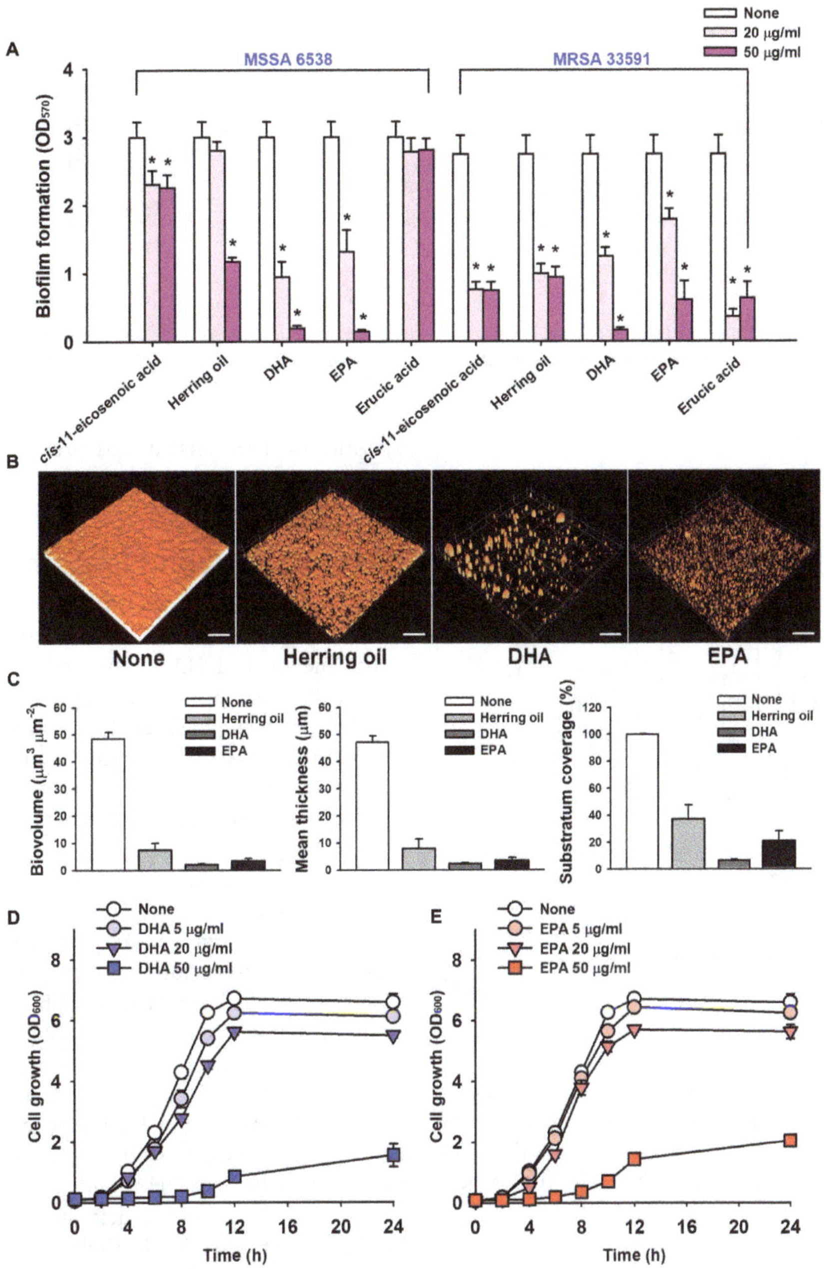


**FIGURE 2 |** Inhibitions of biofilm formation by herring oil, DHA, and EPA. Biofilm formations by the two *S. aureus* strains were quantified in the presence of *cis*-11-eicosenoic acid, herring oil, DHA, EPA, and erucic acid at 20 or 50 μg/ml after incubation for 24 h in 96-well polystyrene plates without agitation **(A)**. Biofilm formation of *S. aureus* MSSA 6538 was observed after 24 h in the presence of herring oil (50 μg/ml), DHA (20 μg/ml), or EPA (20 μg/ml) in 96-well plates by confocal laser scanning microscopy **(B)**. The scale bars represent 100 μm. Biofilm formation was analyzed using COMSTAT **(C)**. Cell growth of *S. aureus* MSSA 6538 was measured in the presence of DHA or EPA **(D,E)**. $^*p < 0.05$ vs. non-treated controls.

## RESULTS AND DISCUSSION

### Effect of Herring Oil on *S. aureus* Biofilm Formation

The anti-biofilm activity of herring oil was investigated against two *S. aureus* strains (MSSA 6538 and MRSA 33591) in 96-well polystyrene plates. The addition of herring oil at the beginning of bacterial culture dose-dependently inhibited *S. aureus* biofilm formation (**Figures 1A,B**). Specifically, herring oil at 100 μg/ml reduced biofilm formation by MSSA 6538 by >75%, whereas 20 μg/ml was required to inhibit biofilm formation by MRSA 33591 by >65%.

Herring oil did not decrease the growth of *S. aureus* strains (MSSA 6538 and MRSA 33591) at concentrations up

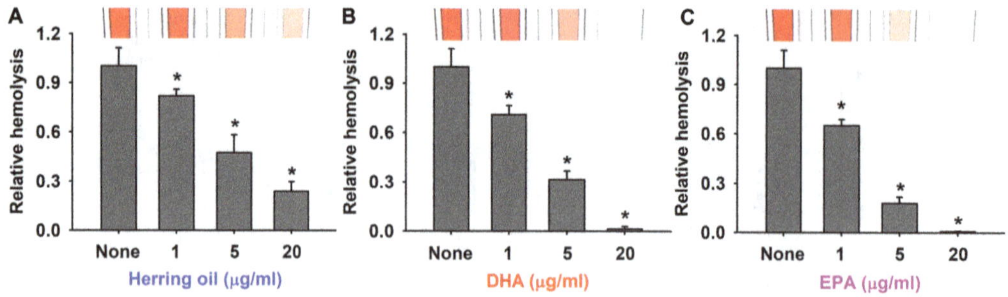


**FIGURE 3 |** Anti-hemolytic activities of herring oil, DHA, and EPA. Human red blood cell hemolysis by *S. aureus* was investigated in the presence of herring oil **(A)**, DHA **(B)**, or EPA **(C)** after culture for 20 h. The images show hemolysis activities in spectrophotometer cuvettes. $^*p < 0.05$ vs. non-treated controls.

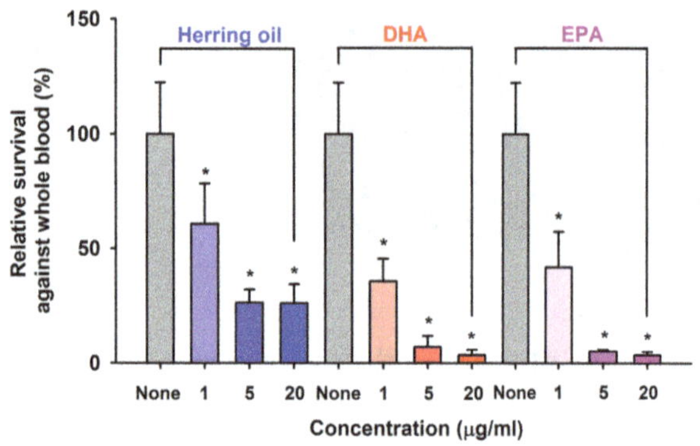


**FIGURE 4 |** Killing of *S. aureus* by whole blood cells in the presence of herring oil, DHA, or EPA. *S. aureus* cells were cultured in the presence of herring oil, DHA, or EPA at 1, 5, and 20 μg/ml for 20 h, then mixed with freshly drawn human whole blood and cultured for 3 h. Percent survival of *S. aureus* treated with or without the test compounds is represented. $^*p < 0.05$ vs. non-treated controls.

to 1000 μg/ml (**Figures 1C,D**), and did not affect planktonic cell numbers of either *S. aureus* strain at concentrations up to 1000 μg/ml (data not shown). These findings show the anti-biofilm activity of herring oil was not due to any bactericidal effects.

## Identification of Main Components in Herring Oil

Gas chromatography-mass spectrometry identified 28 fatty acids in herring oil (**Table 1**). Components that constituted more than 5% of herring oil were; erucic acid (17.49%), *cis*-4,7,10,13,16,19-DHA (11.31%), *cis*-11-eicosenoic acid (9.75%), palmitic acid (8.18%), myristic acid (5.78%), and *cis*-5,8,11,14,17-EPA (5.78%) (**Table 1**). The compositions of herring oil identified by GC-MS analysis concur with previous studies (Lambertsen and Braekkan, 1965). Previously, unsaturated fatty acids, such as, *cis*-11-eicosenoic acid and oleic acid showed strong anti-biofilm effect while saturated fatty acids (myristic acid and palmitic acid) did not have anti-biofilm activity against *S. aureus* (Lee et al., 2017). Therefore, this study was focused on the anti-biofilm activities of three unsaturated predominant omega fatty acids (DHA, EPA, and erucic acid).

## Effect of DHA and EPA on Biofilm Formation by *S. aureus*

The anti-biofilm potencies of four major PUFAs (*cis*-11-eicosenoic acid, DHA, EPA, and erucic acid) were tested against the two *S. aureus* strains (MSSA 6538 and MRSA 33591) in 96-well plates. *cis*-11-Eicosenoic acid, DHA, and EPA at concentrations of 20 μg/ml significantly inhibited biofilm formation by both *S. aureus* strains (**Figure 2A**). DHA and EPA both inhibited biofilm formation by >90% at 50 μg/ml, which was greater than that previously reported for *cis*-11-eicosenoic acid (Lee et al., 2017). In this previous report, relationships between free fatty acids and bacterial biofilm formation were studied. In particular, oleic acid and *cis*-2-decenoic acid were found to suppress biofilm formation of *S. aureus* by blocking bacterial adhesion and dispersion from established biofilms, respectively (Stenz et al., 2008; Davies and Marques, 2009). In addition, it has been suggested that long chain unsaturated fatty acids like *cis*-11-eicosenoic acid (Lee et al., 2017) inhibit the biofilm forming ability of *S. aureus*. However, the present study is the first to report the anti-biofilm activities of DHA and EPA against *S. aureus*. The unsaturated fatty acid erucic acid, which was present in herring oil at high levels (**Table 1**), at 20 μg/ml inhibited biofilm formation by MRSA 33591 by >85%, but did not inhibit biofilm formation by MSSA 6538 (**Figure 2A**). However, higher concentrations of erucic acid at 500 and 1000 μg/ml significantly reduced biofilm formation of MSSA 6538 without affecting planktonic growth (data not shown). Hence, it appears that the effects of erucic acid are dose-dependent and strain dependent.

Confocal laser scanning microscopy was used to quantify biofilm formation by *S. aureus* in the presence of herring oil, DHA, or EPA. Fluorescent stacking 3D images indicated that herring oil (50 μg/ml), DHA (20 μg/ml), or EPA (20 μg/ml) markedly inhibited *S. aureus* biofilm formation (**Figure 2B**), and this, was confirmed by COMSTAT. More specifically, DHA, EPA, and herring oil reduced all three *S. aureus* MSSA 6538 parameters measured (biovolume, mean

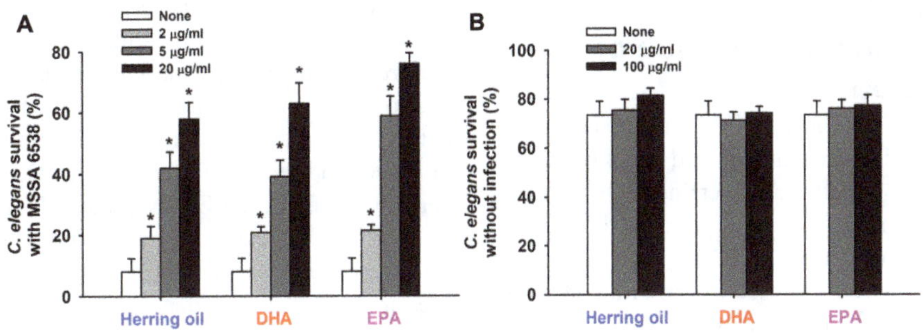


**FIGURE 5 |** Effects of herring oil, DHA, and EPA on nematode survival. *C. elegans fer-15;fem-1* strain survival after infection with *S. aureus* MSSA 6538 in the presence of DHA, EPA, or herring oil (2, 5, or 20 µg/ml) after exposure for 1 day at 25°C **(A)**. Herring oil, DHA, and EPA toxicities were assessed by determining survival rates versus non-infected nematodes **(B)**. Survival was assessed as dead or alive based on movement. $^*p < 0.05$ versus non-treated controls.

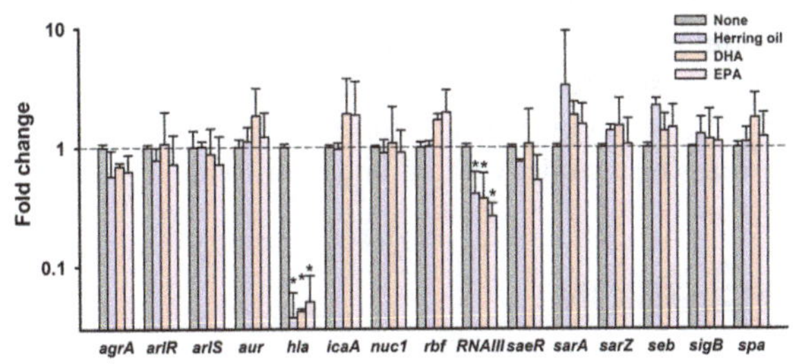


**FIGURE 6 |** Transcriptional profile changes in *S. aureus* after treatment with herring oil, DHA, or EPA. *S. aureus* MSSA 6538 was incubated in LB broth containing herring oil (100 µg/ml), DHA, or EPA (20 µg/ml) for 5 h with agitation at 250 rpm. Relative transcriptional profiles were determined by qRT-PCR with respect to 16s rRNA expression. qRT-PCR was performed in duplicate and fold-changes were calculated using treated versus untreated *S. aureus*. $^*p < 0.05$ vs. non-treated controls.

thickness, and substratum coverage) (**Figure 2C**), actually, DHA and EPA reduced biomass and mean thickness by >90%, respectively. These results show herring oil, DHA, and EPA all effectively reduced biofilm formation on the bottom of 96-well plate.

Mature biofilm detachment by antibiotics, enzymes, and fatty acids is interest due to their resistance to antimicrobial agents (Flemming and Wingender, 2010; Gwisai et al., 2017; Lee et al., 2018). However, herring oil (1000 µg/ml), DHA (100 µg/ml), and EPA (100 µg/ml) could not disperse matured *S. aureus* ATCC 6538 biofilms (data not shown).

## Anti-microbial Effects of DHA and EPA on *S. aureus*

The anti-microbial activities of DHA and EPA were evaluated by determining their minimum inhibitory concentrations (MICs) against *S. aureus* MSSA 6538 and MRSA 33591. Planktonic growth was completely inhibited by DHA and EPA at MICs (200 µg/ml), while MICs of ciprofloxacin and vancomycin are 0.5–1 µg/ml and 4 µg/ml, respectively, which concurs with previously reported values (Desbois and Lawlor, 2013; Gwisai et al., 2017). Notably, these MICs of DHA and EPA were 10 times higher than the concentration (20 µg/ml) required for anti-biofilm activities (**Figure 2A**).

Planktonic cell growths of *S. aureus* MSSA 6538 and MRSA 33591 in the presence of 5 µg/ml DHA or 20 µg/ml EPA were slightly inhibited (**Figures 2D,E**). However, the cell growths of both strains were more than 68% suppressed by DHA or EPA at 50 µg/ml, which indicates both DHA and EPA have anti-bacterial effects at relatively high concentrations (**Figures 2D,E**). These observations suggest DHA and EPA at low concentrations have anti-biofilm effects, but at higher levels these can also suppress the growth of planktonic cells.

## Effects of Herring Oil, DHA, and EPA on Hemolysis by *S. aureus*

*Staphylococcus aureus* produces α-toxin, which is one of the most investigated *S. aureus* cytotoxins. α-Toxin integrates into the membranes of erythrocytes causing hemolysis (Bhakdi et al., 1984; Song et al., 1996), which contributes to biofilm formation (Caiazza and O'Toole, 2003). Thus, the effects of herring oil, DHA, and EPA on human red blood cell hemolysis by *S. aureus* were investigated. As a control, herring oil, DHA, and EPA without *S. aureus* cells did not show any hemolytic activity (data not shown). Interestingly, all three dose-dependently inhibited the hemolytic activity of *S. aureus* (**Figure 3**), and DHA and EPA at 20 µg/ml completely abolished its hemolytic activity, whereas herring oil at 20 µg/ml reduced its hemolytic activity by >75%. Also, herring oil, DHA, and EPA all significantly reduced the hemolytic activity by *S. aureus* even at 1 µg/ml, which is much lower than the concentrations required for anti-biofilm and antimicrobial activities.

These results support that the inhibitions of *S. aureus* biofilm formation by herring oil, DHA, and EPA are associated with the inhibition of hemolysis, and suggest that the genes related to biofilm formation and hemolysis might be responsible for these events. The present study is the first to report that herring oil, DHA, and EPA suppress the hemolysis of human red blood cells by *S. aureus*, which has important implications regarding the control of *S. aureus* virulence.

## Effects of DHA, EPA, and Herring Oil on *S. aureus* Survival in the Presence of Human Whole Blood

*Staphylococcus aureus* characteristically exhibits resistance to phagocytes in humans and other animals, and thus, we used a survival test to investigate the effects of herring oil, DHA, and EPA on *S. aureus* survival in the presence of human whole blood. Herring oil, DHA, or EPA at 1, 5, or 20 μg/ml significantly reduced the survival of *S. aureus* exposed to fresh human whole blood (**Figure 4**), indicating that they weaken the ability of *S. aureus* to resist the human innate immune system.

## Effects of DHA, EPA, and Herring Oil on *S. aureus* Virulence in the Nematode Model

*Staphylococcus aureus* colonizes and replicates in the digestive tract of *C. elegans* and has the ability to kill *C. elegans* by an infection-like process that exhibits remarkable overlap with that observed in mammals (Garsin et al., 2003). Hence, the effects of herring oil, DHA, and EPA on *S. aureus* virulence were investigated by analyzing *C. elegans* survival in the presence of *S. aureus*. Herring oil, DHA, and EPA were found to markedly prolong *C. elegans* survival in the presence of *S. aureus* (**Figure 5A**). For example, nematode survival was only ~10% in the presence of untreated *S. aureus*, whereas in the presence of herring oil, DHA, or EPA at 20 μg/ml more than 55, 60, and 70%, respectively, of worms survived. In other words, the survival rate of *C. elegans* was increased more than seven and ninefold when worms were exposed to *S. aureus* in the presence of DHA or EPA at 20 μg/ml, respectively (**Figure 5A**). In addition, no toxic effects were observed when non-infected worms were exposed to herring oil, DHA, or EPA at concentrations up to 100 μg/ml (**Figure 5B**).

## Transcriptional Changes Induced by DHA, EPA, and by Herring Oil in *S. aureus*

To investigate the molecular mechanisms underlying the inhibitory effects of herring oil, DHA, and EPA against *S. aureus*, expressions of selected biofilm- and virulence-related genes, and important regulatory genes were investigated in *S. aureus* cells by qRT-PCR. Herring oil, DHA, and EPA dramatically reduced the expression of α-hemolysin (*hla*) by 27-, 24-, and 20-fold, respectively (**Figure 6**). Also, herring oil, DHA, and EPA downregulated regulatory RNA molecule (*RNAIII*) that is present upstream of the *agr* operon while the expressions of other genes were not affected (**Figure 6**). It has been reported that RNAIII stimulate *hla* translation (Morfeldt et al., 1995). Hence, *hla* repression is partially due to the down-regulation of RNAIII by herring oil, DHA, and EPA.

α-Hemolysin is known to play a critical role in cell-to-cell interactions during biofilm formation (Caiazza and O'Toole, 2003; Anderson et al., 2012; Scherr et al., 2015). This reduction of α-hemolysin expression has been discovered in recently published articles showing that alizarin (Lee et al., 2016), azithromycin (Gui et al., 2014), flavonoids (Cho et al., 2015), norlichexanthone (Baldry et al., 2016), and stilbenoids (Lee et al., 2014) inhibit both biofilm formation and hemolysis by *S. aureus*. Our findings support that α-hemolysin has a positive relationship with biofilm formation in *S. aureus*. In addition, it has been shown *hla* is essential for *S. aureus* pathogenicity in a nematode model (Sifri et al., 2003, 2006). Notably, neither herring oil, DHA, or EPA significantly affected the expressions of the biofilm-related genes namely, *agrA*, *arlR*, *arlS*, *aur*, *icaA*, *nucl*, *rbf*, *saeR*, *sarA*, *sarZ*, *seb*, *sigB*, or *spa*. Thus, the present study indicates that herring oil, DHA, and EPA attenuate *S. aureus* virulence, as evidenced by reductions in its anti-biofilm (**Figures 1, 2**) and anti-hemolytic (**Figure 3**) activities, and partially by down-regulating the expression of the *hla* gene (**Figure 6**).

These results indicate that herring oil, DHA, and EPA could be used to treat *S. aureus* infections as lone drug or in combination with traditional antibiotics (**Figure 5**). Furthermore, because all three are considered intrinsically safe in animal, they could be used for medicinal purposes or for example, to surface treat in food processing facilities without undue restriction.

## CONCLUSION

The DHA and EPA are long chain omega-3 fatty acids, which have major health benefits in man. More specifically, circulating levels of DHA and EPA are essential part of the body's defense system and play key roles in the inhibitions of inflammation and host immune responses (Calder, 2013). Herring oil was found to contain DHA and EPA at levels of 11.3 and 5.8% by weight, respectively, and inhibit biofilm formation and hemolysis by and the virulence of *S. aureus*. Interestingly, the ability of *S. aureus* to survive exposure to human whole blood was reduced in the presence of DHA or EPA, and exposure to DHA or EPA also increased infected nematode survival. These findings show for the first time that DHA and EPA suppress *S. aureus* biofilm formation and its virulence. Also, herring oil and its constituent omega-3 fatty acids (DHA and EPA) might be useful for the treatment and/or prevention of surface-associated biofilm formation by *S. aureus* (including MRSA strains) and for suppressing its virulence.

## AUTHOR CONTRIBUTIONS

Y-GK, J-HL, CR, and SO performed the experiments and analyzed the data. Y-GK, J-HL, JP, and JL designed the study and wrote the paper. All authors read and approved the final manuscript.

## FUNDING

This research was conducted under the industrial infrastructure program for fundamental technologies (N0000885) which is funded by the Ministry of Trade, Industry and Energy

(MOTIE, South Korea). This research was also supported by the Basic Science Research Program of a National Research Foundation of Korea (NRF) funded by the Korean Ministry of Education (2018R1D1A3B07040699 to J-HL) and (2017R1A6A3A01076089 to Y-GK), and a Priority Research Centers Program (#2014R1A6A1031189).

## REFERENCES

Anderson, M. J., Lin, Y. C., Gillman, A. N., Parks, P. J., Schlievert, P. M., and Peterson, M. L. (2012). Alpha-toxin promotes *Staphylococcus aureus* mucosal biofilm formation. *Front. Cell. Infect. Microbiol.* 2:64. doi: 10.3389/fcimb.2012.00064

Baldry, M., Nielsen, A., Bojer, M. S., Zhao, Y., Friberg, C., Ifrah, D., et al. (2016). Norlichexanthone reduces virulence gene expression and biofilm formation in *Staphylococcus aureus*. *PLoS One* 11:e0168305. doi: 10.1371/journal.pone.0168305

Bhakdi, S., Muhly, M., and Fussle, R. (1984). Correlation between toxin binding and hemolytic activity in membrane damage by staphylococcal alpha-toxin. *Infect. Immun.* 46, 318–323.

Bougnoux, P. (1999). n-3 polyunsaturated fatty acids and cancer. *Curr. Opin. Clin. Nutr. Metab. Care* 2, 121–126. doi: 10.1097/00075197-199903000-00005

Caiazza, N. C., and O'Toole, G. A. (2003). Alpha-toxin is required for biofilm formation by *Staphylococcus aureus*. *J. Bacteriol.* 185, 3214–3217. doi: 10.1128/JB.185.10.3214-3217.2003

Calder, P. C. (2013). Omega-3 polyunsaturated fatty acids and inflammatory processes: nutrition or pharmacology? *Br. J. Clin. Pharmacol.* 75, 645–662. doi: 10.1111/j.1365-2125.2012.04374.x

Chambers, H. F., and Deleo, F. R. (2009). Waves of resistance: *Staphylococcus aureus* in the antibiotic era. *Nat. Rev. Microbiol.* 7, 629–641. doi: 10.1038/nrmicro2200

Cho, H. S., Lee, J.-H., Cho, M. H., and Lee, J. (2015). Red wines and flavonoids diminish *Staphylococcus aureus* virulence with anti-biofilm and anti-hemolytic activities. *Biofouling* 31, 1–11. doi: 10.1080/08927014.2014.991319

Correia, M., Michel, V., Matos, A. A., Carvalho, P., Oliveira, M. J., Ferreira, R. M., et al. (2012). Docosahexaenoic acid inhibits *Helicobacter pylori* growth *in vitro* and mice gastric mucosa colonization. *PLoS One* 7:e35072. doi: 10.1371/journal.pone.0035072

Davies, D. G., and Marques, C. N. (2009). A fatty acid messenger is responsible for inducing dispersion in microbial biofilms. *J. Bacteriol.* 191, 1393–1403. doi: 10.1128/JB.01214-08

Desbois, A. P., and Lawlor, K. C. (2013). Antibacterial activity of long-chain polyunsaturated fatty acids against *Propionibacterium acnes* and *Staphylococcus aureus*. *Mar. Drugs.* 11, 4544–4557. doi: 10.3390/md11114544

Desbois, A. P., Mearns-Spragg, A., and Smith, V. J. (2009). A fatty acid from the diatom *Phaeodactylum tricornutum* is antibacterial against diverse bacteria including multi-resistant *Staphylococcus aureus* (MRSA). *Mar. Biotechnol.* 11, 45–52. doi: 10.1007/s10126-008-9118-5

Flemming, H. C., and Wingender, J. (2010). The biofilm matrix. *Nat. Rev. Microbiol.* 8, 623–633. doi: 10.1038/nrmicro2415

Garsin, D. A., Villanueva, J. M., Begun, J., Kim, D. H., Sifri, C. D., Calderwood, S. B., et al. (2003). Long-lived *C. elegans daf*-2 mutants are resistant to bacterial pathogens. *Science* 300, 1921–1921. doi: 10.1126/science.1080147

Giordano, E., and Visioli, F. (2014). Long-chain omega 3 fatty acids: molecular bases of potential antioxidant actions. *Prostaglandins Leukot. Essent. Fatty Acids* 90, 1–4. doi: 10.1016/j.plefa.2013.11.002

Gui, Z., Wang, H., Ding, T., Zhu, W., Zhuang, X., and Chu, W. (2014). Azithromycin reduces the production of alpha-hemolysin and biofilm formation in *Staphylococcus aureus*. *Indian J. Microbiol.* 54, 114–117. doi: 10.1007/s12088-013-0438-4

Gwisai, T., Hollingsworth, N. R., Cowles, S., Tharmalingam, N., Mylonakis, E., Fuchs, B. B., et al. (2017). Repurposing niclosamide as a versatile antimicrobial surface coating against device-associated, hospital-acquired bacterial infections. *Biomed. Mater.* 12:045010. doi: 10.1088/1748-605X/aa7105

Heydorn, A., Nielsen, A. T., Hentzer, M., Sternberg, C., Givskov, M., Ersboll, B. K., et al. (2000). Quantification of biofilm structures by the novel computer program COMSTAT. *Microbiology* 146, 2395–2407. doi: 10.1099/00221287-146-10-2395

Hirai, A., Hamazaki, T., Terano, T., Nishikawa, T., Tamura, Y., Kamugai, A., et al. (1980). Eicosapentaenoic acid and platelet function in Japanese. *Lancet* 2, 1132–1133. doi: 10.1016/S0140-6736(80)92558-1

Hoffman, L. R., D'Argenio, D. A., MacCoss, M. J., Zhang, Z., Jones, R. A., and Miller, S. I. (2005). Aminoglycoside antibiotics induce bacterial biofilm formation. *Nature* 436, 1171–1175. doi: 10.1038/nature03912

Huang, C. B., and Ebersole, J. L. (2010). A novel bioactivity of omega-3 polyunsaturated fatty acids and their ester derivatives. *Mol. Oral Microbiol.* 25, 75–80. doi: 10.1111/j.2041-1014.2009.00553.x

Kang, H.-S., Jeong, S.-W., Ko, J.-C., Jang, M., and Kim, J.-C. (2011). The quality characteristics of commercial gwamegi by product types. *J. Food Sci. Nutr.* 16, 253–260. doi: 10.3746/jfn.2011.16.3.253

Kim, Y.-G., Lee, J.-H., Gwon, G., Kim, S.-I., Park, J. G., and Lee, J. (2016). Essential oils and eugenols inhibit biofilm formation and the virulence of *Escherichia coli* O157:H7. *Sci. Rep.* 6:36377. doi: 10.1038/srep36377

Kim, Y.-G., Lee, J.-H., Kim, S.-I., Baek, K.-H., and Lee, J. (2015). Cinnamon bark oil and its components inhibit biofilm formation and toxin production. *Int. J. Food Microbiol.* 195, 30–39. doi: 10.1016/j.ijfoodmicro.2014.11.028

Lambertsen, G., and Braekkan, O. R. (1965). The fatty acid composition of herring oils. *Fiskeridirektoratets skrifter Ser. Teknol. Undersøkelser* 4, 13.

Lee, J.-H., Kim, Y.-G., and Lee, J. (2018). Thermostable xylanase inhibits and disassembles *Pseudomonas aeruginosa* biofilms. *Biofouling* 34, 346–356. doi: 10.1080/08927014.2018.1440551

Lee, J.-H., Kim, Y.-G., Park, J. G., and Lee, J. (2017). Supercritical fluid extracts of *Moringa oleifera* and their unsaturated fatty acid components inhibit biofilm formation by *Staphylococcus aureus*. *Food Control* 80, 74–82. doi: 10.1016/j.foodcont.2017.04.035

Lee, J.-H., Kim, Y.-G., Ryu, S. Y., and Lee, J. (2016). Calcium-chelating alizarin and other anthraquinones inhibit biofilm formation and the hemolytic activity of *Staphylococcus aureus*. *Sci. Rep.* 6:19267. doi: 10.1038/srep19267

Lee, J.-H., Park, J.-H., Cho, H. S., Joo, S. W., Cho, M. H., and Lee, J. (2013). Antibiofilm activities of quercetin and tannic acid against *Staphylococcus aureus*. *Biofouling* 29, 491–499. doi: 10.1080/08927014.2013.788692

Lee, K., Lee, J.-H., Ryu, S. Y., Cho, M. H., and Lee, J. (2014). Stilbenes reduce *Staphylococcus aureus* hemolysis, biofilm formation, and virulence. *Foodborne Pathog. Dis.* 11, 710–717. doi: 10.1089/fpd.2014.1758

Lee, J.-W., Cho, K.-H., Yook, H.-S., Jo, C., Kim, D.-H., and Byun, M.-W. (2002). The effect of gamma irradiation on the stability and hygienic quality of semi-dried pacific saury (*Cololabis seira*) flesh. *Radiat. Phys. Chem.* 64, 309–315. doi: 10.1016/S0969-806X(01)00675-2

Liu, C. I., Liu, G. Y., Song, Y., Yin, F., Hensler, M. E., Jeng, W. Y., et al. (2008). A cholesterol biosynthesis inhibitor blocks *Staphylococcus aureus* virulence. *Science* 319, 1391–1394. doi: 10.1126/science.1153018

Lowy, F. D. (1998). Staphylococcus aureus infections. *N. Engl. J. Med.* 339, 520–532. doi: 10.1056/NEJM199808203390806

Menzies, B. E., and Kernodle, D. S. (1996). Passive immunization with antiserum to a nontoxic alpha-toxin mutant from *Staphylococcus aureus* is protective in a murine model. *Infect. Immun.* 64, 1839–1841.

Mil-Homens, D., Bernardes, N., and Fialho, A. M. (2012). The antibacterial properties of docosahexaenoic omega-3 fatty acid against the cystic fibrosis multiresistant pathogen *Burkholderia cenocepacia*. *FEMS Microbiol. Lett.* 328, 61–69. doi: 10.1111/j.1574-6968.2011.02476.x

Morfeldt, E., Taylor, D., von Gabain, A., and Arvidson, S. (1995). Activation of alpha-toxin translation in *Staphylococcus aureus* by the trans-encoded antisense RNA. RNAIII. *EMBO J.* 14, 4569–4577.

Ohlsen, K., Koller, K. P., and Hacker, J. (1997). Analysis of expression of the alpha-toxin gene (hla) of *Staphylococcus aureus* by using a chromosomally encoded hla::lacZ gene fusion. *Infect. Immun.* 65, 3606–3614.

Otto, M. (2014). Staphylococcus aureus toxins. *Curr. Opin. Microbiol.* 17, 32–37. doi: 10.1016/j.mib.2013.11.004

Potera, C. (1999). Forging a link between biofilms and disease. *Science* 283, 1837–1839. doi: 10.1126/science.283.5409.1837

Scherr, T. D., Hanke, M. L., Huang, O., James, D. B., Horswill, A. R., Bayles, K. W., et al. (2015). Staphylococcus aureus biofilms induce macrophage dysfunction through leukocidin AB and alpha-toxin. *MBio* 6, e1021–e1015. doi: 10.1128/mBio.01021-15

Schmidt, E. B., and Dyerberg, J. (1994). Omega-3 fatty acids. Current status in cardiovascular medicine. *Drugs* 47, 405–424. doi: 10.2165/00003495-199447030-00003

Sifri, C. D., Baresch-Bernal, A., Calderwood, S. B., and von Eiff, C. (2006). Virulence of *Staphylococcus aureus* small colony variants in the *Caenorhabditis elegans* infection model. *Infect. Immun.* 74, 1091–1096. doi: 10.1128/IAI.74.2.1091-1096.2006

Sifri, C. D., Begun, J., Ausubel, F. M., and Calderwood, S. B. (2003). Caenorhabditis elegans as a model host for *Staphylococcus aureus* pathogenesis. *Infect. Immun.* 71, 2208–2217. doi: 10.1128/IAI.71.4.2208-2217.2003

Singhal, D., Foreman, A., Jervis-Bardy, J., and Wormald, P. J. (2011). *Staphylococcus aureus* biofilms: Nemesis of endoscopic sinus surgery. *Laryngoscope* 121, 1578–1583. doi: 10.1002/lary.21805

Song, L., Hobaugh, M. R., Shustak, C., Cheley, S., Bayley, H., and Gouaux, J. E. (1996). Structure of staphylococcal α-hemolysin, a heptameric transmembrane pore. *Science* 274, 1859–1866. doi: 10.1126/science.274.5294.1859

Speller, D. C., Johnson, A. P., James, D., Marples, R. R., Charlett, A., and George, R. C. (1997). Resistance to methicillin and other antibiotics in isolates of *Staphylococcus aureus* from blood and cerebrospinal fluid, England and Wales, 1989-95. *Lancet* 350, 323–325. doi: 10.1016/S0140-6736(97)12148-1

Stenz, L., Francois, P., Fischer, A., Huyghe, A., Tangomo, M., Hernandez, D., et al. (2008). Impact of oleic acid (cis-9-octadecenoic acid) on bacterial viability and biofilm production in *Staphylococcus aureus*. *FEMS Microbiol. Lett.* 287, 149–155. doi: 10.1111/j.1574-6968.2008.01316.x

Stewart, P. S., and Costerton, J. W. (2001). Antibiotic resistance of bacteria in biofilms. *Lancet* 358, 135–138. doi: 10.1016/S0140-6736(01)05321-1

Sun, M., Dong, J., Xia, Y., and Shu, R. (2017). Antibacterial activities of docosahexaenoic acid (DHA) and eicosapentaenoic acid (EPA) against planktonic and biofilm growing *Streptococcus mutans*. *Microb. Pathog.* 107, 212–218. doi: 10.1016/j.micpath.2017.03.040

Sun, M., Zhou, Z., Dong, J., Zhang, J., Xia, Y., and Shu, R. (2016). Antibacterial and antibiofilm activities of docosahexaenoic acid (DHA) and eicosapentaenoic acid (EPA) against periodontopathic bacteria. *Microb. Pathog.* 99, 196–203. doi: 10.1016/j.micpath.2016.08.025

Tharmalingam, N., Rajmuthiah, R., Kim, W., Fuchs, B. B., Jeyamani, E., Kelso, M. J., et al. (2018). Antibacterial properties of four novel hit compounds from a methicillin-resistant *Staphylococcus aureus-Caenorhabditis elegans* high-throughput screen. *Microb. Drug Resist.* doi: 10.1089/mdr.2017.0250 [Epub ahead of print].

Thibane, V. S., Kock, J. L., Ells, R., van Wyk, P. W., and Pohl, C. H. (2010). Effect of marine polyunsaturated fatty acids on biofilm formation of *Candida albicans* and *Candida dubliniensis*. *Mar. Drugs* 8, 2597–2604. doi: 10.3390/md8102597

Van Dyke, T. E. (2008). The management of inflammation in periodontal disease. *J. Periodontol.* 79, 1601–1608. doi: 10.1902/jop.2008.080173

Wilke, G. A., and Bubeck Wardenburg, J. (2010). Role of a disintegrin and metalloprotease 10 in *Staphylococcus aureus* α-hemolysin-mediated cellular injury. *Proc. Natl. Acad. Sci. U.S.A.* 107, 13473–13478. doi: 10.1073/pnas.1001815107

9

# Emergence of Carbapenem- and Tigecycline-Resistant *Proteus cibarius* of Animal Origin


*Yan Li[1], Qian Wang[1], Kai Peng[1], Yuan Liu[1,2,3], Ruichao Li[1,2,3]* and Zhiqiang Wang[1,3]**

[1] *College of Veterinary Medicine, Yangzhou University, Yangzhou, China,* [2] *Institute of Comparative Medicine, Yangzhou University, Yangzhou, China,* [3] *Jiangsu Co-innovation Center for Prevention and Control of Important Animal Infectious Diseases and Zoonoses, Yangzhou University, Yangzhou, China*

***Correspondence:**
*Ruichao Li*
*rchl88@yzu.edu.cn*
*Zhiqiang Wang*
*zqwang@yzu.edu.cn*



The emergence of *tet*(X) and carbapenemase genes in Enterobacterales pose significant challenges to the treatment of infectious diseases. Convergence of these two categories of genes in an individual pathogen would deteriorate the antimicrobial resistance (AMR) crisis furthermore. Here, tigecycline-resistant Enterobacterales strains were isolated and detected with carbapenemase genes, characterized by antimicrobial susceptibility testing, PCR, conjugation assay, whole genome sequencing, and bioinformatics analysis. Three tigecycline-resistant isolates consisting of one plasmid-mediated *tet*(X4)-bearing *Escherichia fergusonii* and two chromosomal *tet*(X6)-bearing *Proteus cibarius* were recovered from chicken feces. The *tet*(X4) was located on a conjugative IncX1 plasmid pHNCF11W-tetX4 encoding the identical structure as reported *tet*(X4)-bearing IncX1 plasmids in *Escherichia coli*. Among two *P. cibarius* strains, *tet*(X6) was located on two similar chromosomal MDR regions with genetic contexts IS*26-aac(3)-IVa-aph(4)-Ia*-IS*Ec59-tnpA-tet*(X6)-*orf-orf*-IS*CR2-virD2-floR*-IS*CR2-glmM-sul2* and IS*26-aac(3)-IVa-aph(4)-Ia*-IS*Ec59-tnpA-tet*(X6)-*orf-orf*-IS*CR2-glmM-sul2*. Apart from *tet*(X6), *P. cibarius* HNCF44W harbored a novel transposon Tn*6450b* positive for $bla_{\text{NDM-1}}$ on a conjugative plasmid. This study probed the genomic basis of three *tet*(X)-bearing, tigecycline-resistant strains, one of which coharbored $bla_{\text{NDM-1}}$ and *tet*(X6), and identified *P. cibarius* as the important reservoir of *tet*(X6) variants. Emergence of *P. cibarius* encoding both $bla_{\text{NDM-1}}$ and *tet*(X6) reveals a potential public health risk.



**Keywords: tigecycline resistance, carbapenem resistance, coexistence, plasmid, chromosome**


## INTRODUCTION

Antimicrobial resistance (AMR) is a serious threat to public health globally. Carbapenem and tigecycline are regarded as vital antimicrobials reserved for clinical use due to their broad antibacterial spectrum. However, the increasing spread of carbapenemase-encoding genes has rendered carbapenem-resistant Enterobacteriaceae (CRE) infection a great threat (Du et al., 2018; Tacconelli et al., 2018). Plasmid-mediated resistance genes *tet*(X3) and *tet*(X4) conferring high-level resistance to tigecycline in Enterobacterales and *Acinetobacter* has been found to be ubiquitous in animals and food of animal origin (Bai et al., 2019; He et al., 2019; Sun et al., 2019; Li et al., 2020c). This undermines the efficacy of tigecycline as the last-resort drug in treating MDR bacterial infections, especially those caused by carbapenem-resistant, Gram-negative bacteria, such as CRE.

Initially, *tet*(X) genes were mainly found in *Bacteroides* species and bacteria derived from environmental microbiota (Forsberg et al., 2015; Tian et al., 2019). Alarmingly, novel *tet*(X) variants are being identified from the pathogens of animal, food, and human origins (Li et al., 2019; Wang et al., 2019; He D. et al., 2020; Liu et al., 2020; Peng et al., 2020), which implies that *tet*(X) is expanding from commensals to pathogens (Aminov, 2013). Thus, the convergence of mobile tigecycline-resistant *tet*(X) and carbapenem-resistant genes in Enterobacterales may be inevitable. *Acinetobacter* strains coharboring *tet*(X) and $bla_{NDM-1}$ were identified from samples of waterfowl and dairy cows recently (Cui et al., 2020; He T. et al., 2020), highlighting the potential convergence risk of both critical resistance genes among bacteria. However, Enterobacterales carrying both *tet*(X) and $bla_{NDM-1}$ is unknown, which constitutes a more severe concern. To cover this knowledge gap, we performed a tigecycline-resistant Enterobacterales screening pilot program and identified a *Proteus cibarius* coharboring both *tet*(X6) and $bla_{NDM-1}$, implying that wide surveillance of Enterobacterales conferring resistance to carbapenems and tigecycline among bacteria should be performed worldwide.

# MATERIALS AND METHODS

## Bacterial Isolates

A total of 16 chicken fecal samples were collected from four chicken farms in Henan province, China, in 2019. Tigecycline-resistant Enterobacterales were selected on MacConkey agar plates containing tigecycline (4 mg/L). The species of purified tigecycline-resistant isolates was identified by 16S rRNA gene sequencing and further confirmed by analyzing WGS data. The *tet*(X) and carbapenem-resistant genes were determined by PCR with reported primers (Dallenne et al., 2010; He et al., 2019).

## Antimicrobial Susceptibility Testing

The antimicrobial susceptibility testing (AST) of *tet*(X)-positive tigecycline-resistant strains against 13 antibiotics was performed based on the broth microdilution method with *Escherichia coli* ATCC 25922 as the quality control and interpreted according to CLSI guidelines (CLSI, 2018). The tigecycline non-susceptibility in Enterobacterales was interpreted with an MIC of $\geq$4 mg/L (Marchaim et al., 2014).

## Conjugation Assay and S1-PFGE

A conjugation assay was conducted using rifampicin-resistant *E. coli* C600 ($Rif^r$) as the recipient to investigate the transferability of *tet*(X) and $bla_{NDM-1}$. The donor and recipient strains were mixed at a ratio of 1:4 on a filter, followed by culturing on LB agar plates at 30 and 37°C, respectively, overnight and screening on MacConkey plates containing tigecycline (4 mg/L) or meropenem (2 mg/L) with rifampicin (300 mg/L). Transconjugants were confirmed with PCR. S1 nuclease pulsed-field gel electrophoresis (S1-PFGE) was utilized to characterize the plasmid profiles.

## Whole Genome Sequencing and Bioinformatics Analysis

Genomid DNA (gDNA) was purified with the TIANamp Genomic DNA Kit and quantified by Qubit 4 Fluorometer. Short-read Illumina sequencing and long-read Nanopore sequencing were combined to generate complete genome sequences (Li et al., 2018). The *de novo* assembled sequences were annotated by RAST[1]. Antibiotic resistance genes (ARGs) and plasmid replicon types were determined using the ResFinder and PlasmidFinder[2]. BRIG and Easyfig were used to compare the plasmid and MDR structures (Alikhan et al., 2011; Sullivan et al., 2011).

## Functional Confirmation of *tet*(X6) and Phylogenetic Analysis

To confirm the resistance function of the identified *tet*(X6) variant, TA-cloning and AST were performed. Briefly, the new variant, together with its natural promoter sequence, was amplified by PCR using primers HNCF44W-F/AGCGAACAAGAATATGACTTTACT and HNCF44W-R/CGCCTTTCTGTTTTATAGATTCAT, cloned into a pMD19-T vector and transformed chemically into *E. coli* DH5α. The resistance phenotype of *tet*(X6) was tested by measuring the MICs of different tetracycline antibiotics. Phylogenetic analysis of Tet(X) amino acid sequences were conducted in MEGA X using the neighbor-joining method (Kumar et al., 2018).

## Nucleotide Sequence Accession Numbers

The complete sequences obtained in this study have been deposited in the GenBank database under BioProject number PRJNA625637. The novel $bla_{NDM-1}$-bearing Tn*6450b* was also deposited in the NCBI database (MT701524).

# RESULTS AND DISCUSSION

## Identification of Tigecycline-Resistant Enterobacterales

Three tigecycline-resistant, *tet*(X)-positive Enterobacterales strains were isolated from 16 samples (18.8%), which consisted of *Escherichia fergusonii* HNCF11W carrying *tet*(X4), *P. cibarius* HNCF43W, and HNCF44W positive for a *tet*(X6) variant. Notably, HNCF44W also carried the $bla_{NDM-1}$ gene. Antimicrobial susceptibility testing revealed that the three tigecycline-resistant strains were resistant to multiple antibiotics, including kanamycin, florfenicol, amoxicillin, and tetracyclines, showing high-level resistance to tigecycline (**Supplementary Table S1**). In addition, the NDM-producing strain HNCF44W was also resistant to meropenem (>16 mg/L). S1-PFGE indicated that two plasmids of ca. 130 and 55 kb were observed in *tet*(X4)-bearing *E. fergusonii* HNCF11W, and one plasmid of ca. 140 kb existed in *tet*(X6)-bearing *P. cibarius* HNCF44W, but no plasmid

[1]https://rast.nmpdr.org/

[2]http://www.genomicepidemiology.org/

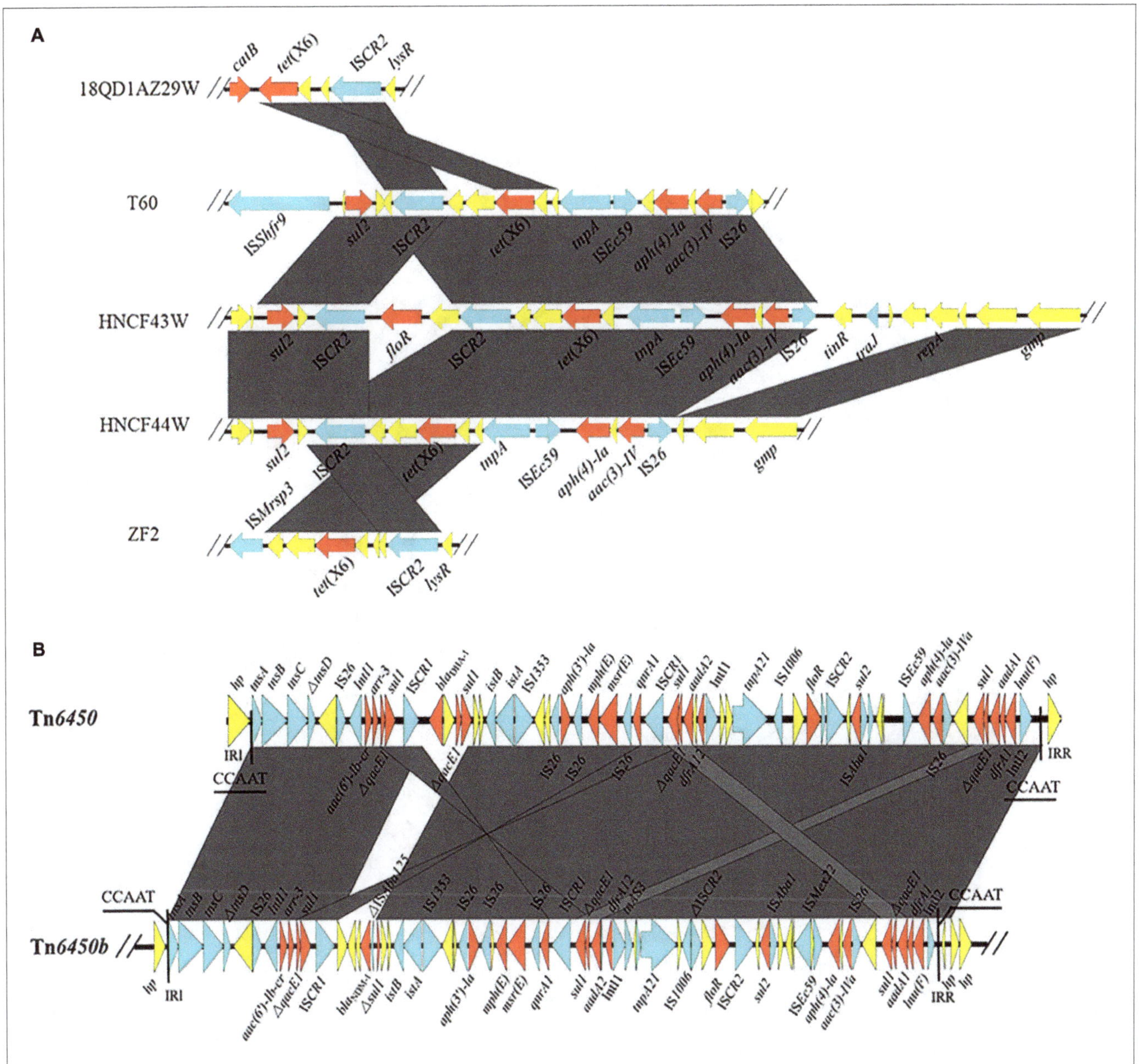


**FIGURE 1 | (A)** Genetic environments of *tet*(X6) from different strains. **(B)** Linear alignment of $bla_{NDM-1}$-bearing Tn*6450b* in pHNCF44W_NDM-1 and reported Tn*6450*. The red arrows denote the resistance genes; the blue arrows represent the mobile elements; the yellow arrows signify other CDSs. The shadow parallelograms stand for homologous genetic regions.

existed in *P. cibarius* HNCF43W (**Supplementary Figure S1**). To uncover the genetic locations of *tet*(X) and $bla_{NDM-1}$, complete genome sequences of the three strains were finished successfully.

## Genome Characterization of Tigecycline-Resistant *E. fergusonii*

The *tet*(X4)-bearing *E. fergusonii* harbored one chromosome (4,584,794 bp, ST10543); one p0111-like plasmid pHNCF11W-130 kb (130,643 bp) harboring *aadA1*, *floR*, *tet*(A), *dfrA14*, $bla_{TEM-209}$, $bla_{OXA-10}$, *cmlA1*, *arr-3*, and *qnrS1*; and one typical IncX1 plasmid pHNCF11W-tetX4 (57,105 bp) encoding *tet*(X4) in the genetic structure of IS*26*-*abh*-*tet*(X4)-IS*CR2*-*virD2*-*floR*-ΔIS*CR2* coupled with *aadA2*, *lnu(F)*, *tet*(A), and $bla_{SHV-12}$. A BLASTn search of pHNCF11W-tetX4 against the nr database retrieved other *tet*(X4)-bearing plasmids p1916D18-1 (59,353 bp), p1916D6-2 (59,351 bp), and pYY76-1-2 (57,104 bp) of swine and cattle origins, sharing nearly identical sequences (**Supplementary Figure S2**). Both pHNCF11W-tetX4 and pHNCF11W-130 kb were transferred into the recipient strain, demonstrating that IncX1-type *tet*(X4)-bearing plasmids were mobilizable and spread in Enterobacterales of animal origin (Chen et al., 2019). Although *tet*(X4) was initially found in plasmids of IncFIB and IncQ1 types (He et al., 2019; Sun et al.,

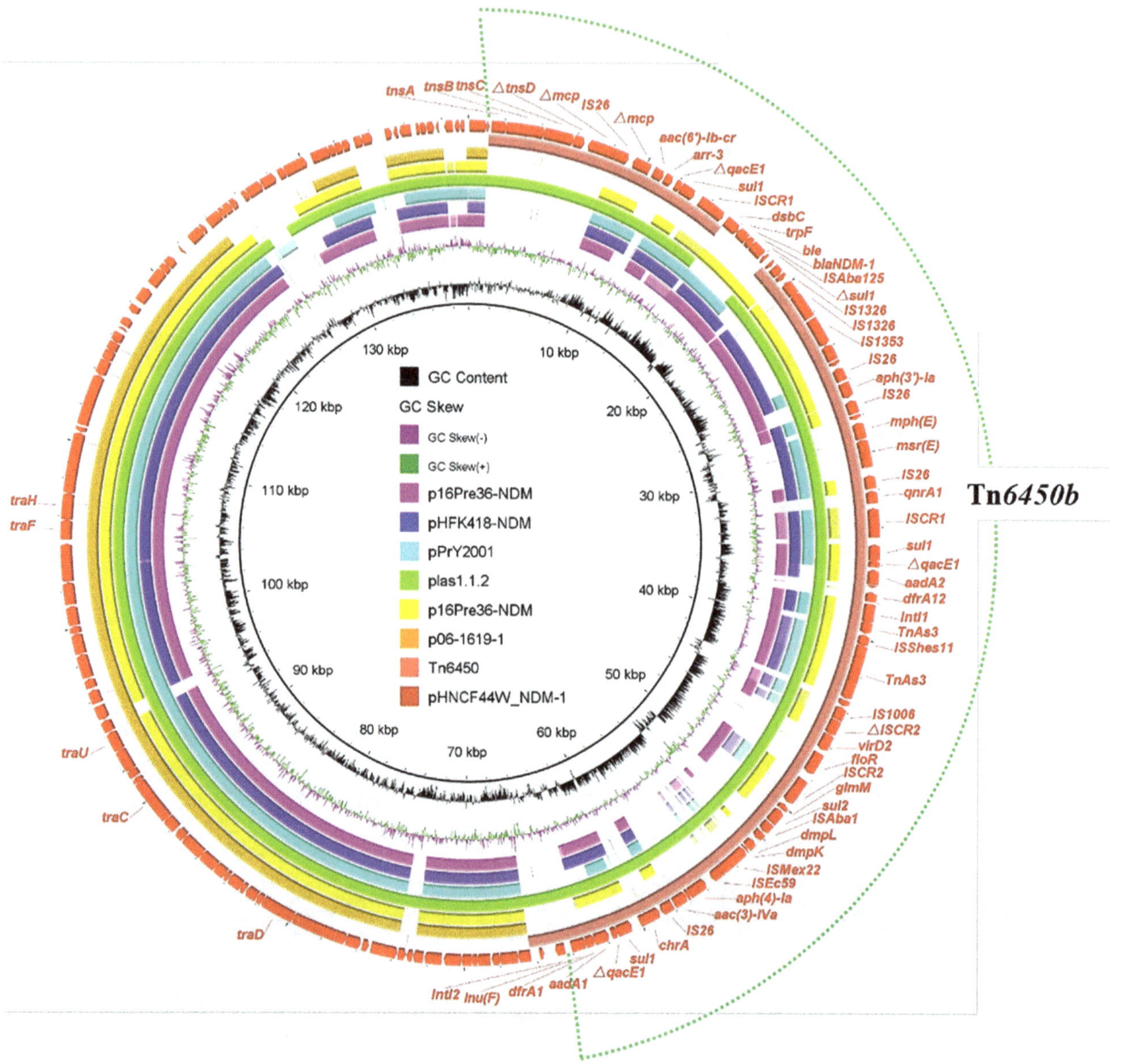


**FIGURE 2 |** Alignment of the plasmid pHNCF44W_NDM-1 identified in this study with other similar plasmids. The outermost red circle denotes the reference plasmid pHNCF44W_NDM-1. The location of Tn*6450b* is highlighted in the dotted circle.

2019), IncX1 plasmids are common in various Enterobacterales and associated with various resistance genes (Dobiasova and Dolejska, 2016; Li et al., 2020b), which potentially increases the transmission of *tet*(X4) between different Enterobacterales.

## Characterization of *Proteus cibarius* Coharboring *tet*(X6) and *bla*$_{\text{NDM-1}}$

HNCF43W harbored a 3,965,977 bp chromosome. HNCF44W contained a 3,929,176 bp chromosome and one *bla*$_{\text{NDM-1}}$-bearing plasmid pHNCF44W_NDM-1 of 139,490 bp in size. A conjugation assay failed to recover transconjugants positive for *tet*(X6). The *tet*(X6) gene was located on large MDR regions (IS*26-aac(3)-IVa-aph(4)-Ia*-IS*Ec59-tnpA-tet*(X6)*-orf-orf*-IS*CR2-virD2-floR*-IS*CR2-glmM-sul2* and IS*26-aac(3)-IVa-aph(4)-Ia*-IS*Ec59-tnpA-tet*(X6)*-orf-orf*-IS*CR2-glmM-sul2,* respectively) embedded in chromosomes of both *P. cibarius* strains (**Figure 1A**), and the MDR regions may derive from recombination of *tet*(X6)-bearing elements and reported plasmids p19110F47-2 (CP046044) and pJXP9 (MK673549) (**Supplementary Figure S3**). The two *tet*(X6)-bearing MDR regions differed by *virD2-floR*-IS*CR2,* which was a potential mobile segment (Doublet et al., 2005). IS*CR2* is the major mobile element associated with *tet*(X3), *tet*(X4), and *tet*(X5) (Bai et al., 2019; He et al., 2019; Sun et al., 2019; Li et al., 2020a). Recently, three reports demonstrated *tet*(X6) could be embedded in ICEs

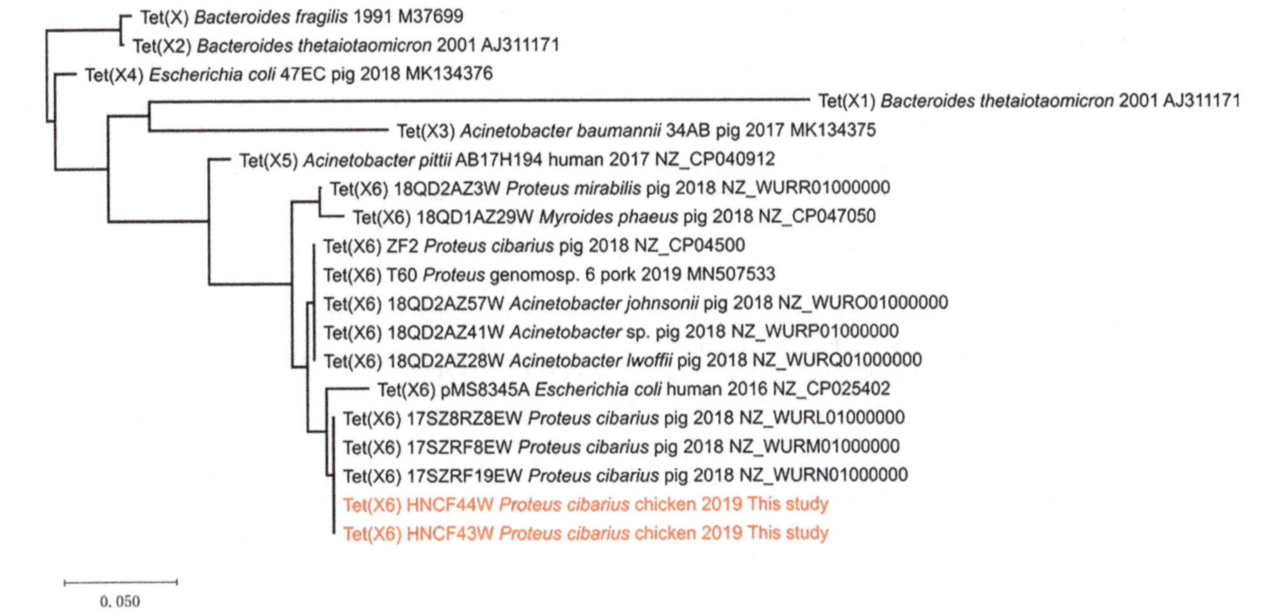


**FIGURE 3** | The phylogenetic tree of Tet(X) variants. The tree is drawn to scale with branch lengths in the same units as those of the evolutionary distances used to infer the phylogenetic tree. The evolutionary distances were computed using MEGA X and are in the units of the number of amino acid substitutions per site.

or other MDR regions, all of which harbor IS*CR2* (He D. et al., 2020; Liu et al., 2020; Peng et al., 2020), suggesting it may facilitate the transfer of *tet*(X6) to other plasmids or chromosomes.

The $bla_{NDM-1}$ gene in HNCF44W was located on an MDR plasmid pHNCF44W_NDM-1 carrying resistance genes *aac(6')-Ib, arr-3, qacE1, sul1, sul2, aph(3')-la, mph(E), msr(E), qnrA1, aadA1, aadA2, dfrA1, dfrA12, floR, aac(3)-IVa,* and *lnu(F)*. No plasmid replicon was identified, but pHNCF44W_NDM-1 was very similar to plasmid plas1.1.2 (CP047114) from *Proteus mirabilis* of swine origin; it differed mainly in the $bla_{NDM-1}$-bearing region (**Figure 2**). The $bla_{NDM-1}$ gene and other resistance genes were found in a 65-kb MDR region, showing high similarity to transposon Tn*6450* but with $bla_{DHA-1}$ replaced by $bla_{NDM-1}$ (Chen et al., 2018), designated as Tn*6450b* here (**Figure 1B**). Other similar plasmids or transposons were found in the nr database, including p16Pre36-NDM from *Providencia rettgeri*, pHFK418-NDM from *P. mirabilis*, pPrY2001 from *P. rettgeri*, p16Pre36-NDM from *P. rettgeri*, p06-1619-1 from *P. rettgeri*, and Tn*6450* from *P. mirabilis*. The plasmid pHNCF44W_NDM-1 carrying $bla_{NDM-1}$ was successfully transferred into *E. coli* EC600 at 30°C. Notably, IS*CR2-lysR-floR-virD2*-ΔIS*CR2* structure in pHNCF44W_NDM-1 was also found in a *tet*(X6)-bearing chromosomal segment, rendering this a Tn*6450b*-bearing plasmid with the potential ability to capture *tet*(X6) under certain circumstances, which warrants further surveillance.

## Functional Analysis of *tet*(X6) and Its Evolution

Recently, several reports have characterized different *tet*(X6) variants from diverse bacteria (He D. et al., 2020; Liu et al., 2020; Peng et al., 2020; Xu et al., 2020). The *tet*(X6) variant carried by HNCF44W and HNCF43W is the same as that reported in *P. cibarius* from swine (Liu et al., 2020). The expression of *tet*(X6) in the cloning vector pMD19-T-tet(X6) in *E. coli* DH5α conferred resistance to tetracycline (64 mg/L) and tigecycline (16 mg/L) with 32-fold increments compared to that of DH5α-pMD19-T, indicating that this *tet*(X6) variant can confer tigecycline resistance (**Supplementary Table S2**). The 1137 bp *tet*(X6) variant encoded 378 amino acids and showed 84.7, 66.3, 84.9, 79.9, 87.8, 93.7, and 98.7% amino acid sequence identity to Tet(X), Tet(X1), Tet(X2), Tet(X3), Tet(X4), Tet(X5), and Tet(X6), respectively (**Figure 3**) with 5, 8, and 16 amino acid substitutions to Tet(X6) (MN507533, T60), Tet(X6) (CP025402, pMS8345A), and Tet(X6) (NZ_CP047050, 18QD1AZ29W).

Phylogenetic analysis of Tet(X) indicated that of all reported Tet(X6) variants clustered in a clade, most related to Tet(X5) (**Figure 3**). Although most *tet*(X6) variants were found in *Proteus* and *Acinetobacter* spp., analysis of the NCBI database shows that *E. coli* positive for *tet*(X6) existed as early as 2003 in Denmark (JWJM01000174), indicating the transmission of *tet*(X6) occurred previously. Furthermore, chromosomal *tet*(X6)-bearing ICEs and MDRs are found in *Proteus, Acinetobacter,* and *Myroides phaeus* (He D. et al., 2020; Liu et al., 2020; Peng et al., 2020). Plasmid-mediated *tet*(X6) in *Proteus, Acinetobacter,* and *E. coli* also emerged according to published reports (Cui et al., 2020; Li et al., 2020c; Xu et al., 2020), implying *tet*(X6) is at the stage of being expanded via different mobile elements. This highlights that *tet*(X6) variants would be the next possible prominent *tet*(X) allele, approaching the widespread situation of *tet*(X4) in *E. coli* (Bai et al., 2019; He et al., 2019; Sun et al., 2019). Nomenclature of *tet*(X) by different allele numbers is not recommended because many of the alleles are 85–100% aa identical[3], but an identical *tet*(X) naming system may not benefit research communications and AMR surveillance, especially as different *tet*(X) alleles possess different resistance phenotypes, genetic contexts, hosts, and evolutionary routes as more research reveals. For example, *tet*(X4) was found to be more common in *E. coli* than *tet*(X6) owing to the fact that *tet*(X4) has merged into conjugative plasmids adapted in *E. coli*. Also, the plasmids coharboring both $bla_{\mathrm{NDM-1}}$ and *tet*(X) in *Acinetobacter* spp. (Cui et al., 2020) could be divided into *tet*(X3)- or *tet*(X6)-bearing plasmids, which could make it difficult to decipher the accurate different genetic contexts if only *tet*(X) represented the two alleles simultaneously. To better investigate the molecular epidemiology, genomic evolution, and functional analysis and avoid confusion in *tet*(X) designations, a clear nomenclature scheme acceptable to researchers worldwide should be proposed as soon as possible. Because *mcr* genes exist in certain bacterial species as housekeeping genes and certain alleles leap over species boundary limits to Enterobacterales via mobile elements like Tn*6330* (Li et al., 2016; Shen et al., 2020), *tet*(X) genes may behave similarly because they exist as core genes in certain bacteria and transfer to Enterobacterales by mobile elements like IS*CR2*. Thus, the *mcr* nomenclature scheme may be a good example when it comes to *tet*(X) designation (Partridge et al., 2018). More research should be performed to put forward a widely accepted *tet*(X) allele numbering system to facilitate research communications.

[3] http://faculty.washington.edu/marilynr/

## CONCLUSION

To conclude, we characterized three *tet*(X)-bearing Enterobacterales strains of chicken origin and found that one *P. cibarius* coharbored both $bla_{\mathrm{NDM-1}}$ and *tet*(X6). To the best of our knowledge, this is the first report of convergence of *tet*(X6) and $bla_{\mathrm{NDM-1}}$ genes in Enterobacterales, highlighting the importance of continuous surveillance of tigecycline- and carbapenem-resistant Enterobacterales of animal origin, which may act as the potential reservoir of clinical Enterobacterales resistant to tigecycline and carbapenems.

## AUTHOR CONTRIBUTIONS

RL and ZW: conceptualization, writing – review and editing, and supervision. YaL and RL: methodology. YaL and QW: investigation. QW, KP, and YuL: data curation and visualization. YaL: writing – original draft preparation. All authors have read and agreed to the published version of the manuscript.

## FUNDING

This work was supported by grants from the Natural Science Foundation of Jiangsu Province (BK20180900), the National Natural Science Foundation of China (31872523), and the Priority Academic Program Development of Jiangsu Higher Education Institutions (PAPD).

## REFERENCES

Alikhan, N. F., Petty, N. K., Ben Zakour, N. L., and Beatson, S. A. (2011). BLAST ring image generator (BRIG): simple prokaryote genome comparisons. *BMC Genomics* 12:402. doi: 10.1186/1471-2164-12-402

Aminov, R. I. (2013). Evolution in action: dissemination of tet(X) into pathogenic microbiota. *Front. Microbiol.* 4:192. doi: 10.3389/fmicb.2013.00192

Bai, L., Du, P., Du, Y., Sun, H., Zhang, P., Wan, Y., et al. (2019). Detection of plasmid-mediated tigecycline-resistant gene tet(X4) in *Escherichia coli* from pork, Sichuan and Shandong Provinces, China, February 2019. *Euro Surveill.* 24:1900340.

Chen, C., Wu, X. T., He, Q., Chen, L., Cui, C. Y., Zhang, Y., et al. (2019). Complete sequence of a tet(X4)-harboring IncX1 plasmid, pYY76-1-2, in *Escherichia coli* from a cattle sample in China. *Antimicrob. Agents Chemother.* 63:e01528-19.

Chen, Y. P., Lei, C. W., Kong, L. H., Zeng, J. X., Zhang, X. Z., Liu, B. H., et al. (2018). Tn6450, a novel multidrug resistance transposon characterized in a *Proteus mirabilis* isolate from chicken in China. *Antimicrob. Agents Chemother.* 62:e02192-17.

CLSI (2018). *Performance Standards for Antimicrobial Susceptibility Testing. 28th ed. CLSI Supplement M100.* Wayne, PA: CLSI.

Cui, C. Y., Chen, C., Liu, B. T., He, Q., Wu, X. T., Sun, R. Y., et al. (2020). Co-occurrence of plasmid-mediated tigecycline and carbapenem resistance in Acinetobacter spp. from waterfowls and their neighboring environment. *Antimicrob. Agents Chemother.* 64:e02502-19.

Dallenne, C., Da Costa, A., Decre, D., Favier, C., and Arlet, G. (2010). Development of a set of multiplex PCR assays for the detection of genes encoding important beta-lactamases in *Enterobacteriaceae*. *J. Antimicrob. Chemother.* 65, 490–495. doi: 10.1093/jac/dkp498

Dobiasova, H., and Dolejska, M. (2016). Prevalence and diversity of IncX plasmids carrying fluoroquinolone and beta-lactam resistance genes in *Escherichia coli* originating from diverse sources and geographical areas. *J. Antimicrob. Chemother.* 71, 2118–2124. doi: 10.1093/jac/dkw144

Doublet, B., Schwarz, S., Kehrenberg, C., and Cloeckaert, A. (2005). Florfenicol resistance gene floR is part of a novel transposon. *Antimicrob. Agents Chemother.* 49, 2106–2108. doi: 10.1128/aac.49.5.2106-2108.2005

Du, X., He, F., Shi, Q., Zhao, F., Xu, J., Fu, Y., et al. (2018). The rapid emergence of tigecycline resistance in blaKPC-2 harboring *Klebsiella pneumoniae*, as mediated in vivo by mutation in tetA during tigecycline treatment. *Front. Microbiol.* 9:648. doi: 10.3389/fmicb.2018.00648

Forsberg, K. J., Patel, S., Wencewicz, T. A., and Dantas, G. (2015). The tetracycline destructases: a novel family of tetracycline-inactivating enzymes. *Chem. Biol.* 22, 888–897. doi: 10.1016/j.chembiol.2015.05.017

He, D., Wang, L., Zhao, S., Liu, L., Liu, J., Hu, G., et al. (2020). A novel tigecycline resistance gene, tet(X6), on an SXT/R391 integrative and conjugative element in a *Proteus* genomospecies 6 isolate of retail meat origin. *J. Antimicrob. Chemother.* 75, 1159–1164. doi: 10.1093/jac/dkaa012

He, T., Li, R., Wei, R., Liu, D., Bai, L., Zhang, L., et al. (2020). Characterization of *Acinetobacter indicus* co-harbouring tet(X3) and blaNDM-1 of dairy cow origin. *J. Antimicrob. Chemother.* 2020:dkaa182.

He, T., Wang, R., Liu, D., Walsh, T. R., Zhang, R., Lv, Y., et al. (2019). Emergence of plasmid-mediated high-level tigecycline resistance genes in animals and humans. *Nat. Microbiol.* 4, 1450–1456. doi: 10.1038/s41564-019-0445-2

Kumar, S., Stecher, G., Li, M., Knyaz, C., and Tamura, K. (2018). MEGA X: molecular evolutionary genetics analysis across computing platforms. *Mol. Biol. Evol.* 35, 1547–1549. doi: 10.1093/molbev/msy096

Li, R., Liu, Z., Peng, K., Liu, Y., Xiao, X., and Wang, Z. (2019). Cooccurrence of Two tet(X) variants in an empedobacter brevis strain of shrimp origin. *Antimicrob. Agents Chemother.* 63:e01636-19.

Li, R., Lu, X., Liu, Z., Liu, Y., Xiao, X., and Wang, Z. (2020a). Rapid detection and characterization of tet(X4)-positive *Escherichia coli* strains with nanopore sequencing. *J. Antimicrob. Chemother.* 75, 1068–1070. doi: 10.1093/jac/dkz528

Li, R., Lu, X., Peng, K., Liu, Z., Li, Y., Liu, Y., et al. (2020b). Deciphering the structural diversity and classification of the mobile tigecycline resistance gene tet (X)-bearing plasmidome among bacteria. *mSystems* 5:e00134-20.

Li, R., Peng, K., Li, Y., Liu, Y., and Wang, Z. (2020c). Exploring tet(X)-bearing tigecycline-resistant bacteria of swine farming environments. *Sci. Total Environ.* 733:139306. doi: 10.1016/j.scitotenv.2020.139306

Li, R., Xie, M., Dong, N., Lin, D., Yang, X., Wong, M. H. Y., et al. (2018). Efficient generation of complete sequences of MDR-encoding plasmids by rapid assembly of MinION barcoding sequencing data. *Gigascience* 7, 1–9.

Li, R., Xie, M., Lv, J., Wai-Chi Chan, E., and Chen, S. (2016). Complete genetic analysis of plasmids carrying mcr-1 and other resistance genes in an *Escherichia coli* isolate of animal origin. *J. Antimicrob. Chemother.* 72, 696–699.

Liu, D., Zhai, W., Song, H., Fu, Y., Schwarz, S., He, T., et al. (2020). Identification of the novel tigecycline resistance gene tet(X6) and its variants in Myroides, Acinetobacter and *Proteus* of food animal origin. *J. Antimicrob. Chemother.* 75, 1428-1431.

Marchaim, D., Pogue, J. M., Tzuman, O., Hayakawa, K., Lephart, P. R., Salimnia, H., et al. (2014). Major variation in MICs of tigecycline in gram-negative *Bacilli* as a function of testing method. *J. Clin. Microbiol.* 52, 1617–1621. doi: 10.1128/jcm.00001-14

Partridge, S. R., Di Pilato, V., Doi, Y., Feldgarden, M., Haft, D. H., Klimke, W., et al. (2018). Proposal for assignment of allele numbers for mobile colistin resistance (mcr) genes. *J. Antimicrob. Chemother.* 73, 2625–2630. doi: 10.1093/jac/dky262

Peng, K., Li, R., He, T., Liu, Y., and Wang, Z. (2020). Characterization of a porcine *Proteus cibarius* strain co-harbouring tet(X6) and cfr. *J. Antimicrob. Chemother.* 75, 1652–1654. doi: 10.1093/jac/dkaa047

Shen, Y., Zhang, R., Schwarz, S., Wu, C., Shen, J., Walsh, T. R., et al. (2020). Farm animals and aquaculture: significant reservoirs of mobile colistin resistance genes. *Environ. Microbiol.* 22, 2469–2484. doi: 10.1111/1462-2920.14961

Sullivan, M. J., Petty, N. K., and Beatson, S. A. (2011). Easyfig: a genome comparison visualizer. *Bioinformatics* 27, 1009–1010. doi: 10.1093/bioinformatics/btr039

Sun, J., Chen, C., Cui, C. Y., Zhang, Y., Liu, X., Cui, Z. H., et al. (2019). Plasmid-encoded tet(X) genes that confer high-level tigecycline resistance in *Escherichia coli*. *Nat. Microbiol.* 4, 1457–1464. doi: 10.1038/s41564-019-0496-4

Tacconelli, E., Carrara, E., Savoldi, A., Harbarth, S., Mendelson, M., Monnet, D. L., et al. (2018). Discovery, research, and development of new antibiotics: the WHO priority list of antibiotic-resistant bacteria and tuberculosis. *Lancet Infect. Dis.* 18, 318–327.

Tian, Z., Liu, R., Zhang, H., Yang, M., and Zhang, Y. (2019). Developmental dynamics of antibiotic resistome in aerobic biofilm microbiota treating wastewater under stepwise increasing tigecycline concentrations. *Environ. Int.* 131:105008. doi: 10.1016/j.envint.2019.105008

Wang, L., Liu, D., Lv, Y., Cui, L., Li, Y., Li, T., et al. (2019). Novel plasmid-mediated tet(X5) gene conferring resistance to tigecycline, eravacycline, and omadacycline in a clinical *Acinetobacter baumannii* isolate. *Antimicrob. Agents Chemother.* 64:e01326-19.

Xu, Y., Liu, L., and Feng, Y. (2020). A new tet(X6) tigecycline resistance determinant co-carried with mcr-1 by a single plasmid. *bioRxiv* [Preprint]. doi: 10.1101/2020.03.06.981738

# 10

# Acquisition of Tigecycline Resistance by Carbapenem-Resistant *Klebsiella pneumoniae* Confers Collateral Hypersensitivity to Aminoglycosides

*Hua-le Chen[1,2†], Yan Jiang[3†], Mei-mei Li[3], Yao Sun[1], Jian-ming Cao[4], Cui Zhou[1], Xiao-xiao Zhang[1], Yue Qu[5*] and Tie-li Zhou[1*]*

*[1] Department of Clinical Laboratory, The First Affiliated Hospital of Wenzhou Medical University, Wenzhou, China, [2] Department of Laboratory Medicine, The Second Affiliated Hospital of Wenzhou Medical University, Wenzhou, China, [3] Department of Infectious Diseases, Sir Run Run Shaw Hospital, Zhejiang University School of Medicine, Hangzhou, China, [4] School of Laboratory Medicine and Life Science, Wenzhou Medical University, Wenzhou, China, [5] Biomedicine Discovery Institute, Department of Microbiology, Faculty of Medicine, Nursing and Health Sciences, Monash University, Clayton, VIC, Australia*

***Correspondence:**
*Tie-li Zhou*
*wyztli@163.com*
*Yue Qu*
*yue.qu@monash.edu*

*† These authors have contributed equally to this work*

Tigecycline is a last-resort antibiotic for infections caused by carbapenem-resistant *Klebsiella pneumoniae* (CRKP). This study aimed to broaden our understanding of the acquisition of collateral hypersensitivity by CRKP, as an evolutionary trade-off of developing resistance to tigecycline. Experimental induction of tigecycline resistance was conducted with tigecycline-sensitive CRKP clinical isolates. Antimicrobial susceptibility testing, microbial fitness assessment, genotypic analysis and full-genome sequencing were carried out for these clinical isolates and their resistance-induced descendants. We found that tigecycline resistance was successfully induced after exposing CRKP clinical isolates to tigecycline at gradually increased concentrations, at a minor fitness cost of bacterial cells. Quantitative reverse transcription-polymerase chain reaction (RT-PCR) found higher expression of the efflux pump gene *acrB* (5.3–64.5-fold) and its regulatory gene *ramA* (7.4–65.8-fold) in resistance-induced strains compared to that in the tigecycline-sensitive clinical isolates. Stable hypersensitivities to aminoglycosides and other antibiotics were noticed in resistance-induced strains, showing significantly lowered MICs (X 4 – >500 times). Full genome sequencing and plasmid analysis suggested the induced collateral hypersensitivity might be multifaceted, with the loss of an antimicrobial resistance (AMR) plasmid being a possible major player. This study rationalized the sequential combination of tigecycline with aminoglycosides for the treatment of CRKP infections.

**Keywords: collateral sensitivity, CRKP, aminoglycosides, tigecycline, antimicrobial resistance**

## INTRODUCTION

Carbapenem-resistant *Klebsiella pneumoniae* (CRKP) has emerged as one of the deadliest causes of hospital-acquired infections and poses a serious therapeutic concern (Petrosillo et al., 2013). Overproduction of various carbapenemases in CRKP, such as *Klebsiella pneumoniae* carbapenemase (KPC) and metallo-β-lactamases (MBLs), renders the bacteria resistant to nearly all β-lactam antibiotics including carbapenems (Petrosillo et al., 2013).

Tigecycline and colistin are the very few options in the antibiotic arsenal for infections caused by carbapenem-resistant Enterobacteriaceae (Stein and Babinchak, 2013; Sun et al., 2013). Resistance to tigecycline of *Klebsiella* or other Enterobacteriaceae has emerged after its wide use in clinical settings, either as a monotherapy or in combination with other antibiotics (Woodford et al., 2007; Poulakou et al., 2009; Hirsch and Tam, 2010; Sekowska and Gospodarek, 2010; Stein and Babinchak, 2013; Sun et al., 2013; Gonzalez-Padilla et al., 2015). Underlying molecular mechanisms of tigecycline resistance are complex, with the upregulation of resistance-nodulation-division (RND) efflux pumps being a major contributor. Efflux pump systems related to tigecycline resistance include AcrAB-TolC and its positive regulators, *ramA*, SoxS, MarA or its negative regulator *ramR* (Hentschke et al., 2010; Roy et al., 2013; Villa et al., 2014; He et al., 2015; Juan et al., 2016; Xu et al., 2016), OqxAB and its positive regulator *rarA* and negative regulator *oqxR* (Zhong et al., 2014; Juan et al., 2016), and KpgABC (Nielsen et al., 2014; Juan et al., 2016). Structural alteration of the 30S ribosomal subunit protein S10 is another important resistance mechanism, mediated by mutations in the *rpsJ* gene and consequential target site modifications (Villa et al., 2014). A unique enzymatic inactivation mechanism mediated by Tet(X3) and Tet(X4), has also been associated with tigecycline resistance of numerous carbapenems-resistant Enterobacteriaceae (He et al., 2019; Sun et al., 2019).

Development of collateral sensitivity is a widespread evolutionary trade-off that occurs in many Gram-negative and Gram-positive bacteria (Barbosa et al., 2017; Lozano-Huntelman et al., 2020). Only a limited number of studies have examined collateral sensitivity in *Klebsiella pneumoniae*. Du et al. (2018) found that *K. pneumoniae* synchronously regained susceptibility to imipenem and meropenem when the patient developed resistance to tigecycline after long-term antibiotic treatment (Du et al., 2018). Villa et al. (2013) reported a reversion to susceptibility to carbapenems of a CRKP clinical isolate under the pressure of tigecycline (Villa et al., 2013). Proposed mechanisms mediating collateral sensitivity include plasticity of mobile elements in the host bacterium (Stohr et al., 2020), change of global gene expression associated with mutations in resistance genes (Maltas and Wood, 2019), amino acid deletions/substitutions that might result in reduced antibiotic hydrolase activity (Frohlich et al., 2019), and resistance mutations in regulatory genes for efflux pumps (Villa et al., 2013; Barbosa et al., 2017). Membrane-potential-altering mutations may also contribute to reversion of bacterial susceptibility to several unrelated classes of antibiotics, by changing the proton-motive force (PMF) and diminishing the activity of PMF-dependent major efflux pumps (Pal et al., 2015; Furusawa et al., 2018).

Recent emergence of CRKP clinical isolates that are resistant to both tigecycline and colistin, and discovery of a plasmid-mediated colistin resistance gene *mcr-1* highlight the pressing need of developing more effective antimicrobial strategies for CRKP infections (Zhang et al., 2018). This study aimed to establish a comprehensive understanding of collateral sensitivity that accompany the development of tigecycline resistance in CRKP, and to rationalize the combination antibiotic therapy using tigecycline and aminoglycosides for CRKP infections.

## MATERIALS AND METHODS

### Bacterial Isolates

Fifty CRKP isolates were from patients visiting the First Affiliated Hospital of Wenzhou Medical University and clinically diagnosed with CRKP infections between December 2013 and 2014. These clinical isolates were identified to a species level using the following tests: the Vitek II Identification System (bioMérieux Vitec Inc., Hazelwood, MO, United States) and MALDI Biotyper Identification System (MALDI-TOF MS, BioMérieux, Craponne, France).

### Pulsed-Field Gel Electrophoresis Analysis

Genomic DNA of *K. pneumoniae* clinical isolates was digested with restriction endonuclease *Xba*I (Takara Bio, Dalian, China). DNA fragments were separated in a Pulsed-field gel electrophoresis (PFGE) CHEF-Mapper XA system (Bio-Rad, Hercules, CA, United States) in 0.5 × Tris-borate-EDTA buffer at 14°C and 120 V for 19 h, with pulse times ranging from 5 s to 35 s. PFGE results were analyzed using Quantity One 1-D Analysis 4.6.9 (Bio-Rad, Hercules, CA, United States) Software.

### Antimicrobial Susceptibility Test

Antimicrobial susceptibility of 50 CRKP isolates to 15 first-line antibiotics were initially tested with the Vitek II Identification System (bioMérieux Vitec Inc., Hazelwood, MO, United States) and then confirmed by the CLSI recommended broth microdilution or agar dilution methods. The MICs of tigecycline for *K. pneumoniae* clinical isolates and resistance-induced strains were interpreted using breakpoints recommended by the European Committee on Antimicrobial Susceptibility Testing (EUCAST) criteria (susceptible, $\leq$1.0 μg/ml; medium, 1.0–2.0 μg/ml; resistant, >2.0 μg/ml) (European Committee on Antimicrobial Susceptibility Testing Steering, 2006). Susceptibility of other antimicrobial agents for *K. pneumoniae* was determined by the agar dilution method according to the Clinical and Laboratory Standards Institute (M100-S24, 2014). *Escherichia coli* ATCC 25922 was used as a quality control.

### *In vitro* Induction of Tigecycline Resistance

Four clinical isolates susceptible to tigecycline (K467, K43, K521, and K428) and one tigecycline-resistant clinical isolate (K537) were used to study tigecycline resistance induction and collateral sensitivity of CRKP. These five clinical isolates were assigned to sequence types by Multilocus sequence typing (MLST), according to the *K. pneumoniae* MLST website.[1] Tigecycline resistance was induced for the tigecycline-susceptible clinical

[1]https://bigsdb.pasteur.fr/klebsiella/klebsiella.html

isolates, by gradually exposing them to tigecycline at serially increasing concentrations at a 24 h interval (1/4 MIC to a higher concentration at which there was no bacterial growth) (Liu et al., 2011).

## Examining General Antimicrobial-Resistance Determinants for Tigecycline Resistance

Polymerase chain reaction (PCR) and sequencing were carried out to examine the presence of common antimicrobial-resistant genes in these 5 CRKP clinical isolates and four resistance-induced strains, including ESBLs genes ($bla_{CTX-M-1}$, $bla_{CTX-M-9}$, $bla_{TEM}$, $bla_{SHV}$, $bla_{VEB}$ and $bla_{PER}$), AmpC genes ($bla_{CMY}$, $bla_{FOX}$, $bla_{MOX}$, $bla_{DHA}$), carbapenemase genes ($bla_{KPC}$, $bla_{SPM}$, $bla_{IMP}$, $bla_{VIM}$, $bla_{GES}$, $bla_{NDM}$, $bla_{OXA-23}$, $bla_{OXA-48}$), PMQR genes (*qnrA, qnrB, qnrC, qnrD, qnrS, qepA, aac(6')-Ib-cr, oqxA, oqxB*), and 16S-RMTase genes (*armA, rmtA, rmtB, rmtC, rmtD, rmtE*). The mutation of chromosomal genes *gyrA* and *parC* was also examined. Primer sequences for PCR assays were adapted from other published studies (Doi and Arakawa, 2007; Dallenne et al., 2010; Park et al., 2012) and are available on request. Nucleotide sequences were compared by BLAST to align drug-resistance gene nucleotide sequences[2].

## Outer Membrane Proteins Analysis

A crude outer membrane fraction of CRKP clinical isolates and resistance-induced strains was obtained by growing the bacteria to a mid-log phase, followed by sonication. Outer membrane proteins (OMPs) were separated by sodium dodecyl sulfate polyacrylamide gel electrophoresis (SDS-PAGE). *K. pneumoniae* ATCC 13883 was used as a control for OMP profiling (Shi et al., 2013). The outer membrane protein encoding genes were further amplified using multiple primer pairs among the 4 paired strains (Zhang et al., 2014).

## Inhibition of Efflux Pumps With CCCP

Efflux pump inhibitor carbonyl cyanide m-chlorophenylhydrazone (CCCP, 10 mg/l) was used to examine the impact of efflux pumps on tigecycline resistance (Zhong et al., 2014). Minimum inhibitory concentrations of tigecycline for CRKP clinical isolates and resistance-induced strains were determined by the broth microdilution method in the presence or absence of CCCP. Four times or greater reduction of tigecycline MICs in the presence of CCCP was adopted as a significant inhibition effect for efflux pumps (He et al., 2015).

## Analysis of *acrR*, *ramR* and *oqxR* Mutations

Efflux pump regulator encoding genes including *acrR*, *ramR* and *oqxR* were amplified by PCR with specific primers (Bialek-Davenet et al., 2011; Lin et al., 2016). The nucleotide sequences of *acrR*, *ramR* and *oqxR* were analyzed using a basic local alignment search tool (BLAST)[3] with *K. pneumoniae* subsp. pneumoniae MGH 78578 as the reference strain (GenBank accession no. CP000647) (Hentschke et al., 2010).

## Quantitative Real-Time PCR

The relative expression levels of genes encoding efflux pumps AcrB and OqxB and their regulators *ramA* and *rarA* were evaluated using a 7500 Real-Time PCR (RT-PCR) system and *rpoB* as the housekeeping gene (Stein and Babinchak, 2013; He et al., 2015). All experiments were performed in triplicate. The relative expression of the target genes was analyzed using the comparative Ct method ($2^{-\Delta \Delta Ct}$) with the Agilent MxPro software.

## Genome Sequencing and Annotation

Whole-genome shotgun sequencing was carried out for 5 CRKP clinical isolates and 4 resistance-induced strains, using a standard run of Illumina HiSeq2000 sequencing using a generating 2 × 100 paired-end libraries (500-bp insert size) sequencing strategy according to the manufacturer's instructions. Clean reads were assembled into scaffolds using Velvet version 1.2.07. Post-Assembly Genome Improvement Toolkit (PAGIT) was then used to extend the initial contiguous sequences (contigs) and correct sequencing errors. Open reading frames (ORFs) were identified using Glimmer version 3.0. Protein-coding sequences were further BLAST-searched against the Antimicrobial Resistance Database (ARDB).

## Plasmid Analysis

Plasmids of 5 CRKP clinical isolates and 4 resistance-induced strains were analyzed by S1-nuclease pulsed-field gel electrophoresis (S1-PFGE). Plasmid DNA was extracted using a QIAGEN Plasmid Midi Kit (Qiagen, shanghai, China) according to the manufacturer's instructions, and was separated by electrophoresis in 0.8% agarose at 120 V for 1 h. The plasmids of *E. coli* V517 served as a size marker.

## Data Analysis and Statistical Methods

One-way ANOVA or a non-parametric test (Mann-Whitney *U* test) was carried out to compare two means, depending on the data distribution. Statistical significance was assumed at *p* value of less than 0.05. Data analysis was performed using Minitab 16 software (Minitab, State College, PA, United States).

# RESULTS

## Microbiological Characteristics of CRKP Clinical Isolates

Pulsed-field gel electrophoresis analysis of 50 CRKP clinical isolates showed five clusters, suggesting clonally distinct nature of these isolates (**Figure 1A**). Antimicrobial susceptibility tests showed that all CRKP isolates were resistant to first-line antibiotics except tigecycline and colistin; one isolate was found to be resistant to tigecycline (K537, MIC 8 mg/L, see **Table 1**). One representative strain from each cluster (designated as K537, K521, K467, K428, and K43) was chosen for further

[2]http://blast.ncbi.nlm.nih.gov/Blast.cgi

[3]http://www.ncbi.nlm.nih.gov/BLAST

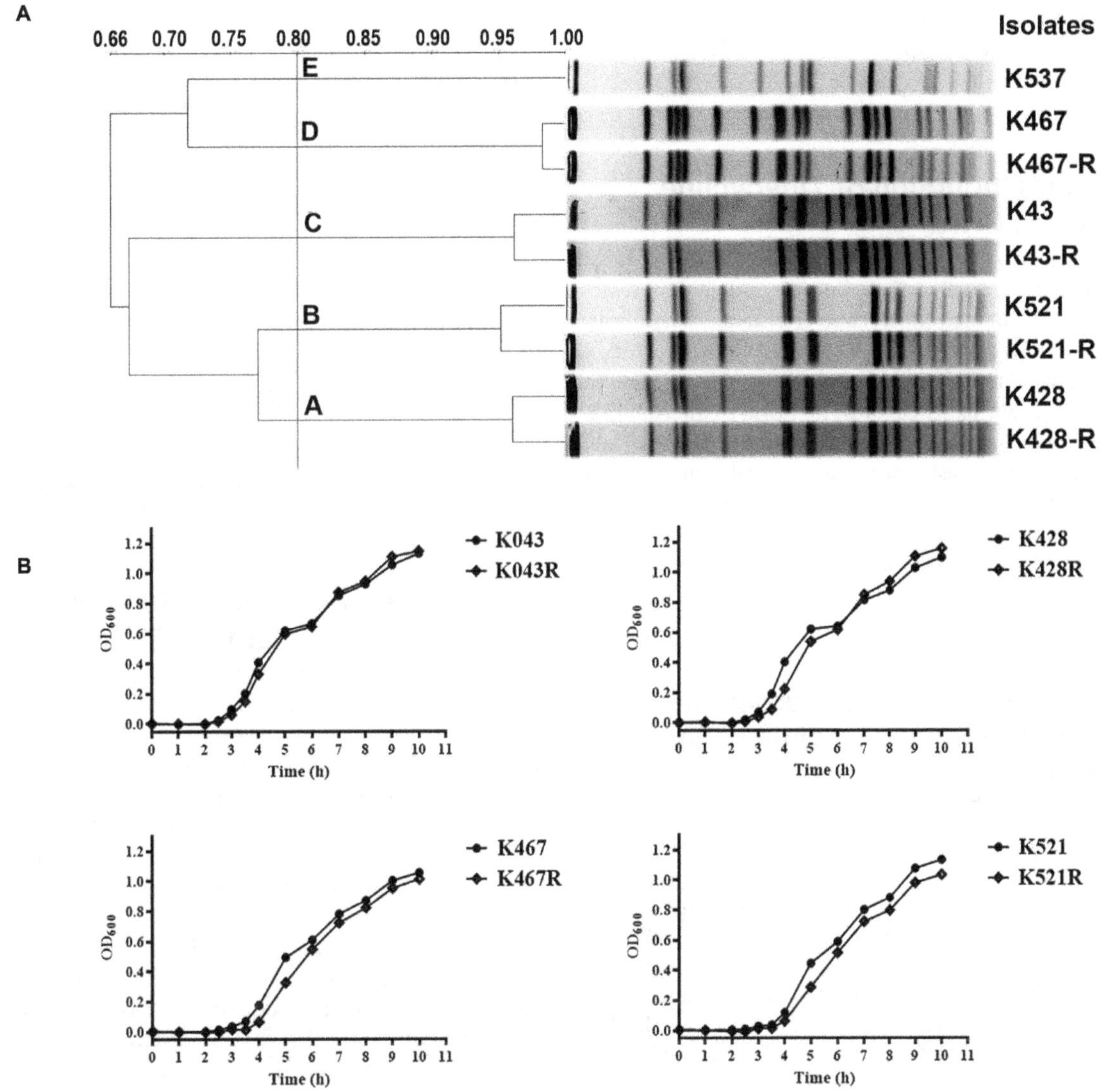


**FIGURE 1 | (A)** Pulsed-field gel electrophoresis (PFGE) analysis of five representative carbapenem-resistant *Klebsiella pneumoniae* (CRKP) clinical isolates and their resistance-induced descendants; **(B)** Growth dynamics of four resistance-induced strains and their parental clinical isolates.

**TABLE 1 |** Antimicrobial susceptibility of five CRKP clinical isolates and four resistance-induced descendant strains.

| **Isolates** | **Minimum inhibitory concentrations (μg/ml)** | | | | | | | | | | | | | | | |
|---|---|---|---|---|---|---|---|---|---|---|---|---|---|---|---|---|
| | **AMK** | **CRO** | **CTX** | **CAZ** | **IPM** | **MEM** | **ETP** | **LEV** | **CIP** | **TOB** | **GEN** | **C** | **FOS** | **PB** | **TGC** | **TGC + CCCP** |
| **K537** | >256 | >256 | >256 | >256 | 64 | 128 | 256 | 16 | 64 | 256 | >128 | >256 | >1024 | 1 | 8 | 4 |
| **K467** | >256 | >256 | >256 | 256 | 128 | 256 | >256 | 16 | 64 | 256 | >128 | >256 | >1024 | 0.5 | 0.5 | 0.5 |
| **K467-R** | <0.25 | 128 | >256 | 128 | 64 | 128 | 128 | 32 | 64 | <0.25 | 0.5 | >256 | 128 | 0.5 | 16 | 4 |
| **K521** | >256 | >256 | >256 | >256 | 128 | 256 | >256 | 16 | 64 | 256 | >128 | >256 | >1024 | 1 | 0.5 | 0.25 |
| **K521-R** | <0.25 | 128 | 256 | 32 | 128 | 128 | >256 | 32 | 64 | <0.25 | <0.25 | >256 | 256 | 1 | 16 | 4 |
| **K428** | >256 | >256 | >256 | >256 | 32 | 128 | >256 | 16 | 64 | 256 | >128 | >256 | >1024 | 1 | 0.5 | 0.5 |
| **K428-R** | 0.5 | 32 | 8 | 256 | 0.25 | 0.25 | 0.25 | 16 | 64 | 128 | 8 | >256 | 4 | 0.5 | 16 | 4 |
| **K43** | >256 | >256 | >256 | 64 | 32 | 256 | 256 | 16 | 64 | 128 | >128 | >256 | >1024 | 1 | 0.5 | 0.5 |
| **K43-R** | <0.25 | 0.25 | 2 | 1 | 0.25 | 1 | 8 | 0.25 | 1 | 0.5 | 1 | >256 | 16 | 1 | 32 | 8 |

*AMK, amikacin; CRO, ceftriaxone; CTX, cefotaxime; CAZ, ceftazidime; IPM, imipenem; MEM, meropenem; ETP, ertapenem; LEV, levofloxacin; CIP, ciprofloxacin; TOB, tobramycinl; GEN, gentamicin; C, chloramphenicol; FOS, fosfomycin; PB, polymyxin B; TGC + CCCP, tigecycline with CCCP.*

studies. MLST found that the tigecycline-resistant clinical isolate K537 and tigecycline-sensitive isolates K521, K467, K428, and K43 belonged to sequence types ST39, ST11, ST11, ST37, and ST3623, respectively.

## Experimental Induction of Tigecycline Resistance in CRKP

Four tigecycline-sensitive clinical isolates (K467, K521, K428, and K43) were treated with tigecycline at gradually increased concentrations to induce tigecycline resistance. Significant increases in the MICs of tigecycline (32- – 64- fold) were achieved for the descendant strains in comparison with their parental clinical isolates (**Table 1**). PFGE analysis further confirmed the origin of the resistance-induced CRKP strains (**Figure 1A**). The induced tigecycline-resistance remained stable after sixteen passages of CRKP in an antibiotic-free growth medium. Comparing the growth dynamics of tigecycline-sensitive clinical isolates and their resistance-induced descendant strains showed a minor but universal fitness loss (**Figure 1B**).

## Molecular Mechanisms Underpinning Experimental Induction of Tigecycline Resistance

We examined the role of adenosine triphosphate (ATP)-driven efflux pumps in the resistance of CRKP to many antibiotics including tigecycline. Using the efflux pump inhibitor CCCP partially restored the susceptibility of all five tigecycline-resistant strains (**Table 1**). Gene expression of pump- and regulator-encoding genes including *acrB*, *ramA*, *oqxB*, and *rarA* was evaluated (**Figure 2**). All tigecycline-resistant strains showed higher expression of *acrB* (6. 9-, 19. 3-, 15. 6-, 5. 3-, 64.5-fold for K537, K467-R, K521-R, K428-R, and K43-R, respectively) and its regulator gene *ramA* (7. 4-, 12. 2-, 13. 5-, 34. 5-, 65.8-fold, respectively). Over-expression of *oqxB* and *rarA* was seen in K43-R (12.5-fold and 2.5-fold) and K521-R (2.7-fold and 5.9-fold).

We also sequenced genes encoding other important regulators of efflux pumps, including *acrR*, *ramR*, and *oqxR*. No mutation was identified in *acrR* and *ramR*. Mutations in *oqxR* were found; no difference between tigecycline-sensitive clinical isolates and their resistance-induced counterparts indicated no direct link between *oqxR* mutation and experimentally induced tigecycline resistance (**Table 2**). SDS-PAGE was carried out to study the role of three major OMPs (ompK34, ompK35, and ompK36) on tigecycline resistance, that may affect the diffusion of tigecycline to its target sites. Using the porin profile of *K. pneumoniae* ATCC 13883 as a control, OmpK36 was missing on SDS-PAGE and amplification of its encoding gene with PCR was unsuccessful (**Figure 3**), suggesting that a deletion and/or rearrangement of its encoding gene might have occurred in strains with clinical background. Same SDS-PAGE results for tigecycline-sensitive clinical isolates and resistance-induced descendant strains, again suggested no direct association between these OMPs and induced tigecycline resistance.

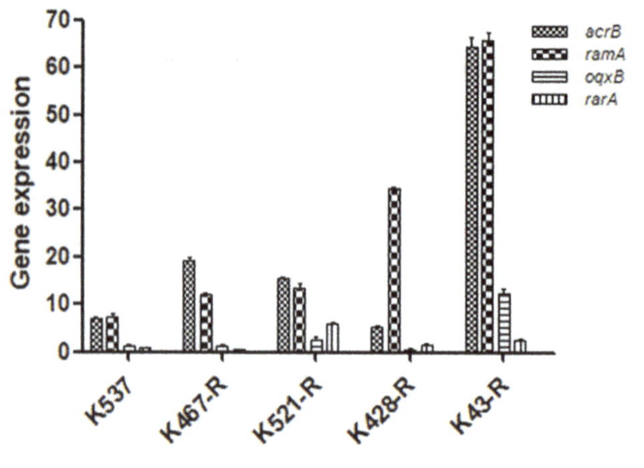


**FIGURE 2 |** Expression of pump and regulator encoding genes including *acrB*, *ramA*, *oqxB*, and *rarA* in five tigecycline-resistant CRKP strains. The values were expressed as mean ± standard deviation (SD).

## Emergence of Collateral Sensitivity in Tigecycline-Resistant CRPK

Interestingly, prolonged exposure of CRKP to tigecycline reversed their resistance to all tested antibiotics except chloramphenicol and tigecycline; significantly lowered MICs of different antibiotics were found for all resistance-induced descendant strains (**Table 1**). The level of acquired hypersensitivity seemed to be antibiotic and strain dependent. Up to 2048-fold decreases in the MIC of cephalosporins and carbapenems were observed when tigecycline-sensitive clinical isolates were converted into tigecycline-resistant descendant strains; up to 64-fold and 512-fold decreases in the MIC were found when fluoroquinolones and fosfomycin were tested, respectively. At least 2 out of 4 tigecycline-sensitive and tigecycline-resistant pairs showed relatively small changes in the MIC of these non-aminoglycoside antibiotics ($\leq$4-fold for cephalosporins and carbapenems, $\leq$2-fold for fluoroquinolones, and $\leq$16-fold for fosfomycin). More significant decreases in the MIC were noticed for aminoglycosides when compared with other antibiotics (**Table 1**). Most resistance-induced strains had MICs of amikacin, tobramycin and gentamicin 250-fold lower than that of their parental clinical isolates. The induced hypersensitivity of CRKP to aminoglycosides and other antibiotics remained stable after regrowth in an antibiotic-free medium for 16 passages.

## Evaluating Common Antibiotic Resistance Determinants for Collateral Hypersensitivity of CRKP

Some common antibiotic resistance determinants were examined for 5 CRKP clinical isolates and 4 resistance-induced descendent strains. All isolates harbored the KPC-2 carbapenemase-encoding gene ($bla_{KPC-2}$) and genes encoding other β-lactamases including SHV (sulf-hydryl variable) and TEM (Temoniera in). Genes encoding CTX-M-type ESBLs were only found in the K467 pairs and K521 pairs. Some other

**TABLE 2 |** Mutations of *acrR*, *ramR* and *oqxR* in five clinical isolates and four resistance-induced descendant strains.

| Strain no. | *acrR* mutation | *ramR* mutation | *oqxR* mutation |
|---|---|---|---|
| K537 | No mutation | No mutation | Missense mutation: R152H, M224T |
| K43 | No mutation | No mutation | Missense mutation: R152H, M224T |
| K43-R | No mutation | No mutation | Missense mutation: R152H, M224T |
| K428 | No mutation | No mutation | Silent mutation: P108P; Missense mutation: R152H, M224T, G317D |
| K428-R | No mutation | No mutation | Silent mutation: P108P; Missense mutation: R152H, M224T, G317D |
| K467 | No mutation | No mutation | Silent mutation: P108P; Missense mutation: R152H, M224T, G317D |
| K467-R | No mutation | No mutation | Silent mutation: P108P; Missense mutation: R152H, M224T, G317D |
| K521 | No mutation | No mutation | Silent mutation: P108P; Missense mutation: R152H, M224T, G317D |
| K521-R | No mutation | No mutation | Silent mutation: P108P; Missense mutation: R152H, M224T, G317D |

common AMR genes conferring antibiotic resistance in CRKP were sequenced, including *gyrA* encoding the DNA gyrase and *parC* encoding DNA topoisomerase that are responsible for fluoroquinolone resistance. An amino acid substitution of S83I was detected in *gyrA* in all 9 strains and S80I was detected in *parC* in the K428, K467, and K521 pairs. *gyrA* mutation D87G was found in the K467 and K521 pairs. The plasmid-carrying quinolone resistance gene *qnrS* was also detected in K537 and K467 pairs. Interestingly, the 16S-rRNA methylase encoding gene *rmtB*, a gene that confers resistance to most clinically relevant aminoglycosides, was found in K467 and K521 but missing in their resistance-induced counterparts.

## Whole Genome Sequencing Broadened Our Understanding of Collateral Sensitivity in CRKP

Common genetic determinants seemed to be inadequate to explain the induced hypersensitivity to aminoglycosides of CRKP. We thus performed a next-generation full genome sequencing for all nine strains selected for this study, intending to identify molecular determinants that differ between the tigecycline-sensitive and tigecycline-resistant groups. Despite the significant difference in the bacterial resistance to multiple antibiotics including aminoglycosides, no obvious chromosome-related genetic difference was found (**Supplementary Figure 1** and **Supplementary Table 1**, for reviewers' information only). Full genome sequencing of CRKP revealed several antibiotic-resistance related mutations that were not unique to the tigecycline-sensitive parental strains or their tigecycline-resistant descendants, including: 1) a 4bp mutation in non-coding region between *ybhN* and *ybhL* in the K428 pairs, 2) a 11bp insertion in the non-coding region between *garK-1* and *tRNA_anti-like,* a 10bp insertion in the non-coding region between *kp467_02292* and *kp467_02293* and a 4bp mutation in the gene encoding DNA polymerase IV (*dinB_4)* in the K467 pairs, 3) and a 12bp insertion in the non-coding region between *kp521_05022* and *kp521_05023* in the K521 pairs (**Table 3**). Several key AMR mobile elements were found in the parental clinical isolates but not the descendants, including *rmtB* (K467 and K521 pairs), $bla_{TEM-1E}$ (K521 pair), *fosA3* (K467 and K521 pairs) (**Supplementary Figure 1**). As *rmtB* and *fosA3* are often co-carried on a large AMR plasmid, we hypothesized that loss of an AMR plasmid might have occurred to compensate the fitness cost. S1-PFGE revealed that all clinical isolates contained multiple plasmids ranging from 2.1 kb to 54.2 kb in size (**Figure 4**). One plasmid of 54.2–5.6 kb was absent in K43-R but present in K43, and one plasmid of approximately 2.1 kb was missing in K467-R but not the parental clinical isolate.

## DISCUSSION

Extended spectrum beta lactamase-producing CRKP are now among the most critical pathogens advised by the recent WHO global priority list of antibiotic-resistant bacteria (WHO, 2020). The overuse of tigecycline and colistin in clinical settings has promoted CRKP to develop resistance to both last-resort antibiotics (Zhang et al., 2018), highlighting a pressing clinical need for alternative strategies such as antibiotic combination therapy. This study intended to increase our understanding of collateral sensitivity in CRKP that tolerates tigecycline treatment, and such knowledge might serve as the foundation of a promising combination therapy for otherwise "untreatable" CRKP infections.

Carbapenem-resistant *Klebsiella pneumoniae* isolates used in this study have distinct PFGE patterns and belong to different sequence types, supporting the non-dominant clonal nature of CRKP encountered in a hospital environment (Chiu et al., 2017). Development of resistance or non-susceptibility to tigecycline has been linked to prolonged use of tigecycline or other antibiotics (Lin et al., 2016). Our mechanistic study of tigecycline resistance only found an association between the reduced tigecycline susceptibility and the overexpression of *acrB/ramA* in CRKP. No significant difference in the expression of *oqxB* and *rarA*, or missense/silent mutations in *oqxR*, *acrR* or *ramR* was found when comparing tigecycline-sensitive clinical isolates and their resistance-induced descendants.

Enterobacteriaceae is known to be able to regain collateral sensitivity to many first-line antibiotics when developing resistance to tigecycline, in particular aminoglycosides (Fang et al., 2016; Barbosa et al., 2017). The underlying mechanisms of collateral sensitivity have been proposed but not been fully disclosed (Barbosa et al., 2017). Barbosa et al. (2017) reported that resistance mutation in the regulatory genes of efflux pumps such as *nalC* or *mexZ* might resensitize β-lactam-adapted bacterial

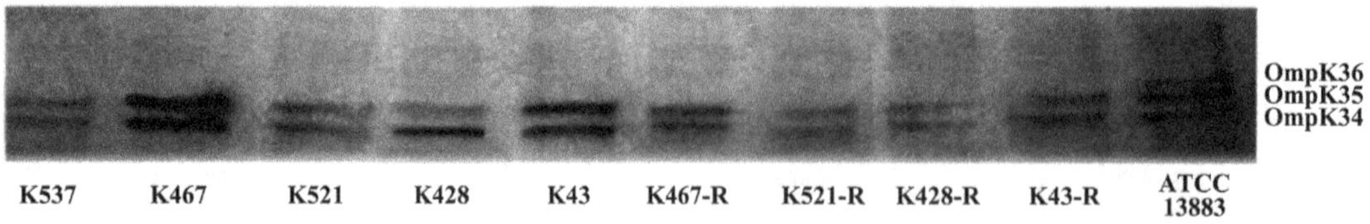


**FIGURE 3 |** Sodium dodecyl sulfate polyacrylamide gel electrophoresis (SDS-PAGE) of outer membrane proteins (OMPs) in five CRKP clinical isolates and four resistance-induced descendants.

**TABLE 3 |** Mutations observed in the four clinical isolates and their resistance-induced descendant strains.

| Strain | Nearest gene(s) | Reference position (nt) | Reference sequence | Mutant sequence | Mutation type | Predicted effect |
|---|---|---|---|---|---|---|
| **K428/ K428-R** | ybhN and ybhL | 171782 | GGGC | AAAT | MNV | Non-coding region |
| **K467/ K467-R** | *garK-1* and *tRNA_anti-like* | 149888 | – | GCTATACCAAA | Insertion | Non-coding region |
| | *kp467_02292* and *kp467_02293* | 1318 | – | CGAAAAATTT | Insertion | Non-coding region |
| | *dinB_4* | 1703 | GGAA | ATCC | MNV | DNA polymerase IV |
| **K521/ K521-R** | *kp521_05022* and *kp521_05023* | 1318 | – | CGAAAAATTTTT | Insertion | Non-coding region |

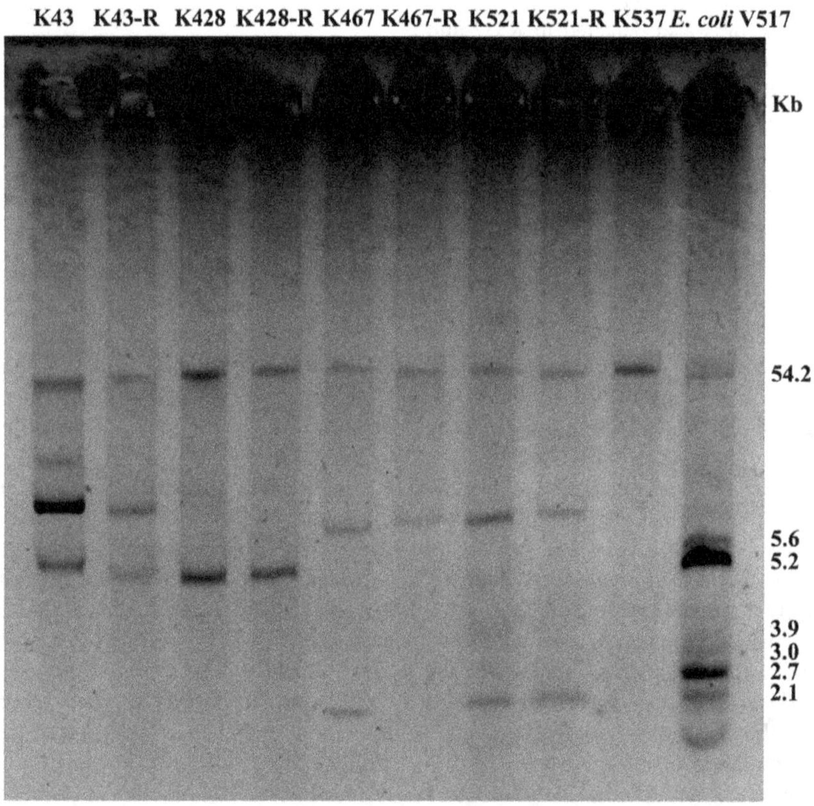


**FIGURE 4 |** Plasmid analysis of five CRKP clinical isolates and four resistance-induced strains. *Escherichia coli* V517 was used as a control.

populations to aminoglycosides (Barbosa et al., 2017). Previously reported collateral sensitivity in *K. pneumoniae* was supported by mild decreases in MICs of several first-line antibiotics, by 2–10 times (Fang et al., 2016). We, however, found dramatic changes in MICs of aminoglycosides (> 100 times) for all 4 experimentally induced tigecycline-resistant strains. Current mechanisms of aminoglycoside resistance do not seem to sufficiently explain the much greater level of collateral sensitivity of CRKP found in this study (Wachino et al., 2020). We hypothesized that accumulative mechanisms drove the development of collateral hypersensitivity of tigecycline-resistant CRKP. We assessed such trade-offs through whole-genome sequencing of clinical isolates and experimentally induced resistant strains. Genomes of our clinical isolates and resistance-induced descendent strains have high similarity to CRKP clinical isolates of different ST (ST15, ST512, ST11 and ST17) sequenced by others (Hua et al., 2014; Villa et al., 2014; Xu et al., 2017; Du et al., 2018); no major chromosome-related genetic difference were found (Fang et al., 2016). We did find loss of a major AMR plasmid in at least two laboratory evolved strains (K43-R and K467-R). It has been proposed that the co-carriage of various important AMR determinants such as $bla_{KPC-2}$, $bla_{TEM-1}$, $bla_{CTX-M-14}$, and *rmtB* on one plasmid could provide evolutionary benefits to bacteria in an antibiotic-rich environment (Sheng et al., 2012). *K. pneumoniae* is an opportunistic pathogen that is well-known for its diversity of antibiotic resistance genes, with significantly more varied DNA composition, and higher plasmid burden than other Gram-negative pathogens (Wyres and Holt, 2018). The high burden of plasmid carriage in *K. pneumoniae*, however, may result in a comparatively lower fitness of the bacterium (Wyres and Holt, 2018). The complex bacterium-plasmid interaction results in not only the adaption of the host to plasmid, but also specific adaption of plasmid to the host. We thus reasoned the voluntary loss of an AMR plasmid under the long-term pressure of tigecycline might also offer survival advantages to the bacterium (Sheng et al., 2012).

Limitations of this study include that only a small number of isolates were used and the structure of the AMR plasmids involved in collateral sensitivity was not further investigated, due to the limited time frame of this study. Another evident limitation is that tigecycline-resistant clinical isolate failed to show any sensitivity to aminoglycoside or other antibiotics and did not provide direct support to the proposed theory. However, theory raised from this experimental study was supported by findings of several recent clinical studies. Stohr et al. (2020) reported loss of the KPC-gene carrying plasmid and plasmid recombination in KPC-producing *K. pneumoniae* clinical isolates from two patients in a hospital outbreak (Stohr et al., 2020). Fang et al. (2016) also isolated tigecycline non-susceptible clinical isolates that had a 2–4-fold decreases in the MICs to aminoglycosides relative to its tigecycline-sensitive ancestral isolates (Fang et al., 2016).

## CONCLUSION

Carbapenem-resistant *Klebsiella pneumoniae* may develop collateral hypersensitivity to aminoglycosides and other antibiotics, accompanying the development of bacterial resistance to tigecycline. This experimental study provides a proof of concept to support the sequentially combinational use of tigecycline and aminoglycosides for the treatment of CRKP infections. Antimicrobial susceptibility tests of CRKP should be frequently repeated to provide more specific and accurate guidance for its treatment (Stohr et al., 2020).

## AUTHOR CONTRIBUTIONS

YQ and T-LZ: conceptualization and supervision. H-LC, YJ, and M-ML: methodology and validation. H-LC, YJ, and YQ: software. H-LC and M-ML: formal analysis, investigation, and writing—original draft preparation. H-LC, J-MC, and CZ: resources. H-LC and YJ: data curation. CZ, X-XZ, and YQ: writing—review and editing. YS, T-LZ, and YQ: funding acquisition. All authors have read and agreed to the published version of the manuscript.

## FUNDING

This work was supported by the National Natural Science Foundation of China (grant number 81802069), the Zhejiang Provincial Natural Science Foundation of China (grant number LY14H190005), the Planned Science and Technology Project of Wenzhou (grant number Y20150312), and Zhejiang Province Program for the Cultivation of High-level Innovative Health Talents.

## ACKNOWLEDGMENTS

We are grateful to the reviewers who helped to improve this paper.

## SUPPLEMENTARY MATERIALS

**Supplementary Figure 1** | Schematic diagram of comparison of chromosome-harboring or plasmid- harboring resistance genes between tigecycline-sensitive and -resistant pairs (K467 and K521 only). The white arrows illustrate the resistance genes among which the red framed arrows indicate the loss of genes in tigecycline-resistant strains.

## REFERENCES

Barbosa, C., Trebosc, V., Kemmer, C., Rosenstiel, P., Beardmore, R., Schulenburg, H., et al. (2017). Alternative evolutionary paths to bacterial antibiotic resistance cause distinct collateral effects. *Mol. Biol. Evol.* 34, 2229–2244. doi: 10.1093/molbev/msx158

Bialek-Davenet, S., Marcon, E., Leflon-Guibout, V., Lavigne, J. P., Bert, F., Moreau, R., et al. (2011). In vitro selection of ramR and soxR mutants overexpressing efflux systems by fluoroquinolones as well as cefoxitin in *Klebsiella pneumoniae*. *Antimicrob. Agents Chemother.* 55, 2795–2802. doi: 10.1128/AAC.00156-11

Chiu, S. K., Chan, M. C., Huang, L. Y., Lin, Y. T., Lin, J. C., Lu, P. L., et al. (2017). Tigecycline resistance among carbapenem-resistant *Klebsiella Pneumoniae*: clinical characteristics and expression levels of efflux pump genes. *PLoS One* 12:e0175140. doi: 10.1371/journal.pone.0175140

Dallenne, C., Da Costa, A., Decre, D., Favier, C., and Arlet, G. (2010). Development of a set of multiplex PCR assays for the detection of genes encoding important beta-lactamases in *Enterobacteriaceae*. *J. Antimicrob. Chemother.* 65, 490–495. doi: 10.1093/jac/dkp498

Doi, Y., and Arakawa, Y. (2007). 16S ribosomal RNA methylation: emerging resistance mechanism against aminoglycosides. *Clin. Infect. Dis.* 45, 88–94. doi: 10.1086/518605

Du, X., He, F., Shi, Q., Zhao, F., Xu, J., Fu, Y., et al. (2018). The rapid emergence of tigecycline resistance in blaKPC-2 harboring *Klebsiella pneumoniae*, as mediated in vivo by mutation in tetA during tigecycline treatment. *Front. Microbiol.* 9:648. doi: 10.3389/fmicb.2018.00648

European Committee on Antimicrobial Susceptibility Testing Steering (2006). EUCAST technical note on tigecycline. *Clin. Microbiol. Infect.* 12, 1147–1149. doi: 10.1111/j.1469-0691.2006.01578.x

Fang, L., Chen, Q., Shi, K., Li, X., Shi, Q., He, F., et al. (2016). Step-wise increase in tigecycline resistance in *Klebsiella pneumoniae* associated with mutations in ramR, lon and rpsJ. *PLoS One* 11:e0165019. doi: 10.1371/journal.pone.0165019

Frohlich, C., Sorum, V., Thomassen, A. M., Johnsen, P. J., Leiros, H. S., and Samuelsen, O. (2019). OXA-48-mediated ceftazidime-avibactam resistance is associated with evolutionary trade-offs. *mSphere* 4:e00024-19. doi: 10.1128/mSphere.00024-19

Furusawa, C., Horinouchi, T., and Maeda, T. (2018). Toward prediction and control of antibiotic-resistance evolution. *Curr. Opin. Biotechnol.* 54, 45–49. doi: 10.1016/j.copbio.2018.01.026

Gonzalez-Padilla, M., Torre-Cisneros, J., Rivera-Espinar, F., Pontes-Moreno, A., Lopez-Cerero, L., Pascual, A., et al. (2015). Gentamicin therapy for sepsis due to carbapenem-resistant and colistin-resistant *Klebsiella pneumoniae*. *J. Antimicrob. Chemother.* 70, 905–913. doi: 10.1093/jac/dku432

He, F., Fu, Y., Chen, Q., Ruan, Z., Hua, X., Zhou, H., et al. (2015). Tigecycline susceptibility and the role of efflux pumps in tigecycline resistance in KPC-producing *Klebsiella pneumoniae*. *PLoS One* 10:e0119064. doi: 10.1371/journal.pone.0119064

He, T., Wang, R., Liu, D., Walsh, T. R., Zhang, R., Lv, Y., et al. (2019). Emergence of plasmid-mediated high-level tigecycline resistance genes in animals and humans. *Nat. Microbiol.* 4, 1450–1456. doi: 10.1038/s41564-019-0445-2

Hentschke, M., Wolters, M., Sobottka, I., Rohde, H., and Aepfelbacher, M. (2010). ramR mutations in clinical isolates of *Klebsiella pneumoniae* with reduced susceptibility to tigecycline. *Antimicrob. Agents Chemother.* 54, 2720–2723. doi: 10.1128/AAC.00085-10

Hirsch, E. B., and Tam, V. H. (2010). Detection and treatment options for *Klebsiella pneumoniae* carbapenemases (KPCs): an emerging cause of multidrug-resistant infection. *J. Antimicrob. Chemother.* 65, 1119–1125. doi: 10.1093/jac/dkq108

Hua, X., Chen, Q., Li, X., Feng, Y., Ruan, Z., and Yu, Y. (2014). Complete genome sequence of *Klebsiella pneumoniae* sequence type 17, a multidrug-resistant strain isolated during tigecycline treatment. *Genome Announc.* 2:e01337-14. doi: 10.1128/genomeA.01337-14

Juan, C. H., Huang, Y. W., Lin, Y. T., Yang, T. C., and Wang, F. D. (2016). Risk factors, outcomes, and mechanisms of tigecycline-nonsusceptible *Klebsiella pneumoniae* bacteremia. *Antimicrob. Agents Chemother.* 60, 7357–7363. doi: 10.1128/AAC.01503-16

Lin, Y. T., Huang, Y. W., Huang, H. H., Yang, T. C., Wang, F. D., and Fung, C. P. (2016). In vivo evolution of tigecycline-non-susceptible *Klebsiella pneumoniae* strains in patients: relationship between virulence and resistance. *Int. J. Antimicrob. Agents* 48, 485–491. doi: 10.1016/j.ijantimicag.2016.07.008

Liu, Y., Li, J., Du, J., Hu, M., Bai, H., Qi, J., et al. (2011). Accurate assessment of antibiotic susceptibility and screening resistant strains of a bacterial population by linear gradient plate. *Sci. China Life Sci.* 54, 953–960. doi: 10.1007/s11427-011-4230-6

Lozano-Huntelman, N. A., Singh, N., Valencia, A., Mira, P., Sakayan, M., Boucher, I., et al. (2020). Evolution of antibiotic cross-resistance and collateral sensitivity in *Staphylococcus epidermidis* using the mutant prevention concentration and the mutant selection window. *Evol. Appl.* 13, 808–823. doi: 10.1111/eva.12903

Maltas, J., and Wood, K. B. (2019). Pervasive and diverse collateral sensitivity profiles inform optimal strategies to limit antibiotic resistance. *PLoS Biol.* 17:e3000515. doi: 10.1371/journal.pbio.3000515

Nielsen, L. E., Snesrud, E. C., Onmus-Leone, F., Kwak, Y. I., Aviles, R., Steele, E. D., et al. (2014). IS5 element integration, a novel mechanism for rapid in vivo emergence of tigecycline nonsusceptibility in *Klebsiella pneumoniae*. *Antimicrob. Agents Chemother.* 58, 6151–6156. doi: 10.1128/AAC.03053-14

Pal, C., Papp, B., and Lazar, V. (2015). Collateral sensitivity of antibiotic-resistant microbes. *Trends Microbiol.* 23, 401–407. doi: 10.1016/j.tim.2015.02.009

Park, K. S., Kim, M. H., Park, T. S., Nam, Y. S., Lee, H. J., and Suh, J. T. (2012). Prevalence of the plasmid-mediated quinolone resistance genes, aac(6')-Ib-cr, qepA, and oqxAB in clinical isolates of extended-spectrum beta-lactamase (ESBL)-producing *Escherichia coli* and *Klebsiella pneumoniae* in Korea. *Ann. Clin. Lab. Sci.* 42, 191–197.

Petrosillo, N., Giannella, M., Lewis, R., and Viale, P. (2013). Treatment of carbapenem-resistant *Klebsiella pneumoniae*: the state of the art. *Expert Rev. Anti Infect. Ther.* 11, 159–177. doi: 10.1586/eri.12.162

Poulakou, G., Kontopidou, F. V., Paramythiotou, E., Kompoti, M., Katsiari, M., Mainas, E., et al. (2009). Tigecycline in the treatment of infections from multi-drug resistant gram-negative pathogens. *J. Infect.* 58, 273–284. doi: 10.1016/j.jinf.2009.02.009

Roy, S., Datta, S., Viswanathan, R., Singh, A. K., and Basu, S. (2013). Tigecycline susceptibility in *Klebsiella pneumoniae* and *Escherichia coli* causing neonatal septicaemia (2007-10) and role of an efflux pump in tigecycline non-susceptibility. *J. Antimicrob. Chemother.* 68, 1036–1042. doi: 10.1093/jac/dks535

Sekowska, A., and Gospodarek, E. (2010). Susceptibility of *Klebsiella* spp. to tigecycline and other selected antibiotics. *Med. Sci. Monit.* 16, BR193–BR196.

Sheng, J. F., Li, J. J., Tu, S., Sheng, Z. K., Bi, S., Zhu, M. H., et al. (2012). blaKPC and rmtB on a single plasmid in *Enterobacter* amnigenus and *Klebsiella pneumoniae* isolates from the same patient. *Eur. J. Clin. Microbiol. Infect. Dis.* 31, 1585–1591. doi: 10.1007/s10096-011-1481-x

Shi, W., Li, K., Ji, Y., Jiang, Q., Wang, Y., Shi, M., et al. (2013). Carbapenem and cefoxitin resistance of *Klebsiella pneumoniae* strains associated with porin OmpK36 loss and DHA-1 beta-lactamase production. *Braz. J. Microbiol.* 44, 435–442. doi: 10.1590/S1517-83822013000200015

Stein, G. E., and Babinchak, T. (2013). Tigecycline: an update. *Diagn. Microbiol. Infect. Dis.* 75, 331–336. doi: 10.1016/j.diagmicrobio.2012.12.004

Stohr, J., Verweij, J. J., Buiting, A. G. M., Rossen, J. W. A., and Kluytmans, J. (2020). Within-patient plasmid dynamics in *Klebsiella pneumoniae* during an outbreak of a carbapenemase-producing *Klebsiella pneumoniae*. *PLoS One* 15:e0233313. doi: 10.1371/journal.pone.0233313

Sun, J., Chen, C., Cui, C. Y., Zhang, Y., Liu, X., Cui, Z. H., et al. (2019). Plasmid-encoded tet(X) genes that confer high-level tigecycline resistance in *Escherichia coli*. *Nat. Microbiol.* 4, 1457–1464. doi: 10.1038/s41564-019-0496-4

Sun, Y., Cai, Y., Liu, X., Bai, N., Liang, B., and Wang, R. (2013). The emergence of clinical resistance to tigecycline. *Int. J. Antimicrob. Agents* 41, 110–116. doi: 10.1016/j.ijantimicag.2012.09.005

Villa, L., Capone, A., Fortini, D., Dolejska, M., Rodriguez, I., Taglietti, F., et al. (2013). Reversion to susceptibility of a carbapenem-resistant clinical isolate of *Klebsiella pneumoniae* producing KPC-3. *J. Antimicrob. Chemother.* 68, 2482–2486. doi: 10.1093/jac/dkt235

Villa, L., Feudi, C., Fortini, D., Garcia-Fernandez, A., and Carattoli, A. (2014). Genomics of KPC-producing *Klebsiella pneumoniae* sequence type 512 clone highlights the role of RamR and ribosomal S10 protein mutations in conferring tigecycline resistance. *Antimicrob. Agents Chemother.* 58, 1707–1712. doi: 10.1128/AAC.01803-13

Wachino, J. I., Doi, Y., and Arakawa, Y. (2020). Aminoglycoside resistance: updates with a focus on acquired 16S Ribosomal RNA methyltransferases. *Infect. Dis. Clin. North Am.* 34, 887–902. doi: 10.1016/j.idc.2020.06.002

WHO (2020). *Essential Medicines and Health Products.* Available online at: http://www.who.int/medicines/publications/global-priority-list-antibiotic-resistant-bacteria (accessed February 15, 2021).

Woodford, N., Hill, R. L., and Livermore, D. M. (2007). In vitro activity of tigecycline against carbapenem-susceptible and -resistant isolates of *Klebsiella* spp. and *Enterobacter* spp. *J. Antimicrob. Chemother.* 59, 582–583. doi: 10.1093/jac/dkl514

Wyres, K. L., and Holt, K. E. (2018). *Klebsiella pneumoniae* as a key trafficker of drug resistance genes from environmental to clinically important bacteria. *Curr. Opin. Microbiol.* 45, 131–139. doi: 10.1016/j.mib.2018.04.004

Xu, H., Zhou, Y., Zhai, X., Du, Z., Wu, H., Han, Y., et al. (2016). Emergence and characterization of tigecycline resistance in multidrug-resistant *Klebsiella pneumoniae* isolates from blood samples of patients in intensive care units in northern China. *J. Med. Microbiol.* 65, 751–759. doi: 10.1099/jmm.0.000299

Xu, J., Gao, M., Hong, Y., and He, F. (2017). Draft genome sequence of a tigecycline-resistant KPC-2-producing *Klebsiella pneumoniae* ST15 clinical isolate from China. *J. Glob. Antimicrob. Resist.* 11, 156–158. doi: 10.1016/j.jgar.2017.10.017

Zhang, R., Dong, N., Huang, Y., Zhou, H., Xie, M., Chan, E. W., et al. (2018). Evolution of tigecycline- and colistin-resistant CRKP (carbapenem-resistant *Klebsiella pneumoniae*) in vivo and its persistence in the GI tract. *Emerg. Microbes Infect.* 7:127. doi: 10.1038/s41426-018-0129-7

Zhang, Y., Jiang, X., Wang, Y., Li, G., Tian, Y., Liu, H., et al. (2014). Contribution of beta-lactamases and porin proteins OmpK35 and OmpK36 to carbapenem resistance in clinical isolates of KPC-2-producing *Klebsiella pneumoniae*. *Antimicrob. Agents Chemother.* 58, 1214–1217. doi: 10.1128/AAC.02045-12

Zhong, X., Xu, H., Chen, D., Zhou, H., Hu, X., and Cheng, G. (2014). First emergence of acrAB and oqxAB mediated tigecycline resistance in clinical isolates of *Klebsiella pneumoniae* pre-dating the use of tigecycline in a Chinese hospital. *PLoS One* 9:e115185. doi: 10.1371/journal.pone.0115185

# 11

# Antimicrobial and Antibiofilm Potential of Acyclic Amines and Diamines against Multi-Drug Resistant *Staphylococcus aureus*

***Gurmeet Kaur, P. Balamurugan, Sahana Vasudevan, Saikiran Jadav and S. A. Princy****

*Quorum Sensing Laboratory, Centre for Research in Infectious Diseases, School of Chemical and Biotechnology, SASTRA University, Thanjavur, India*

***Correspondence:**
*S. A. Princy*
*adlineprinzy@biotech.sastra.edu*

Multi-drug resistant *Staphylococcus aureus* (MDRSA) remains a great challenge despite a decade of research on antimicrobial compounds against their infections. In the present study, various acyclic amines and diamines were chemically synthesized and tested for their antimicrobial as well as antibiofilm activity against MDRSA. Among all the synthesized compounds, an acyclic diamine, (2,2′-((butane-1,4-diylbis(azanediyl)bis(methylene))diphenol) designated as ADM 3, showed better antimicrobial activity (minimum inhibitory concentration at 50 μg/mL) and antibiofilm activity ($MBIC_{50}$ at 5 μg/mL). In addition, ADM 3 was capable of reducing the virulence factors expression (anti-virulence). Confocal laser scanning microscope analysis of the *in vitro* tested urinary catheters showed biofilm reduction as well as bacterial killing by ADM 3. On the whole, our data suggest that acyclic diamines, especially ADM 3 can be a potent lead for the further studies in alternative therapeutic approaches.

**Keywords: biofilm, *Staphylococcus aureus*, multi-drug resistance, antibiofilm, diamines, antibacterial**

## INTRODUCTION

*Staphylococcus aureus*, a Gram-positive, facultative anaerobic cocci bacterium, is one of the most notorious pathogen, causing infections in humans. Their abilities to evade the host immune defense mechanism and resistance to the first and second generation antibiotics has made the pathogen a subject of interest in the scientific community (Fedtke et al., 2004). *S. aureus* is an opportunistic pathogen related to the various types of infectious diseases such as wound infections, catheter-related bloodstream infections (CRBSI), musculoskeletal infections, toxic shock syndrome and, about 20% of population worldwide found to be the long-term carrier as a part of their normal flora (Kluytmans et al., 1997; Cole et al., 2001). Various factors associated with *S. aureus* such as virulence gene expressions, cell to cell signaling mechanism, inactivation of antibiotics, alteration in target sites, efflux pumps, and biofilm formation have led to the emergence of multi-drug resistant *S. aureus* (MDRSA) (Dinges et al., 2000; Becker et al., 2003; Zhu et al., 2008; Arya et al., 2011; Qayyum et al., 2016).

Planktonic microbes attach to a particular substratum and produce an anchoring polymer called as an extracellular polysaccharide (EPS) which leads to the formation of the multicellular microbial community known as biofilm (Flemming et al., 2007). The altered metabolic activity of the cells that are associated with biofilm formation have high rates of EPS production, activation of specific genes associated with biofilm formation and virulence, reduction in the growth rate than their planktonic counterparts (Flemming et al., 2007). Biofilm formation accounts for one of the major reasons for the emergence of multi-drug resistance (MDR) in various pathogenic microbes and is common in bacteria. In the biofilm mode of lifestyle, bacterial population acquires adaptation to tolerate and survive a wide range of diverse environmental stress such as scarce nutritional availability, antibiotics exposure, competition for survival in a multi-species environment (Parsek and Singh, 2003). The antibiotics tolerance ability of the biofilm cells complicates the treatment of various infections in humans, such as, cystic fibrosis, endocarditis, which includes biofilm formation on various biological implants such as, urinary catheters, heart catheters, various joint implants, and replacement of heart valves (Singh et al., 2000). Biofilms pose a threat to the human race because of their persistent nature and plays a major role in certain pathogenic infections (Singh et al., 2000; Ravichandiran et al., 2012; Arya and Princy, 2013; Otto, 2013). Several incidences have been reported with MDRSA strain infections such as CRBSI which is primarily due to either bacterial colonization on a device that may be intraluminal, i.e., formation of biofilm inside the lumen and causing persistent infection (Safdar and Maki, 2004). Similarly, musculoskeletal infections, wound infections, and nosocomial infections have also been reported by MDRSA which are very difficult to treat with the existing drugs (Bascones-Martinez et al., 2011; Abad et al., 2014; Vincze et al., 2014). Antibiofilm compounds are one such alternative option in the recent research focus. These small chemical ligands can independently inhibit bacterial biofilm or disrupt the biofilm matrix at the molecular level via, disturbing their metabolic pathways.

Medicinally important chemical compounds play a crucial role in treating various diseases which pose a threat to human survival at times. From our earlier reports, we have understood that acyclic amines could be promising leads against *S. aureus*, as one of our compounds (SarABI-12, 2-[(methylamino)methyl]phenol) was shown to have target specific interaction with the staphylococcal accessory regulator, SarA (Arya and Princy, 2013). In addition, our *in vitro* studies (Balamurugan et al., 2017) have confirmed the antibiofilm and anti-virulence properties against clinical *S. aureus* strains. The data also showed a significant reduction in the expression of SarA regulated virulence genes like *fnbA*, *hla*, and *hld*. It is also interesting to note that several researchers have reported the potential of cyclic amines and diamines to inhibit MDRSA, *Enterococcus* sp., *Clostridium difficile*, *Escherichia coli*, *Aspergillus oryzae*, *Aspergillus niger* (He et al., 2003; Abdel-Rahman et al., 2004; Hensler et al., 2006). The focus on the use of cyclic amines and diamines for antibacterial, antifungal and anti-proliferative activity has also been implicated (He et al., 2003; Juranić, 2014; Kazakova et al., 2014). Previous reports by Chtchigrovsky et al. (2013) shows the anti-proliferative activity of *trans-N*-heterocyclic carbene–amine–Pt(II) complexes. These complexes have the ability to bind to DNA, leading to intrastrand cross-links between two adjacent guanines and minor interstrand cross links, resulting in DNA damage and cell death (Chtchigrovsky et al., 2013). Similarly, Subík et al. (1977) report the antibacterial and antifungal activity of amine oxides due to their ability to disorganize the cellular membranes leading to cidal effects.

It is expected that similar to cyclic amines, acyclic amines can also have medicinally important biological potentials, supported by our previous works (Arya and Princy, 2013; Balamurugan et al., 2017). Hence, we have investigated the antibiofilm and antibacterial properties of acyclic amines which have not yet been explored against pathogenic bacteria.

## MATERIALS AND METHODS

### Synthesis of Acyclic Amine and Diamine Compounds

The acyclic amines (AAM 1–5) and acyclic diamines (ADM 1–8) compounds were synthesized by a reductive amination process (Ramachandran et al., 2010). The synthesis process of acyclic amine and diamines is shown in the **Figures 1A,B**. For the synthesis of acyclic amines, a solution of the suitable aryl aldehyde (10 mmol) and the suitable acyclic amine (12 mmol) in methanol (5 mL) was stirred at room temperature for 1 h. The reactants

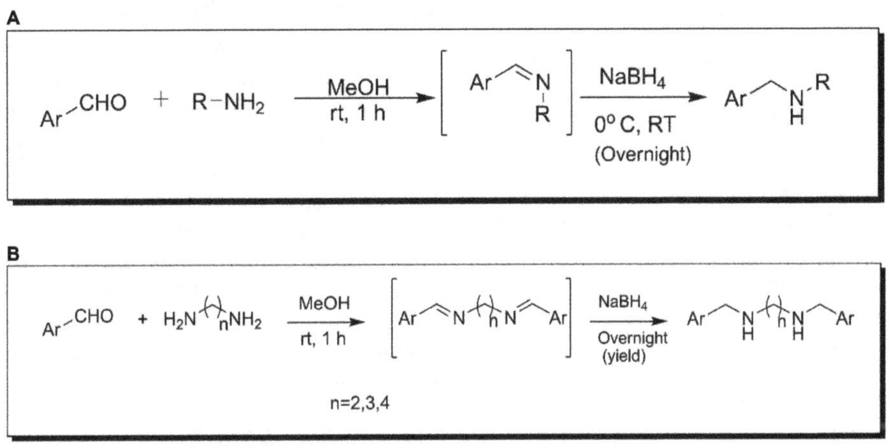


**FIGURE 1** | Schematic representation of the reaction scheme for synthesis of **(A)** acyclic amines **(B)** acyclic diamines.

were shown in Supplementary Table S1. The intermediate imines were reduced to the corresponding acyclic amines and diamines by the addition of sodium borohydride (15 mmol) at the ice-cold condition. After stirring, the reaction mixture was incubated at room temperature overnight and further diluted with water and extracted thrice with dichloromethane. The mixed organic phases were dried with anhydrous sodium sulfate, evaporated to dryness under reduced pressure to obtain the acyclic amines and diamines. The structures of the synthesized products were confirmed by $^{1}$H-NMR spectroscopy.

## Bacterial Strains and Growth Conditions

Clinical isolates of *S. aureus* were received from the rejected urinary catheters, JSS Medical College Mysore with prior approval from the Institutional Ethical Committee (IEC/JSSMC/PG/1050/2015-16). The strains were initially subjected to screening for MDR against the antibiotics: levofloxacin, ampicillin, ciprofloxacin, and methicillin. The *S. aureus* strain (MDRSA - QSL2040) that showed resistance to methicillin as well as other tested antibiotics (**Table 1**) was used as a test strain and the *S. aureus* (ATCC 25923) was used as reference strain (Kumar et al., 2013; Khatkar et al., 2014). These strains were cultured in the cation-adjusted Mueller–Hinton broth (CAMHB) for the minimal drug dose response against the growth and bactericidal actions. For the biofilm assays, the tryptic soy broth (TSB) supplemented with 3% NaCl and 0.5% glucose was used as the biofilm medium.

## Evaluation of Acyclic Amine and Diamine Compounds for MIC, MBC, and MBIC

The minimum inhibitory concentration (MIC), the minimum bactericidal concentration (MBC), and the minimum biofilm inhibitory concentrations (MBIC) of the acyclic amines and diamines were determined according to the Clinical and Laboratory Standards Institute (CLSI) with slight modifications. The *S. aureus* clinical isolate (MDRSA - QSL2040) was grown overnight in TSB. The overnight culture was diluted 1:100 in physiological saline and the bacterial suspensions were adjusted to a final inoculum size of 1 × 10$^{6}$ cells (Issam et al., 2015). The adjusted inoculum was added to the wells of a 96-well microtiter plate containing twofold serial dilutions of the compound (varying concentrations from 2 to 400 μg/mL as individual sets keeping different high concentrations) in CAMHB medium. The plates were incubated at 37°C for 24 h. The setup was carried out as independent experiments (in triplicates) to calculate the effective concentration.

The optical density ($OD_{600}$) was read immediately after inoculation and again after 18 h of incubation at 37°C, in a microtitre plate reader (iMark, Bio-Rad, Japan). The lowest concentration that inhibited growth when compared to the untreated control culture was taken as the MIC. Similarly, MBC was determined by counting the number of colonies (CFU/mL) after 24 h of incubation at 37°C and was defined as the lowest concentration at which the viable cells were reduced to a level by ≥90% in comparison to the untreated control cultures. All independent assays were carried out in triplicates.

For biofilm assay, diluted overnight culture (1:100) was inoculated in TSB and allowed to grow till it reached exponential growth phase (5 h). The culture was tested for 0.5 McFarland unit and followed by inoculation along with varying concentrations of the compounds (2–400 μg/mL) in 96-well microtitre plates. Plates were incubated for 24 h at 37°C without shaking. After incubation, the wells were washed twice with 200 μL of phosphate-buffered saline (PBS) gently to remove the non-adherent cells. Adherent cells in the biofilm were fixed by adding 200 μL of 100% methanol prior to staining with 200 μL of 0.2% (w/v) crystal violet (CV) for 20 min. The excess stain was washed twice with PBS and the plates were air dried. The bound CV in the air dried plates were eluted with 200 μL of 33% acetic acid. The biofilm was quantitatively determined by measuring the absorbance at $OD_{595\ nm}$ in a microtitre plate reader (iMark, Bio-Rad, Japan). The concentration at which the formation of biofilm is inhibited ≥50% when compared to the untreated control culture is defined as $MBIC_{50}$ and ≥90% is $MBIC_{90}$. All the assays were carried out in triplicates.

**TABLE 1** | Antibiotic susceptibility profiling of the two strains used in the study.

| Antibiotics | Strains used | |
|---|---|---|
| | **ATCC 25923** | **QSL2040** |
| Levofloxacin | Sensitive | Resistant |
| Ampicillin | Sensitive | Resistant |
| Ciprofloxacin | Sensitive | Resistant |
| Methicillin | Sensitive | Resistant |
| Amoxicillin | Sensitive | Resistant |
| Penicillin | Sensitive | Resistant |
| Kanamycin | Sensitive | Resistant |
| Gentamicin | Sensitive | Resistant |
| Clindamycin | Sensitive | Intermediate |
| Vancomycin | Sensitive | Resistant |
| Oxacillin | Sensitive | Intermediate |

*Sensitivity/resistance pattern was concluded as per the CLSI guidelines.*

## Anti-virulence Assays

Among the synthesized compounds, ADM 3 was selected as it showed higher antibiofilm activity at minimal concentration. The compound, ADM 3 was tested against the clinical isolate of *S. aureus* with two sub-$MBIC_{50}$ concentrations (i.e., 1/4× $MBIC_{50}$, 1/2× $MBIC_{50}$) and at a higher $MBIC_{50}$ concentration (2× $MBIC_{50}$). *S. aureus* reference strain, untreated with ADM 3 was kept as control. After 24 h, the cultures were centrifuged at 6000 rpm for 10 min at 4°C and filter sterilized in a 0.22 μm filter paper to collect the cell free supernatant. The collected supernatant was stored at 4°C and further used to quantify hemolysin and protease (Pietrow et al., 2013) among the various secreted exotoxins by *S. aureus*.

## Hemolytic Assay

Hemolysin in the culture supernatant was quantified according to the procedure described earlier with slight modifications

(Cheung and Otto, 2012). Briefly, 10 mL of sheep blood was centrifuged at 2400 rpm for 5 min and the pellet obtained was washed twice with 10 mL of PBS. Ten microliters of this erythrocyte suspension was incubated with the cell free supernatant for 1 h at 37°C. Finally, the incubated sample was centrifuged at 2400 rpm for 5 min. Erythrocyte suspension treated with 1% Triton X-100 was used as a positive control. The optical density of the supernatant was read at 540 nm. Water along with the erythrocyte suspension was considered as blank. The percentage (%) hemolysis was calculated using the following formula:

$$\%\text{Hemolysis} = \text{absorbance (sample)} - \text{absorbance (blank)}/\text{absorbance (positive control)}$$

## Proteolysis Assay

Quantitative estimation of the protease was carried out with azocasein assay. A total of 200 μL of the cell free supernatant was incubated with 800 μL of azocasein for 30 min at 37°C. To this, 1200 μL of 1% trichloroacetic acid was added to arrest the enzymatic reaction. The contents were incubated on ice for 30 min and centrifuged at 12,000 rpm for 5 min. To 1600 μL of the supernatant 400 μL of 1.8 N NaOH was added and the optical density was read at 420 nm against the blank (azocasein + TCA + NaOH). The amount of enzyme required to digest 1 mg of azocasein per minute is known as 1 unit of protein activity (Pietrow et al., 2013). The percentage (%) proteolysis was calculated using the following formula:

$$\%\text{Proteolysis} = \text{absorbance (sample)} - \text{absorbance (blank)}/\text{absorbance (control)}$$

## Appraisal of the Therapeutic Challenge of ADM 3 on *S. aureus* Using an *In Vitro* Catheter Model

An *in vitro* catheter model was used to evaluate the effect of ADM 3 on biofilm formation in hydrodynamic conditions (Hancock et al., 2010). Silicone catheter segments of 20 mm length were cut vertically into two halves, sterilized in 0.5% sodium hypochlorite solution followed by washing with sterilized water. The sterilized catheters were placed in a six-well microtitre plate and the surface was coated with human blood plasma by incubation at 37°C for 24 h. Subsequently, the plasma was removed from the wells and the coated catheters were subjected for the establishment of *S. aureus* infection followed by treatment with ADM 3 for 7 days with concentrations of $^1/_4\times$ $MBIC_{50}$, $^1/_2\times$ $MBIC_{50}$, $MBIC_{50}$, and $2\times$ $MBIC_{50}$. The plates were incubated at 37°C for 24 h with shaking at 120 rpm. After 24 h of incubation, the medium was changed along with a fresh dosage of the drug each time and this was repeated for 7 days. Also, at every 24 h interval, the catheters from the wells were removed and analyzed for the viability of cells (Weiss et al., 2009). Briefly, the viability of cells from the catheters was processed by immersing the catheters individually into sterile PBS and followed by sonication. The adherent cells recovered in PBS were plated for colony count in TSB agar plates. Microscopy imaging was used to visually analyze the effect of ADM 3 on biofilm removal. The cells were stained with fluorescein isothiocyanate (5 mg/mL) and ethidium bromide (1.25 mg/mL) prepared by mixing 5 μL each of the dyes in 1 mL of cold 0.9% NaCl solution. The samples were incubated for 10 min, and then the excess dye was removed by washing with 0.9% NaCl. All the stained samples were imaged using Olympus FV 1000 confocal microscope with a 10× objective of numerical aperture 0.3. The stained samples were excited at 488 nm using Multi Argon LASER and images were collected from four randomly chosen spots from the sample surface.

## Cytotoxicity Analysis of ADM 3 on HEp-2 Cells

Cell viability was assessed by MTT assay. The reduction of MTT is catalyzed by mitochondrial dehydrogenase enzymes and thus considered to be a measure of cell viability. HEp-2 cells were seeded to each well in a 96-well microtiter plate ($1 \times 10^5$ cells), in 100 μL of DMEM growth medium and the plate was incubated at 37°C for 24 h. After incubation, the fresh growth medium was replaced in the wells. ADM 3 was diluted from an original stock to obtain a concentration of 200 μg/mL. The HEp-2 cells were incubated with ADM 3 and allowed to adhere for a period of 72 h. A total of 10 μL of MTT solution (5 mg/mL in 1× PBS) was added to each well and the plate was incubated in dark for 4 h at 37°C. Further, the content of the each well was removed and the formazan crystals were dissolved in 200 μL of dimethyl sulfoxide (DMSO) solution per well. The absorbance was measured at 590 nm using ELISA plate reader. Only the interior rows of the microtiter plate were used for these experiments to minimize the variations in cell viability due to medium evaporation at the periphery site. The percentage cell viability was calculated with reference to the untreated control cells. The experiment was conducted twice in quadruplicates.

$$\text{Percentage cell viability} = \frac{\text{OD of drug treated sample} - \text{OD of blank}}{\text{OD of control} - \text{OD of blank}} \times 100$$

## Statistical Analysis

Graph pad prism software (version 6.01) was used for statistical analysis. One-way ANOVA and multiple comparisons were done. The minimum level of significance was set at $P \leq 0.05$. All the assays were conducted in triplicates and the results were expressed as mean ± SD.

# RESULTS

## Synthesis of Acyclic Amines and Diamines

The spectral data of all the synthesized compounds were in full agreement with the proposed structures (Supplementary

Table S1). The $^1$H-NMR data for the synthesized compounds are given below.

**AAM 1: *N*-(naphthalene-2-ylmethyl)butan-1-amine**

Isolated yield = 78%, $^1$H NMR (300 MHz, $CDCl_3$) δ 8.12 (d, *J* = 8.3 Hz, 1H), 7.90–7.83 (m, 1H), 7.77 (d, *J* = 7.9 Hz, 1H), 7.59–7.38 (m, 4H), 4.24 (s, 2H), 2.81–2.71 (m, 2H), 1.61 (s, 1H), 1.52 (dd, *J* = 8.2, 6.1 Hz, 2H), 1.38 (dq, *J* = 14.1, 7.1 Hz, 2H), 0.93 (t, *J* = 7.3 Hz, 3H).

**AAM 2: (*N*-benzylbutan-1-amine)**

Isolated yield = 55%, $^1$H NMR (300 MHz, $CDCl_3$) δ 7.38–7.19 (m, 5H), 3.79 (s, 2H), 2.63 (t, *J* = 7.2 Hz, 2H), 1.76 (s, 1H), 1.50 (dt, *J* = 14.4, 7.0 Hz, 2H), 1.40–1.24 (m, 2H), 0.91 (t, *J* = 7.2 Hz, 3H).

**AAM 3: (*N*-benzylcyclohexanamine)**

Isolated yield = 71%, $^1$H NMR (300 MHz, $CDCl_3$) δ 7.36–7.22 (m, 5H), 3.81 (s, 2H), 2.53–2.44 (m, 1H), 1.31–1.06 (m, 11H).

**AAM 4: 4(*N*-(4-methoxybenzyl)butan-1-amine)**

Isolated yield = 65%, $^1$H NMR (300 MHz, $CDCl_3$) δ 7.28 - 7.22 (m, 2H), 6.91 - 6.81 (m, 2H), 3.79 (s, 3H), 3.74 (s, 2H), 2.66 - 2.58 (m, 2H), 2.49 (s, 1H), 1.52 (ddd, *J* = 14.4, 8.3, 5.9 Hz, 2H), 1.34 (dd, *J* = 15.1, 7.4 Hz, 2H), 0.90 (t, *J* = 7.3 Hz, 3H).

**AAM 5: (*N*-(4-chlorobenzyl)butan-1-amine)**

Isolated yield = 73%, $^1$H NMR (300 MHz, $CDCl_3$) δ 7.33–7.21 (m, 4H), 3.75 (s, 2H), 2.64–2.57 (m, 2H), 1.68 (s, 1H), 1.55–1.43 (m, 2H), 1.40–1.27 (m, 2H), 0.91 (t, *J* = 7.3 Hz, 3H).

**ADM 1: $2,2^1$-((Ethane-1,2-diylbis(azanediyl)bis(methylene)) diphenol**

Yield 72%, $^1$H-NMR (DMSO-$d_6$, 300 MHz): δ 2.51 (s, 4H), 3.79 (s, 4H), 6.68–6.73 (m, 4H), 7.03–7.08 (m, 4H).

**ADM 2: 2,2′-((Propane-1,3-diylbis(azanediyl)bis(methylene)) diphenol**

Yield 79%, $^1$H-NMR (DMSO-$d_6$, 300 MHz): δ 1.63 (quin, *J* = 6.9 Hz, 2H), 2.55 (t, *J* = 6.9 Hz, 4H), 3.80 (s, 4H), 6.67–6.72 (m, 4H), 7.03–7.08 (m, 4H).

**ADM 3: $2,2^1$-((Butane-1,4-diylbis(azanediyl)bis(methylene)) diphenol**

Yield 69%, $^1$H-NMR (DMSO-$d_6$, 300 MHz): δ 1.47 (s, 4H), 2.50 (q, *J* = 1.8 Hz, 4H), 3.81 (s, 4H), 6.66–6.72 (m, 4H), 7.03–7.09 (m, 4H).

**ADM 4: $N^1$,$N^2$-dibenzylethane-1,2-diamine**

Yield 82%, $^1$H-NMR (DMSO-$d_6$, 300 MHz): δ 2.51 (s, 4H), 3.66 (s, 4H), 7.20–7.32 (m, 10H).

**ADM 5: $N^1$,$N^2$-dibenzylpropane-1, 3-diamine**

Yield 73%, $^1$H-NMR ($CDCl_3$, 300 MHz): δ 1.72 (quin, *J* = 6.9 Hz, 2H), 2.69 (t, *J* = 6.9 Hz, 4H), 3.77 (s, 4H), 7.24–7.32 (m, 10H).

**ADM 6: $N^1$,$N^2$-bis(naphthalene-2-ylmethyl)ethane-1,2-diamine**

Yield 76%, $^1$H-NMR (DMSO-$d_6$, 300 MHz): δ 2.75 (s, 4H), 4.11 (s, 4H), 7.40–7.52 (m, 8H), 7.80 (d, *J* = 7.5 Hz, 2H), 7.89–7.92 (m, 2H), 8.13–8.17 (m, 2H).

**TABLE 2** | Antimicrobial and antibiofilm values of acyclic amines and diamines.

| Compound | MIC (μg/mL) | MBC (μg/mL) | MBIC (μg/mL) | |
|---|---|---|---|---|
| | | | 50 | 90 |
| AAM 1 | 200 | 200 | – | – |
| AAM 2 | 200 | 200 | – | – |
| AAM 3 | – | – | – | – |
| AAM 4 | 100 | 200 | – | – |
| AAM 5 | – | 200 | – | – |
| ADM 1 | 200 | 200 | – | – |
| ADM 2 | – | 50 | 10 | – |
| ADM 3 | 50 | 200 | 5 | – |
| ADM 4 | – | – | 25 | – |
| ADM 5 | – | 200 | 20 | – |
| ADM 6 | – | – | 40 | – |
| ADM 7 | – | – | 40 | – |
| ADM 8 | 150 | – | – | – |

**ADM 7: $N^1$,$N^3$-bis(naphthalene-2-ylmethyl)propane-1,3-diamine**

Yield 78%, $^1$H-NMR ($CDCl_3$, 300 MHz): δ 1.61 (t, *J* = 6.3 Hz, 4H), 2.76 (t, *J* = 6.3 Hz, 4H), 4.22 (s, 4H), 7.41–7.55 (m, 8H), 7.76 (d, *J* = 7.5 Hz, 2H), 7.86 (d, *J* = 7.5 Hz, 2H), 8.10 (d, *J* = 7.8 Hz, 2H).

**ADM 8: $N^1$-(naphthalene-2-yl)-$N^4$-(naphthalene-2-ylmethyl) butane-1,4-diamine**

Yield 80%, $^1$H-NMR (DMSO-$d_6$, 300 MHz): δ 1.83 (quin, *J* = 6.9 Hz, 2H), 2.83 (t, *J* = 6.9 Hz, 4H), 4.21 (s, 4H), 7.37–7.52 (m, 8H), 7.76 (dd, *J* = 7.5, 1.8 Hz, 2H), 7.85–7.88 (m, 2H), 8.07–8.11 (m, 2H).

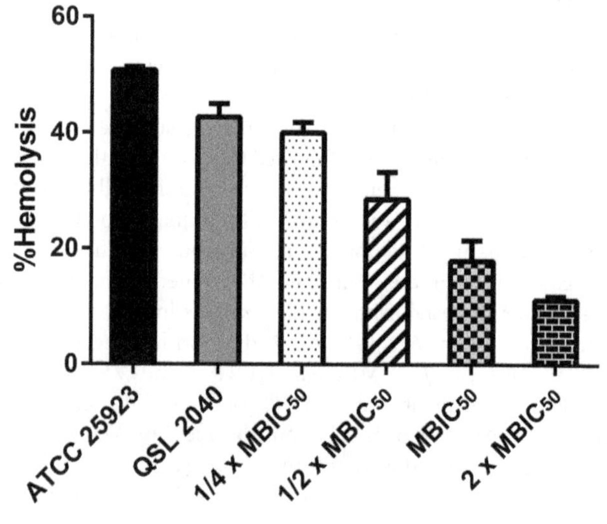


**FIGURE 2** | Effect of ADM 3 on hemolysin production in *S. aureus* (ATCC 25923—reference strain; QSL2040—clinical isolate). The concentrations used were ¼× $MBIC_{50}$ (1.25 μg/mL), ½× $MBIC_{50}$ (2.5 μg/mL), $MBIC_{50}$ (5 μg/mL), and 2× $MBIC_{50}$ (10 μg/mL).

## Antimicrobial and Antibiofilm Activity of Acyclic Amines and Diamines

The MICs, MBCs, and MBICs of acyclic amines and diamines were shown in **Table 2**. In general, acyclic amines were found to have high MIC and MBC values but no antibiofilm activity. Alternatively, the acyclic diamine compounds, particularly ADM 3 was observed to exhibit good antimicrobial as well as antibiofilm activity. The concentration of antimicrobial and antibiofilm activity of ADM 3 was found to be 50 and 5 μg/mL ($MBIC_{50}$) respectively. The biofilm inhibitory concentration for compound ADM 3 was found to be 10-fold lesser than the MIC. Thus, compound ADM 3 acts as a potential antibacterial as well as antibiofilm agent and was considered for further studies.

## Anti-virulence Assays

Percentage hemolysis and proteolysis by ADM 3 on *S. aureus* clinical isolate, MDRSA - QSL2040 are shown in **Figures 2, 3** respectively. ADM 3 exhibited a similar effect on protease as well as on hemolysin production and a dose-dependent reduction was observed in both the cases. Clinical isolate (MDRSA - QSL2040) treated with ADM 3 showed a significant reduction in proteolytic and hemolytic activity when compared with the untreated control.

## *In Vitro* Catheter Model

Live dead staining of *S. aureus* in the presence and absence of ADM 3 revealed that, ADM 3 treatment induced significant loss of viability and colonization of biofilm on catheters as evidenced by the red fluorescence observed in treated samples at day 7. All the captured images were uniform and a representative image is shown in **Figure 4**. Thus, in consonance with our antibiofilm results in microtitre plate experiments, ADM 3 was effective in inhibition of *S. aureus* biofilm in catheters. The treatment of these catheters showed a decrease in the cell count from day 4 onward compared to untreated control (Supplementary Figure S1).

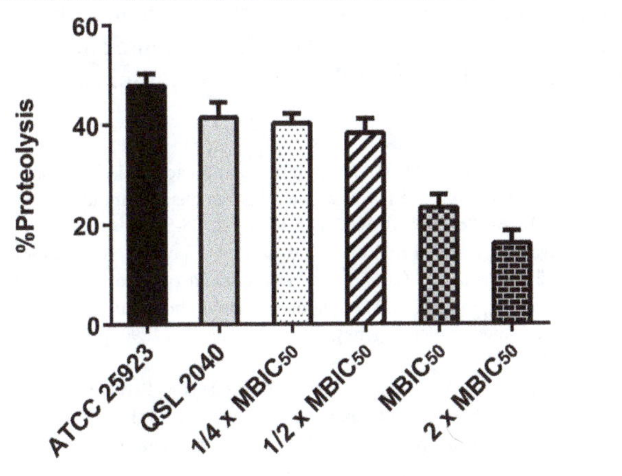


**FIGURE 3** | Effect of ADM 3 on protease production in *S. aureus* (ATCC 25923—reference strain; QSL2040—clinical isolate). The concentrations used were 1/4× $MBIC_{50}$ (1.25 μg/mL), 1/2× $MBIC_{50}$ (2.5 μg/mL), $MBIC_{50}$ (5 μg/mL), and 2× $MBIC_{50}$ (10 μg/mL).

## Cytotoxicity Analysis on HEp-2 Cell Lines

Percentage cell viability of each experimental group was calculated with reference to the untreated control cells and it was observed that cell viability was higher than 85% in all drug doses (**Figure 5**). Statistical analysis was performed using the one way ANOVA and $P \leq 0.001$ was considered significant.

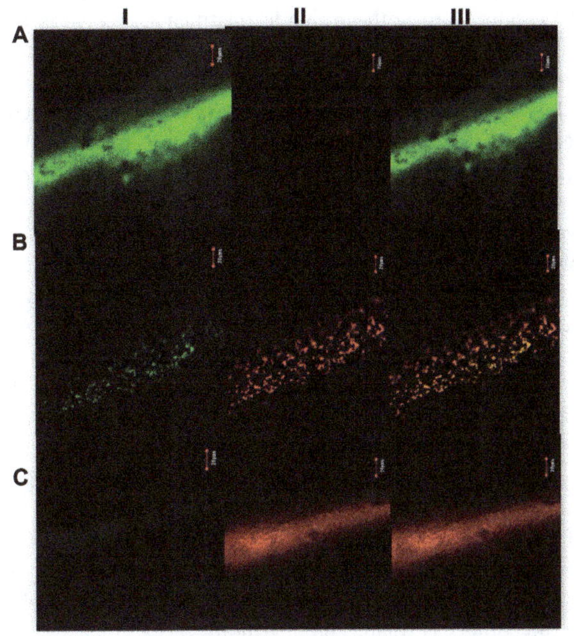


**FIGURE 4** | Confocal laser scanning microscope images of biofilm formed on urinary catheters. I—FITC labeled (green/viable cells); II—ethidium bromide labeled (red/non-viable cells); and III—superimposed images of I and II. **(A)** Control, untreated with ADM 3, **(B)** treated with ADM 3 ($MBIC_{50}$ at 5 μg/mL), and **(C)** treated with ADM 3 (2× $MBIC_{50}$ at 10 μg/mL).

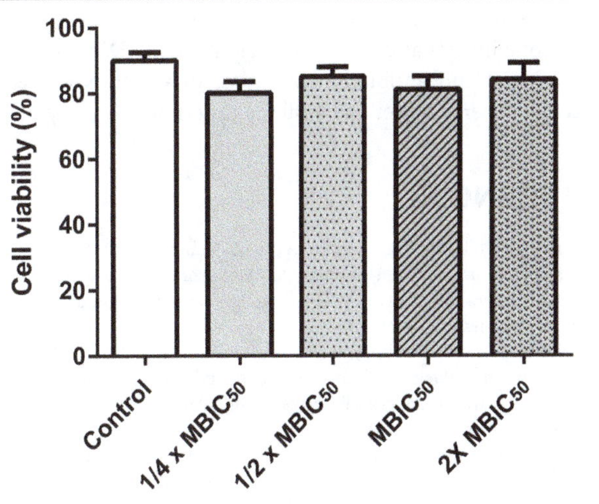


**FIGURE 5** | Effect of ADM 3 on HEp-2 cell lines for cell viability by MTT assay. The concentrations used were 1/4× $MBIC_{50}$ (1.25 μg/mL), 1/2× $MBIC_{50}$ (2.5 μg/mL), $MBIC_{50}$ (5 μg/mL), and 2× $MBIC_{50}$ (10 μg/mL).

## DISCUSSION

The key consequences of biofilm based infections are resistant to antibiotics as well as many other conventional antimicrobial agents. This eventually leads to the development of MDR pathogens with an extreme capacity for evading the host defense mechanisms. It is well known that bacterial biofilm exhibits antibiotic diffusion barrier (Cloete, 2003). In such cases, a large portion of the cells embedded in biofilms might escape from both antibiotic treatments as well as host's immune system responses. Such bacterial cells lead to the replenishment of biofilm at a new site causing are occurrence of infection with high resistance to antibiotics. Consequently, it becomes difficult to treat the infection using bactericidal drugs via systemic administration and demands the need for the evaluation of novel antibiofilm drugs. As an alternative to conventional antibiotic therapy and to control MDR, we hereby report a series of acyclic amines and diamines as potential drug candidates in the light of our earlier studies (Arya and Princy, 2013; Balamurugan et al., 2017). Among these, ADM 3 (2,2′-((butane-1,4-diylbis(azanediyl)bis(methylene))diphenol) showed a significant reduction in bacterial cell count as well as biofilm inhibition.

Targeting virulence factors in bacteria is an alternative approach to antimicrobial therapy that offers promising insights and opportunities to inhibit bacterial pathogenesis (Kauppi et al., 2003; Åberg and Almqvist, 2007). Certain virulence factors have been shown as potential leads for drug design and therapeutic intervention, whereas new possible insights are crucial for exploring others (Projan, 2002). Among the various virulence factors expressed in *S. aureus*, protease, as well as hemolysin production, plays a crucial role in the interaction of bacteria with the host cell for establishing an infection (Kupferwasser et al., 2003). In the present study, ADM 3 that showed effective $MBIC_{50}$ and MIC was also effective in reducing protease as well as hemolysin production.

*In vitro* catheter model showed decreased biofilm as well as increased red fluorescence in the confocal laser scanning microscope images at day 7. This suggests that ADM 3 has both antimicrobial and antibiofilm activities. In addition, decreased cell count observed after day 4 till the experimental study period also suggests the potential of ADM 3. This implies that the ADM 3 was proven to show a potent biofilm inhibiting agent as well as an antimicrobial agent. It is already shown through our *in silico* studies that the hydroxyl and amine groups of the compound SarABI-12, interact with the oxygen atoms of E89 and R90 of SarA protein respectively, to form hydrogen bonds (Arya and Princy, 2013). Moreover, our *in vitro* studies also have confirmed the antibiofilm activities by the target specific interaction with SarA, which is a quorum regulator of *S. aureus*. Since ADM 3 is a derivative of SarABI-12, which carries both the hydroxyl and amine groups, it is speculated that the biofilm inhibition activity also could be of the similar mechanism.

Furthermore, a therapeutic molecule should not have cytotoxic effects if it has to be taken for further clinical trials. Generally, a compound is usually considered to have *in vitro* cytotoxicity if the particular concentration of the drug causes a 50% cell killing. Our data suggest that the compound ADM 3 may act as a potential drug which does not cause any cytotoxicity. To the best of our knowledge, our study is the first to report the antimicrobial and antibiofilm activity of acyclic amines and diamines. Our data also provide an insight that these compounds can act as a potential drug candidate to treat MDRSA. It would be interesting to explore the activity of these organic molecules at the molecular level to depict their mode of action involved in antibiofilm and antibacterial activity.

## AUTHOR CONTRIBUTIONS

All authors listed have made a substantial, direct and intellectual contribution to the work, and approved it for publication.

## ACKNOWLEDGMENTS

We sincerely acknowledge the management and Dr. S. Swaminathan, Dean Sponsored Research of SASTRA University for their support and encouragement throughout this project. The authors are also grateful to the TRR in-house funding scheme of SASTRA University for the purchase of consumables.

## REFERENCES

Abad, C. L., Pulia, M. S., Krupp, A., and Safdar, N. (2014). Reducing transmission of methicillin-resistant *Staphylococcus aureus* and vancomycin-resistant *Enterococcus* in the ICU—an update on prevention and infection control practices. *JCOM* 21, 218–232.

Abdel-Rahman, A. H., Keshk, E. M., Hanna, M. A., and El-Bady, S. M. (2004). Synthesis and evaluation of some new spiro indoline-based heterocycles as potentially active antimicrobial agents. *Bioorg. Med. Chem.* 12, 2483–2488. doi: 10.1016/j.bmc.2003.10.063

Åberg, V., and Almqvist, F. (2007). Pilicides—small molecules targeting bacterial virulence. *Org. Biomol. Chem.* 5, 1827–1834. doi: 10.1039/B702 397A

Arya, R., Kannan, R. V., Shrivastava, S., and Princy, S. (2011). Studies on the effect of amino acids to curb the pathogenesis of multi drug resistant *Staphylococcus aureus*. *Asian J. Chem.* 23, 4295–4298.

Arya, R., and Princy, S. (2013). Computational approach to design small molecule inhibitors and identify SarA as a potential therapeutic candidate. *Med. Chem. Res.* 22, 1856–1865. doi: 10.1007/s00044-012-0185-9

Balamurugan, P., Praveen Krishna, V., Bharath, D., Lavanya, R., Vairaprakash, P., and Adline Princy, S. (2017). *Staphylococcus aureus* quorum regulator SarA targeted compound, 2-[(Methylamino)methyl]phenol inhibits biofilm and down-regulates virulence genes. *Front. Microbiol.* 8:1290. doi: 10.3389/fmicb. 2017.01290

Bascones-Martinez, A., Matesanz-Perez, P., Escribano-Bermejo, M., Gonzalez-Moles, M. A., Bascones-Ilundain, J., and Meurman, J. H. (2011). Periodontal disease and diabetes-review of the Literature. *Med. Oral Patol. Oral Cir. Bucal* 16, e722–e729. doi: 10.4317/medoral.17032

Becker, K., Friedrich, A. W., Lubritz, G., Weilert, M., Peters, G., and Von Eiff, C. (2003). Prevalence of genes encoding pyrogenic toxin superantigens and exfoliative toxins among strains of *Staphylococcus aureus* isolated from blood and nasal specimens. *J. Clin. Microbiol.* 41, 1434–1439. doi: 10.1128/JCM.41.4. 1434-1439.2003

Cheung, G. Y. C., and Otto, M. (2012). The potential use of toxin antibodies as a strategy for controlling acute *Staphylococcus aureus* infections. *Expert Opin. Ther. Targets* 16, 601–612. doi: 10.1517/14728222.2012.682573

Chtchigrovsky, M., Eloy, L., Jullien, H., Saker, L., Ségal-Bendirdjian, E., Poupon, J., et al. (2013). Antitumor trans-N-heterocyclic carbene-amine-Pt(II) complexes: synthesis of dinuclear species and exploratory investigations of DNA binding and cytotoxicity mechanisms. *J. Med. Chem.* 56, 2074–2086. doi: 10.1021/jm301780s

Cloete, T. E. (2003). Resistance mechanisms of bacteria to antimicrobial compounds. *Int. Biodeterior. Biodegradation* 51, 277–282. doi: 10.1016/S0964-8305(03)00042-8

Cole, A. M., Tahk, S., Oren, A., Yoshioka, D., Kim, Y.-H., Park, A., et al. (2001). Determinants of *Staphylococcus aureus* nasal carriage. *Clin. Diagn. Lab. Immunol.* 8, 1064–1069. doi: 10.1128/CDLI.8.6.1064-1069.2001

Dinges, M. M., Orwin, P. M., and Schlievert, P. M. (2000). Exotoxins of *Staphylococcus aureus*. *Clin. Microbiol. Rev.* 13, 16–34. doi: 10.1128/CMR.13.1.16-34.2000

Fedtke, I., Götz, F., and Peschel, A. (2004). Bacterial evasion of innate host defenses–the *Staphylococcus aureus* lesson. *Int. J. Med. Microbiol.* 294, 189–194. doi: 10.1016/j.ijmm.2004.06.016

Flemming, H.-C., Neu, T. R., and Wozniak, D. J. (2007). The EPS matrix: the house of biofilm cells. *J. Bacteriol.* 189, 7945–7947. doi: 10.1128/JB.00858-07

Hancock, V., Dahl, M., and Klemm, P. (2010). Abolition of biofilm formation in urinary tract *Escherichia coli* and *Klebsiella* isolates by metal interference through competition for fur. *Appl. Environ. Microbiol.* 76, 3836–3841. doi: 10.1128/AEM.00241-10

He, Y., Wu, B., Yang, J., Robinson, D., Risen, L., Ranken, R., et al. (2003). 2-Piperidin-4-yl-benzimidazoles with broad spectrum antibacterial activities. *Bioorg. Med. Chem. Lett.* 13, 3253–3256. doi: 10.1016/S0960-894X(03)00661-9

Hensler, M. E., Bernstein, G., Nizet, V., and Nefzi, A. (2006). Pyrrolidine bis-cyclic guanidines with antimicrobial activity against drug-resistant Gram-positive pathogens identified from a mixture-based combinatorial library. *Bioorg. Med. Chem. Lett.* 16, 5073–5079. doi: 10.1016/j.bmcl.2006.07.037

Issam, A.-A., Zimmermann, S., Reichling, J., and Wink, M. (2015). Pharmacological synergism of bee venom and melittin with antibiotics and plant secondary metabolites against multi-drug resistant microbial pathogens. *Phytomedicine* 22, 245–255. doi: 10.1016/j.phymed.2014.11.019

Juranić, I. O., Tošić, A. V., Kolundžija, B., and Drakuliæ, B. J. (2014). Antiproliferative activity of the Michael adducts of aroylacrylic acids and cyclic amines. *Mol. Divers.* 18, 577–592. doi: 10.1007/s11030-014-9528-4

Kauppi, A. M., Nordfelth, R., Uvell, H., Wolf-Watz, H., and Elofsson, M. (2003). Targeting bacterial virulence: inhibitors of type III secretion in *Yersinia*. *Chem. Biol.* 10, 241–249. doi: 10.1016/S1074-5521(03)00046-2

Kazakova, O. B., Giniyatullina, G. V., Medvedeva, N. I., Lopatina, T. V., Baikova, I. P., Tolstikov, G. A., et al. (2014). Synthesis and cytotoxicity of triterpene seven-membered cyclic amines. *Russ. J. Bioorganic Chem.* 40, 198–205. doi: 10.1134/S106816201402006X

Khatkar, A., Nanda, A., Kumar, P., and Narasimhan, B. (2014). Synthesis, antimicrobial evaluation and QSAR studies of p-coumaric acid derivatives. *Arab. J. Chem.* 10, S3804–S3815. doi: 10.1016/j.arabjc.2014.05.018

Kluytmans, J., Van Belkum, A., and Verbrugh, H. (1997). Nasal carriage of *Staphylococcus aureus*: epidemiology, underlying mechanisms, and associated risks. *Clin. Microbiol. Rev.* 10, 505–520.

Kumar, M., Narasimhan, B., Ramasamy, K., Mani, V., Mishra, R. K., and Majeed, A. B. A. (2013). Synthesis, antimicrobial and cytotoxic evaluation of 4-(1-aryl-5-halo-2-oxo-1, 2-dihydro-indol-3-ylideneamino)-N-substituted benzene sulphonamides. *Arab. J. Chem.* 10, S2845–S2852. doi: 10.1016/j.arabjc.2013.11.009

Kupferwasser, L. I., Yeaman, M. R., Nast, C. C., Kupferwasser, D., Xiong, Y.-Q., Palma, M., et al. (2003). Salicylic acid attenuates virulence in endovascular infections by targeting global regulatory pathways in *Staphylococcus aureus*. *J. Clin. Invest.* 112, 222–233. doi: 10.1172/JCI200316876

Otto, M. (2013). Staphylococcal infections: mechanisms of biofilm maturation and detachment as critical determinants of pathogenicity. *Annu. Rev. Med.* 64, 175–188. doi: 10.1146/annurev-med-042711-140023

Parsek, M., and Singh, P. (2003). Bacterial biofilms: an emerging link to disease pathogenesis. *Annu. Rev. Microbiol.* 57, 677–701. doi: 10.1146/annurev.micro.57.030502.090720

Pietrow, O., Panek, A., and Synowiecki, J. (2013). Extracellular proteolytic activity of *Deinococcus geothermalis*. *Afr. J. Biotechnol.* 12, 4020–4027.

Projan, S. J. (2002). New (and not so new) antibacterial targets–from where and when will the novel drugs come? *Curr. Opin. Pharmacol.* 2, 513–522. doi: 10.1016/S1471-4892(02)00197-2

Qayyum, S., Sharma, D., Bisht, D., and Khan, A. U. (2016). Protein translation machinery holds a key for transition of planktonic cells to biofilm state in *Enterococcus faecalis*: a proteomic approach. *Biochem. Biophys. Res. Commun.* 474, 652–659. doi: 10.1016/j.bbrc.2016.04.145

Ramachandran, P., Gagare, P., Sakavuyi, K., and Clark, P. (2010). Reductive amination using ammonia borane. *Tetrahedron Lett.* 51, 3167–3169. doi: 10.1016/j.tetlet.2010.04.014

Ravichandiran, V., Shanmugam, K., Anupama, K., Thomas, S., and Princy, A. (2012). Structure-based virtual screening for plant-derived SdiA-selective ligands as potential antivirulent agents against uropathogenic *Escherichia coli*. *Eur. J. Med. Chem.* 48, 200–205. doi: 10.1016/j.ejmech.2011.12.015

Safdar, N., and Maki, D. G. (2004). The pathogenesis of catheter-related bloodstream infection with noncuffed short-term central venous catheters. *Intensive Care Med.* 30, 62–67. doi: 10.1007/s00134-003-2045-z

Singh, P., Schaefer, A., Parsek, M., and Moninger, T. (2000). Quorum-sensing signals indicate that cystic fibrosis lungs are infected with bacterial biofilms. *Nature* 407, 762–764. doi: 10.1038/35037627

Subík, J., Takácsová, G., Psenák, M., and Devínsky, F. (1977). Antimicrobial activity of amine oxides: mode of action and structure-activity correlation. *Antimicrob. Agents Chemother.* 12, 139–146. doi: 10.1128/AAC.12.2.139

Vincze, S., Stamm, I., Kopp, P. A., Hermes, J., Adlhoch, C., Semmler, T., et al. (2014). Alarming proportions of methicillin-resistant *Staphylococcus aureus* (MRSA) in wound samples from companion animals, Germany 2010–2012. *PLOS ONE* 9:e85656. doi: 10.1371/journal.pone.0085656

Weiss, E. C., Spencer, H. J., Daily, S. J., Weiss, B. D., and Smeltzer, M. S. (2009). Impact of sarA on antibiotic susceptibility of *Staphylococcus aureus* in a catheter-associated in vitro model of biofilm formation. *Antimicrob. Agents Chemother.* 53, 2475–2482. doi: 10.1128/AAC.01432-08

Zhu, J., Lu, C., Standland, M., Lai, E., Moreno, G. N., Umeda, A., et al. (2008). Single mutation on the surface of *Staphylococcus aureus* Sortase A can disrupt its dimerization. *Biochemistry* 47, 1667–1674. doi: 10.1021/bi7014597

12

# Non-Toxigenic *Clostridioides* (Formerly Clostridium) *difficile* for Prevention of *C. difficile* Infection

*Dale N. Gerding*[1*], *Susan P. Sambol*[1,2] *and Stuart Johnson*[1,2]

[1] *Research Service, Edward Hines Jr. VA Hospital, Hines, IL, United States,*

[2] *Department of Medicine, Loyola University Chicago Medical Center, Maywood, IL, United States*

***Correspondence:***
*Dale N. Gerding*
*dale.gerding2@va.gov*

The beneficial effect of colonization of the gastrointestinal tract by non-toxigenic *Clostridioides difficile* (NTCD) strains as a preventive of toxigenic *C. difficile* infection (CDI) has been known since the early 1980s. Investigators in both the USA and United Kingdom demonstrated that prior colonization by randomly selected NTCD strains provided prevention against infection by toxigenic *C. difficile* in hamsters, albeit with limited durability. In the 1980s two patients with multiply recurrent CDI in the UK were treated with vancomycin followed by NTCD to prevent further recurrences, with one success and one failure. Epidemiologic studies of hospitalized patients using weekly rectal swab cultures demonstrated that asymptomatic colonization of patients by toxigenic *C. difficile* was much more common than CDI, but also that the rate of asymptomatic NTCD colonization of patients was unexpectedly high. Development of molecular strain typing of *C. difficile* was instrumental in characterizing different strains of both toxigenic *C. difficile* and NTCD leading to identification of NTCD strains that were effective human colonizers. These strains were reintroduced in hamsters in the 1990s and shown to prevent CDI efficiently and durably when challenged with epidemic toxigenic *C. difficile* strains. One strain of NTCD, NTCD-M3, was manufactured under cGMP standards and was demonstrated to be safe in a phase 1 volunteer trial. NTCD-M3 was then tested in a phase 2 double-blind placebo controlled trial for the prevention of recurrent CDI in patients experiencing their first CDI episode or first CDI recurrence. NTCD-M3 was given at doses of $10^4$ or $10^7$ spores per day orally for 7 or 14 days following successful treatment of CDI with vancomycin and/or metronidazole. CDI recurred in 30% of placebo patients and 11% of all NTCD-M3 patients ($p = 0.006$); recurrence rate for the best dose, $10^7$ spores/d $\times$ 7 days, was 5% ($p = 0.01$ vs. placebo). Detection of colonization predicted prevention success; among the 86 patients who were colonized with NTCD-M3 the recurrence rate was 2% vs. 31% in patients who received NTCD-M3 but were not colonized ($p < 0.001$). Additional trials of NTCD-M3 for primary prevention of CDI and prevention of CDI recurrence seem warranted by these promising results.

**Keywords: non-toxigenic, *Clostridium difficile*, NTCD-M3, prevention, NTCD, colonization, spores, *Clostridioides difficile***

## INTRODUCTION

The purpose of this review is to summarize the experimental, pre-clinical, and clinical data for the use of non-toxigenic *Clostridioides difficile* (NTCD) for prevention of *C. difficile* infection (CDI) caused by toxigenic strains of *C. difficile*. NTCD strains in which the pathogenicity locus (PaLoc) for the main *C. difficile* virulence factors, toxin A and B is replaced by a 115 bp sequence occur naturally. Multiple investigators have published convincing results of experiments over the last 35 years that demonstrate the efficacy of NTCD as a colonizing bacterial agent that prevents infection with toxigenic strains of *C. difficile* in animals and humans. Although a definitive mechanism for this protection remains to be determined, the effectiveness of this approach in multiple animal models and human clinical observations and trials suggests that it is a safe and effective biotherapeutic strategy that could be used for both primary prevention of CDI and prevention of CDI recurrence.

### Background Bench Discoveries in the 1980s

The concept of NTCD inhibiting or interfering with the infectivity of a toxigenic strain of *C. difficile* was first reported by Wilson and Sheagren (1983) in the hamster model in 1983. They demonstrated that following cefoxitin administration, colonization with NTCD prior to challenge with toxigenic *C. difficile* increased hamster survival from 21% to 93%, however, durability of prevention was not determined. Simultaneous administration of the NTCD strain and a toxigenic *C. difficile* strain did not increase survival. Borriello and Barclay (1985) extended these observations by colonization of hamsters with three different strains of NTCD, M-1, D-1 and S-1 administered at doses ranging from $3 \times 10^6$ to $3 \times 10^9$ organisms followed by challenge 5 days later with a toxigenic strain B-1 at a dose of $3 \times 10^7$ organisms. Results of these experiments showed at 25 days post toxigenic challenge survival of 13 of 18 (72%) vs. 0/21 (0%) hamsters not given an NTCD strain. Additional experiments showed (1) that protection was dependent upon live NTCD organisms; heat-killed NTCD did not protect hamsters, (2) that protection was dependent upon NTCD colonization; decolonization with vancomycin resulted in no protection against toxigenic challenge, and (3) that protection was specific to *C. difficile*; attempts to colonize with *C. perfringens*, *C. bifermentans*, and *C. beijerincki*, failed, and *C. sporogenes* colonized but failed to protect against toxigenic *C. difficile* challenge.

Borriello and Barclay (1985) also attempted to identify the mechanism by which NTCD protected against toxigenic *C. difficile*. They showed that NTCD did not degrade or alter the potency of *C. difficile* toxin. They investigated the mucosal association of NTCD by harvesting cecum samples from three NTCD-colonized hamsters at day 51 of colonization, washing them eight times with brain heart infusion (BHI) broth and saline, then homogenizing the tissue and doing quantitative culture of the homogenate. They found association of NTCD with the cecal mucosa ranging from $6 \times 10^3$ to $3 \times 10^5$ cfu/g tissue, suggesting there may be association of NTCD with the cecal mucosa or alternatively, they suggested competition for essential nutrients. However, in the discussion they report that after day 25 death occurred in most animals and that toxigenic *C. difficile* and cytotoxin could be detected in the cecum of these animals. Sequential analysis of the fecal pellets in these animals detected a change over time from only NTCD recovery to recovery of toxigenic *C. difficile* or both. This was of concern and the authors speculated that the presence of toxin enabled toxigenic strains of *C. difficile* to have a colonization advantage over NTCD. In a subsequent publication, Borriello et al. (1988) showed that a virulent toxigenic strain B-1 of *C. difficile* was more adherent to mucosa of small and large bowel in the hamster than NTCD strain M-1. They also showed that injection of toxin into the cecum of hamsters enhanced colonization of M-1 in the colon, but not in the small bowel or cecum when compared to toxigenic strain B-1.

Similar observations of protection against toxigenic *C. difficile* by NTCD were shown in gnotobiotic mice by Corthier and Muller (1988). NTCD protected against toxigenic challenge from 18h to 10 days following NTCD in 100% of gnotobiotic mice. If there was no delay in administration of the toxigenic strain following NTCD, 60% of mice survived. Survival of mice beyond 10 days was not recorded.

These early bench and animal studies were not further pursued beyond the 1980s, most likely because the protective effect in hamsters did not appear to be durable. However, these observations provide a valuable early insight into the potential utility of NTCD as a preventive strategy for CDI.

### Bedside Clinical Observations

The first published report of the use of NTCD in patients was by Seal et al. (1987). Two patients with multiple recurrences of CDI were treated orally with a BHI culture of NTCD strain M-1 previously shown by Borriello and Barclay (1985) to prevent CDI in hamsters transiently. One ml of the 24h culture was diluted in 50 ml of milk (final concentration $\sim 1 \times 10^7$ cfu/ml) which was administered once daily for 3 days. **Patient A**, age 88 years, was treated for her first CDI episode with metronidazole and for episodes two and three with oral vancomycin. Although successfully treated with resolution of symptoms, she had persistent *C. difficile* in her stool for at least 3 days following the last vancomycin treatment but was negative on stool culture just prior to receiving NTCD. Following NTCD her stool cultures were positive for NTCD for 14 days with no toxigenic *C. difficile* detected, and she had no further CDI recurrences for at least 4 months. **Patient B**, age 76, was also treated for her first CDI episode with metronidazole and for episodes two and three with vancomycin. She was treated successfully for her diarrhea symptoms with vancomycin, but had high counts of toxigenic *C. difficile* in her stool for the first 3 days of NTCD administration (5.9–7.5 $\log_{10}$/gm stool) with no NTCD detected. NTCD did not appear in the stool until day 6 at which time there were $\sim 10^7$ cfu/gm stool of both NTCD and toxigenic *C. difficile*, but on days 9 and 10 only toxigenic *C. difficile* was found at a concentration of $\sim 10^5$ cfu/gm stool. Starting on day 17 she had 2 days of self-limited diarrhea with both toxigenic *C. difficile* and NTCD at $\sim 10^3$ cfu/gm stool and stool toxin detected. On day

28 counts of both toxigenic *C. difficile* and NTCD had declined to ~$10^2$ cfu/gm and on day 45 neither were detected in stool. The patient died 1 month later of an unrelated cause but had no further diarrhea. In view of the mild recurrence of diarrhea with stool toxin detected at day 17 it is likely that this patient failed preventive treatment with NTCD, whereas patient A was a success. No further patient treatments with NTCD were reported until well into the 21st century, however, considerable clinical information on detection of NTCD in patients was obtained in the interim.

In the 1980s it became apparent that CDI was a healthcare associated infection (Gerding et al., 1986; McFarland et al., 1989), and typing systems for identification of specific *C. difficile* strains were developed (Kuijper et al., 1987; McFarland et al., 1989; Clabots et al., 1993) based not only on isolates from patients with CDI, but also from specimens collected from asymptomatic patients using rectal swabs (McFarland et al., 1989; Johnson et al., 1990; Clabots et al., 1992). McFarland et al. (1989) were the first to detect the presence of large numbers of patients in hospital that were asymptomatically colonized with *C. difficile.* They demonstrated that transmission of *C. difficile* was frequent in the hospital setting using immunoblot organism typing and space/time relations. They found that nearly 2/3 of patients that acquired *C. difficile* remained asymptomatic whereas just over 1/3 had symptomatic CDI (McFarland et al., 1989).

The use of restriction endonuclease analysis (REA) typing of *C. difficile* markedly enhanced the epidemiologic investigation of CDI in hospitals (Kuijper et al., 1987; Clabots et al., 1993). Early in the development of REA there were 75 distinct groups identified by letters of the alphabet, 43 cytotoxin positive groups, 28 NTCD groups, and 4 groups that included both cytotoxin positive and negative isolates. Isolates for typing were obtained from CDI patients, rectal swabs of asymptomatic patients and multiple environmental sites. In comparison with other typing systems then in use REA demonstrated greater sensitivity than immunoblot typing, bacteriophage-bacteriocin typing and ribotyping (Clabots et al., 1993). Remarkably, the most frequently isolated REA group was the NTCD group M which was found more commonly than any toxigenic groups and may be a reflection of the inclusion of large numbers of isolates collected from asymptomatic patients using rectal swabs.

Using a similar weekly rectal swab methodology used by McFarland et al. (1989) to detect *C. difficile* asymptomatic colonization coupled with REA typing of *C. difficile* (Kuijper et al., 1987; Clabots et al., 1993), Johnson et al. (1990) showed that 21% of patients hospitalized on three wards were culture-positive for *C. difficile*, the majority 51 of 60 (85%) were asymptomatic. All of the 9 cases of CDI were caused by two closely related toxigenic REA types, B and B2, and none occurred among the 51 asymptomatic colonized patients, 9 of whom were colonized with the B or B2 strain types but remained asymptomatic. Fifteen of the 17 patients with the B or B2 isolates were located on the same surgical ward suggesting transmission on that ward. Among the 18 different REA type *C. difficile* isolates found on the 3 study wards, 10 were toxigenic and 8 (44%) were non-toxigenic including 7 distinct REA groups of NTCD, groups A, C, M, P, S, T, and U. This was the first indication that NTCD strains were carried frequently by hospital patients. In addition, it was found that asymptomatic *C. difficile* colonization occurred in approximately the same frequency on all 3 hospital wards, ranging from 12.2 to 19.3% of patients, all of whom had relatively long hospital stays. All the patients with toxigenic *C. difficile* or NTCD in their stool remained asymptomatic.

A larger similar study using rectal swab cultures was conducted on a single surgical ward with a historically high rate of CDI by Clabots et al. (1992). The study was conducted over 9 months and enrolled 634 (94%) of 678 admissions to this ward, obtaining rectal swab cultures on admission and weekly thereafter. Of the 634 ward admissions, 65 (10.3%) were either asymptomatically culture-positive for *C. difficile* (61 patients) or had CDI (4 patients). Twelve additional asymptomatic admissions were positive for *C difficile* when first sampled, but were not sampled within 48 h of admission and were indeterminate as to whether they acquired *C. difficile* on the ward or were already colonized when admitted. The majority of admissions (355, 56%) were admitted from home and had not been hospitalized within the previous 30 days. Twenty-two (7%) of these home admissions were culture-positive for *C. difficile* indicating the high potential for introduction of *C. difficile* strains to the hospital from the community. Of the 557 admissions to the ward that were not culture-positive for *C. difficile*, 54 (9.7%) acquired *C difficile* while on the ward, but only 3 had CDI. REA typing identified 58 different distinct types during the study. Of the top seven most frequently isolated REA types, three were NTCD types and constituted 23/68 (34%) of these isolates. The most commonly isolated NTCD strain type was M3 which subsequently, together with types M23 and T7, was selected for laboratory trials in hamsters for prevention of CDI.

Low rates of CDI among patients previously asymptomatically colonized with *C. difficile* were observed in several trials utilizing weekly rectal swab cultures and suggested that colonization might be protective against CDI if symptoms did not develop relatively quickly following toxigenic *C. difficile* exposure, or if patients were colonized by NTCD. Data from four such prospective studies were combined in a random effects model by Shim et al. (1998). All four studies employed similar weekly rectal swab cultures for *C. difficile* in asymptomatic hospitalized patients and utilized stool cultures for *C. difficile* if CDI symptoms developed. Patients recovering from prior CDI were excluded as they have a high colonization rate with toxigenic *C. difficile* post treatment and are prone to recurrences of CDI. Asymptomatic patients were included if they had at least two consecutive weekly *C. difficile* rectal swab cultures and were classified as either colonized or not colonized. Colonized patients were further categorized as colonized with a toxigenic *C. difficile* strain or NTCD. All isolates underwent REA typing as well as toxin testing. Among the 618 non-colonized patients, 22 (3.6%) developed CDI whereas only 2 (1%) of 192 colonized patients developed CDI (pooled risk difference −2.3%, $p = 0.021$, **Figure 1**). When the analysis was confined only to patients who had received antibiotics within 14–21 days of the start of the sampling or during sampling, the pooled risk difference was −3.2%, $p = 0.024$. Greater exposure to antibiotics in non-colonized patients could explain the increased rate of CDI, but

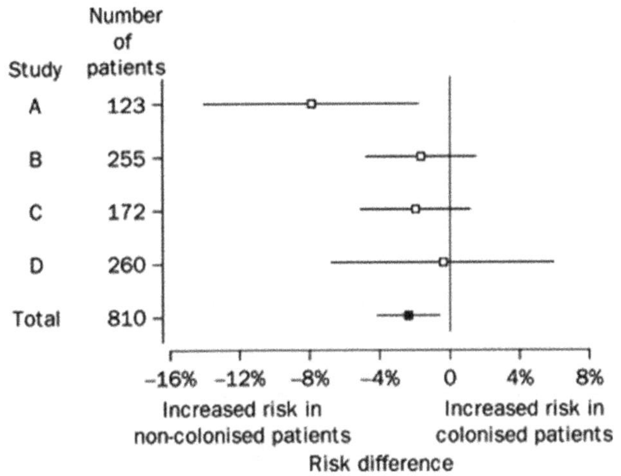


**FIGURE 1** | Risk difference (95% CI) for CDI among patients initially colonized and non-colonized with *C difficile* in four studies. Risk difference pooled across studies with a random effects model is shown in bottom row (Total). From Shim et al. (1998).

antibiotic exposure was lower (79%) in non-colonized patients compared to colonized patients (92%). The mechanism by which colonization prevents CDI is unknown, and toxigenic strains of *C. difficile* as typed by REA that caused CDI were also found to be carried asymptomatically suggesting that strain type did not explain prevention. In these 4 studies there was a very high proportion (44%) of patients that were colonized by NTCD. There were 15 different REA groups of NTCD found among the 76 NTCD isolates, but the majority of NTCD were in two REA groups, M (49%) and T (19%). No CDI occurred among NTCD colonized patients and may account at least partially for the reduced CDI rates in colonized patients.

Taken together these clinical observations documented the relatively high rate of colonization of hospitalized patients by non-toxigenic strains of *C. difficile* and documented a very low rate of CDI among all colonized patients. Furthermore, REA typing demonstrated the ability to group and type NTCD strains in a manner similar to toxigenic *C. difficile* and identified two dominant groups of NTCD, the M and T groups by REA typing.

## Back to Bench Investigation: Pre-clinical NTCD Development

Bedside clinical and epidemiologic observations coupled with the evolution of molecular typing of *C. difficile* prompted further laboratory testing of *C. difficile*, particularly in animal models. Of specific interest was whether strains of *C. difficile* responsible for hospital outbreaks were more virulent than other strains that were found to asymptomatically colonize patients more often than they caused CDI. Sambol et al. (2001) tested three toxigenic epidemic *C. difficile* strains, REA types B1, J9, and K14 in the hamster model and compared them to toxigenic REA type Y2 which was found to commonly colonize patients but caused little CDI. A fifth strain, toxin variant REA type CF2, which is toxin A-negative, toxin B-positive and associated with CDI outbreaks was also included. The hamster protocol was similar to that of Borriello and Barclay (Borriello and Barclay, 1985), but differed in that only spores of *C. difficile* were administered by gavage 5 days following a single oral clindamycin dose of 30 mg/kg. A minimum infective dose for each *C. difficile* strain was predetermined to be 100 spores to mimic a postulated low inoculum exposure. The epidemic strains B1, J9, and K14 infected hamsters within 24–48 h of administration and caused 100% mortality by 48 h. REA type Y2 infected 9 of 10 hamsters over a range of 1–4 days, somewhat more slowly than the epidemic strains, but eventually all 9 infected hamsters died. Toxin variant strain CF2 infected only 6 of 10 hamsters over a range of 1 to 10 days and only 3 of the 6 died; the remaining 3 hamsters were colonized through study termination at day 79 and appeared to have no symptoms. The study documented differences in virulence of *C. difficile* strains in the hamster model and served as a basis on which to test preventive strategies with NTCD in the hamster model.

### NTCD Prevention

To test the effectiveness of NTCD as a preventive of infection with toxigenic *C. difficile*, the above described hamster model was used (Sambol et al., 2002). Three NTCD strains were selected from among isolates collected with rectal swabs from asymptomatic hospitalized patients; M3, M23, and T7, all of which were isolated at high frequency from patients (**Figure 2**). The NTCD inoculum was $10^6$ spores by oral gavage on day 2 following clindamycin 30 mg/kg orally. Toxigenic *C. difficile* challenge with strains B1, J9, or K14 with 100 spores by oral gavage occurred on day 5 following clindamycin (3 days after the NTCD inoculum). Prevention of CDI mortality ranged from 87 to 97% (**Figure 3**) and correlated closely with detection of NTCD colonization of the stool prior to challenge with toxigenic *C. difficile* strains. Colonization with NTCD persisted in these surviving hamsters until end of study which varied from 55 to 106 days and there was no late mortality from toxigenic *C. difficile*.

### NTCD Prevention Durability

Durability of protection against late challenge with toxigenic *C. difficile* was performed with M3 and M23 NTCD. In the first of these studies M3 colonized 5 of 5 hamsters on day 4 following inoculation on day 2 following clindamycin. All 5 hamsters lost colonization between days 23 and 44. The uncolonized hamsters were challenged with 100 spores of toxigenic B1 *C. difficile* on day 62 and survived until day 153 end of study. In a second M3 experiment 3 of 4 hamsters were colonized on day 3 following inoculation on day 2 post clindamycin and were challenged on day 63 with 100 spores of toxigenic J9 and all survived with 3 of 4 remaining colonized with M3 until end of study day 125. In a third experiment, 12 hamsters were given clindamycin on day 0; 10 received NTCD strain M23 on day 2 and became colonized by day 5. All 12 hamsters were challenged with toxigenic strain B1 on day 41 and all survived (10 colonized with M23 and 2 uncolonized). All 10 remained colonized until day 49 when the study ended. These studies suggest that hamsters apparently recover colonization resistance following clindamycin by days

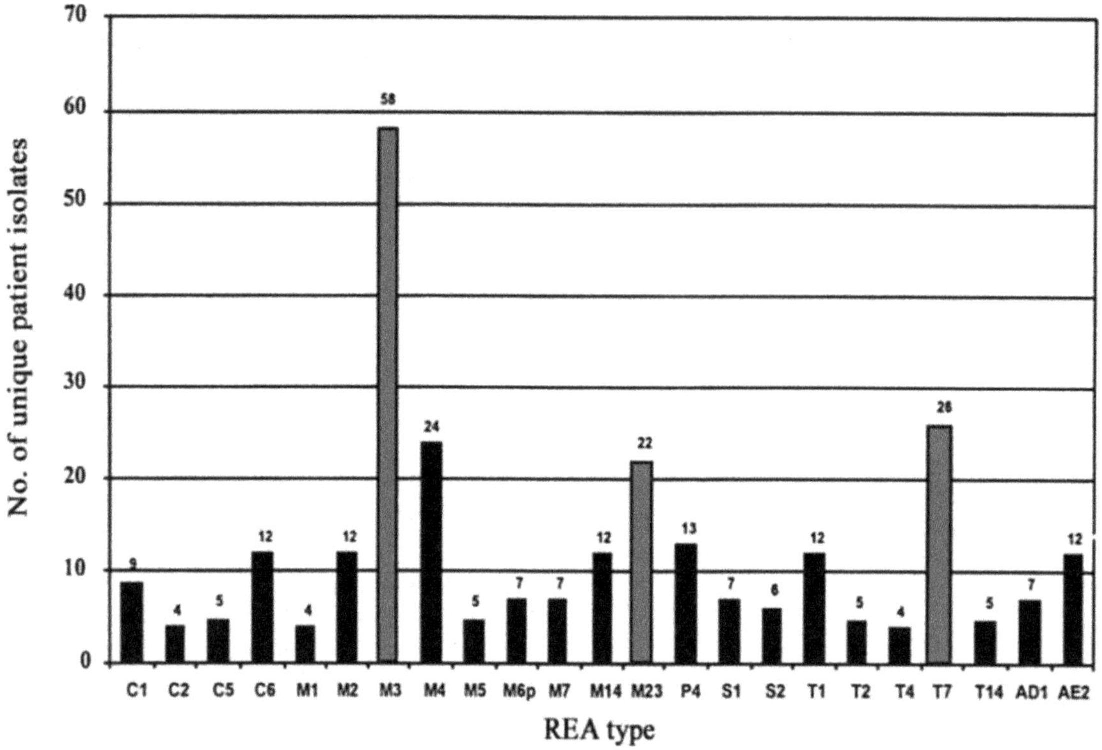


**FIGURE 2 |** Frequency of isolation of *Clostridium difficile* nontoxigenic restriction endonuclease analysis (REA) types from individual patients during 1982–1993. Gray bars indicate frequency of REA types used in hamster prevention trials. From Sambol et al. (2002) with permission.

41–62 and are protected from late challenge with toxigenic *C. difficile* whether colonized with NTCD or not.

Patients are occasionally treated with a single antibiotic dose, as for example when undergoing surgical prophylaxis, and would be representative of the experiments with hamsters following a single dose of antibiotic. However, most infection treatment is carried out using multiple doses, often on the same day and for multiple days at a time. This raises the question of how NTCD might be employed to prevent CDI since many of the antibiotics used systemically will be active against NTCD and presumably prevent it from colonizing the patient. NTCD REA types M3, M23, and T7 are susceptible to most antibiotics including ampicillin, clindamycin, erythromycin, tetracycline, trimethoprim-sulfamethoxazole and metronidazole, but resistant to ciprofloxacin and ceftriaxone (Sambol et al., 2002), patterns that are typical of most *C. difficile* isolates. Resistance to clindamycin, tetracyclines, carbapenems and erythromycins as well as very high-level resistance to fluoroquinolones is known to occur in *C. difficile* and may be transferrable. Whereas use of a highly antibiotic resistant strain of NTCD would favor more frequent colonization, it would also increase the risk of antibiotic resistance transfer to other bacteria in the gastrointestinal tract.

## Effect of Daily Clindamycin and Resistance in NTCD

To assess the effect of antibiotic resistance of NTCD on colonization and prevention of infection by toxigenic *C. difficile*, Merrigan et al. (2003) conducted experiments in hamsters treated with daily oral doses (30 mg/kg) of clindamycin for 5 consecutive days. Two strains of NTCD, REA type M3 (clindamycin susceptible at 0.5 mcg/ml), REA type M13 (clindamycin resistant at >256 mcg/ml) and a toxigenic strain of *C. difficile*, REA type B1 (clindamycin resistant at >256 mcg/ml) were used. Clindamycin resistance in type M13 and B1 was determined to be due to presence of the *erm*(B) gene. M3 was negative for *erm*(B). Colonization experiments with M3 and M13 were conducted in groups of 5 hamsters by administering (1) a single dose of $1 \times 10^6$ spores on day 3 of clindamycin, (2) a daily dose of $1 \times 10^6$ spores on days 3–5 of clindamycin or (3) a daily dose of $1 \times 10^6$ spores on days 3–7. Colonization occurred with all doses of resistant strain M13 within 1.25 days of the first dose. No colonization occurred following the single dose of susceptible strain M3, but following the 3-day and 5-day administrations all 10 hamsters eventually became colonized but after a mean lag time of 6.4 to 6.6 days following the first dose. When the experiment was repeated with challenge with toxigenic strain B1, 100 spores orogastrically, on day 5, day 7, or day 9, all hamsters were protected by all doses of clindamycin resistant M13. Clindamycin susceptible M3 gave no protection against challenge with B1 on day 5, but protected 1 of 5 hamsters challenged on day 7, and 5 of 5 challenged on day 9. The results of the experiment clearly show the advantage of an antibiotic resistant NTCD strain in preventing CDI, but also suggest that an antibiotic susceptible strain can be effective if administered daily past the end of antibiotic administration,

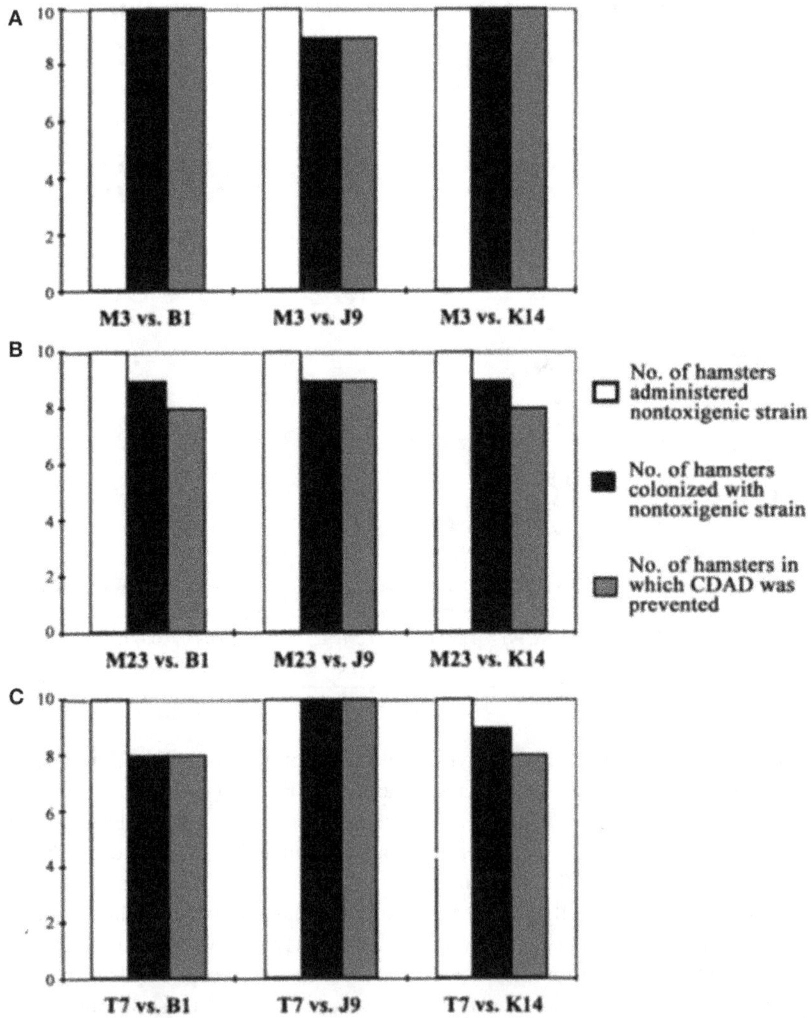


**FIGURE 3 |** Colonization by nontoxigenic restriction endonuclease analysis (REA) types and prevention of *Clostridium difficile*-associated disease (CDAD) in hamsters. Bars indicate number of animals colonized by nontoxigenic *C. difficile* REA type M3 **(A)**, type M23 **(B)**, and type T7 **(C)** and challenged with 3 different toxigenic *C. difficile* REA types (B1, J9, and K14). From Sambol et al. (2002) with permission.

albeit without as many days of prevention due to the longer time required to establish colonization in the presence of an antibiotic to which it is susceptible. Obviously, a toxigenic *C. difficile* strain resistant to the antibiotic being given has an advantage over susceptible NTCD while the antibiotic is being given, an advantage that is lost within a few days of stopping the antibiotic.

## NTCD Prevention After Daily Exposure to Antibiotics Other Than Clindamycin

Similar experiments were conducted to determine NTCD protection during continuous daily administration of ampicillin or ceftriaxone (Merrigan et al., 2009) with the exception that the dose of the toxigenic challenge strain was raised to $1 \times 10^6$ spores to further test NTCD prevention. Most strains of *C. difficile* are resistant to cephalosporins including ceftriaxone, and are susceptible to penicillins such as ampicillin. In the ceftriaxone experiments the antibiotic was given intraperitoneally (60 mg/kg) daily for 5 days and NTCD strains M3, M23, or T7 were given to groups of 5 hamsters orogastrically at a dose of $1 \times 10^6$ spores 3 h following the first ceftriaxone dose. The toxigenic challenge strain (REA type J9, $1 \times 10^6$ spores orogastrically) was responsible for multiple outbreaks of CDI in U.S. hospitals in the 1990s (Johnson et al., 1999). All the strains used were resistant to ceftriaxone; M3 and M23 MIC = 128 mg/mL; T7 MIC = 96 mg/mL; and J9 MIC = >256 mg/mL. Results are shown in **Figure 4** and demonstrate colonization within 48h for all NTCD strains and protection from J9 challenge on day 3 in all hamsters. A single control animal died within 48h as expected with J9 challenge.

Protection against daily administration of an antibiotic such as ampicillin to which NTCD and toxigenic *C. difficile* are both susceptible poses a different challenge (Merrigan et al., 2009). In these experiments NTCD REA type M3 (ampicillin MIC=2.0 mcg/ml) was utilized for prevention ($1 \times 10^6$ spores daily) and challenged at intervals of 2 days with $1 \times 10^6$ spores of toxigenic

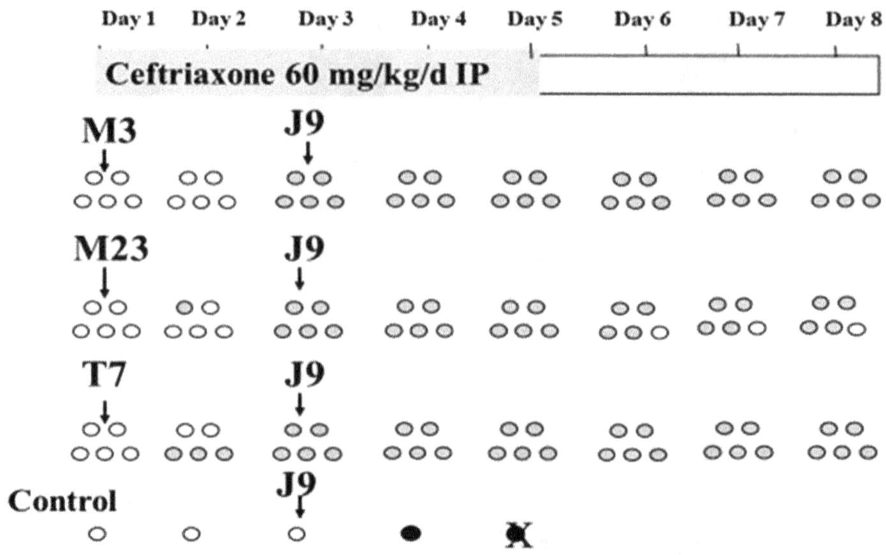


**FIGURE 4 |** Colonization of non-toxigenic *Clostridium difficile* strains M3, M23, or T7 and subsequent challenge with toxigenic strain J9 during daily ceftriaxone administration. Animals are indicated by ovals: open ovals indicate no detection of *C. difficile* in stool; gray-shaded ovals indicate detection of non-toxigenic *C. difficile* in stool; black ovals indicate detection of toxigenic strain J9 in stool. An X superimposed over an oval indicates the day of death. IP, intraperitoneally. From Merrigan et al. (2009).

strain J9 (ampicillin MIC = 0.75 mcg/ml). Ampicillin was given orogastrically (60 mg/kg daily) to groups of 4 hamsters for 5 days. As expected based on pilot studies, neither M3 or J7 colonized during ampicillin administration, but were able to establish colonization by day 8 if given near the end of the ampicillin course, indicating that following fecal excretion of the inhibitory antibiotic colonization could be established. Experiments were then designed to determine if NTCD M3 administered daily for 5 days to 3 groups of 4 hamsters beginning on day 1, day 3, and day 5 could protect against toxigenic J9 challenges on the middle day of each 5-day M3 course, days 3, 5, and 7, with both strains administered orogastrically at $1 \times 10^6$ spores. The study was designed to simulate periodic exposure to toxigenic *C. difficile* while being given NTCD daily. The experiment is shown schematically in **Figure 5** and demonstrates absence of J9 infection despite no colonization by either strain during the 5 days of ampicillin, followed by progressive colonization by M3 on days 7 and 8 in all hamsters. Results of these experiments suggest that in the presence of daily administration of an antibiotic to which NTCD is susceptible, that NTCD should be given daily and for several days after cessation of the antibiotic to attain successful colonization. Toxigenic *C. difficile* is not likely to infect during antibiotic administration and daily NTCD prophylaxis unless the toxigenic strain is resistant to the antibiotic and NTCD is susceptible.

## NTCD Prevention Against the Highly Virulent BI Strain of C. difficile

Early in the twenty first century it became apparent that CDI rates, morbidity and mortality were increasing in North America and were attributed at least in part to the presence of an epidemic strain characterized as BI group by REA, NAP1 by pulsed field gel electrophoresis, and 027 by PCR ribotyping and referred to as NAP1/BI/027 (Loo et al., 2005; McDonald et al., 2005). This strain spread throughout the United States and Canada as well as the United Kingdom and much of Europe as CDI rates rose precipitously in these countries. NAP1/BI/027 carries a third toxin, binary toxin and when compared to historic isolates of the same type it was apparent that high-level fluoroquinolone resistance had been acquired (McDonald et al., 2005). This prompted study of these strains in the hamster model by Razaq et al. (2007) who compared epidemic BI strains BI6 and BI17 to historic non-epidemic BI strain BI1 and 2 standard toxigenic strains, K14 and 630 (REA type R23). In these studies groups of 10 hamsters were given 100 spores of each strain of *C. difficile* orogastrically 5 days following a single clindamycin dose (30 mg/kg orally). Although group BI strains were not more rapidly fatal than standard toxinotype 0 strain K14, they were more rapidly fatal than strain 630 and epidemic strain BI6 was the most rapidly fatal of all the strains tested.

The widespread clinical presence of epidemic strain NAP1/BI/027 raised the question of whether NTCD strains would be effective in preventing disease due to BI strains in the hamster model. Nagaro et al. (2013) gave groups of 12 hamsters oral clindamycin (30 mg/kg orally) followed 2 days later by $1 \times 10^6$ spores of NTCD strains M3 or T7 in 10 hamsters, and on day 5 challenged all 12 with 100 spores of historic strain BI1 or epidemic strain BI6. All hamsters colonized with M3 or T7 and were protected against challenge with historic strain BI1. NTCD strain M3 colonized 9 of 10 hamsters and protected against BI6 challenge in the 9 colonized hamsters, but not the uncolonized animal. However, epidemic strain BI6 proved more difficult for protection by NTCD strain T7. For the first time in these hamster experiments we found NTCD colonization

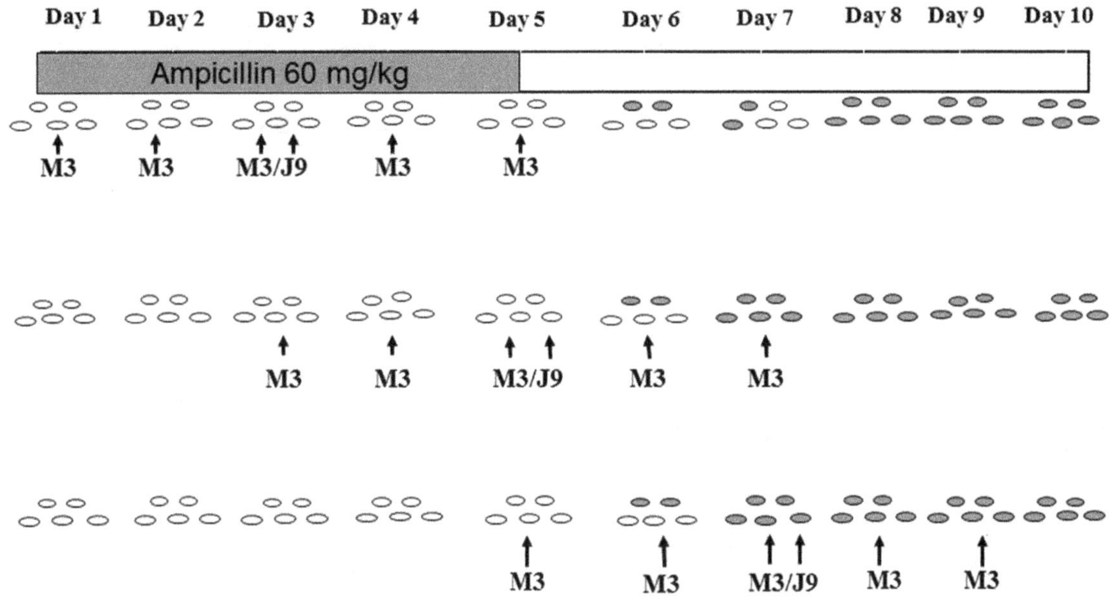


**FIGURE 5 |** Colonization with non-toxigenic *Clostridium difficile* M3 and challenge with toxigenic strain J9 during daily oral ampicillin administration for 5 days. Both J9 and M3 are susceptible to ampicillin. Animals are indicated by ovals: open ovals indicate no detection of *C. difficile* in stool; gray-shaded ovals indicate detection of non-toxigenic M3 in stool. PO, orally. From Merrigan et al. (2009).

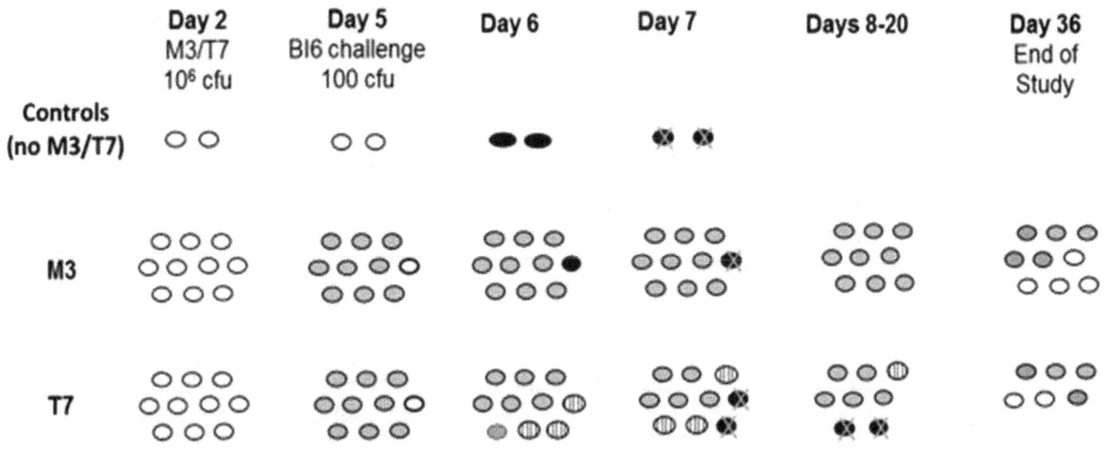


**FIGURE 6 |** Hamsters ($n = 10$/group) challenged with epidemic toxigenic BI6 *Clostridium difficile*. Day 2 = 2 days post-clindamycin treatment. *White ovals*; uncolonized hamsters. *Gray ovals*; non-toxigenic colonized hamsters. *Striped ovals*; hamsters co-colonized with non-toxigenic and toxigenic *C. difficile*. *Black ovals with "X"*; hamster death from toxigenic BI6. From Nagaro et al. (2013).

displaced by the toxigenic strain (**Figure 6**). Five of 10 hamsters were co-colonized with T7 and BI6 on day 7 and 4 of the 5 died. The remaining co-colonized hamster lost BI6 colonization on day 21 and survived. These results suggest that toxigenic and NTCD strains of *C. difficile* compete for colonization and that certain strains such as BI6 (but not its historic predecessor BI1) despite their lower inoculum and later administration are able to compete more effectively than other toxigenic strains against NTCD strain T7, but not against strain M3. Thus, differences in colonization efficiency are evident for both toxigenic strains of *C. difficile* as well as NTCD strains.

## Possible Mechanism of NTCD Prevention

The mechanism by which *C. difficile* strains establish colonization is not established. One possibility is that strains differ in their ability to adhere to colonic mucosal cells or mucus. Merrigan et al. (2013) utilized a derivative of the Caco-2-derived human intestinal epithelial cell-line to assess adherence of 33 strains of toxigenic *C. difficile* (with an emphasis on epidemic NAP1/BI/027 and ribotype 078 strains) and 3 NTCD strains (REA types M3, M23, and T7) in this assay with a focus on differences in surface layer protein A (SlpA) in the strains. The average adherence range of vegetative cells was approximately 8–11% for

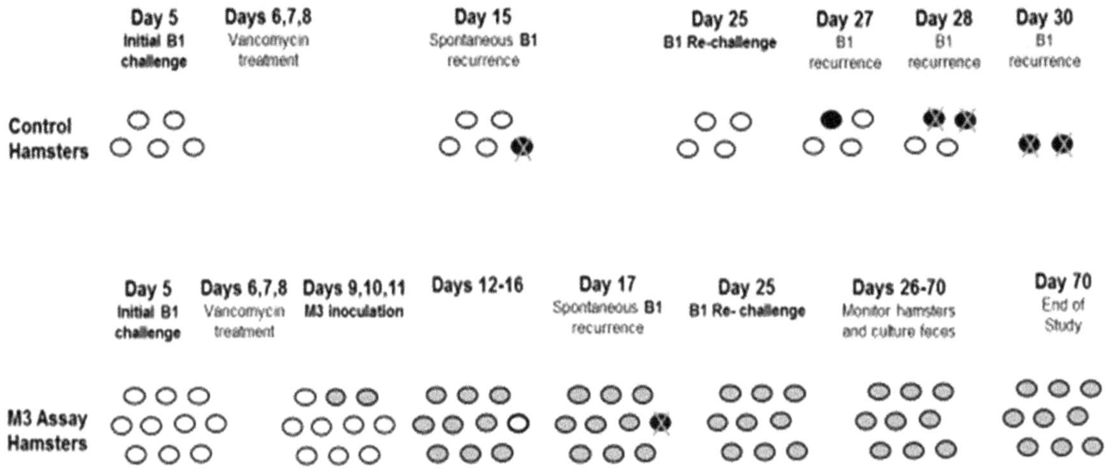


**FIGURE 7 |** Prevention of recurrence with NTCD-M3 following vancomycin treatment of toxigenic B1 *C. difficile* infection in hamsters. Day 5 = 5 days post-clindamycin treatment. *White ovals*: uncolonized hamsters. *Black ovals*: toxigenic infected hamsters. *Gray ovals*: non-toxigenic colonized hamsters. *Black ovals with "X"*: hamster death from toxigenic B1. From Sambol et al. (2004).

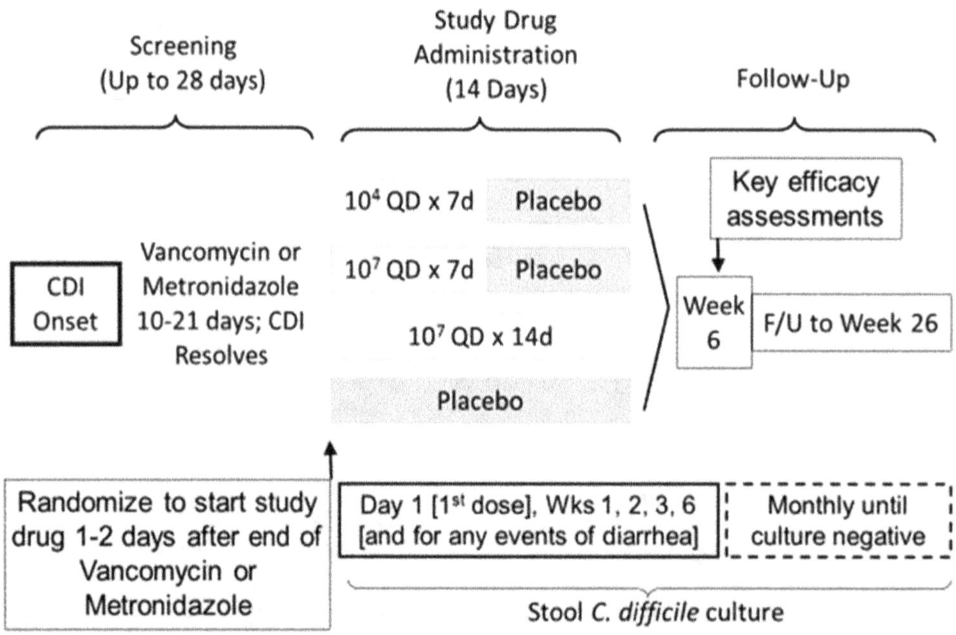


**FIGURE 8 |** Trial Design for Phase 2 clinical trial of study drug NTCD-M3, spores of non-toxigenic *C. difficile* strain M3 (Gerding et al., 2015).

strain 630, 2–4% for strain K14, 5–9% for strain BI17, 8–14% for NTCD strain M3, and 9–12% for NTCD strain T7. As a group, BI/NAP1/027 strains exhibited a mean adherence value of 4.6%. Further experiments showed that pretreatment of cell layers with surface layer protein (SLP) preparations inhibited *C. difficile* adherence up to 80% with the maximum SLP dose. SLP inhibition was not strain specific; NTCD M3 SLP inhibited M3 and BI17 adherence equally, and BI17 SLP inhibited BI17 and M3 adherence equally. Sequence analysis of the SlpA proteins for both the high molecular weight and low molecular weight subunits was compared among strains. One might postulate that there would be a high degree of conservation of amino acid sequences among highly competitive strains, yet NTCD strain M3 displayed the least sequence conservation, especially in the low molecular weight subunit, compared not only to epidemic toxigenic strains, but also when compared to NTCD strain T7.

## NTCD Prevention of Recurrent CDI

Patients who have CDI incur about a 20–30% risk of having a recurrence of their symptoms following successful treatment. If

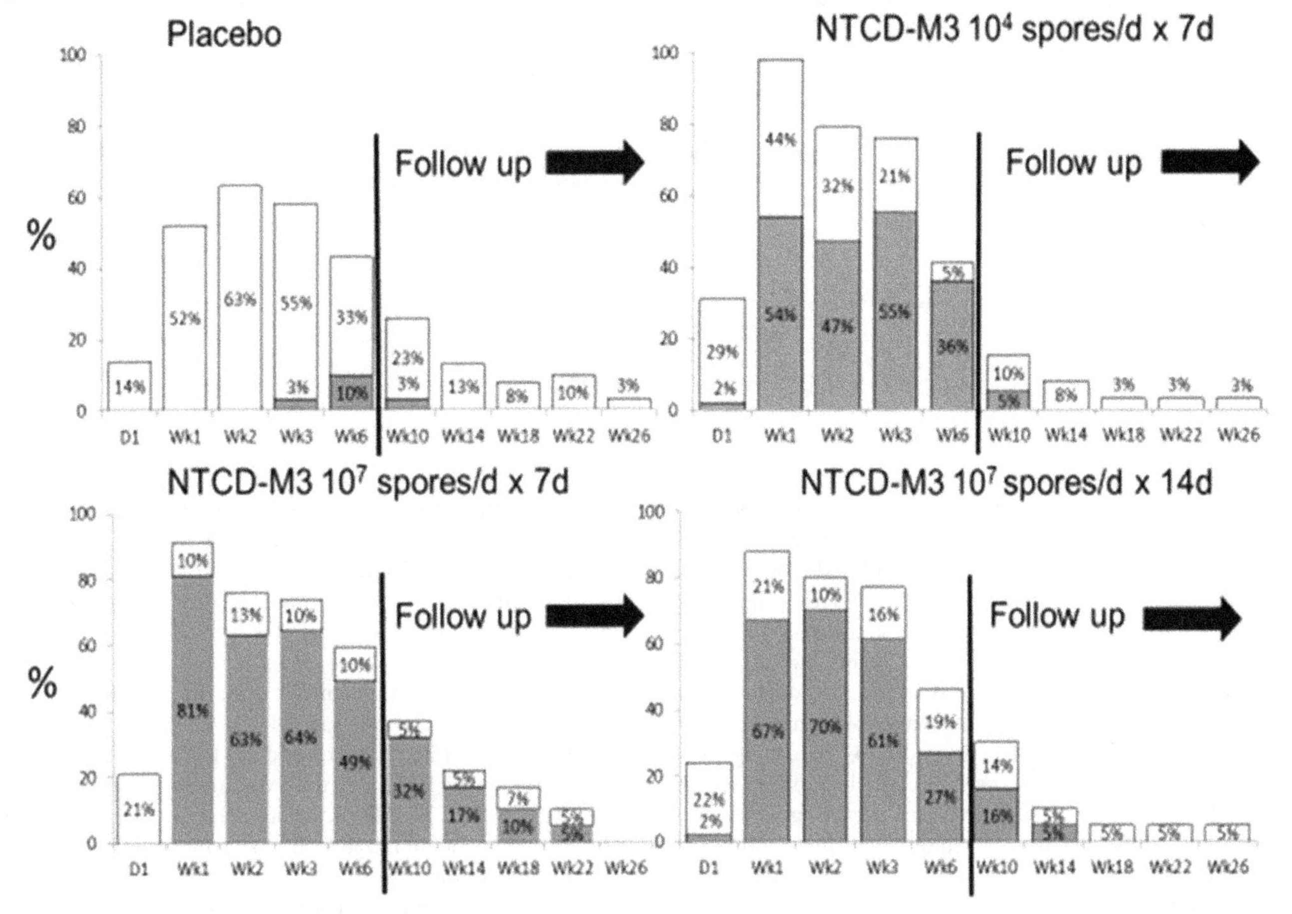


**FIGURE 9** | Proportion of patients with positive *Clostridium difficile* stool cultures at specified visits through week 6 and during follow-up (weeks 10–26) by treatment group for the intent-to-treat safety population. White bars: culture positive for toxigenic *C. difficile*. Gray bars: culture positive for NTCD. NTCD, non-toxigenic *C. difficile*. From Gerding et al. (2015) (Supplementary Material) with permission.

such patients could be colonized with NTCD following antibiotic treatment of CDI, it could prevent subsequent recurrence. To test this possibility, the CDI treatment model in hamsters that demonstrated late recurrence of CDI mortality following treatment with vancomycin was modified to administer NTCD M3 following vancomycin treatment (Swanson et al., 1991; Sambol et al., 2004). Sambol et al. (2004) gave a group of 15 hamsters oral clindamycin (30 mg/kg) followed 5 days later by $1 \times 10^4$ spores of epidemic strain B1. Vancomycin was administered orogastrically in doses of 100 mg/kg daily for 3 consecutive days on Days 6, 7, and 8 with the first dose administered within 14 h of the initial B1 challenge. On Days 9, 10, and 11, NTCD strain M3 was orally administered to 10 of the 15 hamsters at $1 \times 10^6$ spores/day per hamster (5 control hamsters did not receive NTCD). On Day 25, all surviving hamsters were given a re-challenge dose of $1 \times 10^4$ toxigenic B1 spores to simulate re-exposure to the toxigenic strain (**Figure 7**). Of the control hamsters, one out of 5 was infected with B1 three days after vancomycin treatment, and died on Day 15, a spontaneous B1 recurrence. After the B1 re-challenge on Day 25, 4 of 4 surviving control hamsters became infected with B1 between Days 27 and 30, and died by Day 30.

Of the hamsters given NTCD, 9 of 10 colonized with M3 between Days 10–16; one hamster remained uncolonized until Day 17, when it became infected with epidemic strain B1 and died, a spontaneous CDI recurrence. After the B1 re-challenge on Day 25, all 9 surviving hamsters remained colonized with M3 until study end on Day 70 with no evidence of B1 infection. These results demonstrate that NTCD colonization following vancomycin treatment is successful and will prevent recurrent *C. difficile* infection.

## Potential for NTCD Acquisition of Toxin Genes

Concern has been raised that in clinical use NTCD strains may acquire the toxin A and B pathogenicity locus (PaLoc) and become pathogenic. Brouwer et al. (2013) have shown *in vitro* that toxigenic strain 630Δerm can transfer the PaLoc to NTCD strain CD37, which is REA type T18. PaLoc-containing transconjugants were obtained at a frequency of $7.5 \times 10^{-9}$ transconjugants per donor in filter matings. DNA fragments containing the PaLoc ranged in size from 66,034 to 272,977 bp.

**TABLE 1 |** *C. difficile* recurrence and any diarrhea event by treatment arm in a phase 2 clinical trial of NTCD-M3 administered at two different doses of $10^4$ and $10^7$ spores for 7 or 14 days vs. placebo for 14 days (Gerding et al., 2015).

| | | Placebo | $10^4$ x 7d | $10^7$ x 7d | $10^7$ x 14d | All NTCD |
|---|---|---|---|---|---|---|
| Number of patients, n | | 43 | 41 | 43 | 41 | 125 |
| CDI recurrence, n (%) | | 13 (30) | 6 (15) | 2 (5) | 6 (15) | 14 (11) |
| | *p*-value* | | 0.11 | 0.01 | 0.10 | 0.006 |
| CDI recurrence defined by antibacterial use for CDI treatment, n (%) | | 14 (33) | 6 (15) | 4 (9) | 7 (17) | 17 (14) |
| | *p*-value* | | 0.07 | 0.02 | 0.14 | 0.009 |
| Any event of diarrhea (of any severity) or CDI, n (%) | | 33 (77) | 23 (56) | 25 (58) | 23 (56) | 71 (57) |
| | *p*-value* | | 0.05 | 0.09 | 0.02 | 0.020 |

**p-values adjusted for pre-specified parameters: use of metronidazole vs. vancomycin, and primary episode vs. first recurrence.*

Transfers from 630Δerm to two other NTCD isolates, PCR ribotypes 138 and 140, were also successful demonstrating that PaLoc transfer is not restricted to a specific donor-recipient pair. Supernatants of recipient strain CD37 following PaLoc transfer were found to cause cell rounding in the cell cytotoxicity assay that was neutralized by toxin B antibodies indicating that the PaLoc transfer resulted in functional toxin production. The mechanism by which PaLoc transfer takes place has not been precisely defined, but transfer via a cell-to-cell conjugation-like transfer mechanism has been proposed (Brouwer et al., 2016). The likelihood of such transfers occurring *in vitro* is unknown, but would presumably require high concentrations of a toxigenic *C. difficile* strain and NTCD in close proximity in the gastrointestinal tract of a host. In the hamster model, we have demonstrated that vancomycin administered daily for 3 days will eliminate NTCD detection in stool, and would presumably be effective in managing CDI if PaLoc transfers were to occur in patients.

## Back Again to Bedside: Clinical Trials

The above pre-clinical data were used to file investigational new drug applications with agencies in the US, Canada and Europe. Manufacturing of spores of NTCD-M3 under cGMP was undertaken successfully by ViroPharma, Inc. and the spores prepared in liquid suspension for safety testing in healthy volunteers at doses of $10^4$, $10^6$, and $10^8$ spores/dose or placebo (Villano et al., 2012). NTCD-M3 was found to be safe in younger volunteers age 18–45 years at all three single doses given in the absence of any antibiotic pre-treatment. To better simulate the likely age of patients with CDI, volunteers age >60 years (age range 60–73 years) were given single doses of $10^4$, $10^6$, and $10^8$ spores or placebo safely. Volunteers >60 years were then given the highest dose, $10^8$ spores twice daily for 5 days and tolerated this safely. This was the only group in which NTCD could be detected in the stools of the volunteers in the absence of prior antibiotic administration. Stool cultures first became positive on days 2–4 and were positive in 6 of 8 volunteers at day 7 but in none at day 14 and 21 suggesting the possibility that this may have been pass-through of NTCD spores and not colonization.

Finally, groups of 12 >60 year old volunteers were pre-treated with 5 days of oral vancomycin 125 mg 4 × daily to simulate patients being treated for CDI to determine if colonization with NTCD would occur post vancomycin treatment. Each group of 9 NTCD and 3 placebo subjects was given $10^4$ or $10^6$ or $10^8$ spores of NTCD-M3 or placebo daily for 14 days beginning the day following the last vancomycin dose. In each group the 9 volunteers given NTCD-M3 had NTCD detected in their stools during the 14-day administration and in 4 to 5 volunteers on days 21 and 28 following NTCD. In the 3 volunteers receiving placebo in the $10^4$ and $10^6$ NTCD-M3 spore cohorts one volunteer in each cohort became colonized with a toxigenic strain of *C. difficile* but remained asymptomatic. In the cohort receiving $10^8$ spores of NTCD-M3 the 3 placebo patients all became colonized with NTCD-M3, indicating that at this highest dose of NTCD-M3 there was transmission of NTCD-M3 from the active recipient group or the environment to the placebo group who were housed on the same clinical trial facility. No safety issues were identified in the volunteers receiving NTCD-M3.

For the first time since Seal et al. (1987) reported the treatment of 2 CDI patients with NTCD in 1987, NTCD was again administered in a Phase 2 double blind, randomized, dose-ranging, placebo controlled trial of NTCD for prevention of recurrent CDI in patients who have had their first episode or first recurrence of CDI. The primary outcome of the study was safety, with fecal colonization rate, CDI recurrence rate, and optimal dosing of NTCD-M3 as exploratory secondary outcomes. The study design shown in **Figure 8** compared 2 doses, $10^4$ and $10^7$ spores given orally in liquid once daily for 2 durations, 7 days ($10^7$ spores) and 14 days ($10^4$ and $10^7$ spores) compared to placebo for 14 days. NTCD-M3 was begun 1–2 days following completion of successful treatment of CDI with vancomycin or metronidazole (Gerding et al., 2015). A total of 168 patients were randomized and treated and 157 completed treatment. The four arms of the study were well balanced in terms of patient age (range 18–94 years) with 39% >65 years old. Most patients were having their primary CDI episode (83%), were outpatients (76%), and were treated with metronidazole (60%). Vancomycin was used for treatment in 20% of subjects and 20% were treated with both vancomycin and metronidazole.

Safety results indicated that participants who received NTCD-M3 had fewer treatment emergent adverse events and fewer serious adverse events than placebo patients with the exception of headache which occurred in 10% of NTCD-M3 recipients and 2% of placebo (Gerding et al., 2015). No serious adverse events were considered treatment related. Colonization by NTCD-M3 was defined as detection of NTCD-M3 in stool at any time following completion of treatment. **Figure 9** demonstrates that colonization with toxigenic *C. difficile* following antibiotic treatment of CDI is common (63% of placebo subjects at week 2) whereas with administration of NTCD-M3, much of the toxigenic *C. difficile* colonization was replaced by NTCD-M3; 71% of participants who received $10^7$ spores and 63% who received $10^4$ spores. Colonization with NTCD-M3 was maximal in weeks 1–3 and slowly declined thereafter until last detected in week 22. A small number of participants still harbored toxigenic *C. difficile* at 26 weeks, the last time stools were sampled.

Prevention of recurrence of CDI is summarized in **Table 1**. Using the protocol definition of recurrence of CDI at 6 weeks, recurrence rate was 13 (30%) of 43 placebo subjects and 14 (11%) of 125 NTCD-M3 subjects (odds ratio [OR], 0.28; 95%CI, 0.11–0.69; $P = 0.006$); the lowest recurrence was in 2 of 43 (5%) patients receiving $10^7$ spores/day for 7 days (OR, 0.1; 95%CI, 0.0–0.6; $P = 0.01$ vs. placebo). Using an alternate definition of recurrent CDI defined as use of antibacterial treatment for CDI, the recurrence rate was 14 of 43 (33%) placebo subjects and 17 of 125 (14%) NTCD-M3 subjects ($p = 0.009$). NTCD-M3 also reduced all-cause diarrhea from 77% in placebo subjects to 57% of NTCD-M3 subjects ($p = 0.020$). There was good correlation of CDI prevention with colonization by NTCD-M3; among subjects who received NTCD-M3 and became colonized, the CDI recurrence rate was 2 of 86 (2%) vs. 12 of 39 (31%) subjects who received NTCD-M3 and were not colonized ($p < 0.001$). Dose-ranging indicated that $10^7$ spores were more effective than $10^4$ spores, and there was no advantage to extending treatment to 14 days vs. 7 days for the $10^7$ dose. In summary, NTCD-M3 was safe and effective in preventing CDI in patients who were experiencing their first CDI episode or first recurrence of CDI.

## SUMMARY

NTCD has a long history of basic laboratory and clinical experience that suggests it is a safe and very effective preventive for recurrent CDI (hamster and human data) and as a preventive for first episode CDI if used in subjects receiving antibiotics (hamster data only). Further development is required with phase 3 clinical trials for recurrent CDI prevention and for phase 2 and 3 primary CDI prevention clinical trials.

## AUTHOR CONTRIBUTIONS

DG wrote the first manuscript draft and designed the experiments described from his laboratory and provided funding. SJ and SS edited the manuscript, contributed text and figures, and were instrumental in designing and carrying out the described experiments in the DG laboratory.

## FUNDING

This work has been supported by multiple Merit Review grants from the Department of Veterans Affairs Research Service.

## REFERENCES

Borriello, S. P., and Barclay, F. E. (1985). Protection of hamsters against *Clostridium difficile* ileocaecitis by prior colonization with non-pathogenic strains. *J. Med. Microbiol.* 19, 339–350. doi: 10.1099/00222615-19-3-339

Borriello, S. P., Welch, A. R., Barclay, F. E., and Davies, H. A. (1988). Mucosal association by *Clostridium difficile* in the hamster gastrointestinal tract. *J. Med. Microbiol.* 25, 191–196. doi: 10.1099/00222615-25-3-191

Brouwer, M. S., Mullany, P., Allan, E., and Roberts, A. P. (2016). Investigating transfer of large chromosomal regions containing the pathogenicity locus between clostridium difficile strains. *Methods Mol. Biol.* 1476, 215–222. doi: 10.1007/978-1-4939-6361-4_16

Brouwer, M. S., Roberts, A. P., Hussain, H., Williams, R. J., Allan, E., Mullany, P., et al. (2013). Horizontal gene transfer converts non-toxigenic Clostridium difficile strains into toxin producers. *Nat. Commun.*4:2601. doi: 10.1038/ncomms3601

Clabots, C. R., Johnson, S., Bettin, K. M., Mathie, P. A., Mulligan, M. E., Schaberg, D. S., et al. (1993). Development of a rapid and efficient endonuclease analysis typing system for *Clostridium difficile* and correlation with other typing systems. *J. Clin. Microbiol.* 31, 1870–1895.

Clabots, C. R., Johnson, S., Olson, M. M., Peterson, L. R., and Gerding, D. N. (1992). Acquisition of *Clostridium difficile* by hospitalized patients: evidence for colonized new admissions as a source of infection. *J. Infect. Dis.* 166, 561–567.

Corthier, G., and Muller, M. C. (1988). Emergence in gnotobiotic mice of nontoxinogenic clones of *Clostridium difficile* from a toxinogenic one. *Infect. Immunity* 56, 1500–1504.

Gerding, D. N., Meyer, T., Lee, C., Cohen, S. H., Murthy, U. K., Poirier, A., et al. (2015). Administration of spores of nontoxigenic *Clostridium difficile* strain M3 for prevention of recurrent *C. difficile* infection: a randomized clinical trial. *J. Am. Med. Assoc.* 313, 1719–1727. doi: 10.1001/jama.2015.3725

Gerding, D. N., Olson, M. M., Peterson, L. R., Teasley, D. G., Gebhard, R. L., Schwartz, M. L., et al. (1986). *Clostridium difficile* associateddiarrhea and colitis in adults. *Arch. Intern. Med.* 146, 95–100.

Johnson, S., Clabots, C. R., Linn, F. V., Olson, M. M., Peterson, L. R., and Gerding, D. N. (1990). Nosocomial *Clostridium difficile* colonization and disease. *Lancet* 336, 97-100.

Johnson, S., Samore, M. H., Farrow, K. A., Killgore, G. E., Tenover, F. C., Lyras, D.,et al. (1999). Epidemics of diarrhea caused by a clindamycin-resistant strain of *Clostridium difficile* in four hospitals. *N. Engl. J. Med.* 341, 1645–1651. doi: 10.1056/NEJM199911253412203

Kuijper, E. J., Oudbier, J. H., Stuifbergen, W. N. H. M., Jansz, A., and Zanen, H. C. (1987). Application of whole-cell DNA restriction endonuclease profiles to the epidemiology of *Clostridium difficile*-induced diarrhea. *J. Clin. Microbiol.* 25, 751–753.

Loo, V. G., Poirier, L., Miller, M. A., Oughton, M., Libman, M. D., Michaud, S., et al. (2005). A predominantly clonal multi-institutional outbreak of *Clostridium difficile*-associated diarrhea with high morbidity and mortality. *N. Engl. J. Med.* 353, 2442–2449. doi: 10.1056/NEJMoa051639

McDonald, L. C., Killgore, G. E., Thompson, A., Owens, R. C. Jr, Kazakova, S. V., Sambol, S. P., et al. (2005). Emergence of an epidemic, toxin gene variant strain of *Clostridium difficile* responsible for outbreaks in the United States between 2000 and 2004. *N. Engl. J. Med.* 353, 2433–2441. doi: 10.1056/NEJMoa051590

McFarland, L. V., Mulligan, M. E., Kwok, R. Y. Y., and Stamm, W. E. (1989). Nosocomial acquisition of *Clostridium difficile* infection. *N. Engl. J. Med.* 320, 204–210. doi: 10.1056/NEJM198901263200402

Merrigan, M. M., Sambol, S. P., Johnson, S., and Gerding, D. N. (2003). Prevention of fatal *Clostridium-difficile*-associated disease during continuous administration of clindamycin in hamsters. *J. Infect. Dis.* 188, 1922–1927. doi: 10.1086/379836

Merrigan, M. M., Sambol, S. P., Johnson, S., and Gerding, D. N. (2009). New approach to the management of *Clostridium difficile* Infection: colonization with Non-toxigenic *C. difficile* during daily ampicillin or ceftriaxone administration. *Int. J. Antimicrob. Agents* 33, S46–S50. doi: 10.1016/S0924-8579(09)70017-2

Merrigan, M. M., Venugopal, A. A., Roxas, J. L., Anwar, F., Mallozzi, M. J., Gerding, D. N., et al. (2013). Surface-layer protein A (SlpA) is a major contributor to host-cell adherence of the diarrheagenic pathogen *Clostridium difficile*. *PLoS ONE* 8:e78404. doi: 10.1371/journal.pone.0078404

Nagaro, K. J., Phillips, S. T., Cheknis, A. K., Sambol, S. P., Zukowski, W. E., Johnson, S., et al. (2013). Non-toxigenic *Clostridium difficile* protects hamsters against challenge with historic and epidemic toxigenic BI/NAP1/027 *C. difficile*. *Antimicrob. Agents Chemother.* 57, 5266–5270. doi: 10.1128/AAC.00580-13

Razaq, N., Sambol, S., Nagaro, K., Zukowski, W., Cheknis, A., Johnson, S., et al. (2007). Infection of hamsters with historic and epidemic "BI" Types of *Clostridium difficile*. *J. Infect. Dis.* 196, 1813–1819. doi: 10.1086/523106

Sambol, S. P., Merrigan, M. M., Johnson, S. J., and Gerding, D. N. (2004). "Susceptibility of hamsters to colonization by toxigenic or non-toxigenic *Clostridium difficile* (CD) following treatment with vancomycin or metronidazole," in *Anaerobe 2004 Meeting of the Anaerobe Society of the Americas* (Annapolis, MD).

Sambol, S. P., Merrigan, M. M., Tang, J. K., Johnson, S., and Gerding, D. N. (2002). Colonization for the prevention of *Clostridium difficile* disease in hamsters. *J. Infect. Dis.* 186, 1781–1789 doi: 10.1086/345676

Sambol, S. P., Tang, J. K., Merrigan, M. M., Johnson, S., and Gerding, D. N. (2001). Infection of hamsters with epidemiologically important strains of *Clostridium difficile*. *J. Infect. Dis.* 183, 1760–1766. doi: 10.1086/320736

Seal, D., Borriello, S. P., Barclay, F., Welch, A., Piper, M., and Bonnycastle, M. (1987). Treatment of relapsing *Clostridium difficile* diarrhoea by administration of a non-toxigenic strain. *Eur. J. Clin. Microbiol.* 6, 51–53. doi: 10.1007/BF02097191

Shim, J. K., Johnson, S., Samore, M. H., Bliss, D. Z., and Gerding, D. N. (1998). Primary symptomless colonization by *Clostridium difficile* and decreased risk of subsequent diarrhoea. *Lancet* 351, 633–636. doi: 10.1016/S0140-6736(97)08062-8

Swanson, R. N., Hardy, D. J., Shipkowitz, N. L., Hanson, C. W., Ramer, N. C., Fernandes, P. B., et al. (1991). *In vitro* and *in vivo* evaluation of tiacumicins B and C against *Clostridium difficile*. *Antimicrob. Agents Chemother.* 35, 1108–1111. doi: 10.1128/AAC.35.6.1108

Villano, S. A., Seiberling, M., Tatarowicz, W., Monnot-Chase, E., and Gerding, D. N. (2012). Evaluation of an oral suspension of VP20621, spores of nontoxigenic *Clostridium difficile* strain M3, in healthy subjects. *Antimicrob. Agents Chemother.* 56, 5224–5229. doi: 10.1128/AAC.00913-12

Wilson, K. H., and Sheagren, J. N. (1983). Antagonism of toxigenic *Clostridium difficile* by nontoxigenic C. difficile. *J. Infect. Dis.* 147, 733–736. doi: 10.1093/infdis/147.4.733

13

# Whole-Genome Sequencing of Clinically Isolated Carbapenem-Resistant Enterobacterales Harboring *mcr* Genes in Thailand, 2016–2019

***Wantana Paveenkittiporn[1], Watcharaporn Kamjumphol[1], Ratchadaporn Ungcharoen[2] and Anusak Kerdsin[2]****

*[1] National Institute of Health, Department of Medical Sciences, Ministry of Public Health, Nonthaburi, Thailand,*

*[2] Faculty of Public Health, Kasetsart University, Nakhon, Thailand*

***Correspondence:***
*Anusak Kerdsin*
*Anusak.ke@ku.th*

Mobile colistin-resistant genes (*mcr*) have become an increasing public health concern. Since the first report of *mcr-1* in Thailand in 2016, perspective surveillance was conducted to explore the genomic characteristics of clinical carbapenem-resistant Enterobacterales (CRE) isolates harboring *mcr* in 2016–2019. Thirteen (0.28%) out of 4,516 CRE isolates were found to carry *mcr* genes, including 69.2% (9/13) of *E. coli* and 30.8% (4/13) of *K. pneumoniae* isolates. Individual *mcr-1.1* was detected in eight *E. coli* (61.5%) isolates, whereas the co-occurrence of *mcr-1.1* and *mcr-3.5* was seen in only one *E. coli* isolate (7.7%). No CRE were detected carrying *mcr-2, mcr-4,* or *mcr-5* through to *mcr-9*. Analysis of plasmid replicon types carrying *mcr* revealed that IncX4 was the most common (61.5%; 8/13), followed by IncI2 (15.4%; 2/13). The minimum inhibitory concentration values for colistin were in the range of 4–16 μg/ml for all CRE isolates harboring *mcr*, suggesting they have 100% colistin resistance. Clermont phylotyping of nine *mcr*-harboring carbapenem-resistant *E. coli* isolates demonstrated phylogroup C was predominant in ST410. In contrast, ST336 belonged to CC17, and the KL type 25 was predominant in carbapenem-resistant *K. pneumoniae* isolates. This report provides a comprehensive insight into the prevalence of *mcr*-carrying CRE from patients in Thailand. The information highlights the importance of strengthening official active surveillance efforts to detect, control, and prevent *mcr*-harboring CRE and the need for rational drug use in all sectors.

**Keywords: *mcr*, carbapenem-resistant Enterobacterales, Thailand, colistin, genome**

## INTRODUCTION

The global spread of carbapenem-resistant Enterobacterales (CRE) has become a leading public health concern. The lack of accessible treatment has resulted in the use of colistin, an outmoded antibiotic, as a last-resort therapeutic drug for human infections by gram-negative bacteria. The widespread use of colistin in humans and animals has led to the emergence of colistin resistance in gram-negative bacteria, and the rates of resistance are continuously increasing

(Kempf et al., 2016; Elbediwi et al., 2019). In 2017, the World Health Organization acknowledged that CRE are a serious priority in a published list of globally important of 12 antimicrobial-resistant pathogens (World Health Organization, 2017). Of particular concern is the spread of *mcr* genes into CRE, which would create strains that are potentially pan-drug resistant (PDR).

A common mechanism of colistin resistance is thought to be associated with chromosomal mediation (Meletis and Skoura, 2018). The discovery of the first plasmid-mediated colistin resistance gene *mcr-1* in an *Escherichia coli* strain isolated from a pig in China led to an increasing number of reports on the identification of *mcr* in many bacterial species worldwide (Liu et al., 2016; Elbediwi et al., 2019). Thus far, 10 variants of *mcr* (*mcr-1* through to *mcr-10*) have been reported (Gharaibeh and Shatnawi, 2019; Wang et al., 2020). The *mcr* gene has been shown to encode a phosphoethanolamine transferase that alters lipid A in the lipopolysaccharide of the bacterial outer membrane by adding a phosphoethanolamine (Gharaibeh and Shatnawi, 2019). This reduces the attachment of colistin to the bacterial outer membrane and, therefore, prevents cell lysis.

The presence of *mcr* has been reported in different gram-negative bacteria isolated worldwide from animal and human sources (Elbediwi et al., 2019; Gharaibeh and Shatnawi, 2019). In Thailand, the first reported *mcr-1*-harboring *E. coli* were isolated from the stool of an asymptomatic person in 2012 (Olaitan et al., 2016). There has since been documentation of *mcr- 1-*, *mcr- 2-*, and *mcr-3*-carrying *E. coli* and *Klebsiella pneumoniae* strains isolated from patients (Paveenkittiporn et al., 2017; Srijan et al., 2018; Kamjumphol et al., 2019; Malchione et al., 2019). The current study investigated the genomic characterization of antimicrobial resistance genes and antimicrobial susceptibility of CRE isolated from patients in Thailand during a laboratory-based surveillance program in 2016–2019.

## MATERIALS AND METHODS

### Identification of CRE and Detection of Antimicrobial Resistance Genes

In total, 6,996 multidrug-resistant (MDR) bacterial isolates were collected from individuals during 2016–2019 from a hospital network in 24 provinces throughout Thailand (**Figure 1**). There were 666, 2,763, 2,618, and 949 MDR isolates surveyed in 2016–2019, respectively. Conventional biochemical tests described elsewhere were used for the species identification of Enterobacterales (Abbott, 2011). The presence of carbapenemase ($bla_{IMP}$, $bla_{KPC}$, $bla_{NDM}$, and $bla_{OXA-48-like}$) and *mcr-1* genes was determined using multiplex PCR (Hatrongjit et al., 2018). The *mcr* genes (*mcr-1* to *mcr-9*) were detected using PCR, as described elsewhere (Rebelo et al., 2018; Wang et al., 2018; Yang et al., 2018; Yuan et al., 2019). All *mcr*-positive isolates were subjected to whole-genome sequencing.

### Antimicrobial Susceptibility Testing

Analysis of the minimal inhibitory concentration (MIC) of antimicrobials for *mcr*-harboring CRE isolates was performed using the Epsilometer test (*E* test) and interpreted according to the 2020 Clinical and Laboratory Standards Institute guidelines (Clinical and Laboratory Standards Institute, 2020), and *E. coli* ATCC 25922 was used as the control. The *E* test was based on ampicillin, amoxicillin-clavulanate, ampicillin-sulbactam, piperacillin-tazobactam, cefazolin, cefepime, cefotaxime, cefoxitin, ertapenem, meropenem, imipenem, gentamicin, amikacin, ciprofloxacin, levofloxacin, trimethoprim, fosfomycin, nitrofurantoin, chloramphenicol, tetracycline, aztreonam, and azithromycin. Additionally, a modified carbapenem inactivation method (mCIM) was applied to all CRE isolates according to 2020 CLSI M100-S30.

Broth microdilution was used to determine the MIC of colistin using colistin sulfate (Merck, Germany) at 1, 2, 4, 8, 16, and 32 μg/ml, respectively. According to 2020 CLSI M100-S30, an MIC of $\leq 2$ μg/ml was interpreted as intermediate susceptibility, whereas an MIC of $\geq 4$ μg/ml was considered to indicate resistance.

### Whole-Genome Sequencing and Analysis

DNA from 13 *mcr*-carrying CRE isolates was extracted from nutrient agar plate cultures using a DNeasy blood & tissue kit (Qiagen, Hilden, Germany) following the manufacturer's recommendations, and the concentration was determined using the Qubit dsDNA BR assay kit (Invitrogen, Oregon, United States). Sequence libraries were prepared using a Qiagen QIAseq FX DNA library kit (Qiagen, Hilden, Germany) according to the manufacturer's protocol. The prepared libraries were sequenced on the Illumina Miseq platform with Illumina MiSeq 2X 250 base paired-end chemistry (Illumina, CA, United States) according to the manufacturer's instructions. The genomes for each strain were *de novo* assembled using CLC Genomics Workbench v12.0.2 (Qiagen, Aarhus, Denmark) with mostly default settings, except that the minimum contig size threshold was set to 500 bp.

Analysis of the whole-genome sequence data was performed as described elsewhere (Kerdsin et al., 2019). Briefly, the isolates were identified to species level using KmerFinder 3.1 (Larsen et al., 2014)[1]. Antimicrobial resistance genes were identified using ResFinder 4.1 (Zankari et al., 2012)[2] and the Comprehensive Antibiotic Resistance Database (CARD) (Alcock et al., 2020)[3]. We investigated chromosome-mediated colistin resistance by analyzing the *mgrB*, *phoPQ*, *pmrAB*, *crrB*, and *rpoN* genes. The gene sequences were analyzed using local BLAST + and Clustal W, including *K. pneumoniae* MGH78578 (GenBank accession number NC_009648.1) and *E. coli* K12 sub-strain MG1655 (GenBank accession number U00096) genomes as colistin-susceptible references.

Plasmid replicons were analyzed using PlasmidFinder (Carattoli et al., 2014)[4]. Phylogrouping for *E. coli* and

[1]https://cge.cbs.dtu.dk/services/KmerFinder/
[2]https://cge.cbs.dtu.dk/services/ResFinder/
[3]https://card.mcmaster.ca/
[4]https://cge.cbs.dtu.dk/services/PlasmidFinder/

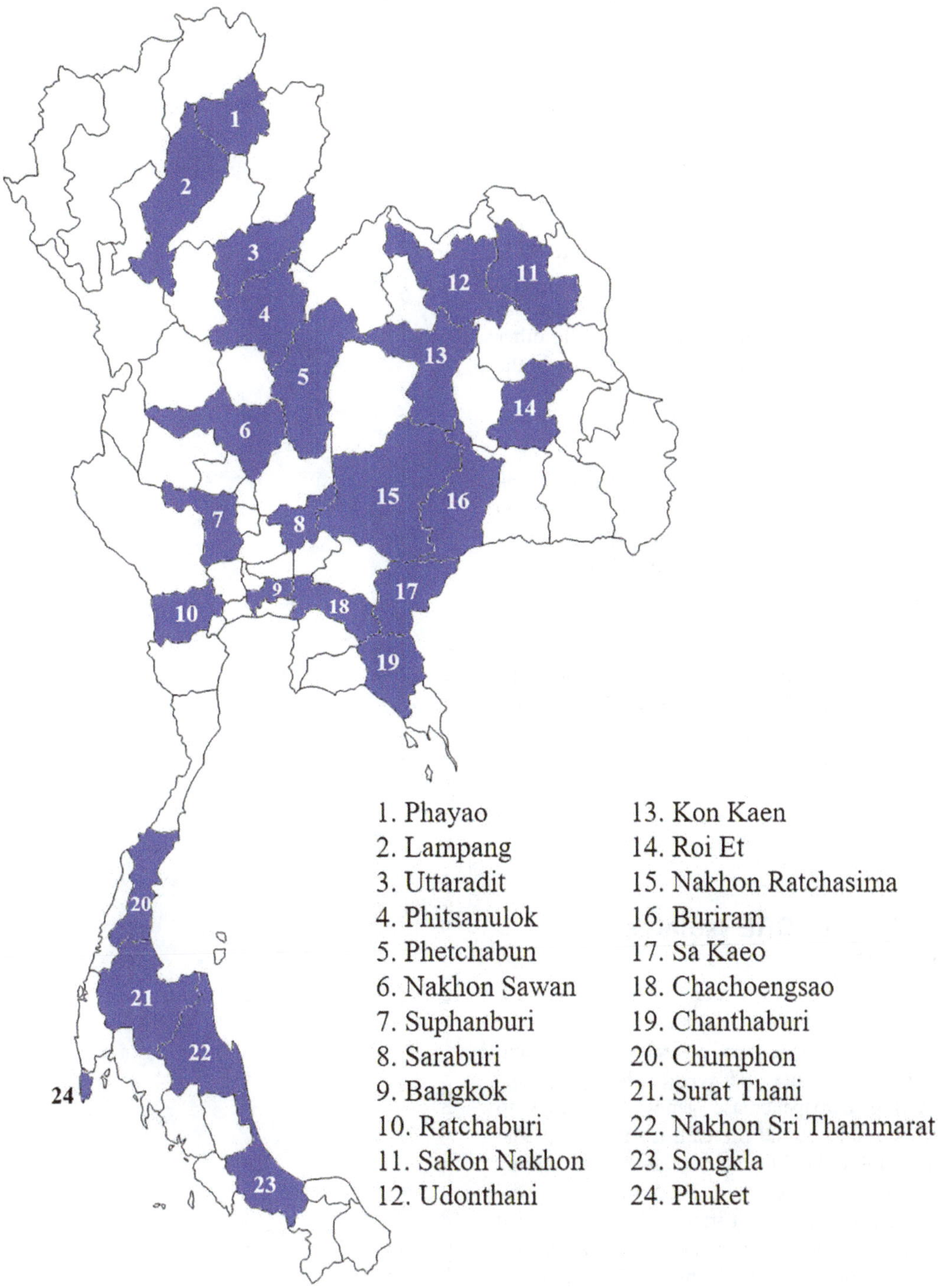


**FIGURE 1** | Location of hospital network in 24 provinces throughout Thailand.

the KL type of *K. pneumoniae* were based on analysis using ClermonTyping (Beghain et al., 2018)[5] and Kaptive (Wick et al., 2018)[6]. The virulence genes of *E. coli* and *K. pneumoniae* were analyzed using VirulenceFinder 2.0 (Joensen et al., 2014)[7] and Institut Pasteur[8], respectively.

For multilocus sequence typing (MLST) analysis of the sequence types (STs) of *E. coli* and *K. pneumoniae*, we used MLST

[5]http://clermontyping.iame-research.center/

[6]http://kaptive.holtlab.net

[7]https://cge.cbs.dtu.dk/services/VirulenceFinder/

[8]https://bigsdb.pasteur.fr/klebsiella/klebsiella.html

2.0 (Larsen et al., 2012)[9]. The genomic comparison of 13 *mcr*-harboring CRE isolates was conducted using a modular Single Genome Analysis to search for the genetically closest relatives in the database following the single nucleotide polymorphism (SNP) approach with BacWGSTdb (Feng et al., 2020)[10]. A phylogenetic tree was constructed using REALPHY and MEGA X via the neighbor-joining method with 500 bootstrap replicates by applying the Tamura three-parameter model (Bertels et al., 2014; Kumar et al., 2018). The tree was visualized and annotated using Interactive Tree of Life (ITOL) V4 (Letunic and Bork, 2016). *E. coli* K12 substrain MG1655 (accession no. U00096) and *K. pneumoniae* HS11286 (accession no. CP003200) were used as the reference sequences for SNP analysis. Details of the other genomes used for comparison with our isolates are shown in the **Supplementary Materials**.

## Statistical Analysis

The associations between *mcr* genes, *mcr*-harboring *E. coli* isolates, and non-*E. coli* isolates were analyzed by calculating the odds ratios (OR) and *p*-values using the STATA version 14 software package, with $p < 0.05$ considered to be statistically significant.

### Accession Number

The assembled genomic sequences were deposited under the BioProject accession number PRJNA525849 with BioSample accessions: SAMN15497997-SAMN15498009. The accession numbers for each *mcr-1*-harboring CRE isolate are provided in **Table 2**.

# RESULTS

## Genomic Analysis of CRE Isolates Harboring *mcr* Genes

Of the 6,996 MDR isolates, 4,516 were identified as CRE (64.5%). Of these, 4,235 (93.7%) isolates were classified as carbapenemase-producing Enterobacterales (CPE) and carried carbapenemase genes ($bla_{NDM}$, $bla_{OXA-48-like}$, $bla_{IMP}$, or coexisting carbapenemase genes) according to the mCIM and PCR results. Of all the CPE isolates, 13 (0.3%) carried *mcr* genes (**Table 1**). The *mcr*-carrying rates among carbapenemase-producing *E. coli* and *K. pneumoniae* were 1.03 and 0.12%, respectively. Statistical analysis revealed a strong association between *mcr* and carbapenemase-producing *E. coli*, with the OR being 11.06 (95% CI, 3.07–49.23) and statistically significant ($p < 0.0001$) (**Table 1**).

The proportions of *E. coli* and *K. pneumoniae* isolates showing *mcr* genes were 69.2% (9/13) and 30.8% (4/13), respectively. Individual *mcr-1.1* genes were detected in eight *E. coli* (61.5%) from 13 *mcr*-carrying CRE isolates, whereas the co-occurrence of *mcr-1.1* and *mcr-3.5* was found in only one *E. coli* isolate (7.7%) (**Table 2**). However, *mcr-2*, *mcr-4*, and *mcr-5* through to

[9]https://cge.cbs.dtu.dk/services/MLST/

[10]http://bacdb.org/BacWGSTdb/

**TABLE 1** | Distribution of *mcr* and carbapenemase genes in carbapenemase-producing Enterobacterales (CPE) during 2016–2019.

| Species | Total | $bla_{NDM}$ | $bla_{OXA-48-like}$ | $bla_{IMP}$ | $bla_{NDM}$ + $bla_{OXA-48-like}$ | $bla_{IMP}$ + $bla_{NDM}$ | $bla_{IMP}$ + $bla_{OXA-48-like}$ | $bla_{NDM}$ + *mcr* | $bla_{OXA-48-like}$ + *mcr* | *mcr*-carrying rate | *p*-value | Odd ratio (95% CI) |
|---|---|---|---|---|---|---|---|---|---|---|---|---|
| *Escherichia coli* | 868 | 695 | 54 | 1 | 108 | 1 | | 8 | 1 | 1.03% | <0.0001 | 11.06 (3.07–49.23) |
| *Escherichia* sp. | 2 | 1 | 1 | | | | | | | | | |
| *Klebsiella pneumoniae* | 3129 | 1206 | 1341 | 46 | 529 | 1 | 2 | 3 | 1 | 0.12% | | |
| *Klebsiella aerogenes* | 11 | 5 | 6 | | | | | | | | | |
| *Klebsiella oxytoca* | 3 | 3 | | | | | | | | | | |
| *Enterobacter cloacae* | 189 | 108 | 24 | 37 | 12 | 3 | 5 | | | | | |
| *Enterobacter* sp. | 1 | 1 | | | | | | | | | | |
| *Citrobacter freundii* | 10 | 9 | | | 1 | | | | | | | |
| *Citrobacter* sp. | 1 | 1 | | | | | | | | | | |
| *Morganella morganii* | 1 | 1 | | | | | | | | | | |
| *Pantoea agglomerans* | 4 | 3 | | | 1 | | | | | | | |
| *Proteus mirabilis* | 7 | 5 | | 1 | 1 | | | | | | | |
| *Proteus vulgaris* | 2 | 2 | | | | | | | | | | |
| *Providencia* sp. | 3 | 1 | 1 | | 1 | | | | | | | |
| *Salmonella enterica* | 4 | 2 | | 2 | | | | | | | | |
| | 4235 | 2043 | 1427 | 87 | 653 | 5 | 7 | 11 | 2 | 0.31% | | |

**TABLE 2** | Distribution of sequence types and antimicrobial resistant genes in carbapenem-resistant *E. coli* and *K. pneumoniae* carrying *mcr* genes.

| Strain no. | Genome accession | Species | Isolation year | Sex | Age | Isolation source | Province/Region in Thailand | CC | ST | Clermont phylogroup | KL type | Virulence genes | Plasmid replicon types | Plasmid carrying-*mcr* | *mcr* |
|---|---|---|---|---|---|---|---|---|---|---|---|---|---|---|---|
| 53037 | JACGZL000000000 | *E. coli* | 2016 | F | 74 | Urine | Bangkok/ Central | 23 | 410 | C | | *fyuA, gad, hlyF, iroN, irp2, iss, iucC, iutA, lpfA, neuC, ompT, sitA, terC, traT* | IncFIB, IncFII, IncN2, IncX1, IncX4, IncY | IncX4 | 1.1 |
| 53360 | JACGZM000000000 | *E. coli* | 2016 | M | 63 | Urine | Phetchabul/ North | 23 | 410 | C | | *hra, lpfA, papA, terC, traT* | Col, IncC, IncFIA, IncFIB, IncFII, IncQ1, IncX1, IncX4 | IncX4 | 1.1 |
| 56511 | JACGZN000000000 | *E. coli* | 2017 | M | 68 | Urine | Saraburi/ Central | 23 | 410 | C | | *gad, lpfA, terC* | Col, Col440I, IncFIA, IncFIB, IncFII, IncX4, IncY | IncX4 | 1.1 |
| 58967 | JACGZO000000000 | *E. coli* | 2018 | M | 67 | Sputum | Phitsanulok/ North | 23 | 410 | C | | *fyuA, irp2, lpfA, terC* | Col, IncC, IncFIA, IncFIB, IncFII, IncQ1, IncX4 | IncX4 | 1.1 |
| 62122 | JACGZP000000000 | *E. coli* | 2018 | M | 41 | Urine | Buriram/ Northeast | 23 | 410 | C | | *fyuA, hra, irp2, lpfA, terC* | Col, IncC, IncFIA, IncFIB, IncFII, IncQ1, IncX4, IncY | IncX4 | 1.1 |
| 54881 | JACGZQ000000000 | *E. coli* | 2017 | F | 55 | Rectal swab | Nan/ North | 38 | 3052 | D | | *air, chuA, eilA, iss, kpsE, ompT, papA, terC, traT* | Col, IncFII, IncI2, IncN2 | IncI2 | 1.1 |
| 54882 | JACGZR000000000 | *E. coli* | 2017 | F | 50 | Rectal swab | Nan/ North | 38 | 3052 | D | | *air, chuA, eilA, iss, kpsE, ompT, papA, terC, traT* | Col, IncFII, IncI2, IncN2 | IncI2 | 1.1 |
| 60000 | JACGZS000000000 | *E. coli* | 2018 | F | 66 | Rectal swab | Nan/ North | 10 | 10 | A | | *gad, mcbA, terC, traT* | IncFIB, IncL, IncX1, IncX4, p0111, IncB/O/K/Z | IncX4 | 1.1 |
| 54715 | JACGZT000000000 | *E. coli* | 2017 | M | 54 | Sputum | Bangkok/ Central | 10 | 1287 | A | | *cia, fyuA, gad, irp2, iss, iucC, iutA, sitA, terC, traT* | IncFIA, IncFIB, IncFII, IncI1-I, IncI2 | Unknown | 1.1+3.5 |
| 59990 | JACXSU000000000 | *K. pneumoniae* | 2018 | F | 69 | Sputum | Phuket/ South | 17 | 336 | | K25 | *fyuA, irp1, irp2, mrk locus, ybt locus* | ColRNAI, IncFIB, IncFII, IncN2, IncR, IncX4 | IncX4 | 1.1 |
| 61843 | JACGZU000000000 | *K. pneumoniae* | 2018 | F | 76 | Urine | Phuket/ South | 17 | 336 | | K25 | *fyuA, irp1, irp2, mrk locus, ybt locus* | ColRNAI, IncFIB, IncFII, IncI2, IncN2 | Unknown | 1.1 |
| 2514-18 | JADCQU000000000 | *K. pneumoniae* | 2018 | F | 61 | Urine | Phuket/ South | 17 | 336 | | K25 | *fyuA, irp1, irp2, mrk locus, ybt locus* | ColRNAI, IncFIB, IncFII, IncI2, IncN2 | Unknown | 1.1 |
| 60220 | JACGZV000000000 | *K. pneumoniae* | 2018 | M | 71 | Ascitic fluid | Khon Kaen/ Northeast | 258 | 340 | | K15 | *fyuA, irp1, irp2, mrk locus, ybt locus* | Col440I, ColKP3, IncFIB, IncFII, IncR, IncX3, IncX4 | IncX4 | 1.1 |

| Strain no. | *mgrB* mutation | *pmrA* mutation | *pmrB* mutation | *phoP* mutation | *phoQ* mutation | *crrB* mutation | *rpoN* mutation | $bla_{NDM}$ | $bla_{OXA-48-like}$ | $bla_{CTX-M}$ | $bla_{CMY}$ | $bla_{TEM}$ | $bla_{OXA-1}$ | $bla_{SHV}$ | *aac(6')-Ib-cr* | *aac(3)-IId* | *aadA* |
|---|---|---|---|---|---|---|---|---|---|---|---|---|---|---|---|---|---|
| 53037 | | S29G, G144S | D283G, Y358N | | | | E150D, I165M | 1 | | 55 | | 1B | | | | | |
| 53360 | | S29G, G144S | D283G, Y358N | | | | E150D, I165M | 1 | | 15 | 2 | 1B | | | | | 5 |
| 56511 | | S29G, G144S | D283G, Y358N | | | | E150D, I165M | 5 | | 15 | 2 | 1B | | | | | 2,5 |
| 58967 | | S29G, G144S | D283G, Y358N | | | | E150D, I165M | 5 | | 15 | 2 | 1B | | | | | 2,5 |
| 62122 | | S29G, G144S | D283G, Y358N | | | | E150D, I165M | 5 | | 15 | 2 | 1B | | | | | 2,5 |
| 54881 | | S29G | H2R, D283G | I44L | | | E150D, I165M | 1 | | 15 | | 1C | | | | | 16 |
| 54882 | | S29G | H2R, D283G | I44L | | | E150D, I165M | 1 | | 15 | | 1C | | | | | 16 |
| 60000 | | S29G | | | | | R217G | 1 | | 3 | | 1B | | 12 | | | 2,5 |
| 54715 | | S29G | | | L343V | | | | 48 | | | | | | | | 1,2b |
| 59990 | | E57G | T246A | | | L296Q | F304Y | 1 | | | | | | 12 | | | |
| 61843 | | E57G | T246A | | | L296Q | F304Y | 1 | | | | | | 11 | | | |
| 2514-18 | | E57G | T246A | | | L296Q | F304Y | 1 | | | | | | 11 | | | |
| 60220 | | | T246A, R256G | | | L296Q | | | 181 | 15 | | 1B | | 182 | | | 2 |

| Strain no. | *aac(3)-VIa* | *aph(3')-Ia* | *aph(3'')-Ib* | *aph(3')-VI* | *aph(6)-Id* | *mdf(A)* | *mph(A)* | *mef(B)* | *erm(42)* | *lnu(F)* | *catB3* | *floR* | *cmlA1* | *oqxA,B* | *qnrB6* | *qnrS1* | *ARR-3* | *sul* | *tet* | *dfrA* | *fosA* |
|---|---|---|---|---|---|---|---|---|---|---|---|---|---|---|---|---|---|---|---|---|---|
| 53037 | | | | | | | | | | | | | | | | | | 2 | A | | |
| 53360 | | | | | | | | | | | | | | | | | | 1,2 | B | 17 | |
| 56511 | | | | | | | | | | | | | | | | | | 1 | B | 12,17 | |
| 58967 | | | | | | | | | | | | | | | | | | 1,2 | B | 12,17 | |
| 62122 | | | | | | | | | | | | | | | | | | 1,2 | B,X4 | 12,17 | |
| 54881 | | | | | | | | | | | | | | | | | | 1,2 | A,B | 27 | |
| 54882 | | | | | | | | | | | | | | | | | | 1,2 | A,B | 27 | |
| 60000 | | | | | | | | | | | | | | | | | | 1,2 | A,X4 | 17 | |
| 54715 | | | | | | | | | | | | | | | | | | 3 | A | 12 | |
| 59990 | | | | | | | | | | | | | | | | | | | D | | |
| 61843 | | | | | | | | | | | | | | | | | | | A,D | 12 | |
| 2514-18 | | | | | | | | | | | | | | | | | | | A,D | 12 | |
| 60220 | | | | | | | | | | | | | | | | | | 1 | D | 12,14 | |

*mcr-9* were not detected. Analysis of the plasmid replicon types carrying *mcr* revealed that IncX4 was the most common (61.5%; 8/13), followed by IncI2 (15.4%; 2/13), as shown in **Table 2**. However, three isolates were unidentified. Six carbapenem-resistant *E. coli* isolates harboring *mcr* carried IncX4, whereas two isolates contained IncI2. Of the four carbapenem-resistant *K. pneumoniae* isolates harboring *mcr*, two carried IncX4 and the other two had unknown plasmid replicon types. The genetic organization of the *mcr* genes in these 13 isolates is outlined in **Figure 2**. A common gene found downstream of *mcr-1.1* in all isolates encoded the PAP2 family protein, whereas the upstream genes varied. However, a DUF2726-domain-containing protein-encoding gene was commonly found in 8 of the 13 isolates (seven *E. coli* and one *K. pneumoniae*). Furthermore, the upstream and downstream genetic organization of *mcr-3.5* was quite different from that of *mcr-1.1*.

As shown in **Table 2**, chromosomal-mediated colistin resistance gene mutations, including those in *mgrB*, *pmrAB*, *phoPQ*, *crrB*, and *rpoN*, were analyzed. We detected substitutions in *pmrAB* and *rpoN* in almost *mcr*-harboring CRE isolates, whereas *phoPQ* substitutions were found in three isolates, and no mutations were detected in *mgrB*. Substitutions were commonly found in the *pmrA* genes of 12 out of 13 *mcr*-harboring isolates, while *pmrB* and *rpoN* substitutions were detected in 11 isolates. The isolates 54881 and 54882 contained more mutations in the chromosomal-mediated colistin resistance genes than other isolates. Substitution at S29G and E57G in *pmrA* was predominant in *E. coli* and *K. pneumoniae*, respectively. The *pmrB* substitution at D283G was commonly found in *E. coli*, whilst all four *mcr-1*-harboring *K. pneumoniae* contained a T246A substitution. Only one substitution in *phoP* (I44L) and one in *phoQ* (L343V) were detected in *mcr-1*-carrying *E. coli*. Substitution at E150D and I165M in *rpoN* was predominant in *E. coli* isolates, in contrast to those at F304Y which was commonly found in *K. pneumoniae* isolates. In addition, one *crrB* substitution (L296Q) was found in all *K. pneumoniae* isolates. Insertion or deletion in those described genes was not detected in all *mcr-1*-harboring CRE isolates.

As shown in **Table 2**, of the 13 isolates, five and three *mcr*-harboring *E. coli* isolates carried $bla_{NDM-1}$ and $bla_{NDM-5}$, respectively. Only one *E. coli* isolate contained $bla_{OXA-48}$. Three and one *mcr-1.1*-harboring *K. pneumoniae* isolates carried $bla_{NDM-1}$ and $bla_{OXA-181}$, respectively. Among the β-lactamase genes, $bla_{CTX-M}$, $bla_{SHV}$, or $bla_{TEM}$ were detected in almost all isolates (92.3%, 12/13), and only one *E. coli* isolate had no β-lactamase genes. The predominant $bla_{CTX-M}$ was $bla_{CTX-M-15}$, which was detected in 53.8% (7/13) of all isolates. The gene $bla_{SHV}$ was found in all *K. pneumoniae* and one isolate of *E. coli* (**Table 2**). Among the ampC β-lactamase genes, $bla_{CMY-2}$ only was detected in four *E. coli* isolates (28.6%). The other antimicrobial resistance genes in the *mcr*-carrying CRE isolates, including those for fluoroquinolones, aminoglycosides, rifampicin, macrolides, chloramphenicol, sulfonamide, tetracycline, fosfomycin, and trimethoprim, are shown in **Table 2**.

## Antimicrobial Susceptibility of CRE Isolates Harboring *mcr* Genes

As shown in **Table 3**, the colistin MIC values for the *mcr*-harboring isolates were in the range of 4–16 μg/ml. According to the 2020 CLSI M100-S30 guidelines, a microbe with a colistin MIC value of $\geq$4 μg/ml is resistant, whereas MIC $\leq$ 2 μg/ml indicates intermediate resistance. Thus, the results indicate that 100% of the *mcr*-carrying CRE isolated from patients were resistant to colistin. The highest MIC value for colistin (16 μg/ml) was found in two carbapenem-resistant *K. pneumoniae* isolates. Most of the *mcr*-harboring *E. coli* had colistin MIC values of 4 μg/ml (8/9; 88.8%).

More than 50% of the *mcr*-harboring CRE isolates were susceptible to amikacin (11/13), fosfomycin (12/13), and nitrofurantoin (7/13). Of the 13 CRE-harboring *mcr* isolates, four *E. coli* isolates and one *K. pneumoniae* isolate were extensively drug-resistant (XDR; 38.5%). Details of the antimicrobial resistance profiles of the 13 isolates are provided in **Table 3**. Moreover, 12 of the 13 *mcr*-harboring CRE isolates were resistant to ciprofloxacin. As shown in **Table 2**, ciprofloxacin resistance may result from the presence of quinolone resistance genes: *oqxA*, *oqxB*, *qnrS1*, *qnrB6*, and *aac(6′)-Ib-cr*.

## Molecular Typing of *mcr*-Harboring CRE Isolates

As summarized in **Table 2**, Clermont phylotyping of nine *mcr*-harboring carbapenem-resistant *E. coli* isolates demonstrated that phylogroup C (5/9; 55.6%) was predominant, followed by phylogroups A (2/9; 22.2%) and D (2/9; 22.2%). The Clermont phylogroup was concordant with clonal complexes (CC). Phylogroup C was concordant with CC23, which contained only ST410. Phylogroup D was concordant with CC38, which consisted of ST3052, whereas phylogroup A was concordant with CC10, which contained either ST10 or ST1287. Four carbapenem-resistant *K. pneumoniae* isolates harboring *mcr* were predominantly ST336 (3/4; 75%) and one was ST340 (1/4; 25%). ST336 belonged to CC17 and KL type 25, whereas ST340 belonged to CC258 and KL type 15.

The genetic relationships based on the SNPs of these *mcr*-harboring isolates are demonstrated in **Figures 3**, **4**. Five *E. coli* ST410 isolates were widely distributed in several sub-clusters of the ST410 cluster. Strain no. 53360 was closely related to the strain AMA1167 from Denmark, whereas strain no. 56511 clustered with strains from Norway, India, Lebanon, China, and Denmark (**Figure 3**). Strains no. 58967 and no. 62122 were related to strain KBN10P04869 from South Korea. Strain no. 53037 clustered with strains from Norway, the United States, Brazil, and Germany. Two ST3052 isolates (nos. 54881 and 54882) were closely related to the strain WCHEC020028 from China; they had similar characteristics and were from different individuals in the same hospital ward, indicating that they were likely to have originated from the same source. Strain no. 54715 (ST1287) was related to a strain from the United States (ST617), and these were clustered together with strain no. 6000 (ST10) (**Figure 3**).

**TABLE 3 |** Antimicrobial susceptibility of *mcr*-harboring carbapenem-resistant *E. coli* and *K. pneumoniae*.

| No. | | 1 | 2 | 3 | 4 | 5 | 6 | 7 | 8 | 9 | 10 | 11 | 12 | 13 |
|---|---|---|---|---|---|---|---|---|---|---|---|---|---|---|
| Isolate No. | | 53360 | 54881 | 54882 | 56511 | 58967 | 62122 | 60000 | 54715 | 53037 | 59990 | 60220 | 61843 | 2514-18 |
| Organism | | *E. coli* | *E. coli* | *E. coli* | *E. coli* | *E. coli* | *E. coli* | *E. coli* | *E. coli* | *E. coli* | *K. pneumoniae* | *K. pneumoniae* | *K. pneumoniae* | *K. pneumoniae* |
| Classification | | XDR | XDR | MDR | MDR | MDR | XDR | XDR | MDR | MDR | MDR | XDR | MDR | MDR |
| Penicillin | AMP (μg/ml) | >256 (R) | >256 (R) | >256 (R) | >256 (R) | >256 (R) | >256 (R) | >256 (R) | >256 (R) | >256 (R) | >256 (R) | >256 (R) | >256 (R) | >256 (R) |
| β-lactam combination | AMC (μg/ml) | >256 (R) | >256 (R) | >256 (R) | >256 (R) | >256 (R) | >256 (R) | >256 (R) | >256 (R) | >256 (R) | >256 (R) | >256 (R) | >256 (R) | >256 (R) |
| | SAM (μg/ml) | >256 (R) | >256 (R) | >256 (R) | >256 (R) | >256 (R) | >256 (R) | > 256 (R) | > 256 (R) | > 256 (R) | > 256 (R) | > 256 (R) | > 256 (R) | > 256 (R) |
| | TZP (μg/ml) | > 256 (R) | >256 (R) | > 256 (R) | >256 (R) | > 256 (R) | >256 (R) | > 256 (R) | 64 (I) | > 256 (R) | >256 (R) | > 256 (R) | >256 (R) | > 256 (R) |
| 13rd generation Cephalosporins | KZ (μg/ml) | >256 (R) | >256 (R) | >256 (R) | >256 (R) | >256 (R) | >256 (R) | >256 (R) | 32 (R) | >256 (R) | >256 (R) | >256 (R) | >256 (R) | >256 (R) |
| | FEP (μg/ml) | >256 (R) | >256 (R) | >256 (R) | >256 (R) | >256 (R) | >256 (R) | >256 (R) | 0125 (S) | >256 (R) | >256 (R) | >256 (R) | 96 (R) | 96 (R) |
| | CTX (μg/ml) | >32 (R) | >32 (R) | >32 (R) | >32 (R) | >32 (R) | >32 (R) | >32 (R) | 0.25 (S) | >32 (R) | >32 (R) | >32 (R) | >32 (R) | >32 (R) |
| | FOX (μg/ml) | >256 (R) | >256 (R) | >256 (R) | >256 (R) | >256 (R) | >256 (R) | >256 (R) | 8 (S) | >256 (R) | >256 (R) | >256 (R) | >256 (R) | >256 (R) |
| Carbapenems | ERT (μg/ml) | >32 (R) | >32 (R) | >32 (R) | >32 (R) | >32 (R) | >32 (R) | >32 (R) | 0.75 (I) | 32 (R) | >32 (R) | >4(R) | >32 (R) | >32 (R) |
| | MER (μg/ml) | >32 (R) | >32 (R) | >32 (R) | 12(R) | 12 (R) | 8 (R) | >32 (R) | 0.5 (S) | 8 (R) | >32 (R) | >8(R) | >32 (R) | >32 (R) |
| | IMP (μg/ml) | >32 (R) | >32 (R) | >32 (R) | 1.5 (I) | 8 (R) | 8 (R) | >32 (R) | 0.25 (S) | 4 (R) | 32 (R) | >8 (R) | >32 (R) | >32 (R) |
| Aminoglycoside | CN (μg/ml) | 64 (R) | 32 (R) | 0.38 (S) | 0.75 (S) | 32 (R) | 16 (R) | >256 (R) | 24 (R) | 0.75 (S) | 0.5 (S) | 0.75 (S) | 0.75 (S) | 0.75 (S) |
| | AK (μg/ml) | 32 (I) | 4 (S) | 4 (S) | 8 (S) | 6 (S) | 3 (S) | 3 (S) | 2 (S) | 3 (S) | 2 (S) | 32 (I) | 4 (S) | 6 (S) |
| Quinolone | CIP (μg/ml) | >32 (R) | >32 (R) | 3 (R) | >32 (R) | >32 (R) | >32 (R) | >32 (R) | >32 (R) | >32 (R) | 0.094 (S) | >32 (R) | 1.5 (R) | 1 (R) |
| | LEV (μg/ml) | >32 (R) | >32 (R) | 0.75 (S) | >32 (R) | >32 (R) | >32 (R) | >32 (R) | >32 (R) | >32 (R) | 0.125 (S) | >32 (R) | 0.5 (S) | 0.25 (S) |
| Folate | SXT (μg/ml) | >32 (R) | >32 (R) | >32 (R) | >32 (R) | >32 (R) | >32 (R) | >32 (R) | >32 (R) | 0.38 (S) | 0.38 (S) | >32 (R) | 4 (R) | >32 (R) |
| Fosfomycin | FOT (μg/ml) | 0.75 (S) | 6 (S) | 0.75 (S) | 0.75 (S) | 1 (S) | 1.5 (S) | 0.75 (S) | 0.5 (S) | 0.38 (S) | 24 (S) | 64 (S) | 96 (S) | >256 (R) |
| Nitrofuran | N (μg/ml) | 32 (S) | 16 (S) | 16 (S) | 24 (S) | 48 (S) | 64 (I) | 64 (I) | 32 (S) | 16 (S) | 128 (R) | >512 (R) | 96 (R) | >256 (R) |
| Phenicol | C (μg/ml) | 24 (I) | >256 (R) | 16 (I) | 12 (S) | 24 (I) | 64 (R) | >256 (R) | 128 (R) | 6 (S) | 32 (R) | 96 (R) | 8 (S) | 3 (S) |
| Tetracycline | TE (μg/ml) | >256 (R) | >256 (R) | >256 (R) | >256 (R) | >256 (R) | >256 (R) | 96 (R) | 48 (R) | 64 (R) | >256 (R) | >256 (R) | >256 (R) | >256 (R) |
| Monobactam | ATM (μg/ml) | >256 (R) | >256 (R) | >256 (R) | >256 (R) | >256 (R) | >256 (R) | >256 (R) | 0.047 (S) | 48 (R) | 96 (R) | >256 (R) | 0.064 (S) | 0.125 (S) |
| Macrolide | AZM (μg/ml) | 32 (R) | >256 (R) | >256 (R) | 32 (R) | >256 (R) | >256 (R) | >256 (R) | 32 (R) | >256 (R) | >256 (R) | >256 (R) | >256 (R) | 32 (R) |
| Colistin | COL (μg/ml) | 4 (R) | 4 (R) | 4 (R) | 4 (R) | 4 (R) | 4 (R) | 8 (R) | 4 (R) | 8 (R) | 8 (R) | 8 (R) | 16 (R) | 16 (R) |

*AMP, ampicillin; AMC, amoxicillin/clavulanic acid; SAM, ampicillin-sulbactam; TZP, piperacillin-tazobactam; KZ, Cefazolin; FEP, cefepime; CTX, cefotaxime; FOX, Cefoxitin; ERT, ertapenem; MER, meropenem; IMP, imipenem; CN, gentamicin; AK, amikacin; CIP, ciprofloxacin; LEV, levofloxacin; SXT, trimethoprim; FOT, Fosfomycin; N, nitrofurantoin; C, chloramphenicol; TE, tetracycline; ATM, aztreonam; AZM, azithromycin; COL colistin.*

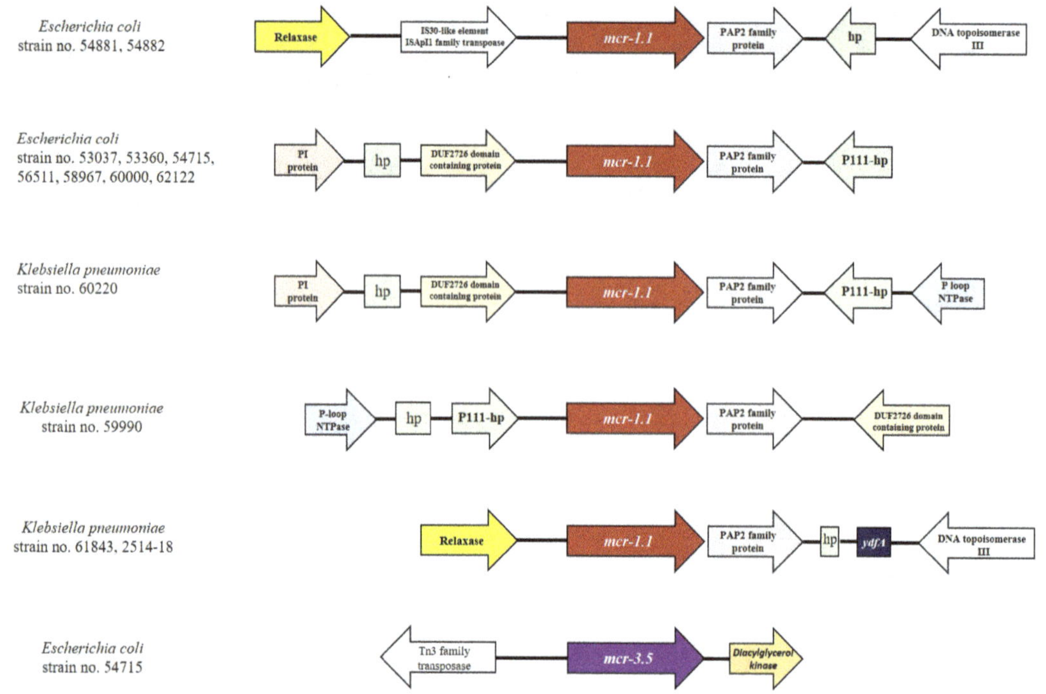


**FIGURE 2 |** Comparison of the genetic organization of the *mcr* genes in 13 CRE isolates. The schematic shows the genes flanking the *mcr* genes in the isolates.

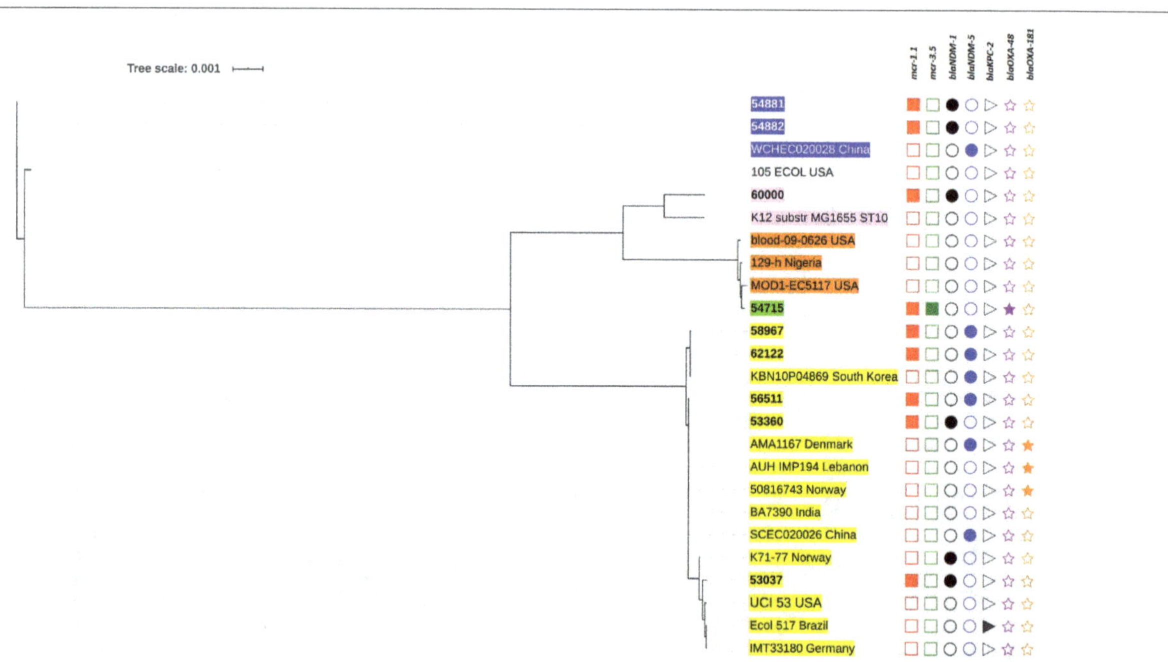


**FIGURE 3 |** Phylogenetic tree based on single nucleotide polymorphisms (SNP) in *E. coli* using the neighbor-joining method. The tree was visualized and annotated using Interactive Tree of Life (iToL). The tree is annotated based on sequence types (STs; color highlight), *mcr* (square), $bla_{NDM}$ (circle), $bla_{KPC}$ (right triangle), and $bla_{OXA-48-like}$ (star). Presentation of the genes is shown by filled symbols. STs 410, 1287, 617, 10, and 3052 are highlighted in yellow, green, brown, pink, and blue, respectively. The isolates used in this study are shown in bold.

Among the *K. pneumoniae* isolates, the ST336 isolates were closely related and clustered with other ST336 strains isolated in Thailand (**Figure 4**). Interestingly, the Thai-ST336 isolates were in a different cluster from that containing the ST336 isolates from other countries. Similarly, isolate no. 60220 (ST340) in this study was

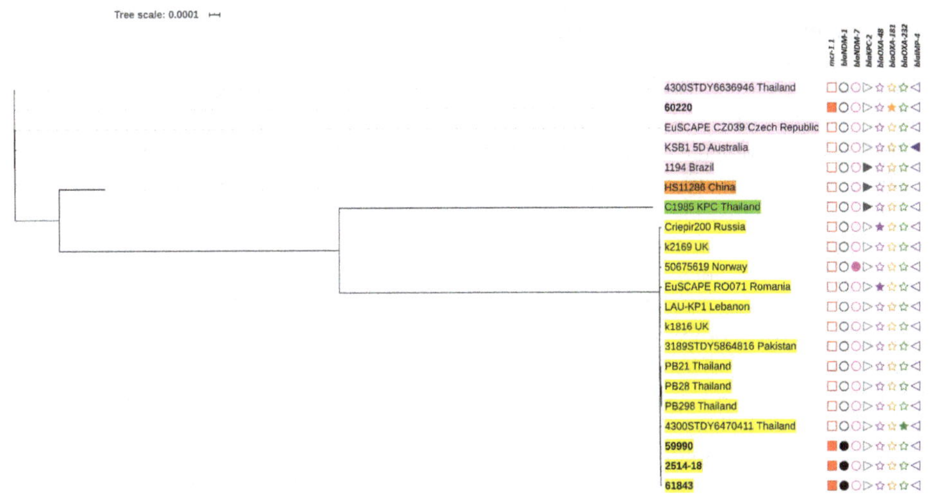

FIGURE 4 | Phylogenetic tree based on single nucleotide polymorphisms (SNP) in *K. pneumoniae* using the neighbor-joining method. The tree was visualized and annotated using Interactive Tree of Life (iToL). The tree is annotated based on sequence types (STs; color highlight), *mcr* (square), $bla_{NDM}$ (circle), $bla_{KPC}$ (right triangle), $bla_{OXA-48-like}$ (star), and $bla_{IMP}$ (left triangle). Presentation of the genes is revealed by filled symbols. STs 336, 340, 11, and 4008 are highlighted in yellow, pink, and brown, and green, respectively. The isolates used in this study are shown in bold.

closely related to strain 4300STDY6636946 circulating in Thailand (**Figure 4**).

## DISCUSSION

The discovery that plasmid-mediated colistin resistance is encoded by *mcr* genes and the high prevalence of human isolates harboring these genes are of global concern. A recent report revealed the overall average prevalence of *mcr* genes to be 4.7% (0.1–9.3%) in 47 countries across six continents (Elbediwi et al., 2019), and as many as 10 *mcr* genes (*mcr-1* through to *mcr-10)* have been reported (Gharaibeh and Shatnawi, 2019; Wang et al., 2020). A study of the global prevalence of *mcr* genes revealed that *mcr-1* (4917/5191; 94.7%) is a common gene and has a wider distribution compared with *mcr*-2 through to *mcr-8* (Elbediwi et al., 2019). Human infections with both CRE and non-CRE isolates carrying *mcr-1* have been widely reported (Liu et al., 2016; Mediavilla et al., 2016; Paveenkittiporn et al., 2017; Quan et al., 2017; Mendes et al., 2018; Srijan et al., 2018; Zhong et al., 2018; Elbediwi et al., 2019).

The coexistence of *mcr* and carbapenemase genes, such as $bla_{NDM}$, $bla_{OXA-48-like}$, and $bla_{IMP}$, in CRE isolates has been described in countries worldwide (Mediavilla et al., 2016; Arabaci et al., 2019; Huang et al., 2020; Kananizadeh et al., 2020). The current study found the predominant *mcr* gene to be *mcr-1*, which more frequently coexists with $bla_{NDM}$ than $bla_{OXA48-like}$, highlighting the potential dissemination of *mcr-1* and $bla_{NDM}$ among CRE isolates in Thailand. This concurs with a study in China (Huang et al., 2020), where *mcr-1* and $bla_{NDM-5}$ were predominant (78.6%, 11/14). In this study, *mcr-1* and $bla_{NDM-1}$ were the most prevalent resistance genes (61.5%, 8/13). A previous study showed that *mcr-3* had a wide distribution in water, animals, food, and human isolates (Elbediwi et al., 2019). We found a 7.7% (1/13) prevalence for *mcr-3.5*, which co-occurred with *mcr-1* and $bla_{OXA-48}$ in *E. coli.* The phenomenon of double *mcr* genes has been reported in isolates from humans, with *K. pneumoniae* harboring *mcr-3* and *mcr-8* being isolated from the stool of a healthy individual in Laos (Hadjadj et al., 2019).

Our study revealed that the most common type of plasmid replicon carrying *mcr* was IncX4. Previous reports have shown IncX4, IncI2, and IncHI2 to be the major plasmid types driving the global dissemination of *mcr-1* (Wu et al., 2018). A study in Thailand revealed two predominant plasmid types (IncX4 and IncI2) carrying *mcr-1* in CRE (Shanmugakani et al., 2019). This suggests that IncX4 bearing *mcr-1* mediates the transmission of CRE and may promote its circulation throughout Thailand. IncX4 and IncI2 acting as vehicles for *mcr-1* propagation enhance host fitness and provide a competitive advantage over strains with other plasmid replicon types, resulting in greater plasmid stability (Wu et al., 2018).

On the basis of the Clermont phylotyping scheme, *E. coli* species can be divided into eight main phylogroups, termed A, B1, B2, C, D, E, F, and G (Clermont et al., 2019). The nine carbapenem-resistant *E. coli* isolates carrying *mcr* (55.6%) in this study belonged to phylogroup C, whereas the rest belonged to phylogroups A and D (22.2% each). The *E. coli* strains responsible for extra-intestinal infection were more likely to be members of phylogroups B2 or D, which show greater pathogenesis than A, B1, or C (Clermont et al., 2013). Strains belonging to phylogroups A, B1, and C are commonly commensal, suggesting that more than half of the *E. coli* harboring *mcr* isolated from patients in this study were commensal strains.

Our study revealed seven carbapenem-resistant STs that carry *mcr*, of which *E. coli* ST410 (35.7%) and *K. pneumoniae* ST336 (21.4%) isolates were predominant. Elbediwi et al. (2019) reported that *E. coli* ST101 carrying *mcr-1* have been found in environmental samples, animals, and humans. However, ST10 was the most globally common ST of *E. coli* carrying *mcr-1* (Elbediwi et al., 2019). In Asia, ST116 was found to be the predominant ST that carries *mcr*-1 isolated from humans, followed by ST117, ST10, ST38, ST101, and ST156 (Elbediwi et al., 2019). *E. coli* ST410 is internationally considered a new high-risk clone that can cause several types of infection; it is highly resistant and has a global distribution (Roer et al., 2018). This ST has been described in Southeast Asia following multiple introductions through several independent events and differs from clones detected in Europe and North America (Nadimpalli et al., 2019). SNP phylogenetic analysis in this study revealed that the ST410 isolates were diverse or not closely related to other strains. Instead, they were shown to be related to strains from countries other than Thailand. This adds support to the assumption that there have been multiple dissemination events into this area.

*Klebsiella pneumoniae* ST336 (CC17) is considered an international clone (Rodrigues et al., 2014; Novović et al., 2017; Palmieri et al., 2020) and has been frequently associated with the worldwide spread of $bla_{\text{CTX-M-15}}$ and $bla_{\text{OXA-48-like}}$ (Rodrigues et al., 2014; Novović et al., 2017; Palmieri et al., 2020). Interestingly, all ST336 isolates in the current study carried $bla_{\text{NDM-1}}$, but not any $bla_{\text{CTX-M}}$ genes, suggesting that they may be from different lineages. To the best of our knowledge, the carbapenem-resistant ST336 isolates in this study are the first to be described as having *mcr-1*. Previous studies revealed that colistin-resistant ST336 resulted from an *mgrB* mutation, and no *mcr* genes have been detected in this ST (Novović et al., 2017; Palmieri et al., 2020). SNP phylogenetic analysis allocated the ST336 isolates to the same cluster as other Thai-ST336 isolates, and this cluster was independent from another ST336 cluster consisting of isolates from other countries. This suggests that Thai-ST336 isolates circulate throughout our country by clonal expansion.

The colistin MIC values (4–16 μg/ml) for our isolates indicated they have 100% resistance. Combinations of *mcr* and chromosome-mediated colistin resistant genes (*pmrAB*, *phoPQ*, *crrB*, or *recN*) contributed to the colistin resistance of our isolates. It is interesting that substitutions in *pmrAB* and *crrB* in *mcr-1*-carrying *K. pneumoniae* are quite different from previous reports (Olaitan et al., 2014a,b; Wright et al., 2015; Cheng et al., 2016). In addition, substitution of *phoPQ* was not found in our *K. pneumoniae* isolates comparing to those studies (Olaitan et al., 2014a,b; Wright et al., 2015; Cheng et al., 2016). On the other hand, substitutions of *pmrA* (G144S), *pmrB* (H2R, D283G, Y358N), and *phoP* (I44L) in our *mcr-1*-harboring *E. coli* are similar to a study previously described (Choi et al., 2020). In case of *rpoN*, inactivation of this gene resulting in polymyxin resistance has been observed in *Salmonella enterica* (Barchiesi et al., 2009). However, polymyxin resistance via *rpoN* inactivation or substitution is not yet reported in either *E. coli* or *K. pneumoniae*. Although our study detected substitution of *rpoN*, but its role on polymyxin resistance remain to be investigated.

Several studies have shown *mcr-1*-carrying CRE isolated from humans to have high frequencies of colistin resistance, such as 71.4% in China (Huang et al., 2020), 100% in the United States (Mediavilla et al., 2016), and 100% in Turkey (Arabaci et al., 2019). A previous study in Thailand reported colistin resistance rates of 75.0 and 79.1% in carbapenem-resistant *E. coli* and *K. pneumoniae* isolates, respectively (Eiamphungporn et al., 2018). The 13 carbapenem-resistant *mcr-1*-harboring CRE isolates described here showed a high susceptibility (>50%) to the antibiotics amikacin, fosfomycin, and nitrofurantoin. In contrast, the human *mcr-1*-harboring CRE isolate from China was reported to be highly susceptible only to tigecycline, amikacin, and aztreonam (Huang et al., 2020), whereas the isolate from the United States was susceptible to more antibiotics, including amikacin, aztreonam, gentamicin, nitrofurantoin, tigecycline, and trimethoprim-sulfamethoxazole (Mediavilla et al., 2016).

Polymyxins, including colistin, were reintroduced into human medical practice by the WHO in 2012 (World Health Organization, 2012). In China, this antibiotic was approved for clinical use in the treatment of bacterial infections in 2017. Since then, the relative prevalence of CRE carrying *mcr* genes increased from 0.41 to 1.38% (Huang et al., 2020). A study in Singapore revealed that prior exposure to polymyxin (adjusted OR, 21.31; 95% CI, 3.04–150.96) and carbapenem (OR 3.74; CI 1.13–12.44) were independent risk factors for polymyxin-resistant CRE among hospitalized patients (Teo et al., 2019). A study in Thailand demonstrated that chronic kidney diseases (OR 3.95; CI 1.26–12.32) and exposure to antimicrobials for less than 3 months (OR 2.29; CI 0.29–18.21) were risk factors associated with infections by *mcr-1*-carrying Enterobacteriaceae (Shanmugakani et al., 2019). In patients infected with polymyxin-resistant CRE, the 30-day all-cause in-hospital mortality was 50.0% compared with a 38.1% mortality in patients with polymyxin-susceptible CRE (Teo et al., 2019). Therefore, minimizing the use of polymyxin and carbapenem is strongly recommended.

The findings of the current study provide comprehensive insights into the prevalence of *mcr*-carrying CRE in patients in Thailand. In general, *mcr-1* was present in *E. coli* and *K. pneumoniae* isolates. The co-occurrence of two *mcr* genes was also demonstrated in CRE isolated from patients. To slow the emergence of XDR or PDR strains, priority should be given to strengthening official surveillance, active control, and prevention efforts as well as minimizing the dissemination of *mcr* genes among CRE isolates in humans.

## ETHICS STATEMENT

The Human Research Ethics Committee of Department of Medical Sciences, Ministry of Public Health, reviewed this study and judged that the protocol constituted routine public health activities and therefore did not involve human subject research. Written informed consent for participation was not required for this study in accordance with the national legislation and the institutional requirements.

## AUTHOR CONTRIBUTIONS

WP and AK conceived and designed the study, performed the data analysis, drafted the manuscript, and performed critical revisions of the manuscript for intellectual content. WK performed the laboratory experiments and analyzed the data. RU performed the statistical analysis and critical revision of the manuscript for intellectual content. All the authors read, edited, and approved the final manuscript.

## FUNDING

This work was supported by the National Institute of Health, Department of Medical Sciences, Ministry of Public Health, Thailand, and the Division of Global Health Protection, Thailand MoPH–U.S. CDC Collaboration.

## ACKNOWLEDGMENTS

We would like to thank Dr. Charatdao Bunthi, Division of Global Health Protection, Thailand MoPH–U.S. CDC Collaboration for critical review of the manuscript and the Kasetsart University Research and Development Institute (KURDI), Bangkok, Thailand for English-editing assistance. We also thank Suzanne Leech, Ph.D., from Edanz Group (https://en-author-services.edanzgroup.com/ac) for editing the draft of this manuscript.

## REFERENCES


Abbott, S. (2011). "*Klebsiella, Enterobacter, Citrobacter, Serratia, Plesiomonas,* and other Enterobacteriaceae," in Manual of Clinical Microbiology, 10th Edn, Vol. 2, eds J. Versalovic, K. C. Carroll, G. Funke, J. H. Jorgensen, M. L. Landry, and D. W. Warnock, (Washington, DC: ASM Press), 639–657.

Alcock, B. P., Raphenya, A. R., Lau, T., Tsang, K. K., Bouchard, M., Edalatmand, A., et al. (2020). CARD 2020: antibiotic resistome surveillance with the comprehensive antibiotic resistance database. *Nucleic Acids Res.* 48, D517–D525. doi: 10.1093/nar/gkz935

Arabaci, Ç, Dal, T., Başyiğit, T., Genişel, N., and Durmaz, R. (2019). Investigation of carbapenemase and *mcr-1* genes in carbapenem-resistant *Klebsiella pneumoniae* isolates. *J. Infect. Dev. Ctries* 13, 504–509. doi: 10.3855/jidc.11048

Barchiesi, J., Espariz, M., Checa, S. K., and Soncini, F. C. (2009). Downregulation of RpoN-controlled genes protects *Salmonella* cells from killing by the cationic antimicrobial peptide polymyxin B. *FEMS Microbiol. Lett.* 291, 73–79. doi: 10.1111/j.1574-6968.2008.01437.x

Beghain, J., Bridier-Nahmias, A., Le Nagard, H., Denamur, E., and Clermont, O. (2018). ClermonTyping: an easy-to-use and accurate in silico method for *Escherichia* genus strain phylotyping. *Microb. Genom.* 4:e000192. doi: 10.1099/mgen.0.000192

Bertels, F., Silander, O. K., Pachkov, M., Rainey, P. B., and van Nimwegen, E. (2014). Automated reconstruction of whole-genome phylogenies from short-sequence reads. *Mol. Biol. Evol.* 31, 1077–1088. doi: 10.1093/molbev/msu088

Carattoli, A., Zankari, E., García-Fernández, A., Voldby Larsen, M., Lund, O., Villa, L., et al. (2014). In silico detection and typing of plasmids using PlasmidFinder and plasmid multilocus sequence typing. *Antimicrob. Agents Chemother.* 58, 3895–3903. doi: 10.1128/AAC.02412-14

Cheng, Y. H., Lin, T. L., Lin, Y. T., and Wang, J. T. (2016). Amino acid substitutions of CrrB responsible for resistance to colistin through CrrC in *Klebsiella pneumoniae. Antimicrob. Agents Chemother.* 60, 3709–3716. doi: 10.1128/AAC.00009-16

Choi, Y., Lee, J. Y., Lee, H., Park, M., Kang, K., Lim, S. K., et al. (2020). Comparison of fitness cost and virulence in chromosome- and plasmid-mediated colistin-resistant *Escherichia coli. Front. Microbiol.* 11:798. doi: 10.3389/fmicb.2020.00798

Clermont, O., Christenson, J. K., Denamur, E., and Gordon, D. M. (2013). The clermont *Escherichia coli* phylo-typing method revisited: improvement of specificity and detection of new phylo-groups. *Environ. Microbiol. Rep.* 5, 58–65. doi: 10.1111/1758-2229.12019

Clermont, O., Dixit, O. V. A., Vangchhia, B., Condamine, B., Dion, S., Bridier-Nahmias, A., et al. (2019). Characterization and rapid identification of phylogroup G in *Escherichia coli*, a lineage with high virulence and antibiotic resistance potential. *Environ. Microbiol.* 21, 3107–3117. doi: 10.1111/1462-2920.14713

Clinical and Laboratory Standards Institute, (2020). *Performance Standards for Antimicrobial Susceptibility Testing:* CLSI Document M100-S30, 30th Edn. Wayne, PA: Clinical and Laboratory Standards Institute.

Eiamphungporn, W., Yainoy, S., Jumderm, C., Tan-Arsuwongkul, R., Tiengrim, S., and Thamlikitkul, V. (2018). Prevalence of the colistin resistance gene *mcr-1* in colistin-resistant *Escherichia coli* and *Klebsiella pneumoniae* isolated from humans in Thailand. *J. Glob. Antimicrob. Resist.* 15, 32–35. doi: 10.1016/j.jgar.2018.06.007

Elbediwi, M., Li, Y., Paudyal, N., Pan, H., Li, X., Xie, S., et al. (2019). Global burden of colistin-resistant bacteria: mobilized colistin resistance genes study (1980-2018). *Microorganisms.* 7:E461. doi: 10.3390/microorganisms7100461

Feng, Y., Zou, S., Chen, H., Yu, Y., and Ruan, Z. (2020). BacWGSTdb 2.0: a one-stop repository for bacterial whole-genome sequence typing and source tracking. *Nucleic Acids Res.* 3:gkaa821. doi: 10.1093/nar/gkaa821

Gharaibeh, M. H., and Shatnawi, S. Q. (2019). An overview of colistin resistance, mobilized colistin resistance genes dissemination, global responses, and the alternatives to colistin: a review. *Vet. World* 12, 1735–1746. doi: 10.14202/vetworld.2019

Hadjadj, L., Baron, S. A., Olaitan, A. O., Morand, S., and Rolain, J. M. (2019). Co-occurrence of variants of *mcr-3* and *mcr-8* Genes in a *Klebsiella pneumoniae* isolate from Laos. *Front. Microbiol.* 10:2720. doi: 10.3389/fmicb.2019.02720

Hatrongjit, R., Kerdsin, A., Akeda, Y., and Hamada, S. (2018). Detection of plasmid-mediated colistin-resistant and carbapenem-resistant genes by multiplex PCR. *MethodsX* 5, 532–536. doi: 10.1016/j.mex.2018.05.016

Huang, H., Dong, N., Shu, L., Lu, J., Sun, Q., Chan, E. W., et al. (2020). Colistin-resistance gene *mcr* in clinical carbapenem-resistant *Enterobacteriaceae* strains in China, 2014-2019. *Emerg. Microbes Infect.* 9, 237–245. doi: 10.1080/22221751.2020.1717380

Joensen, K. G., Scheutz, F., Lund, O., Hasman, H., Kaas, R. S., Nielsen, E. M., et al. (2014). Real-time whole-genome sequencing for routine typing, surveillance, and outbreak detection of verotoxigenic *Escherichia coli. J. Clin. Microbiol.* 52, 1501–1510. doi: 10.1128/JCM.03617-13

Kamjumphol, W., Wongboot, W., Suebwongsa, N., Kluabwang, P., Chantaroj, S., and Okada, K. (2019). Draft genome sequence of a colistin-resistant *Escherichia coli* ST226: a clinical strain harbouring an *mcr-1* variant. *J. Glob. Antimicrob. Resist.* 16, 168–169. doi: 10.1016/j.jgar.2019.01.009

Kananizadeh, P., Oshiro, S., Watanabe, S., Iwata, S., Kuwahara-Arai, K., Shimojima, M., et al. (2020). Emergence of carbapenem-resistant and colistin-susceptible *Enterobacter cloacae* complex co-harboring $bla_{IMP-1}$ and *mcr-9* in Japan. *BMC Infect. Dis.* 20:282. doi: 10.1186/s12879-020-05021-7

Kempf, I., Jouy, E., and Chauvin, C. (2016). Colistin use and colistin resistance in bacteria from animals. *Int. J. Antimicrob. Agents* 48, 598–606. doi: 10.1016/j.ijantimicag.2016.09.016

Kerdsin, A., Deekae, S., Chayangsu, S., Hatrongjit, R., Chopjitt, P., Takeuchi, D., et al. (2019). Genomic characterization of an emerging $bla_{KPC-2}$ carrying *Enterobacteriaceae* clinical isolates in Thailand. *Sci. Rep.* 9:18521. doi: 10.1038/s41598-019-55008-x

Kumar, S., Stecher, G., Li, M., Knyaz, C., and Tamura, K. (2018). Mega X: molecular evolutionary genetics analysis across computing platforms. *Mol. Biol. Evol.* 35, 1547–1549. doi: 10.1093/molbev/msy096

Larsen, M. V., Cosentino, S., Lukjancenko, O., Saputra, D., Rasmussen, S., Hasman, H., et al. (2014). Benchmarking of methods for genomic taxonomy. *J. Clin. Microbiol.* 52, 1529–1539. doi: 10.1128/JCM.02981-13

Larsen, M. V., Cosentino, S., Rasmussen, S., Friis, C., Hasman, H., Marvig, R. L., et al. (2012). Multilocus sequence typing of total-genome-sequenced bacteria. *J. Clin. Microbiol.* 50, 1355–1361. doi: 10.1128/JCM.06094-11

Letunic, I., and Bork, P. (2016). Interactive tree of life (iTOL) v3: an online tool for the display and annotation of phylogenetic and other trees. *Nucleic Acids Res.* 44, W242–W245. doi: 10.1093/nar/gkw290

Liu, Y. Y., Wang, Y., Walsh, T. R., Yi, L. X., Zhang, R., Spencer, J., et al. (2016). Emergence of plasmid-mediated colistin resistance mechanism MCR-1 in animals and human beings in China: a microbiological and molecular biological study. *Lancet Infect. Dis.* 16, 161–168. doi: 10.1016/S1473-3099(15)00424-7

Malchione, M. D., Torres, L. M., Hartley, D. M., Koch, M., and Goodman, J. L. (2019). Carbapenem and colistin resistance in *Enterobacteriaceae* in Southeast Asia: review and mapping of emerging and overlapping challenges. *Int. J. Antimicrob. Agents* 54, 381–399. doi: 10.1016/j.ijantimicag.2019.07.019

Mediavilla, J. R., Patrawalla, A., Chen, L., Chavda, K. D., Mathema, B., Vinnard, C., et al. (2016). Colistin- and carbapenem-resistant *Escherichia coli* harboring *mcr-1* and $bla_{NDM-5}$, causing a complicated urinary tract infection in a patient from the United States. *mBio* 7:e01191-16. doi: 10.1128/mBio.01191-16

Meletis, G., and Skoura, L. (2018). Polymyxin resistance mechanisms: from intrinsic resistance to *mcr* genes. *Recent Pat. Antiinfect. Drug Discov.* 13, 198–206. doi: 10.2174/1574891X14666181126142704

Mendes, A. C., Novais, Â, Campos, J., Rodrigues, C., Santos, C., Antunes, P., et al. (2018). *mcr-1* in carbapenemase-producing *Klebsiella pneumoniae* with hospitalized patients, Portugal, 2016-2017. *Emerg. Infect. Dis.* 24, 762–766. doi: 10.3201/eid2404.171787

Nadimpalli, M. L., de Lauzanne, A., Phe, T., Borand, L., Jacobs, J., Fabre, L., et al. (2019). *Escherichia coli* ST410 among humans and the environment in Southeast Asia. *Int. J. Antimicrob. Agents* 54, 228–232. doi: 10.1016/j.ijantimicag.2019.05.024

Novović, K., Trudić, A., Brkić, S., Vasiljević, Z., Kojić, M., Medić, D., et al. (2017). Molecular epidemiology of colistin-resistant, carbapenemase-producing *Klebsiella pneumoniae* in Serbia from 2013 to 2016. *Antimicrob. Agents Chemother.* 61:e02550-16. doi: 10.1128/AAC.02550-16

Olaitan, A. O., Chabou, S., Okdah, L., Morand, S., and Rolain, J. M. (2016). Dissemination of the *mcr-1* colistin resistance gene. *Lancet Infect. Dis.* 16:147. doi: 10.1016/S1473-3099(15)00540-X

Olaitan, A. O., Diene, S. M., Kempf, M., Berrazeg, M., Bakour, S., Gupta, S. K., et al. (2014a). Worldwide emergence of colistin resistance in *Klebsiella pneumoniae* from healthy humans and patients in Lao PDR, Thailand, Israel, Nigeria and France owing to inactivation of the PhoP/PhoQ regulator mgrB: an epidemiological and molecular study. *Int. J. Antimicrob. Agents* 44, 500–507. doi: 10.1016/j.ijantimicag.2014.07.020

Olaitan, A. O., Morand, S., and Rolain, J. M. (2014b). Mechanisms of polymyxin resistance: acquired and intrinsic resistance in bacteria. *Front. Microbiol.* 5:643. doi: 10.3389/fmicb.2014.00643

Palmieri, M., D'Andrea, M. M., Pelegrin, A. C., Mirande, C., Brkic, S., Cirkovic, I., et al. (2020). Genomic epidemiology of carbapenem- and colistin-resistant *Klebsiella pneumoniae* isolates from Serbia: predominance of ST101 strains carrying a novel OXA-48 plasmid. *Front. Microbiol.* 11:294. doi: 10.3389/fmicb.2020.00294

Paveenkittiporn, W., Kerdsin, A., Chokngam, S., Bunthi, C., Sangkitporn, S., and Gregory, C. J. (2017). Emergence of plasmid-mediated colistin resistance and New Delhi metallo-β-lactamase genes in extensively drug-resistant *Escherichia coli* isolated from a patient in Thailand. *Diagn. Microbiol. Infect. Dis.* 87, 157–159. doi: 10.1016/j.diagmicrobio.2016.11.005

Quan, J., Li, X., Chen, Y., Jiang, Y., Zhou, Z., Zhang, H., et al. (2017). Prevalence of *mcr-1* in *Escherichia coli* and *Klebsiella pneumoniae* recovered from bloodstream infections in China: a multicentre longitudinal study. *Lancet Infect. Dis.* 17, 400–410. doi: 10.1016/S1473-3099(16)30528-X

Rebelo, A. R., Bortolaia, V., Kjeldgaard, J. S., Pedersen, S. K., Leekitcharoenphon, P., Hansen, I. M., et al. (2018). Multiplex PCR for detection of plasmid-mediated colistin resistance determinants, *mcr-1, mcr-2, mcr-3, mcr-4* and *mcr-5* for surveillance purposes. *Euro. Surveill.* 23:17-00672. doi: 10.2807/1560-7917.ES.2018.23.6.17-00672

Rodrigues, C., Machado, E., Ramos, H., Peixe, L., and Novais, Â (2014). Expansion of ESBL-producing *Klebsiella pneumoniae* in hospitalized patients: a successful story of international clones (ST15, ST147, ST336) and epidemic plasmids (IncR, IncFIIK). *Int. J. Med. Microbiol.* 304, 1100–1108. doi: 10.1016/j.ijmm.2014.08.003

Roer, L., Overballe-Petersen, S., Hansen, F., Schønning, K., Wang, M., Røder, B. L., et al. (2018). *Escherichia coli* sequence type 410 is causing new international high-risk clones. *mSphere* 3:e00337-18. doi: 10.1128/mSphere.00337-18

Shanmugakani, R. K., Akeda, Y., Sugawara, Y., Laolerd, W., Chaihongsa, N., Sirichot, S., et al. (2019). PCR-dipstick-oriented surveillance and characterization of *mcr-1*- and carbapenemase-carrying *Enterobacteriaceae* in a Thai hospital. *Front. Microbiol.* 10:149. doi: 10.3389/fmicb.2019.00149

Srijan, A., Margulieux, K. R., Ruekit, S., Snesrud, E., Maybank, R., Serichantalergs, O., et al. (2018). Genomic characterization of nonclonal *mcr-1*-positive multidrug-resistant *Klebsiella pneumoniae* from clinical samples in Thailand. *Microb. Drug Resist.* 24, 403–410. doi: 10.1089/mdr.2017.0400

Teo, J. Q., Chang, C. W., Leck, H., Tang, C. Y., Lee, S. J., Cai, Y., et al. (2019). Risk factors and outcomes associated with the isolation of polymyxin B and carbapenem-resistant *Enterobacteriaceae* spp.: a case-control study. *Int. J. Antimicrob. Agents* 53, 657–662. doi: 10.1016/j.ijantimicag.2019.03.011

Wang, C., Feng, Y., Liu, L., Wei, L., Kang, M., and Zong, Z. (2020). Identification of novel mobile colistin resistance gene *mcr-10*. *Emerg. Microbes Infect.* 9, 508–516. doi: 10.1080/22221751.2020.1732231

Wang, X., Wang, Y., Zhou, Y., Li, J., Yin, W., Wang, S., et al. (2018). Emergence of a novel mobile colistin resistance gene, *mcr-8*, in NDM-producing *Klebsiella pneumoniae*. *Emerg. Microbes Infect.* 7:122. doi: 10.1038/s41426-018-0124-z

Wick, R. R., Heinz, E., Holt, K. E., and Wyres, K. L. (2018). Kaptive Web: user-friendly capsule and lipopolysaccharide serotype prediction for *Klebsiella* genomes. *J. Clin. Microbiol.* 56:e00197-18. doi: 10.1128/JCM.00197-18

World Health Organization, (2012). *Critically Important Antimicrobials for Human Medicine, 3rd Revision*. Geneva: WHO.

World Health Organization, (2017). *Global Priority List of Antibiotic-Resistant Bacteria to Guide Research, Discovery, and deveLopment of New Antibiotics*. Geneva: WHO.

Wright, M. S., Suzuki, Y., Jones, M. B., Marshall, S. H., Rudin, S. D., van Duin, D., et al. (2015). Genomic and transcriptomic analyses of colistin-resistant clinical isolates of *Klebsiella pneumoniae* reveal multiple pathways of resistance. *Antimicrob. Agents Chemother.* 59, 536–543. doi: 10.1128/AAC.04037-14

Wu, R., Yi, L. X., Yu, L. F., Wang, J., Liu, Y., Chen, X., et al. (2018). Fitness advantage of *mcr-1*-bearing IncI2 and IncX4 plasmids *in vitro*. *Front. Microbiol.* 9:331. doi: 10.3389/fmicb.2018.00331

Yang, Y. Q., Li, Y. X., Lei, C. W., Zhang, A. Y., and Wang, H. N. (2018). Novel plasmid-mediated colistin resistance gene *mcr-7.1* in *Klebsiella pneumoniae*. *J. Antimicrob. Chemother.* 73, 1791–1795. doi: 10.1093/jac/dky111

Yuan, Y., Li, Y., Wang, G., Li, C., Xiang, L., She, J., et al. (2019). Coproduction of *mcr-9* and NDM-1 by colistin-resistant *Enterobacter hormaechei* isolated from bloodstream infection. *Infect. Drug Resist.* 12, 2979–2985. doi: 10.2147/IDR.S217168

Zankari, E., Hasman, H., Cosentino, S., Vestergaard, M., Rasmussen, S., Lund, O., et al. (2012). Identification of acquired antimicrobial resistance genes. *J. Antimicrob. Chemother.* 67, 2640–2644. doi: 10.1093/jac/dks261

Zhong, L. L., Phan, H. T. T., Shen, C., Vihta, K. D., Sheppard, A. E., Huang, X., et al. (2018). High rates of human fecal carriage of mcr-1-positive multidrug-resistant *Enterobacteriaceae* emerge in China in association with successful plasmid families. *Clin. Infect. Dis.* 66, 676–685. doi: 10.1093/cid/cix885

# 14

# *In Vitro* Antimicrobial Activity of Green Synthesized Silver Nanoparticles Against Selected Gram-Negative Foodborne Pathogens

*Yuet Ying Loo[1]*, Yaya Rukayadi[1], Mahmud-Ab-Rashid Nor-Khaizura[1], Chee Hao Kuan[2], Buong Woei Chieng[3,4], Mitsuaki Nishibuchi[5] and Son Radu[1,6]*

[1] *Department of Food Science, Faculty of Food Science and Technology, Universiti Putra Malaysia, Selangor, Malaysia,* [2] *Department of Agricultural and Food Science, Faculty of Science, Universiti Tunku Abdul Rahman, Kampar, Malaysia,* [3] *Department of Chemistry, Faculty of Science, Universiti Putra Malaysia, Selangor, Malaysia,* [4] *Materials Processing and Technology Laboratory, Institute of Advanced Technology, Universiti Putra Malaysia, Selangor, Malaysia,* [5] *Center for Southeast Asian Studies, Kyoto University, Kyoto, Japan,* [6] *Laboratory of Food Safety and Food Integrity, Institute of Tropical Agriculture and Food Security (ITAFoS), Universiti Putra Malaysia, Selangor, Malaysia*

***Correspondence:**
*Yuet Ying Loo*
*yuetying88@gmail.com*

Silver nanoparticles (AgNPs) used in this study were synthesized using pu-erh tea leaves extract with particle size of 4.06 nm. The antibacterial activity of green synthesized AgNPs against a diverse range of Gram-negative foodborne pathogens was determined using disk diffusion method, resazurin microtitre-plate assay (minimum inhibitory concentration, MIC), and minimum bactericidal concentration test (MBC). The MIC and MBC of AgNPs against *Escherichia coli*, *Klebsiella pneumoniae*, *Salmonella* Typhimurium, and *Salmonella* Enteritidis were 7.8, 3.9, 3.9, 3.9 and 7.8, 3.9, 7.8, 3.9 μg/mL, respectively. Time-kill curves were used to evaluate the concentration between MIC and bactericidal activity of AgNPs at concentrations ranging from 0×MIC to 8×MIC. The killing activity of AgNPs was fast acting against all the Gram-negative bacteria tested; the reduction in the number of CFU $mL^{-1}$ was >3 $Log_{10}$ units (99.9%) in 1–2 h. This study indicates that AgNPs exhibit a strong antimicrobial activity and thus might be developed as a new type of antimicrobial agents for the treatment of bacterial infection including multidrug resistant bacterial infection.

**Keywords: silver nanoparticles, tea leave extracts, antimicrobial activity, foodborne pathogens, Gram-negative, time-kill curves**

## INTRODUCTION

Recently, nanotechnology has emerged as a dynamically developing area of scientific interest in the world. Nanoparticles are defined as a nanoscale particle of size ranging from 1 to 100 nm. Among the metallic nanoparticles, silver nanoparticles (AgNPs) have gained increasingly attention due to its unique physical, biological and chemical properties. AgNPs are well-known to exhibit a strong antimicrobial activity against various microorganisms such as bacteria, viruses, and fungi due to its smaller in size and large surface area (Franci et al., 2015). AgNPs are also widely used as anti-fungal (Medda et al., 2015), anti-inflammatory (Hebeish et al., 2014), and anti-viral properties (Bekele et al., 2016).

Green synthesis of AgNPs employing either biological microorganisms or plant extracts has emerged as a simple and alternative to chemical synthesis. Green synthesis method provides advancements over chemical methods as it is environmental friendly and cost effective. Plant extracts-mediated synthesis of AgNPs can be advantageous compared with other biological processes as it does not require the process of maintaining the cell cultures and aseptic environments (Loo et al., 2012). Several studies on the green synthesis of AgNPs using plant extracts have been reported (Medda et al., 2015; Ahmed et al., 2016; Dhand et al., 2016; Selvam et al., 2017).

Foodborne illnesses have emerged as a major public health concern around the world. WHO (2014) reported that there is about 30% of the population in industrialized countries affected by foodborne diseases every year. The consumption of foods contaminated with foodborne pathogens such as bacteria, fungi, viruses, and toxins are often recognized as the main source of foodborne illness in humans. Food especially minimal-processed food can be contaminated during pre-harvesting, post-harvesting, processing, transport, handling, or preparation. The most common foodborne pathogens found in food are *Salmonella* spp. (Lee et al., 2015; D'Ostuni et al., 2016), *Listeria* spp. (Ferreira et al., 2014; Välimaa et al., 2015), *Escherichia coli* O157 (Heiman et al., 2015), *Campylobacter* spp. (Kaakoush et al., 2015), and *Clostridia* spp. (Chukwu et al., 2016).

The presence of multidrug resistance pathogens have increased the number of infectious disease and became the main cause of death in the world (WHO, 2000; Tanwar et al., 2014). Widely misuse and abuse of antibiotics are the leading cause of antibiotic resistance in the bacteria (O'Bryan et al., 2018). Multidrug resistant bacteria infection may lead to several impacts including increase of mortality and morbidity rates, prolong of hospitalization period, and economic loss (Patel et al., 2008). Woh et al. (2017) detected multi-drug resistant non-typhoidal *Salmonella* among migrant food handlers, which may cause cross-contamination to the food products. Thus, the development of a new and natural antimicrobial agent is needed as there is a growing concern in multidrug resistant foodborne pathogens.

The aim of this study is to determine the antibacterial activity of green synthesized AgNPs against a diverse range of Gram-negative foodborne pathogens by using disk diffusion method, resazurin microtitre-plate assay minimum inhibitory concentration (MIC), minimum bactericidal concentration test (MBC), and time-kill curve assay.

## MATERIALS AND METHODS

### Preparation of Silver Nanoparticles

The synthesis of AgNPs using pu-erh tea leaves extracts was done using the method as described previously (Loo et al., 2012). Ten gram of tea leaves was weighed in a beaker. The tea leaves was added with 100 mL of distilled water and maintained at 60°C for 10 min. After 10 min, the tea extract was filtered using 0.45 μm Millipore membrane filter and followed by 0.2 μm Millipore membrane filter. For synthesis of AgNPs, 12 mL of tea extracts was added into 100 mL of $AgNO_3$ (1 mM) in Erlenmeyer flask at room temperature. Color changes of the solution were observed. The synthesized AgNPs were characterized by UV-vis spectroscopy, X-ray diffraction (XRD), Fourier transform infrared (FTIR) spectroscopy, and transmission electron microscopy (TEM).

### Bacteria Strains Preparation

*Escherichia coli* ATCC 25922 (*E. coli*), *Klebsiella pneumoniae* ATCC 13773 (*K. pneumoniae*), *Salmonella* Typhimurium ATCC 14028 (*S.* Typhimurium), and *Salmonella* Enteritidis ATCC 13076 (*S.* Enteritidis) were obtained from the American Type Culture Collection (Rockville, MD, United States). All the bacteria strains were cultured in Mueller Hinton broth (MHB) (Merck, Germany) at 37°C for 24 h with 200 rpm agitation.

### Preparation of Resazurin Solution

The resazurin solution was prepared at 0.02% (wt/vol) according to Khalifa et al. (2013). A 0.002 g of resazurin salt powder was dissolved in 10 mL of distilled water and vortexed. The mixture was filtered by Millipore membrane filter (0.2 μm). The resazurin solution can be kept at 4°C for 2 weeks.

### *In Vitro* Susceptibility Test

#### Disk Diffusion Method

The antibacterial activity of AgNPs against the selected Gram-negative foodborne pathogens was carried out using Kirby–Bauer Disk Diffusion Susceptibility Test method (Bauer et al., 1966). The bacteria strains were spread on the Mueller-Hinton agar (MHA) (Merck, Germany) using sterile cotton swab. Sterile blank antimicrobial susceptibility disk was used in the test. The disks were loaded with 10 μL of tea leaves extracts, silver nitrate solution (1 mM), and solution containing tea leaves mediated synthesized AgNPs separately. The disks were then placed on the agar plate and incubated at 37°C for 24 h. The zone of inhibition was observed after 24 h of incubation.

#### Minimum Inhibitory Concentration (MIC) and Minimum Bactericidal Concentration (MBC) Evaluation

The MIC and MBC of green synthesized AgNPs were done using the method described in the guideline of CLSI (2012). The MIC test was performed in 96-well round bottom microtiter plate using standard broth microdilution methods while the MBC test was performed on the MHA plates. The bacterial inoculums were adjusted to the concentration of $10^6$ CFU/mL. For the MIC test, 100 μL of the synthesized AgNPs stock solution (500 μg/mL) was added and diluted twofold with the bacterial inoculums in 100 μL of MHB started from column 12 to column 3. Column 12 of the microtiter plate contained the highest concentration of AgNPs, while column 3 contained the lowest concentration. Column 1 served as negative control (only medium) and the column 2 served as positive control (medium and bacterial inoculums). Each well of the microtiter plate was added with 30 μL of the resazurin solution and incubated at 37°C for 24 h. Any color changes were observed. Blue/purple color indicated no bacterial growth while pink/colorless indicated bacterial growth.

The MIC value was taken at the lowest concentration of antibacterial agents that inhibits the growth of bacteria (color remained in blue).

The MBC was defined as the lowest concentration of the antibacterial agents that completely kill the bacteria. MBC test was performed by plating the suspension from each well of microtiter plates into MHA plate. The plates were incubated at 37°C for 24 h. The lowest concentration with no visible growths on the MHA plate was taken as MBC value.

### Time-Kill Curve

Time-kill assay was done in MHB medium as described by Zainin et al. (2013) and Lau et al. (2014). The bacterial inoculums were adjusted to $10^6$ CFU/mL. The AgNPs solution was diluted with MHB media containing bacterial inoculums to obtain the final concentration of 0× MIC, 0.5× MIC, 1× MIC, 2× MIC, 4× MIC, and 8× MIC for each type of bacteria in the total final volume of 1 mL. The cultures were then incubated at 37°C with 150 rpm agitation. The cultures (100 μL) were spread on MHA plates at time 0, 0.25, 0.5, 1, 2, and 4 h. The experiment was carried out in triplicate. The number of colonies on the MHA plates was quantified in CFU/mL after incubation at 37°C for 24 h. For statistical analysis, SPSS (v.19) statistical package was used to determine the significant ($P < 0.05$) difference among the tested foodborne pathogens.

## RESULTS AND DISCUSSION

This study was aimed to determine the antibacterial effect of green synthesized AgNPs. The green synthesized AgNPs used in this study were characterized by UV-vis spectroscopy, XRD, FTIR spectroscopy, and TEM. The XRD patterns for synthesized AgNPs showed that five main characteristic diffraction peaks for Ag were observed at $2\theta$ = 38.4, 44.5, 64.8, 77.7, and 81.7, which correspond to the (111), (200), (220), (311), and (222) crystallographic planes of face-centered cubic (fcc) Ag crystals. The UV-vis absorption spectrum of the synthesized AgNPs showed a broad peak at 436 nm which is a characteristic band for Ag. Three infrared bands were observed at 3,271, 1,637, and 386 $cm^{-1}$ in FTIR measurement. The band at 3,271 and 1,637 $cm^{-1}$ indicated that the presence of protein as capping agent for AgNPs which increases the stability of the nanoparticles, while the broad peak at 386 $cm^{-1}$ corresponded to the Ag metal. TEM image revealed that the AgNPs is spherical with the particle size of 4.06 nm (Loo et al., 2012).

The antibacterial activity of AgNPs was determined against four species of Gram-negative foodborne pathogens: *E. coli* ATCC 25922, *K. pneumoniae* ATCC 13773, *S.* Typhimurium ATCC 14028, and *S.* Enteritidis ATCC 13076. The results for disk diffusion test, MIC and MBC of the AgNPs are summarized in **Table 1**. For the disk diffusion test, the presence of clear zone around the AgNPs disk suggesting that the AgNPs possessed antibacterial activity which is able to inhibit the growth of the Gram-negative foodborne pathogens. As previous study by Guzman et al. (2012), reported that AgNPs employed antibacterial activity on Gram-negative bacteria. The visible clear zone produced by AgNPs against four different species of Gram-negative bacteria is showed in **Figure 1**.

Disk diffusion test was described as the preliminary study in screening the antibacterial activity of an antimicrobial agent; therefore, a further evaluation in determining the antibacterial activity of AgNPs using MIC value was needed (Burt, 2004). MIC was defined as the lowest concentration of the antibacterial agent to inhibit the growth of bacteria by serial dilution. As showed in **Table 1**, the MIC values of AgNPs against the foodborne pathogens were ranged from 3.9 to 7.8 μg/mL. *K. pneumonia*, *S.* Typhimurium and *S.* Enteritidis showed the MIC value of 3.9 μg/mL while *E. coli* showed the MIC value of 7.8 μg/mL. MBC is the lowest concentration of antibacterial agent to kill the bacteria (showed no growth on the agar plate). In the study, MBC for *K. pneumoniae* and *S.* Enteritidis were 3.9 μg/mL while *S.* Typhimurium and *E. coli* showed the MBC value of 7.8 μg/mL. The MIC and MBC value of *E. coli* showed that *E. coli* was less susceptible to AgNPs. This may due to the positive charges of AgNPs trapped and blocked by lipopolysaccharide, thus make *E. coli* less susceptible to AgNPs (Lara et al., 2010b).

Resazurin dye was used in the study as an indicator in the determination of cell growth, especially in cytotoxicity assays (McNicholl et al., 2007). Oxidoreductases within viable cells reduced the resazurin salt to resorufin and changed the color from blue non-fluorescent to pink and fluorescent. According to McNicholl et al. (2007), resazurin dye has been applied for decades to check for the bacterial and yeast contamination in milk.

The time kill activity of four foodborne pathogens is shown in **Figure 2**. The bactericidal activity of AgNPs is effective against the selected Gram-negative pathogens; the reduction in the number of CFU/mL was ≥3 Log units (99%). The bactericidal endpoint of AgNPs for *E. coli* was reached after 2 h of incubation at 4× MIC (31.2 μg/mL) and 8× MIC (62.4 μg/mL); while for *K. pneumoniae*, the bacteria was killed after 2 h of incubation at 2× MIC (7.8 μg/mL), 4× MIC (15.6 μg/mL), and 8× MIC (31.2 μg/mL). *S.* Typhimurium was killed after 1 h of incubation at 4× MIC (15.6 μg/mL) and 8× MIC (31.2 μg/mL). The bactericidal endpoint of AgNP for *S.* Enteritidis was reached after 2 h of incubation at 2× MIC (7.8 μg/mL) and 4× MIC (15.6 μg/mL); however, the end point reached faster after 1 h of incubation at 8× MIC (31.2 μg/mL). No significant differences ($P > 0.05$) were found among the tested Gram-negative foodborne pathogens. This indicates that AgNPs are

**TABLE 1** | The diameter of zone inhibition (mm), MIC value (μg/mL), and MBC value (μg/mL).

| Bacteria | Diameter of inhibition zone (mm) | MIC (μg/mL) | MBC (μg/mL) |
|---|---|---|---|
| *Escherichia coli* | 15 | 7.8 | 7.8 |
| *Klebsiella pneumoniae* | 10 | 3.9 | 3.9 |
| *Salmonella* Typhimurium | 20 | 3.9 | 7.8 |
| *Salmonella* Enteritidis | 20 | 3.9 | 3.9 |

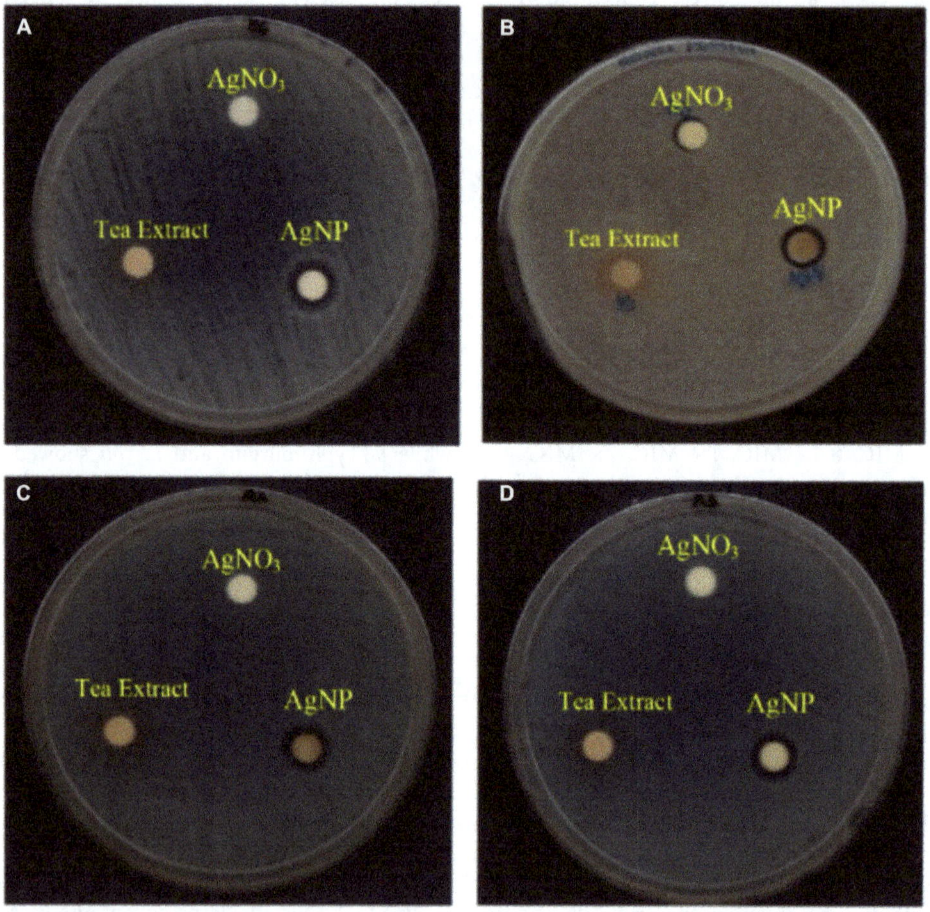


**FIGURE 1** | Visible clear zone produced by tea leaves extract mediated AgNP against four species of foodborne pathogens: **(A)** *E. coli* ATCC 25922, **(B)** *K. pneumoniae* ATCC 13773, **(C)** *S.* Typhimurium ATCC 14028, and **(D)** *S.* Enteritidis ATCC 13076.

broad spectrum antimicrobial agents which exert the same effect to all Gram-negative bacteria strains.

Silver nanoparticles are well-known as the most universal antimicrobial substances due to their strong biocidal effect against microorganisms, which has been used for over the past decades to prevent and treat various diseases (Oei et al., 2012). AgNPs are also widely used as anti-fungal (Kim et al., 2009), anti-inflammatory (Nadworny et al., 2010), and anti-viral properties (Lara et al., 2010a). Recently, non-hazardous AgNPs can easily be synthesized using a cost-effective method and tested as a new type of antimicrobial agents.

In this study, the application of AgNPs as an antimicrobial agent was tested against selected Gram-negative bacteria on agar plate and liquid medium. The results showed that the tested bacteria could completely inhibit by AgNPs. The inhibition of bacteria growth was reported affected by the concentration of AgNPs and bacteria used in the experiments (Sondi and Salopek-Sondi, 2004). The green synthesized AgNPs in this study are able to inhibit the high concentration of bacteria (approximately $10^6$ CFU/mL). This indicated that AgNPs showed an excellent antimicrobial effect as the high CFU concentration of bacteria used in this study are rarely appeared in real-life systems.

The antibacterial activity of AgNPs has been reported by many researchers. However, the MIC values from the previous studies showed the range through a large extent of variation. Therefore, the comparison of the results is difficult as there is no standard method for determination of antibacterial activity of AgNPs and different methods have been applied by the researchers (Zarei et al., 2014). In this study, AgNPs exhibit a good antibacterial activity against the tested foodborne pathogens. Based on the results, the tested bacteria were able to kill in a shorter time at low concentration of AgNPs. This may due to the cell wall structure of Gram-negative bacteria. The characteristic cell wall structure of Gram-negative bacteria is different from Gram-positive bacteria. Gram-negative bacteria have a cytoplasmic membrane, a thin peptidoglycan layer, and an outer membrane containing lipopolysaccharide. There is a space between the cytoplasmic membrane and the outer membrane called the periplasmic space or periplasm. The periplasmic space contains the loose network of peptidoglycan chains known as the peptidoglycan layer.

The rapid reproduction time of bacteria is one of the main causes of bacteria's infectivity (Lara et al., 2010b). However, the reproduction time of the bacteria could be an ideal way to prevent the viable infection as AgNPs were effective in inhibiting

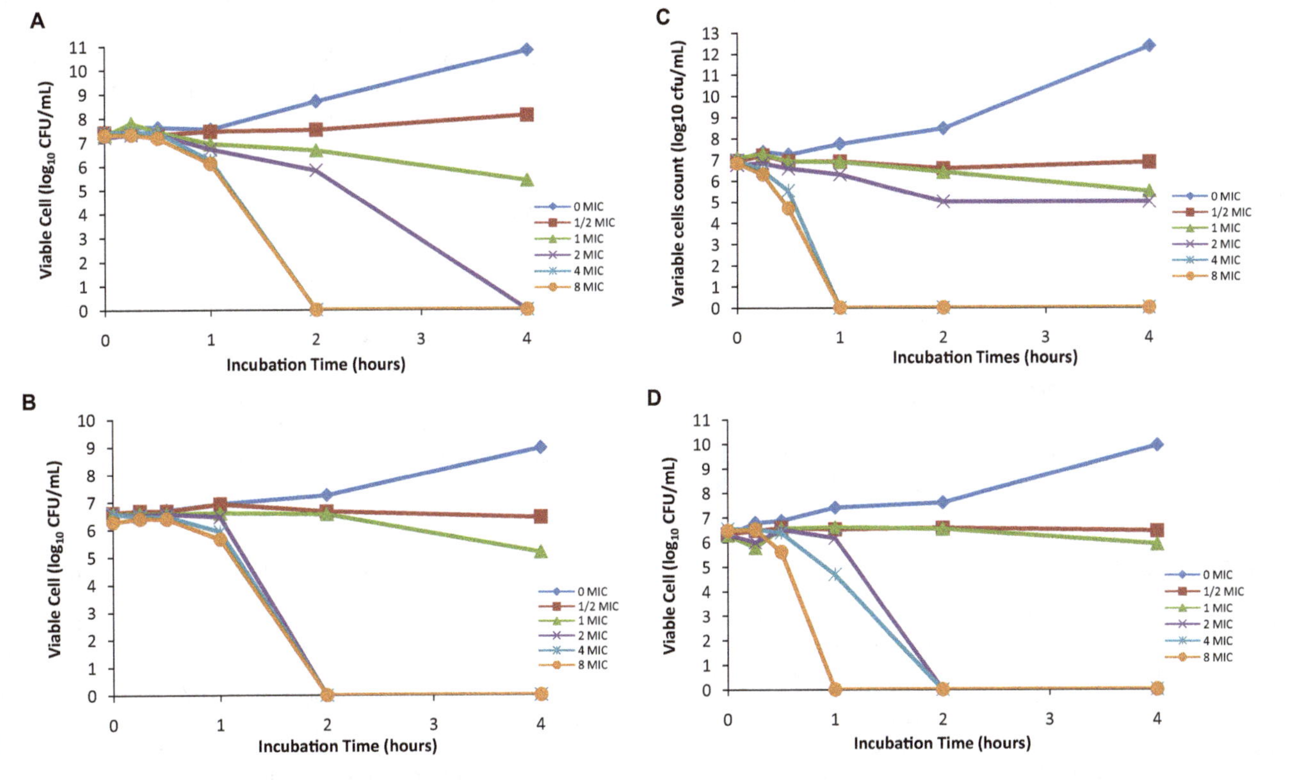


**FIGURE 2 |** Time-kill plots of AgNPs against **(A)** *E. coli* ATCC 25922, **(B)** *K. pneumoniae* ATCC 13773, **(C)** *S.* Typhimurium ATCC 14028, and **(D)** *S.* Enteritidis ATCC 13076 at different concentration and time-length.

and killing the bacteria in a dose and time dependent manner as shown in the time-kill assays. Zhang et al. (2016) reported that the smaller size of AgNPs could cause more toxicity to the bacteria and show better bactericidal effect compared to the larger particles as they have larger surface area. Previous study by Agnihotri et al. (2014) found that the antibacterial efficacy was increased for the AgNPs with less than 10 nm size. They also concluded that AgNPs with the size of 5 nm have the fastest antibacterial activity compared to others size of AgNPs.

Silver nanoparticles have emerged as antimicrobial agents against multidrug resistant bacteria due to their high surface-area-to-volume ration and unique chemical and physical properties. AgNPs have particle size ranging from 1 to 100 nm. The surface area-to-volume ratio of AgNPs increases as the particles size decreases. Morones et al. (2005) reported that AgNPs with the size of 10-100 nm showed strong antimicrobial effect against both Gram-positive and negative bacteria. The small particle size enables AgNPs to adhere to the cell wall and penetrate into the bacteria cell easily, which in turn improves their antimicrobial activity against bacteria. The antimicrobial effects of AgNPs against multidrug resistant bacteria have been studied by many researchers and it was proved that AgNPs are effective against multidrug resistant bacteria such as multidrug resistant *E. coli* (Paredes et al., 2014; Kar et al., 2016), multidrug resistant strain of *Pseudomonas aeruginosa* (Durairaj et al., 2012), methicillin-resistant *Staphylococcus aureus* (MRSA) (Paredes et al., 2014; Yuan et al., 2017), and extended-spectrum β-lactam (ESBL) producing bacteria (Doudi et al., 2013; Subashini et al., 2014).

On the other hands, AgNPs are advantageous compared to conventional chemical antimicrobial agents as the major problem caused by the conventional chemical antimicrobial agents is multidrug resistance. The effectiveness of the chemical antimicrobial agents depends on the specific binding of the microorganisms with the surface and metabolites of the antimicrobial agents. However, the chemical antimicrobial agents are limited to use especially in medical field as various microorganisms have developed multiple resistance traits over a period of generations. Thus, the development of AgNPs could be an alternative way to overcome the multidrug resistance microorganisms as bacteria are less likely to develop resistance to metal nanoparticles compared to the conventional antibiotics.

The exact mechanisms of AgNPs against bacteria still remain unknown. However, there are some researchers proposed that the action of AgNPs on bacteria may due to its ability to penetrate into the cell (Sondi and Salopek-Sondi, 2004), the formation of free radicals (Danilczuk et al., 2006; Kim et al., 2007), the inactivation of proteins in the cell by silver ions (Rai et al., 2012) and the production of reactive oxygen species (ROS) (Dakal et al., 2016). Besides that, there are also some factors in affecting the bactericidal mechanisms of AgNPs such as the concentration of AgNPs and bacteria class (Kim et al., 2007; Zhang et al., 2014), shape (Pal et al., 2007; Meire et al., 2012), size

(Martinez-Castanon et al., 2008), and the combination of various antibiotics (Fayaz et al., 2010; Singh et al., 2013).

## CONCLUSION

Silver nanoparticles showed significant antibacterial activity against the selected Gram-negative foodborne pathogens. Thus, AgNPs might be a good alternative to develop as antibacterial agent against the multidrug-resistant strains of bacteria. The applications of AgNPs may lead to valuable findings in various fields such as medical devices and antimicrobial systems.

## AUTHOR CONTRIBUTIONS

YL, BC, YR, and RS developed the study design. YL and CK carried out the confirmation for the selected foodborne pathogens. MN provided culture media and technical advice in the study. YL interpreted the data, drafted the manuscript, and revised the manuscript. YR, M-A-RN-K, CK, BC, and RS checked on the manuscript. All authors read and approved the final version of the manuscript.

## FUNDING

This research was funded by a Research University Grant Scheme Initiative Six (RUGS 6) of Universiti Putra Malaysia (GP-IPS 9438703) and Fundamental Research Grant Scheme (FRGS) of Ministry of Higher Education (MOHE), Malaysia (02-01-14-1475FR) and, in part, by the Kakenhi Grant-in-Aid for Scientific Research (KAKENHI 24249038), Japan Society for the Promotion of Sciences and grant-in-aid of Ministry of Health, Labor and Welfare, Japan.

## REFERENCES

Agnihotri, S., Mukherji, S., and Mukherji, S. (2014). Size-controlled silver nanoparticles synthesized over the range 5–100 nm using the same protocol and their antibacterial efficacy. *RSC Adv.* 4, 3974–3983. doi: 10.1039/C3RA44507K

Ahmed, S., Ahmad, M., Swami, B. L., and Ikram, S. (2016). A review on plants extract mediated synthesis of silver nanoparticles for antimicrobial applications: a green expertise. *J. Adv. Res.* 7, 17–28. doi: 10.1016/j.jare.2015.02.007

Bauer, A. W., Kirby, W. M., Sherris, J. C., and Turck, M. (1966). Antibiotic susceptibility testing by a standardized single disk method. *Am. J. Clin. Pathol.* 45, 493–496. doi: 10.1093/ajcp/45.4_ts.493

Bekele, A. Z., Gokulan, K., Williams, K. M., and Khare, S. (2016). Dose and size-dependent antiviral effects of silver nanoparticles on feline calicivirus, a human norovirus surrogate. *Foodborne Pathog. Dis.* 13, 239–244. doi: 10.1089/fpd.2015.2054

Burt, S. (2004). Essential oils: their antibacterial properties and potential applications in foods—a review. *Int. J. Food Microbiol.* 94, 223–253. doi: 10.1016/j.ijfoodmicro.2004.03.022

Chukwu, E. E., Nwaokorie, F. O., Coker, A. O., Avila-Campos, M. J., Solis, R. L., Llanco, L. A., et al. (2016). Detection of toxigenic *Clostridium perfringens* and *Clostridium botulinum* from food sold in Lagos, Nigeria. *Anaerobe* 42, 176–181. doi: 10.1016/j.anaerobe.2016.10.009

CLSI (2012). *Performance Standards for Antimicrobial Susceptibility Testing; Twenty-Second Informational Supplement.* Wayne, PA: The Clinical and Laboratory Standards Institute.

Dakal, T. C., Kumar, A., Majumdar, R. S., and Yadav, V. (2016). Mechanistic basis of antimicrobial actions of silver nanoparticles. *Front. Microbiol.* 7:1831. doi: 10.3389/fmicb.2016.01831

Danilczuk, M., Lund, A., Sadlo, J., Yamada, H., and Michalik, J. (2006). Conduction electron spin resonance of small silver particles. *Spectrochim. Acta A Mol. Biomol. Spectrosc.* 63, 189–191. doi: 10.1016/j.saa.2005.05.002

Dhand, V., Soumya, L., Bharadwaj, S., Chakra, S., Bhatt, D., and Sreedhar, B. (2016). Green synthesis of silver nanoparticles using *Coffea arabica* seed extract and its antibacterial activity. *Mater. Sci. Eng. C* 58, 36–43. doi: 10.1016/j.msec.2015.08.018

D'Ostuni, V., Tristezza, M., De Giorgi, M. G., Rampino, P., Grieco, F., and Perrotta, C. (2016). Occurrence of *Listeria monocytogenes* and *Salmonella* spp. in meat processed products from industrial plants in Southern Italy. *Food Control* 62, 104–109.

Doudi, M., Naghsh, N., and Setorki, M. (2013). Comparison of the effects of silver nanoparticles on pathogenic bacteria resistant to beta-lactam antibiotics (ESBLs) as a prokaryote model and Wistar rats as a eukaryote model. *Med. Sci. Monit. Basic Res.* 19, 103–110. doi: 10.12659/MSMBR.883835

Durairaj, R., Amirulhusni, A. N., Palanisamy, N. K., Mohd-Zain, Z., and Ping, L. J. (2012). Antibacterial effect of silver nanoparticles on multi drug resistant *Pseudomonas aeruginosa. World Acad. Sci. Eng. Technol.* 6, 210–213. doi: 10.12659/MSMBR.883835

Fayaz, A. M., Balaji, K., Girilal, M., Yadav, R., Kalaichelvan, P. T., and Venketesan, R. (2010). Biogenic synthesis of silver nanoparticles and their synergistic effect with antibiotics: a study against Gram-positive and Gram-negative bacteria. *Nanomedicine* 6, 103–109. doi: 10.1016/j.nano.2009.04.006

Ferreira, V., Wiedmann, M., Teixeira, P., and Stasiewicz, M. (2014). *Listeria monocytogenes* persistence in food-associated environments: epidemiology, strain characteristics, and implications for public health. *J. Food Prot.* 77, 150–170. doi: 10.4315/0362-028X.JFP-13-150

Franci, G., Falanga, A., Galdiero, S., Palomba, L., Rai, M., Morelli, G., et al. (2015). Silver nanoparticles as potential antibacterial agents. *Molecules* 20, 8856–8874. doi: 10.3390/molecules20058856

Guzman, M., Dille, J., and Godet, S. (2012). Synthesis and antibacterial activity of silver nanoparticles against gram-positive and gram-negative bacteria. *Nanomedicine* 8, 37–45. doi: 10.1016/j.nano.2011.05.007

Hebeish, A., El-Rafie, M., El-Sheikh, M., Seleem, A. A., and El-Naggar, M. E. (2014). Antimicrobial wound dressing and anti-inflammatory efficacy of silver nanoparticles. *Int. J. Biol. Macromol.* 65, 509–515. doi: 10.1016/j.ijbiomac.2014.01.071

Heiman, K. E., Mody, R. K., Johnson, S. D., Griffin, P. M., and Gould, L. H. (2015). *Escherichia coli* O157 outbreaks in the United States, 2003–2012. *Emerg. Infect. Dis.* 21, 1293–1301. doi: 10.3201/eid2108.141364

Kaakoush, N. O., Castaño-Rodríguez, N., Mitchell, H. M., and Man, S. M. (2015). Global epidemiology of *Campylobacter* infection. *Clin. Microbiol. Rev.* 28, 687–720. doi: 10.1128/CMR.00006-15

Kar, D., Bandyopadhyay, S., Dimri, U., Mondal, D. B., Nanda, P. K., Das, A. K., et al. (2016). Antibacterial effect of silver nanoparticles and capsaicin against MDR-ESBL producing *Escherichia coli*: an in vitro study. *Asian Pac. J. Trop. Dis.* 6, 807–810. doi: 10.1016/S2222-1808(16)61135-0

Khalifa, R. A., Nasser, M. S., Gomaa, A. A., Osman, N. M., and Salem, H. M. (2013). Resazurin Microtiter Assay Plate method for detection of susceptibility of multidrug resistant *Mycobacterium tuberculosis* to second-line anti-tuberculous drugs. *Egypt. J. Chest Dis. Tuberc.* 62, 241–247. doi: 10.1016/j.ejcdt.2013.05.008

Kim, J. S., Kuk, E., Yu, K. N., Kim, J.-H., Park, S. J., Lee, H. J., et al. (2007). Antimicrobial effects of silver nanoparticles. *Nanomedicine* 3, 95–101. doi: 10.1016/j.nano.2006.12.001

Kim, K.-J., Sung, W. S., Suh, B. K., Moon, S.-K., Choi, J.-S., Kim, J. G., et al. (2009). Antifungal activity and mode of action of silver nano-particles on *Candida albicans. Biometals* 22, 235–242. doi: 10.1007/s10534-008-9159-2

Lara, H. H., Ayala-Nuñez, N. V., Ixtepan-Turrent, L., and Rodriguez-Padilla, C. (2010a). Mode of antiviral action of silver nanoparticles against HIV-1. *J. Nanobiotechnol.* 8:1. doi: 10.1186/1477-3155-8-1

Lara, H. H., Ayala-Núnez, N. V., Turrent, L. D. C. I., and Padilla, C. R. (2010b). Bactericidal effect of silver nanoparticles against multidrug-resistant bacteria. *World J. Microbiol. Biotechnol.* 26, 615–621. doi: 10.1007/s11274-009-0211-3

Lau, K., Zainin, N., Abas, F., and Rukayadi, Y. (2014). Antibacterial and sporicidal activity of *Eugenia polyantha* Wight against *Bacillus cereus* and *Bacillus subtilis*. *Int. J. Curr. Microbiol. Appl. Sci.* 3, 499–510.

Lee, K.-M., Runyon, M., Herrman, T. J., Phillips, R., and Hsieh, J. (2015). Review of *Salmonella* detection and identification methods: aspects of rapid emergency response and food safety. *Food Control* 47, 264–276. doi: 10.1016/j.foodcont.2014.07.011

Loo, Y. Y., Chieng, B. W., Nishibuchi, M., and Radu, S. (2012). Synthesis of silver nanoparticles by using tea leaf extract from *Camellia sinensis*. *Int. J. Nanomed.* 7, 4263–4267. doi: 10.2147/IJN.S33344

Martinez-Castanon, G., Nino-Martinez, N., Martinez-Gutierrez, F., Martinez-Mendoza, J., and Ruiz, F. (2008). Synthesis and antibacterial activity of silver nanoparticles with different sizes. *J. Nanopart. Res.* 10, 1343–1348. doi: 10.1007/s11051-008-9428-6

McNicholl, B. P., McGrath, J. W., and Quinn, J. P. (2007). Development and application of a resazurin-based biomass activity test for activated sludge plant management. *Water Res.* 41, 127–133. doi: 10.1016/j.watres.2006.10.002

Medda, S., Hajra, A., Dey, U., Bose, P., and Mondal, N. K. (2015). Biosynthesis of silver nanoparticles from *Aloe vera* leaf extract and antifungal activity against *Rhizopus* sp. and *Aspergillus* sp. *Appl. Nanosci.* 5, 875–880. doi: 10.1007/s13204-014-0387-1

Meire, M., Coenye, T., Nelis, H., and De Moor, R. (2012). Evaluation of Nd: YAG and Er: YAG irradiation, antibacterial photodynamic therapy and sodium hypochlorite treatment on *Enterococcus faecalis* biofilms. *Int. Endod. J.* 45, 482–491. doi: 10.1111/j.1365-2591.2011.02000.x

Morones, J. R., Elechiguerra, J. L., Camacho, A., Holt, K., Kouri, J. B., Ramírez, J. T., et al. (2005). The bactericidal effect of silver nanoparticles. *Nanotechnology* 16, 2346–2353. doi: 10.1088/0957-4484/16/10/059

Nadworny, P. L., Wang, J., Tredget, E. E., and Burrell, R. E. (2010). Anti-inflammatory activity of nanocrystalline silver-derived solutions in porcine contact dermatitis. *Int. J. Inflamm.* 7:13. doi: 10.1186/1476-9255-7-13

O'Bryan, C. A., Crandall, P. G., and Ricke, S. C. (2018). *Antimicrobial Resistance in Foodborne Pathogens. Food and Feed Safety Systems and Analysis*. New York, NY: Elsevier.

Oei, J. D., Zhao, W. W., Chu, L., DeSilva, M. N., Ghimire, A., Rawls, H. R., et al. (2012). Antimicrobial acrylic materials with in situ generated silver nanoparticles. *J. Biomed. Mater. Res. B Appl. Biomater.* 100, 409–415. doi: 10.1002/jbm.b.31963

Pal, S., Tak, Y. K., and Song, J. M. (2007). Does the antibacterial activity of silver nanoparticles depend on the shape of the nanoparticle? A study of the Gram-negative bacterium *Escherichia coli*. *Appl. Environ. Microbiol.* 73, 1712–1720. doi: 10.1128/AEM.02218-06

Paredes, D., Ortiz, C., and Torres, R. (2014). Synthesis, characterization, and evaluation of antibacterial effect of Ag nanoparticles against *Escherichia coli* O157: H7 and methicillin-resistant *Staphylococcus aureus* (MRSA). *Int. J. Nanomed.* 9, 1717–1729. doi: 10.2147/IJN.S57156

Patel, G., Huprikar, S., Factor, S. H., Jenkins, S. G., and Calfee, D. P. (2008). Outcomes of carbapenem-resistant *Klebsiella pneumoniae* infection and the impact of antimicrobial and adjunctive therapies. *Infect. Control Hosp. Epidemiol.* 29, 1099–1106. doi: 10.1086/592412

Rai, M., Deshmukh, S., Ingle, A., and Gade, A. (2012). Silver nanoparticles: the powerful nanoweapon against multidrug-resistant bacteria. *J. Appl. Microbiol.* 112, 841–852. doi: 10.1111/j.1365-2672.2012.05253.x

Selvam, K., Sudhakar, C., Govarthanan, M., Thiyagarajan, P., Sengottaiyan, A., Senthilkumar, B., et al. (2017). Eco-friendly biosynthesis and characterization of silver nanoparticles using *Tinospora cordifolia* (Thunb.) Miers and evaluate its antibacterial, antioxidant potential. *J. Radiat. Res. Appl. Sci.* 10, 6–12. doi: 10.1016/j.jrras.2016.02.005

Singh, R., Wagh, P., Wadhwani, S., Gaidhani, S., Kumbhar, A., Bellare, J., et al. (2013). Synthesis, optimization, and characterization of silver nanoparticles from *Acinetobacter calcoaceticus* and their enhanced antibacterial activity when combined with antibiotics. *Int. J. Nanomed.* 8, 4277–4290. doi: 10.2147/IJN.S48913

Sondi, I., and Salopek-Sondi, B. (2004). Silver nanoparticles as antimicrobial agent: a case study on *E. coli* as a model for Gram-negative bacteria. *J. Colloid Interface Sci.* 275, 177–182. doi: 10.1016/j.jcis.2004.02.012

Subashini, J., Khanna, V. G., and Kannabiran, K. (2014). Anti-ESBL activity of silver nanoparticles biosynthesized using soil *Streptomyces* species. *Bioprocess Biosyst. Eng.* 37, 999–1006. doi: 10.1007/s00449-013-1070-8

Tanwar, J., Das, S., Fatima, Z., and Hameed, S. (2014). Multidrug resistance: an emerging crisis. *Interdiscip. Perspect. Infect. Dis.* 2014: 541340. doi: 10.1155/2014/541340

Välimaa, A.-L., Tilsala-Timisjärvi, A., and Virtanen, E. (2015). Rapid detection and identification methods for *Listeria monocytogenes* in the food chain–a review. *Food Control* 55, 103–114. doi: 10.1016/j.foodcont.2015.02.037

WHO (2000). *Overcoming Antimicrobial Resistance*. Geneva: World Health Organization.

WHO (2014). *Initiative to Estimate the Global Burden of Foodborne Diseases: Information and Publications*. Geneva: World Health Organization.

Woh, P. Y., Thong, K. L., Behnke, J. M., Lewis, J. W., and Zain, S. N. M. (2017). Characterization of nontyphoidal *Salmonella* isolates from asymptomatic migrant food handlers in Peninsular Malaysia. *J. Food Prot.* 80, 1378–1383. doi: 10.4315/0362-028X.JFP-16-342

Yuan, Y.-G., Peng, Q.-L., and Gurunathan, S. (2017). Effects of silver nanoparticles on multiple drug-resistant strains of *Staphylococcus aureus* and *Pseudomonas aeruginosa* from mastitis-infected goats: an alternative approach for antimicrobial therapy. *Int. J. Mol. Sci.* 18:E569. doi: 10.3390/ijms18030569

Zainin, N., Lau, K., Zakaria, M., Radu, S., Razis, A., Faizal, A., et al. (2013). Antibacterial activity of *Boesenbergia rotunda* (L.) Mansf. A. extract against *Escherichia coli*. *Int. Food Res. J.* 20, 3319–3323.

Zarei, M., Jamnejad, A., and Khajehali, E. (2014). Antibacterial effect of silver nanoparticles against four foodborne pathogens. *Jundishapur J. Microbiol.* 7, 8720–8723. doi: 10.5812/jjm.8720

Zhang, M., Zhang, K., De Gusseme, B., Verstraete, W., and Field, R. (2014). The antibacterial and anti-biofouling performance of biogenic silver nanoparticles by *Lactobacillus fermentum*. *Biofouling* 30, 347–357. doi: 10.1080/08927014.2013.873419

Zhang, X.-F., Liu, Z.-G., Shen, W., and Gurunathan, S. (2016). Silver nanoparticles: synthesis, characterization, properties, applications, and therapeutic approaches. *Int. J. Mol. Sci.* 17:E1534. doi: 10.3390/ijms17091534

# 15

# Antimicrobial Potential of Epiphytic Bacteria Associated with Seaweeds of Little Andaman, India

*Perumal Karthick* and Raju Mohanraju*

*Department of Ocean Studies and Marine Biology, Pondicherry University, Port Blair, India*

***Correspondence:***
*Perumal Karthick*
*karthickmicrobes@gmail.com*

Seaweeds of the intertidal regions are a rich source of surface associated bacteria and are potential source of antimicrobial molecules. In the present study, 77 epiphytic isolates from eight different algae collected from Little Andaman were enumerated. On testing for their antimicrobial activities against certain pathogens twelve isolates showed positive and six of them showed significant antimicrobial inhibition zone against *Shigella boydii* type 1, *Shigella flexneri* type 2a, *Shigella dysenteriae* type 5, Enterotoxigenic *Escherichia coli* O115, Enteropathogenic *E. coli* serotype O114, *Vibrio cholera*; O1 Ogawa, *Aeromonas hydrophila, Klebsiella pneumoniae, Staphylococcus aureus.* Based on the activity these six isolates (G1C, G2C, G3C, UK, UVAD, and Tor1) were identified by 16S rRNA gene sequence and were found to belong to the phyla Firmicutes and Proteobacteria. Purified antimicrobial compounds obtained from these isolates were identified by GC-MS. Furan derivatives were identified from G2C *Pseudomonas stutzeri* KJ849834, UVAD *Alcanivorax dieselolei* KJ849833, UK *Vibrio* sp. KJ849837, Tor1 *Exiguobacterium profundum* KJ849838. While 2-Pyrrolidinone, Phenol, 2, 4-bis (1, 1-dimethylethyl) were from G3C *Vibrio owensii* KJ849836 and (1-Allylcyclopropyl) methanol from the extracts of G1C *Bacillus* sp. KJ849835. The results of the present study shows that these six potent isolates isolated from the seaweeds are found to be a source of antimicrobial compounds.

**Keywords:** ***Alcanivorax dieselolei*, Little Andaman, Furan, *Gracilaria corticata*, seaweeds**

## INTRODUCTION

Marine eukaryotes such as seaweeds are one of the primary producers which offers nutrient rich environment for microbial communities (Egan et al., 2008; Wahl, 2008). Biofilm forming bacteria isolated from the surface of seaweeds release certain compounds (Zheng et al., 2005) which serve as nutrient supplement for the algae (Croft et al., 2005), such compounds protect the host plant from the fouling communities (Rao et al., 2007). Surface associated marine organisms such as bacteria, fungi, diatoms, larval forms of marine invertebrate's have been reported to be associated with the thallus of seaweeds (Goecke et al., 2010; Burke et al., 2011; Murthy et al., 2016; Karthick and Mohan, 2017). Such host association particularly epiphytic bacteria are sources of certain natural compounds (Singh et al., 2011; Ali et al., 2012; Martin et al., 2014). Importance of microbial diversity of seaweeds, particularly bacterial genus are highly host specific with novel species, which have emerged from these algal environment (Goecke et al., 2013).

The secondary metabolites produced by these bacteria are highly recognized for their importance in the field of biomedical applications (Armstrong et al., 2001; Kelecom, 2002; Burgess et al., 2003). Antimicrobial activity of the epiphytic bacterial communities from seaweeds have been reported (Kanagasabhapathy et al., 2006, 2008; Vijayalakshmi et al., 2008; Ravisankar et al., 2013; Horta et al., 2014; Martin et al., 2014; Karthick et al., 2015a), similarly anti-diatom activity have also been observed by Kumar et al. (2011). In the Andaman Islands, luxuriant growth of all the three groups of seaweeds are available throughout the year. Some studies on taxonomy of seaweeds have been carried out in this region but information on the epiphytic interaction and its potentiality has not been undertaken. Based on the occurrence of seaweeds in Little Andaman and their bacterial association, the present study has been undertaken to describe the isolation of epiphytic bacterial, screening, optimization, evaluation and identification of potential isolates and their antimicrobial activity against different pathogens as test organisms.

## MATERIALS AND METHODS

### Isolation of Marine Bacteria

Eight different seaweeds representing all the three groups were handpicked from the intertidal region of Harminder Bay Bridge, Little Andaman, Andaman Islands, India. Among these, six species *Gracilaria corticata, Acanthophora spicifera* (red algae), *Ulva lactuca* (green algae), *Sargassum swartzii, Turbinaria ornata,* and *Padina tetrastromatica* (brown algae) are common and other two species *Mastophora rosea* (red algae) and *Caulerpa microphysa* (green algae) were found to be rare in occurrence in these islands. The collected samples were placed in sterile plastic bags and transported to the laboratory. These were washed thrice with autoclaved seawater to remove loosely bounded epiphytes, sand particles and other attached settlements on the surface of thallus. After rinsing, firmly attached epiphytic bacteria from thallus region were swabbed with sterile cotton buds and these were then swabbed on Zobell marine agar plate (Himedia). Plates were incubated for 5 days at 32°C (Lemos et al., 1985). After incubation, colonies were picked and restreaked for the isolation of individual colonies and the purity of the isolates were checked under the microscope for single morphology. These pure cultures obtained were stored at −20°C in marine broth supplemented with 20% glycerol.

### Antimicrobial Assay of Epiphytic Bacteria

The antagonistic activity of epiphytic bacteria obtained were studied on solid media by cross streaking and double-layer method described Lemos et al. (1985) and agar well diffusion method by Karthick et al. (2013b).

### Extraction of Antimicrobial Compounds

All the 77 isolates were cultured on 100ml marine broth, Luria broth and minimal media by modifying the methodology slightly by decreasing the incubation time and by increasing the temperature for obtaining better results. The culture broth was centrifuged at 10000 rpm for 30 s to remove the cells and cell free broth was extracted thrice with 100 ml of ethyl acetate. All the solvents were removed under reduced pressure at 40°C (Zheng et al., 2005). Crude extracts obtained were stored at −20°C until usage for the antimicrobial assay against targeted pathogens. Sterile media without culture being adjusted to pH 7 were used as control.

### Minimal Medium

All the potential isolates were cultured in inorganic salt medium referred to as minimal medium for the extraction of secondary metabolites (Jafarzade et al., 2013).

### Inoculum Preparation

Potential cultures were cultivated in 100 ml minimal medium supplemented with 3% NaCl, 1% glucose and 1% yeast extract as carbon and nitrogen sources in a 250 ml Erlenmeyer flask and incubated at 32°C for 24 h in an incubator shaker. Five milliliter of this culture was used as bacterial (Starter) culture (Jafarzade et al., 2013).

### Effect of pH

1 ml of starter cultures were grown with minimal media supplemented with 3% NaCl, 1% glucose, and 1% yeast extract prepared and inoculated with minimal media supplemented with 0.75% of sodium chloride, 1% of glucose and yeast extract for the production of antimicrobial compounds with various pH levels (6–8) at 32°C for 5 days. After incubation, supernatant was extracted three times with ethyl acetate (EtOAc). The sterile media without the culture adjusted to pH was used as control. The extracts were then tested for antimicrobial activity.

### Effect of Sodium Chloride Concentration

100 ml of minimal medium was dispensed into 250 ml Erlenmeyer flasks and sterilized. Yeast extract (1%) and glucose (1%) were filter sterilized and added as nitrogen and carbon sources just prior to inoculation. One milliliter of the starter culture was inoculated into the sterilized medium. Effect of salinity in the production of antimicrobial properties at various concentrations of sodium chloride ranging from 1 to 3% with constant pH of 7 at 32°C for 5 days was experimented. After incubation cell free supernatant was extracted three times with ethyl acetate (EtOAc). Sterile media without the inoculum adjusted with various concentration of sodium chloride was used as control (Jafarzade et al., 2013). The extracts were then tested for antimicrobial activity.

### Effect of Different Concentrations of Glucose and Yeast Extract

Effect of different concentration (1–3%) of glucose and yeast extract for the production of antimicrobial compound by the epiphytic bacterial isolates was studied using 1 ml of the starter culture inoculated into the minimal medium. Other parameters such as pH 7 and 0.75% sodium chloride were maintained at optimum level during the primary screening at

32°C for 5 days. After incubation supernatant was extracted three times with ethyl acetate (EtOAc). The sterile medium containing glucose, yeast extract and sodium chloride was used as control. The extracts were then tested for antimicrobial activity.

## Test Microorganisms

Eighteen bacterial pathogens namely *Escherichia coli* MTCC 443, *Klebsiella pneumoniae* MTCC 109, *Salmonella typhi* MTCC 733, *Staphylococcus aureus* MTCC 96, *Shigella flexneri* MTCC 1457, *Shigella flexneri* type2a 503004, *Shigella boydii* type 1 NK2379, *Shigella sonnei* NK4010, *Shigella dysenteriae* type 5 NK2440, Enterotoxic *E. coli* serotype 0115, Enteropathogenic *E. coli* serotype 0114, Shiga toxin producing *E. coli* serotype O157:H7 VT3, *Vibrio fluvialis* IDH 02036, *Vibrio parahaemolyticus* serovar O3: K6 K5030, *Vibrio cholera* O139, *Vibrio cholera* 01, Ogawa Eltor, *Aeromonas hydrophila* IDH1585, *Salmonella enterica* serovar typhi C6953 and three fungal strains *Aspergillus niger, Aspergillus flavus* and *Rhizopus* sp. were used for studying the antibacterial and antifungal assay.

## Determine Minimum Inhibitory Concentration of TLC Purified Metabolites

Minimum inhibitory concentration (MIC) of TLC purified metabolites of potential six isolates (G1C, G2C, G3C, UK, UVAD, and Torl) was tested against *Klebsiella pneumoniae* and *Staphylococcus aureus* and it was determined by well diffusion assay. 50 mg of TLC purified extracts was dissolved in 1 ml DMSO. 50 and 100 µl/ml concentration of 50 mg/ml concentration of purified extracts was transferred into the well prepared (9 mm) with well cutter. Gentamicin was used as a positive control and Dimethyl sulfoxide (DMSO) was used as a negative control. Growth inhibition zone formed after the incubation was examined with measuring the diameter (mm) and results were recorded. All the assay was performed in triplicates.

## Partial Purification and GC-MS Analysis

Concentrated fractions were fractioned by Thin Layer Chromatography (TLC) using Silica gel plates with different solvents in a ratio of 2:2:1 ethyl acetate, chloroform and methanol. Bands was scraped from the plates and screened for antimicrobial assay. Active fraction was collected and analyzed by Gas Chromatography and Mass spectrometry GC-MS QP 2010 Shimadzu Corp (Japan). One µl of purified fractioned extract was loaded into the DB-5 Column with Helium as a carrier gas at a flow rate of 1 ml/min. Split Injection mode of the ratio of 1:20 was adopted. Temperature programming was from 75°C for 2 min further increased to 175°C with 15°C/min and then increased up to 280°C at the rate of 5°C/min. Sample run time was maintained upto 10 min. The peaks representing mass to charge ratio characteristic of the antimicrobial fractions were compared with those in the mass spectrum of NIST library identifying the corresponding organic antimicrobial compounds.

## Phenotypic Characterization

Phenotypic characterization of all the seventy seven bacterial isolates were identified following as described in the Bergey's manual of systemic Bacteriology (Brenner et al., 2005).

## Molecular Identification by 16S rDNA Sequencing

Genomic DNA was prepared from the bacterial isolates by following the method of Mohandass et al. (2012). PCR amplification of 16S rRNA gene was conducted in a final volume of 25 µl with the bacterial consensus universal forward and reverse 16S rDNA primers 27F and 1492R (Lane, 1991). The reaction mixture contained 1x PCR buffer (Sigma, United States), 2.5 mM $MgCl_2$, 200 µM DNTP's, 1U of Taq DNA polymerase, 25 picomol of each forward and reverse oligonucleotide primers and approximately 20 ng of genomic DNA. The amplification profile consisted of an initial denaturation at 94°C for 3 min, followed by 35 cycles at 94°C for 1 min, 55°C for 1 min and 72°C for 1 min. This was followed by a final extension step of 72°C for 5 min. The samples were held at 4°C until further analysis. The PCR products were sequenced by an automated Sequencer (Applied Biosystems, Foster City, CA, United States) at the National Institute of Oceanography, Goa, India. The sequences were submitted to Gen Bank for which accession numbers were assigned.

## BLAST Search and Phylogenetic Analysis

The PINTAIL program (Ashelford et al., 2005) was used to check chimera formations. The partial 16S rRNA gene sequences of the potential isolates were compared with those available in the public databases. Identification upto the species level was determined by a 16S rDNA sequence similarity of more than 99% with that of the prototype sequence in GenBank. Sequence alignment and comparison were performed using the multiple sequence alignment program Clustal X 1.81 (Thompson et al., 1997). Sequences were edited manually to remove the gaps. Neighbor-joining method was employed to construct the Phylogenetic tree using MEGA4 software (Tamura et al., 2007) and the maximum likelihood method was adopted for calculating the evolutionary distance (Tamura et al., 2004).

## Bacterial Identification Based on Fatty Acid Methyl Ester (FAME)

Young pure cultures of SG107, 108, 114, 115, 120, and Tor6 were grown on Trypticase Soy Broth Agar (TSBA) for 24 or 48 h at 28°C. The Gas chromatographic analysis of whole cell fatty acid methyl ester (FAME) was performed for further identification and grouping of isolates. FAME extraction were performed using the standard procedures of extraction, purification, and methylation (Sasser, 1990). Fatty acid profiles generated were compared against an inbuilt Sherlock TSBA Library Version 6.0B [S/N 160284] (MIDI Inc., Newark, DE, United States). A similarity index of more than 0.500 was used for clustering of isolates at species level. Cellular fatty acid composition analysis was done at Regional center of Kochi, National Institute of Oceanography.

# RESULTS

## Identification of Epiphytic Bacterial Isolates

All the seventy seven cultivable epiphytic bacterial isolates obtained from the thallus of eight different seaweeds were plated on Marine agar. These isolates were purified and based on by phenotypic characterization were assigned to belong to the phylum Firmicutes and Proteobacteria (**Table 1**). Among these isolates, six of them (G1C, G2C, G3C, UK, UVAD, and Torl) showed wide range of activities against pathogens with an range of 10–30 mm zone of inhibition and were identified by partial 16S rRNA gene sequences (**Table 2**). The isolate G1C showed 99% similarity as *Bacillus* sp., G2C as *Pseudomonas stutzeri*, G3C and UK were identified as *Vibrio owensii* and *Vibrio* sp., respectively. The Isolate UVAD was identified as *Alcanivorax dieselolei* with 99% similarity and Torl strain was identified with 99.7% similarity as *Exiguobacterium profundum* (**Figure 1**).

Six other isolates showed moderate to less activity activities against the pathogens with a range of 5–10 mm zone of inhibition and were identified by FAME analysis. Among them three isolates SG107 as *Bacillus* sp., SG108 *Paenibacillus lentimorbus* and SG115 as *Bacillus sphaericus* belonged to phylum Firmicutes. The other three isolates *Pantoea agglomerans,* SG 120 was *Vibrio aestuarianus* and TR was identified as *Klebsiella pneumoniae ozaena* and were assigned to phylum Proteobacteria, SG114 (**Table 3**).

**TABLE 1** | List of bacterial isolates obtained from different seaweeds.

| S. no | Name of seaweeds | Number of isolates obtained |
|---|---|---|
| | **Red algae** | |
| 1 | *Gracilaria corticata* (J. Agardh) Agardh 1852 | 9 |
| 2 | *Acanthophora spicifera* (M.Vahl) Borgesen 1910 | 11 |
| 3 | *Mastophora rosea* (C.Agardh) Setchell 1943 | 6 |
| | **Green algae** | |
| 4 | *Ulva lactuca* Linn 1753 | 14 |
| 5 | *Caulerpa microphysa* (Weber van Bosse) J. Feldman | 6 |
| | **Brown algae** | |
| 6 | *Sargassum swartzii* (Turner) C. Agardh 1820 | 14 |
| 7 | *Turbinaria ornata* (Turner) J. Agardh 1848 | 7 |
| 8 | *Padina tetrastromatica* Hauck 1887 | 10 |

## Antimicrobial Activity of Epiphytic Bacteria

Antimicrobial activity for all the 77 bacterial isolates were tested by adopting three different methods (Agar overlay, cross streaking and agar well diffusion technique) against 21 pathogens. Among these larger zones of inhibition were observed in agar well diffusion assay and this assay was chosen for further antimicrobial activity test. All the isolates were cultured in three different media (marine broth, luria broth and minimal medium) among the medium used minimal media showed broad range of antimicrobial activity (**Table 4**). Based on the preliminary activity only six potential isolates (G1C, G2C, G3C, UK, UVAD, and Tor1) were optimized in minimal medium for the production of antimicrobial compounds.

## Zone of Inhibitory Activity With Optimized Bacterial Isolates

Isolate G1C showed strong inhibitory activity against *Shigella boydii* (31 mm), Enterotoxigenic *E. coli* (28 mm), Enteropathogenic *E. coli* and *Aeromonas hydrophila* (23 mm) and this higher inhibition zones were obtained with minimal media supplemented with 1 and 2% Sodium chloride, 1% of glucose and yeast extract with pH in the range of 7–8. Isolate G2C was more effective against Shigatoxin *E. coli* (26 mm), *Aeromonas hydrophila* and *Salmonella typhi* (24 mm) observed from minimal medium containing only 1% of sodium chloride, glucose and yeast extract with pH in the range of 6–7. Isolate G3C was effective against *Salmonella enterica* serovar *typhimurium* (26 mm), *Vibrio cholerae* Eltor and *Shigella dysenteriae* (24 mm) and antimicrobial activity was observed with minimal media with 1 and 2% of sodium chloride, glucose and 1% of yeast extract with pH in the range of 6–7. Isolate TOR1 exhibited broad range of antibacterial activity against *Klebsiella pneumoniae, Shigella dysenteriae* (31 mm), *Shigella sonnei* (25 mm). UVAD isolate showed maximum zone of inhibitory activity against *Staphylococcus aureus* (30 mm), *Salmonella enterica* serovar *typhimurium* (29 mm) and *Shigella dysenteriae* (27 mm) and isolate UK displayed maximum zone of inhibition against *Aeromonas hydrophila* (29 mm), *Shigella flexneri* 2A and *Shigella flexneri* (24 mm), respectively. All these six bacterial isolates showed maximum inhibitory activity against most of the tested pathogens (**Table 4**).

**TABLE 2** | 16S rRNA gene sequence identity of six potential bacterial isolates obtained from different seaweeds.

| Isolate | Seaweed | Accession number | Identified bacteria | % identity | Phylum |
|---|---|---|---|---|---|
| G1C | *Gracilaria corticata* | KJ849835 | *Bacillus* sp. | 99 | Firmicutes |
| G2C | *Gracilaria corticata* | KJ849834 | *Pseudomonas stutzeri* | 99 | Proteobacteria |
| G3C | *Gracilaria corticata* | KJ849836 | *Vibrio owensii* | 100 | Proteobacteria |
| UK | *Mastophora rosea* | KJ849837 | *Vibrio* sp. | 99 | Proteobacteria |
| UVAd | *Ulva lactuca* | KJ849833 | *Alcanivorax dieselolei* | 100 | Proteobacteria |
| Tor1 | *Turbinaria ornata* | KJ849838 | *Exiguobacterium profundum* | 100 | Firmicutes |

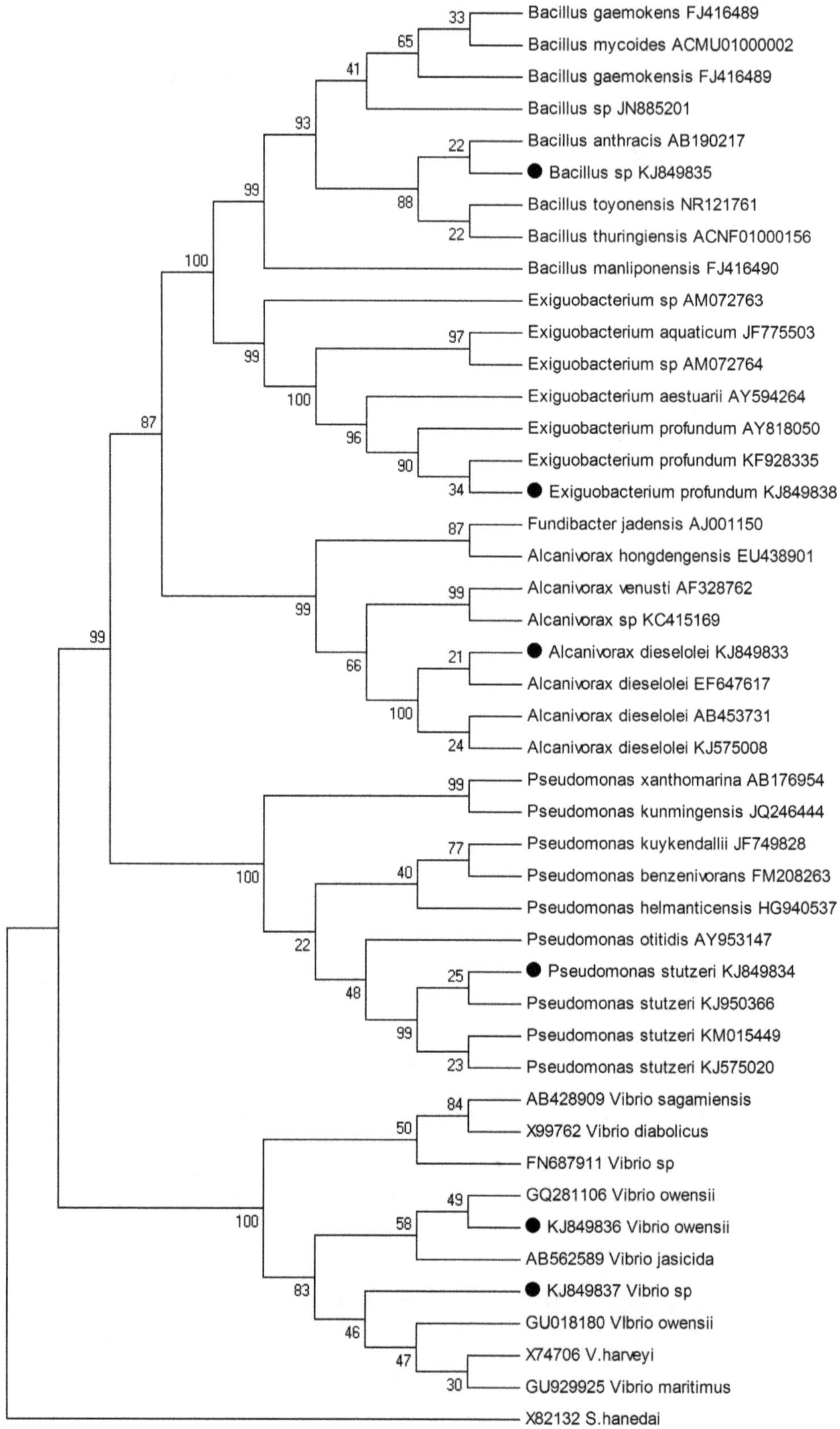


**FIGURE 1 |** Neighbor-joining phylogenetic tree based on 16S rRNA gene sequences showing the relationship of six potential strains with its closest neighbors. Bootstrap values (50%) are shown at branch points in value and *S. hanedai* X82132 were used as outgroup.

**TABLE 3 |** Comparison of cellular fatty acid composition of 6 moderate activity identified from brown algae (1) SG107 *Bacillus* sp, (2) SG108 *Paenibacillus lentimorbus*, (3) SG114 *Pantoea agglomerans*, (4) SG115 *Bacillus sphaericus*, (5) SG120 *Vibrio aestuarianus*, (6) Tor6 *Klebsiella pneumoniae ozaenae*.

| Fatty acid | SG107 | SG108 | SG114 | SG115 | SG120 | Tor6 |
|---|---|---|---|---|---|---|
| **Straight-chain saturated** | | | | | | |
| 14:00 | 1.99 | 3.03 | 0.81 | 0.75 | 5.10 | 9.31 |
| 15:00 | – | – | – | – | – | – |
| 16:00 | 8.01 | 16.57 | 35.53 | 1.62 | 18.34 | 31.44 |
| 17.00 | – | – | 0.27 | – | 0.44 | – |
| 18:00 | 1.08 | 2.48 | 1.40 | 0.29 | 1.33 | 0.78 |
| **Terminally branched saturated** | | | | | | |
| 13:0 iso | 0.28 | 0.43 | – | 0.11 | 0.07 | – |
| 14:0 iso | 8.56 | 4.58 | – | 5.67 | – | – |
| 15:0 iso | 27.43 | 22.96 | – | 52.57 | 0.08 | – |
| 16:0 iso | 6.11 | 2.93 | – | 10.20 | 0.19 | – |
| 17:0 iso | 4.50 | 5.57 | 0.13 | 3.75 | – | – |
| 18:0 iso | 0.28 | 0.28 | – | – | – | – |
| 19:0 iso | – | – | 0.51 | – | – | 0.50 |
| 15:0 anteiso | 26.59 | 24.25 | – | 9.39 | – | – |
| 17:0 anteiso | 5.57 | 4.65 | – | 2.98 | – | – |
| **Mono-unsaturated** | | | | | | |
| 16:1w7c alcohol | 2.11 | 0.69 | – | 6.43 | – | – |
| 16:1w11c | 4.55 | 6.41 | – | 1.71 | – | – |
| Sum of 18:2 w6,9c/18:0 ante | – | 0.3 | – | – | – | – |
| Sum of 18:1 w7c | – | 0.1 | – | – | 0.08 | – |
| Sum of 18:1w9c | – | 0.20 | – | 0.16 | 0.31 | – |

**TABLE 4 |** Antimicrobial activity of six potential epiphytic bacterial isolates.

| Clinical pathogens | G1C | G2C | G3C | UK | UVAD | Tor1 |
|---|---|---|---|---|---|---|
| *Shigella boydii* type 1 | + | ++ | ++ | +++ | +++ | ++ |
| *Shigella sonnei* | + | ++ | ++ | – | +++ | ++ |
| *Shigella flexneri* | ++ | – | – | +++ | ++ | ++ |
| *Shigella flexneri* type 2a | ++ | ++ | ++ | +++ | ++ | ++ |
| *Shigella dysenteriae* type 5 | – | ++ | ++ | +++ | +++ | +++ |
| *Salmonella typhi* | + | + | – | + | ++ | ++ |
| *Salmonella enterica* serovar typhi | + | ++ | +++ | + | ++ | + |
| *Escherichia coli* | ++ | + | + | ++ | – | – |
| Enterotoxigenic *Escherichia coli* O115 | ++ | ++ | ++ | +++ | ++ | + |
| Enteropathogenic *Escherichia coli* serotype O114 | ++ | ++ | ++ | +++ | ++ | + |
| Shiga toxin *Escherichia coli*O157:H7 | + | ++ | ++ | – | ++ | + |
| *Aeromonas hydrophila* | + | ++ | ++ | +++ | ++ | + |
| *Vibrio cholera*; O1 Ogawa | ++ | ++ | ++ | – | ++ | ++ |
| *Vibrio cholera* O139 | – | – | – | – | – | – |
| *Vibrio fluvialis* | – | – | – | ++ | + | – |
| *Vibrio parahaemolyticus* serovar O3: K6 | – | – | – | ++ | – | – |
| *Klebsiella pneumoniae* | + | + | ++ | | +++ | +++ |
| *Staphylococcus aureus* | + | + | ++ | +++ | +++ | ++ |

*(+) > 10 mm, (++) 10–20 mm, (+++), 20–30 mm, (–) No inhibition zone observed.*

## Identification of Compounds From Purified Extract

Cell free supernatant of the six potential isolates (G1C, G2C, G3C, UK, UVAD, and Tor1) that showed antimicrobial activity were purified by TLC. Results of minimum inhibitory concentration of TLC purified metabolites of all the six potential isolates at 50 mg/mL concentration diluted in 50 and 100 μl/ml concentration showed the positive results against *K. pneumoniae* and *S. aureus*. 50 μl/ml concentration of potential extracts exhibited inhibitory activity against the tested pathogens. Maximum zone of inhibition 10 mm was measured against *K. pneumoniae* by UK, UVAD, Tor1, G1C, and G3C extract at

100 μl concentration. 9 mm zone of inhibition was measured against *S. aureus* by 100 μl concentration of G2C, G3C, UK, and Tor1. Based on the inhibitory growth of bacteria at 50 μl concentration of purified metabolites, it can be concluded that minimum inhibitory concentration was observed at 2.5 mg/mL. Based on the activity purified compounds obtained from these six isolates were characterized and identified. Furan derivatives were found to be present in four of the isolates namely G2C *Pseudomonas stutzeri*, Tor1 *Exiguobacterium profundum*. UVAD *Alcanivorax dieselolei* and UK *Vibrio* sp. While 2-Pyrrolidinone, Phenol, 2, 4-bis (1, 1-dimethylethyl) were identified from the isolate G3C *Vibrio owensii* and (1-Allylcyclopropyl) methanol from G1C *Bacillus* sp.

## DISCUSSION

Seaweed biomass were found in large quantities in both intertidal and subtidal regions of all the regions of Andaman Island and in Little Andaman's (Karthick et al., 2013a,b). Good hemolytic activity in certain seaweeds of these Island has been reported recently (Punnam Chander et al., 2014). Besides these studies Karthick et al. (2015b) had reported on antimicrobial activity of certain seaweeds against pathogenic bacterial and fungal stains. Several authors suggested that macro algal associated bacteria were found to be an efficient producer of antimicrobial compounds (Burgess et al., 1999; Lee et al., 2006; Kanagasabhapathy et al., 2008; Karthick et al., 2015a; Ismail et al., 2016). On the other hand, certain brown algae also produced biologically active compounds which inhibited the settlement of bacterial colonies on the thallus (Nagayama et al., 2002).

In the present study it was observed that higher number of epiphytic bacteria were isolated from brown and red algae, certainly the proportion of higher isolates were from brown rather than green and red algae. On surface colonization non-pigmented bacterial isolates were found dominant in most of the seaweeds used in this study. Epiphytic bacteria from marine macro algae have been well studied in reference to their ecological importance with host organisms (Croft et al., 2005) with a dominance of Gram-negative bacteria. Similarly in the present study 46 Gram-negative bacterial isolates were isolated in comparison to 31 being Gram-positive. Bacteria belonging to genus the *Bacillus* were dominant with 20 isolates followed by other genus such as *Vibrio*, *Aeromonas*, and *Pseudomonas*.

Ravisankar et al. (2013) observed that the surface of the brown algae *Hypnea valentiae* and *Padina tetrastromatica* contained more number of non-pigmented bacterial colonies which are similar to our studies wherein 10 isolates were obtained from Padina *tetrastromatica*. Similar observations were observed in Tunisian waters, where 17 isolates were obtained from the thallus of *Ulva intestinalis* (Ali et al., 2010) and 10 isolates were reported from *Ulva lactuca* in Fiji waters, of which majority of the isolates were efficient antimicrobial producers (Kumar et al., 2011).

In the present study twelve isolates (15.7%) of the total 77 isolated exhibited antimicrobial activity and six isolates showed broad spectrum of activity against both bacterial and fungal pathogens. Similarly (Jayanth et al., 2002) isolated 14.52% of associated bacteria from the red algae *Gracilaria* with antagonistic properties against certain human pathogens. On the other hand 11% of associated bacteria isolated from seaweeds were reported to have antagonistic nature against *Bacillus subtilis, E. coli, S. aureus, Agrobacterium tumefaciens,* and *Saccharomyces cerevisiae* (Zheng et al., 2005).

The 16S rRNA sequences of bacterial isolates obtained from the surface of green algae *Ulva australis* and *Delisea pulchra,* belonged to the representative's classes of *Alpha* and *Gammaproteobacteria* and interestingly *Actinobacteria, Firmicutes,* and *Bacteroidetes* were observed as antimicrobial producers (Penesyan et al., 2009). Ali et al. (2012) on 16S rRNA sequence of the isolates obtained from the surface of coralline red algae *Jania rubens* found them belong to the group Proteobacteria. Similar observation made by Singh et al. (2015) also highlighted that bacterial isolates belonged to the order *Bacillales, Pseudomonadales, Alteromonadales,* and *Vibrionales* were dominant in green algae *Ulva lactuca, U. fasciata,* and red algae *Gracilaria corticata* and *G. dura.* In this study also it's evident that all the 77 bacterial isolates were closely related to the phylum Proteobacteria and Firmicutes. These findings substantiate that these groups are more specific to the macro algal surface. Similarly species belonging to the genera *Bacillus* and *Vibrio* were found to be strong antimicrobial producers colonizing more on the surface of seaweeds.

Genus *Bacillus* predominantly colonizes on the surface of marine niche and several studies have been reported *Bacillus* from different marine sources particularly associated with brown algae (Thakur and Anil, 2000) and from the thallus surface of different red algae (Kanagasabhapathy et al., 2008). Apart from their association with seaweeds *Bacillus* were previously isolated from sediments and seaweeds with antimicrobial properties (Prieto et al., 2012). So far, more than 800 metabolites have been reported with various biological activities from the *Bacillus* genera. Recently, cell free supernatant extracted from *Bacillus* associated with a nematode were found to be very effective against multidrug resistant *Staphylococcus aureus* (Susilowati et al., 2015). As observed in the present study one potential isolate G1C identified as *Bacillus* sp. showed remarkable activity against most of the tested pathogens, in particular against toxin producing pathogens like *Shigella boydii*, Enterotoxigenic *E. coli*, Shigatoxin *E. coli* Enteropathogenic *E. coli,* and *Aeromonas hydrophila* etc. Similarly SG107 *Bacillus* sp. and SG115 *Bacillus sphaericus* obtained from the brown algae *Sargassum swartzii* also showed moderate to less activity against few pathogens.

*Vibrios* being truly marine and they are widespread in various marine niches and are known to produce secondary metabolites for their survival. Earlier genus *Vibrio* sp., *Pseudomonas* sp., and *Bacillus pumilus* were reported to be a probiotic bacteria used in aquaculture (Hill et al., 2009). Kanagasabhapathy et al. (2008) reported that Vibrio strain isolated from red algae showed certain biological activities. In the present study, two potential *Vibrio* isolates GC3 *Vibrio owensii* and UK *Vibrio* sp. were obtained from the surface of red algae *Gracilaria corticata* and *Mastophora rosea,* respectively, and these isolates exhibited wider range of antimicrobial activity against most of the tested pathogens like *Salmonella typhi, Shigella dysenteriae, Vibrio cholerae,* and

*Staphylococcus aureus*. Similarly, Pawar et al. (2015) extracted antibacterial compounds from marine *Vibrio* sp. which were found to be active against numerous pathogens.

In our study of 14 bacterial isolates were obtained green algae *Ulva lactuca* among these one isolate UVAD *Alcanivorax dieselolei* was found to possess higher range of antimicrobial activity. Previously this species *Alcanivorax dieselolei* has been reported to be isolated from the deep sea sediment involved in degrading alcanes (Liu and Shao, 2005), and petroleum products (Brito et al., 2006). Ali et al. (2010) reported that two epiphytic bacteria obtained from green alga *U. intestinalis* showed potent antimicrobial activity. These studies suggest that green algae *Ulva* species attracts novel bacterial colonization on their surface with potential microbial communities and these isolates produce various compounds to protect the host from the predators and other micro and macro fouling colonization.

*Pseudomonas stutzeri* has been reported to have wide range of biological activity by the production of secondary metabolites. Previously *Pseudomonas stutzeri* isolated from fish gut exhibited antimicrobial activity (Uzair et al., 2008), hydrocarbon degradation (Vazquez et al., 2009), and reported as uncommon opportunistic pathogen (Park et al., 2013), controlling biofilm formation (Wu et al., 2016). In this study *Pseudomonas stutzeri* isolated from the red algae *Gracilaria corticata* produced antimicrobial compounds which showing potent activity against numerous toxin producing pathogens *S. aureus, Shigella boydii, S. flexneri 2A, S. dysenteriae, K. pneumoniae, Et. E. coli, St. E. coli, V. cholerae* Eltor, *A. hydrophila*.

Earlier *Exiguobacterium* sp. showed antimicrobial properties (Shatila et al., 2013) and this bacterium also known to produce antifouling compound and thus protected the host organisms from fouling communities (Jain et al., 2013). In the present study Tor1 *Exiguobacterium profundum* isolate obtained from *Turbinaria ornata,* showed antibacterial activity against clinical pathogens *S. aureus, Shigella boydii, S. flexneri, S. flexneri 2A, S. dysenteriae, K. pneumoniae, Et. E. coli,* and *St. E. coli.* The same genus was identified in earlier studies from different seaweeds occurring in different geographical locations showing various biological activities. In the present study 6 potential isolates obtained from seaweeds were found to be good antimicrobial producers. The same genus was identified in earlier studies from

**TABLE 5 |** Biological activities of associated bacteria isolated from seaweeds.

| Seaweeds | Associated bacteria | Biological activity | Reference |
|---|---|---|---|
| *Jania rubens* | *Bacillus firmicutes* | Antimicrobial | Ali et al., 2012 |
| *Plocamium telfairiae* | *Bacillus anthracis* | Antimicrobial | Kanagasabhapathy et al., 2008 |
| *Gelidium amansii* | *Bacillus cereus* | Antimicrobial | Kanagasabhapathy et al., 2008 |
| *Grateloupia filicina* | *Bacillus cereus* | Antimicrobial | Kanagasabhapathy et al., 2008 |
| *Porphyra yezoensis* | *Bacillus pumilus* | Antimicrobial | Kanagasabhapathy et al., 2008 |
| *Lomentaria catenata* | *Bacillus clausii* | Antimicrobial | Kanagasabhapathy et al., 2008 |
| *Chondrus ocellatus* | *Bacillus pumilus* | Antimicrobial | Kanagasabhapathy et al., 2008 |
| *Laminaria saccharina* | *Bacillus* sp. | Antibacterial | Wiese et al., 2009 |
| *Sargassum thunbergii* | *Bacillus* sp. | Antimicrobial | Zheng et al., 2005 |
| *Ulva lactuca* | *Bacillus* sp. | Antidiatom | Kumar et al., 2011 |
| *Padina pavonica* | *Bacillus pumilus* | Antimicrobial | Ismail et al., 2016 |
| *Sargassum* sp. | *Bacillus pumilus* | Antibacterial | Susilowati et al., 2015 |
| *Gracilaria corticata* | *Bacillus* sp. | Antimicrobial | In this study* |
| *Plocamium telfairiae* | *Vibrio* sp. | Antimicrobial | Kanagasabhapathy et al., 2008 |
| *Ulva lactuca* | *Vibrio* | Antidiatom | Kumar et al., 2011 |
| *Stoechospermum polypodioides* | *Vibrio* sp. | Antifouling | Jain et al., 2013 |
| *Laminaria saccharina* | *Vibrio* sp. | Antibacterial | Wiese et al., 2009 |
| *Stoechospermum polypodioides* | *Vibrio* sp. | Antifouling | Jain et al., 2013 |
| *Ulva reticulata* | *Vibrio* sp. | Antifouling | Harder et al., 2004 |
| *Gracilaria corticata* | *Vibrio owensii* | Antimicrobial | In this study* |
| *Mastophora rosea* | *Vibrio* sp. | Antimicrobial | In this study* |
| *Laminaria saccharina* | *Pseudomonas* sp. | Antibacterial | Wiese et al., 2009 |
| *Padina pavonica* | *Pseudomonas* sp. | Antimicrobial | Ismail et al., 2016 |
| *Sargassum sp* | *Pseudomonas koreensis* | Antioxidant | Pawar et al., 2015 |
| *Chaetomorpha media* | *Pseudomonas argentinensis* | Antioxidant | Pawar et al., 2015 |
| *Ulva reticulata* | *Pseudomonas stutzeri* | Antimicrobial | Dhanya et al., 2016 |
| *Gracilaria corticata* | *Pseudomonas stutzeri* | Antimicrobial | In this study* |
| *Stoechospermum polypodioides* | *Exiguobacterium* sp. | Antifouling | Jain et al., 2013 |
| *Turbinaria ornata* | *E. profundum* | Antimicrobial | In this study* |
| *Ulva lactuca* | *Alcanivorax dieselolei* | Antimicrobial | In this study* |

**Indicates the species identified in this study.*

different seaweeds occurring in different geographical locations showing various biological activities (**Table 5**).

In earlier studies Furan derivatives were reported to have antimicrobial properties (Kirilmis et al., 2009; Joshi et al., 2010; Ramasamy and Balasubramanian, 2012), cytotoxic agent (Wang et al., 2008) and were observed to have a wide range of biological activities like antiproliferative, antiviral, antifungal, immunosuppressive, anti-platelet, anti-oxidative, insecticidal, anti-inflammatory, anti-feedant, and cancer preventative activity (Venkateshwarlu et al., 2013). In our present study we have identified Furan compounds from four potential isolates (G2C, UVAD, Tor1, and UK). Apart from antimicrobial properties, these compounds are being used for other pharmacological properties (Bober et al., 2012). In this study G3C *Vibrio owensii* produced antimicrobial compounds such as 2-Pyrrolidinone, Phenol, 2, 4-bisdimetyl ethyl)-ester and Pyrrolo [1,2-a] pyrazine-1,4-dione. Earlier, these compounds were reported to have antimicrobial properties (Sutariya et al., 2012; Khatiwora et al., 2013; Padmavati et al., 2014; Dhanya et al., 2016). Marine *Vibrio* sp. is highly capable of producing Phenol, pyrrolo [1,2-a]pyrazine-1,4-dione, Pyrrolidinone derivative compounds containing pharmacological properties (Pawar et al., 2015). Based on earlier findings and as observed in the present study Vibrios are efficient producer of Phenol and Pyrrolidinone derivatives. In conclusion based on the findings of the present study, the compounds produced from six potential isolates (G1C, G2C, G3C, UK, UVAD, and Tor1) having effective antimicrobial properties, could be further studied for other activities. These isolates could prove to be potential candidates for the production of novel antimicrobial compounds in order to control the pathogens.

## AUTHOR CONTRIBUTIONS

PK designed the work, performed all the experiments, analyzed and wrote the manuscript. RM contributed the designation of research work and evaluated the manuscript.

## ACKNOWLEDGMENTS

The authors are greatful to Dr. C. Mohandass, Chief Scientist, National Institute of Oceanography (NIO), Goa for sequencing studies, Dr. Anas Abdulaziz, Scientist, Marine Microbial Reference Facility (NIO) RC, Kochi, Dr. R. Babu Rajendran, Professor, Department of Environmental Biotechnology, Bharathidasan University for GC-MS facilities. The authors also thank personally to their colleagues Dr. K. N. Murthy, Dr. C. H. Ramesh, Dr. Sumantha Narayana for their support during field collection and Pondicherry University authorities for providing the facilities.

## REFERENCES

Ali, A. I., Bour, M. E., Ktari, L., Bolhuis, H., Ahmed, A., Boudabbous, A., et al. (2012). *Jania rubens*-associated bacteria: molecular identification and antimicrobial activity. *J. Appl. Phycol.* 24, 525–534. doi: 10.1007/s10811-011-9758-0

Ali, I. B., Ktari, L., Bolhuis, H., Boudabbous, A., Stal, L. J., and Bour, M. E. L. (2010). *Ulva intestinalis* associated bacteria: molecular identification and antimicrobial potential. *Rap. Comm. Int. Mer. Medit.* 39:372.

Armstrong, E., Yan, L., Boyd, K. G., Wright, P. C., and Burgess, J. G. (2001). The symbiotic role of marine microbes on living surfaces. *Hydrobiologia* 461, 37–40. doi: 10.1023/A:1012756913566

Ashelford, K. E., Chuzhanova, N. A., Fry, J. C., Jones, A. J., and Weightman, A. J. (2005). At least 1 in 20 16S rRNA sequence records currently held in public repositories is estimated to contain substantial anomalies. *Appl. Environ. Microbiol.* 71, 7724–7736. doi: 10.1128/AEM.71.12.7724-7736.2005

Bober, L., Kawczak, P., and Baczek, T. (2012). Pharmacological classification and activity evaluation of furan and thiophene amide derivatives applying semi-empirical ab initio molecular modeling methods. *Int. J. Mol. Sci.* 13, 6665–6678. doi: 10.3390/ijms13066665

Brenner, D. J., Krieg, N. R., and Staley, J. T. (eds). (2005). *Bergeys Manual of Systematic Bacteriology*. New York, NY: Springer.

Brito, E. M., Guyoneaud, R., Urizza, M., Ranchou-Peyruse, A., Verbaere, A., Crapez, M. C., et al. (2006). Characterization of hydrocarbonoclastic bacterial communities from mangrove sediments in Guanabara Bay, Brazil. *Res. Microbiol.* 157, 752–762. doi: 10.1016/j.resmic.2006.03.005

Burgess, J. G., Boyd, K. G., Armstrong, E., Jiang, Z., Yan, L., Berggren, M., et al. (2003). The development of a marine natural product-based antifouling paint. *Biofouling* 19, 197–205. doi: 10.1080/0892701031000061778

Burgess, J. G., Mearns-Spragg, A., Jordan, E. M., Bregu, M., and Boyd, K. G. (1999). Microbial antagonism: a neglected avenue of natural products research. *J. Biotechnol.* 70, 27–32. doi: 10.1016/S0168-1656(99)00054-1

Burke, C., Thomas, T., Lewis, M., Steinberg, P., and Kjelleberg, S. (2011). Composition, uniqueness and variability of the epiphytic bacterial community of the green alga *Ulva australis*. *ISME J.* 5, 590–600. doi: 10.1038/ismej.2010.164

Croft, M. T., Lawrence, A. D., Raux-Deery, E., Warren, M. J., and Smith, A. G. (2005). Algae acquire vitamin B12 through a symbiotic relationship with bacteria. *Nature* 438, 90–93. doi: 10.1038/nature04056

Dhanya, K. I., Swati, V. I., Vanka, K. S., and Osborne, W. J. (2016). Antimicrobial activity of *Ulva reticulata* and its endophytes. *J. Ocean Univ. China* 15, 363–369.

Egan, S., Thomas, T., and Kjelleberg, S. (2008). Unlocking the diversity and biotechnological potential of marine surface associated microbial communities. *Curr. Opin. Microbiol.* 11, 219–225. doi: 10.1016/j.mib.2008.04.001

Goecke, F., Labes, A., Wiese, J., and Imhoff, J. F. (2010). Chemical interactions between marine macroalgae and bacteria. *Mar. Ecol. Prog. Ser.* 409, 267–299. doi: 10.3354/meps08607

Goecke, F., Thiel, V., Wiese, J., Labes, A., and Imhoff, J. (2013). Algae as an important environment for bacteria – phylogenetic relationships among new bacterial species isolated from algae. *Phycologia* 52, 14–24. doi: 10.2216/12-24.1

Harder, T., Dobretsov, S., and Qian, P.-Y. (2004). Waterborne polar macromolecules act as algal antifoulants in the seaweed *Ulva reticulata*. *Mar. Ecol. Prog. Ser.* 274, 131–141. doi: 10.3354/meps274133

Hill, J. E., Baiano, J. C. F., and Barnes, A. C. (2009). Isolation of a novel strain of *Bacillus pumilus* from penaeid shrimp that is inhibitory against marine pathogens. *J. Fish Dis.* 32, 1007–1016. doi: 10.1111/j.1365-2761.2009.01084.x

Horta, A., Pinteus, S., Alves, C., Fino, N., Silva, J., Fernandez, S., et al. (2014). Antioxidant and antimicrobial potential of the *Bifurcaria bifurcata* epiphytic bacteria. *Mar. Drugs* 12, 1676–1689. doi: 10.3390/md12031676

Ismail, A., Ktari, L., Ahmed, M., Bolhuis, H., Boudabbous, A., Stal, L. J., et al. (2016). Antimicrobial activities of bacteria associated with the brown alga *Padina pavonica*. *Front. Microbiol.* 7:1072. doi: 10.3389/fmicb.2016.01072

Jafarzade, M., Shayesteh, F., Usup, G., and Ahmad, A. (2013). Influence of culture conditions and medium composition on the production of antibacterial compounds by marine *Serratia* sp. WPRA3. *J. Microbiol.* 51, 373–379. doi: 10.1007/s12275-013-2440-2

Jain, S. C., Sivakumar, A. J., and Pandian, P. M. (2013). Surface associated bacteria of marine algae in Kovalam beach, Chennai, had screened for its antifouling activity. *Indian J. Geomarine Sci.* 42, 498–502.

Jayanth, K., Jeyasekaran, G., and Shakila, R. J. (2002). Isolation of marine bacteria, antagonistic to human pathogens. *Ind. J. Mar. Sci.* 31, 39–44.

Joshi, S. D., Ashwini, J., and Gadaginamath, G. S. (2010). Synthesis and antimicrobial evaluation of some new pyrrolylnaphtho [2, 1-b] furan derivatives. *Ind. J. Pharm. Educ. Res.* 44, 148–155.

Kanagasabhapathy, M., Sasaki, H., Haldar, S., Yamasaki, S., and Nagata, S. (2006). Antibacterial activities of marine epibiotic bacteria isolated from brown algae of Japan. *Ann. Microbiol.* 56, 167–173. doi: 10.1007/BF03175000

Kanagasabhapathy, M., Sasaki, H., and Nagata, S. (2008). Phylogenetic identification of epibiotic bacteria possessing antimicrobial activities isolated from red algal species of Japan. *World J. Microbiol. Biotechnol.* 24, 2315–2321. doi: 10.1007/s11274-008-9746-y

Karthick, P., and Mohan, P. M. (2017). Associated epiphytic faunal distribution on brown algae *Sargassum wightii* Greville ex J.Agardh, in the environments, off South Andaman. *J. Terr. Mar. Res.* 1, 41–44.

Karthick, P., Mohanraju, R., Murthy, K. N., and Ramesh, C. H. (2013a). Seaweed potential of Little Andaman, India. *Seaweed Res. Utilin.* 35, 17–21.

Karthick, P., Mohanraju, R., Ramesh, C. H., Murthy, K. N., and Narayana, S. (2013b). Distribution and diversity of seaweeds in North and South Andaman Island. *Seaweed Res. Utilin.* 35, 8–16.

Karthick, P., Mohanraju, R., Mohandass, C., and Rajasabapathy, R. (2015a). Antimicrobial activity of Serratia sp isolated from the coralline red algae *Amphiroa anceps. Indian J. Geomarine Sci.* 44, 1857–1866.

Karthick, P., Mohanraju, R., Murthy, K. N., and Ramesh, C. H. (2015b). Antibacterial activity of seaweeds collected from South Andaman, India. *J. Algal Biomass Util.* 6, 33–36.

Kelecom, A. (2002). Secondary metabolites from marine microorganisms. *An. Acad. Bras. Cienc.* 74, 151–170. doi: 10.1590/S0001-37652002000100012

Khatiwora, E., Adsula, V. B., Kulkarni, M., Deshpande, N. R., and Kashalkar, R. V. (2013). Isolation and characterization of substituted dibutyl phthalate from Ipomoea carnea stem. *Der Pharma Chemica* 5, 5–10.

Kirilmis, C., Koca, M., Servi, S., and Gur, S. (2009). Synthesis and antimicrobial activity of dinaphtho[2,1-b]furan-2-yl-methanone and their oxime derivatives. *Turkish J. Chem.* 33, 375–384.

Kumar, V., Rao, D., Thomas, T., Kjelleberg, S., and Egan, S. (2011). Antidiatom and antibacterial activity of epiphytic bacteria isolated from *Ulva lactuca* in tropical waters. *World J. Microbiol. Biotechnol.* 27, 1543–1549. doi: 10.1007/s11274-010-0606-1

Lane, D. J. (1991). "16S/23S rRNA sequencing," in *Nucleic Acid Techniques in Bacterial Systematics*, eds E. Stackebrandt and M. Goodfellow (New York, NY: John Wiley & Sons Inc), 115–175.

Lee, Y. K., Jung, H. J., and Lee, H. K. (2006). Marine bacteria associated with the Korean brown alga, *Undaria pinnatifida. J. Microbiol.* 44, 694–698.

Lemos, M. L., Toranzo, A. E., and Barja, J. L. (1985). Antibiotic activity of epiphytic bacteria isolated from intertidal seaweeds. *Microbial. Ecol.* 11, 149–163. doi: 10.1007/BF02010487

Liu, C., and Shao, Z. (2005). *Alcanivorax dieselolei* sp. nov., a novel alkane-degrading bacterium isolated from sea water and deep-sea sediment. *Int. J. Syst Evol. Microbiol.* 55, 1181–1186. doi: 10.1099/ijs.0.63443-0

Martin, M., Portetelle, D., Michel, G., and Vandenbol, M. (2014). Microorganisms living on macroalgae: diversity, interactions, and biotechnological applications. *Appl Microbiol. Biotechnol.* 98, 2917–2935. doi: 10.1007/s00253-014-5557-2

Mohandass, C., Rajasabapathy, R., Ravindran, C., Colaco, A., and Meena, R. M. (2012). Bacterial diversity and their adaptations in the shallow water hydrothermal vent at D. Joao de Castro Seamount (DJCS), Azores, Portugal. *Cah. Biol. Mar.* 53, 65–76.

Murthy, K. N., Mohanraju, R., Karthick, P., and Ramesh, C. H. (2016). Phenotypic and molecular characterization of epiphytic Vibrios from the marine macro algae of Andaman Islands, India. *Indian J. Mar. Sci.* 45, 304–309.

Nagayama, K., Iwamura, Y., Shibata, T., Hirayama, I., and Nakamura, T. (2002). Bactericidal activity of phlorotannins from the brown alga *Ecklonia kurome. J. Antimicrob. Chemother.* 50, 889–893. doi: 10.1093/jac/dkf222

Padmavati, A. R., Abinaya, B., and Pandian, S. K. (2014). Phenol, 2,4-bis(1,1-dimethylethyl) of marine bacterial origin inhibits quorum sensing mediated biofilm formation in the uropathogen *Serratia marcescens. Biofouling* 30, 1111–1122. doi: 10.1080/08927014.2014.972386

Park, S. W., Back, J. H., Lee, S. W., Song, J. H., Shin, C. H., Kim, G. E., et al. (2013). Successful antibiotic treatment of *Pseudomonas stutzeri*-induced peritonitis without peritoneal dialysis catheter removal in continuous ambulatory peritoneal dialysis. *Kidney Res. Clin. Pract.* 32, 81–83. doi: 10.1016/j.krcp.2013.04.004

Pawar, R., Mohandass, C., Sivaperumal, E., Sabu, E., Rajasabapathy, R., and Jagtap, T. (2015). Epiphytic marine pigmented bacteria: a prospective source of antioxidants. *Braz. J. Microbiol.* 46, 29–39. doi: 10.1590/S1517-838246120130353

Penesyan, A., Marshall-Jones, Z., Holmstrom, C., Kjelleberg, S., and Egan, S. (2009). Antimicrobial activity observed among cultured marine epiphytic bacteria reflects their potential as a source of new drugs. *FEMS Microbiol. Ecol.* 69, 113–124. doi: 10.1111/j.1574-6941.2009.00688.x

Prieto, M., Sullivan, L. O., McLoughlin, P., Hughes, H., O'Connor, P. M., and Gardiner, G. E. (2012). Assessment of the bacteriocinogenic potential of marine bacteria reveals lichenicidin production by seaweed-derived *Bacillus* spp. *Mar. Drugs* 10, 2280–2299. doi: 10.3390/md10102280

Punnam Chander, M., Sachithanandam, V., and Vijayachari, P. (2014). Antimicrobial and hemolytic activity of seaweed *Padina gymnospora* from South Andaman, Andaman and Nicobar Islands of India. *Int. J. Curr. Microbiol. App. Sci.* 3, 364–369.

Ramasamy, M., and Balasubramanian, U. (2012). Identification of bioactive compounds and antimicrobial activity of marine clam *Anadara granosa* (LINN.). *Int. J. Sci. Nat.* 3, 263–266.

Rao, D., Webb, J. S., Holmstrom, C., Case, R., Low, A., Steinberg, P., et al. (2007). Low densities of epiphytic bacteria from the marine alga *Ulva australis* inhibit settlement of fouling organisms. *Appl. Environ. Microbiol.* 73, 7844–7852. doi: 10.1128/AEM.01543-07

Ravisankar, A., Gnanambal, M. E., and Sundaram, L. R. (2013). A newly isolated *Pseudomonas* sp., epibiotic on the seaweed, *Padina tetrastromatica*, off Southeastern Coast of India, reveals antibacterial action. *Appl. Biochem. Biotechnol.* 171, 1968–1985. doi: 10.1007/s12010-013-0473-y

Sasser, M. (1990). "Identification of bacteria through fatty acid analysis," in *Methods in Phytobacteriology*, eds Z. Klement, K. Rudolph, and D. C. Sands (Budapest: Akademiai Kiado).

Shatila, F., Yusef, H., and Beirut, H. H. (2013). Pigment production by *Exiguobacterium aurantiacum* FH, a novel Lebanese isolate. *Int. J. Curr. Microbiol. App. Sci.* 2, 176–191.

Singh, R. P., Baghel, R. S., Reddy, C. R. K., and Jha, B. (2015). Effect of quorum sensing signals produced by seaweed-associated bacteria on carpospore liberation from *Gracilaria dura. Front. Plant Sci.* 6:117. doi: 10.3389/fpls.2015.00117

Singh, R. P., Mantri, V. A., Reddy, C. R. K., and Jha, B. (2011). Isolation of seaweed-associated bacteria and their morphogenesis-inducing capability in axenic cultures of the green alga *Ulva fasciata. Aquat. Biol.* 12, 13–21. doi: 10.3354/ab00312

Susilowati, R., Sabdono, A., and Widowati, I. (2015). Isolation and characterization of bacteria associated with brown algae *Sargassum* spp. from Panjang Island and their antibacterial activities. *Procedia Environ. Sci.* 23, 240–246. doi: 10.1016/j.proenv.2015.01.036

Sutariya, S. D., Parmar, K. A., and Kharadi, G. J. (2012). Synthesis, spectral studies and antibacterial screening of some novel derivatives of 2-pyrrolidinones based on Schiff base. *Der Chem. Sin.* 3, 854–859.

Tamura, K., Dudley, J., Nei, M., and Kumar, S. (2007). MEGA4: molecular evolutionary genetics analysis (MEGA) software version 4.0. *Mol. Biol. Evol.* 24, 1596–1599. doi: 10.1093/molbev/msm092

Tamura, K., Nei, M., and Kumar, S. (2004). Prospects for inferring very large phylogenies by using the neighbor-joining method. *Proc. Natl. Acad. Sci. U.S.A.* 101, 11030–11035. doi: 10.1073/pnas.0404206101

Thakur, N. L., and Anil, A. C. (2000). Antibacterial activity of the sponge Ircinia ramosa: importance of its surface-associated bacteria. *J. Chem. Ecol.* 26, 57–71. doi: 10.1023/A:1005485310488

Thompson, J. D., Plewniak, F., Jeanmougin, F., and Higgins, D. G. (1997). The Clustal X windows interface: flexible strategies for multiple sequence alignment aided by quality analysis tools. *Nucleic Acids Res.* 24, 4876–4882. doi: 10.1093/nar/25.24.4876

Uzair, B., Ahmed, N., and Edwards, D. H. (2008). The isolation, purification and biological activity of a novel antibacterial compound produced by *Pseudomonas stutzeri*. *FEMS Microbiol. Lett.* 279, 243–250. doi: 10.1111/j.1574-6968.2007.01036.x

Vazquez, S., Nogales, B., Ruberto, L., Hernandez, E., Christie-Oleza, J., Lo Balbo, A., et al. (2009). Bacterial community dynamics during bioremediation of diesel oil-contaminated Antarctic soil. *Microb. Ecol.* 57, 598–610. doi: 10.1007/s00248-008-9420-9

Venkateshwarlu, T., Ravindernath, A., and Chennapragada, K. P. (2013). Synthesis and antimicrobial activity of novel benzo[b]furan derivatives. *Der Pharma Chemica* 5, 229–234.

Vijayalakshmi, S., Santhanaramasamy, M., Murugesh, S., and Murugan, A. (2008). Isolation and screening of marine associated bacteria from Tamil Nadu, Southeast coast of India for potential antibacterial activity. *Ann. Microbiol.* 58, 605–609. doi: 10.1007/BF03175564

Wahl, M. (2008). Ecological lever and interface ecology: epibiosis modulates the interactions between host and environment. *Biofouling* 24, 427–438. doi: 10.1080/08927010802339772

Wang, J., Zhang, H., Yang, X., Zhou, Y., Wang, H., and Bai, H. (2008). HS071, a new furan-type cytotoxic metabolite from *Streptomyces* sp. HS-HY-071. *J. Antibiot.* 61, 623–626. doi: 10.1038/ja.2008.82

Wiese, J., Thiel, V., Nagel, K., Staufenberger, T., and Imhoff, J. F. (2009). Diversity of antibiotic-active bacteria associated with the brown alga *Laminaria saccharina* from the Baltic Sea. *Mar. Biotechnol.* 11, 287–300. doi: 10.1007/s10126-008-9143-4

Wu, S., Liu, G., Jin, W., Xiu, P., and Sun, C. (2016). Antibiofilm and anti-Infection of a marine bacterial exopolysaccharide against *Pseudomonas aeruginosa*. *Front. Microbiol.* 7:102. doi: 10.3389/fmicb.2016.00102

Zheng, L., Han, X., Chen, H., Lin, W., and Yan, X. (2005). Marine bacteria associated with marine macroorganisms: the potential antimicrobial resources. *Ann. Microbiol.* 55, 119–124.

16

# The Emergence of Novel Sequence Type Strains Reveals an Evolutionary Process of Intraspecies Clone Shifting in ICU-Spreading Carbapenem-Resistant *Klebsiella pneumoniae*

*Dongdong Zhao[1,2,3]†, Qiucheng Shi[4]†, Dandan Hu[1,2,3], Li Fang[1,2,3], Yihan Mao[1,2,3], Peng Lan[1,2,3], Xinhong Han[1,2,3], Ping Zhang[1,2,3], Huangdu Hu[1,2,3], Yanfei Wang[1,2,3], Jingjing Quan[1,2,3], Yunsong Yu[1,2,3] and Yan Jiang[1,2,3]**

[1] Department of Infectious Diseases, Sir Run Run Shaw Hospital, Zhejiang University School of Medicine, Hangzhou, China, [2] Key Laboratory of Microbial Technology and Bioinformatics of Zhejiang Province, Hangzhou, China, [3] Regional Medical Center for National Institute of Respiratory Diseases, Sir Run Run Shaw Hospital, Zhejiang University School of Medicine, Hangzhou, China, [4] Department of Clinical Laboratory, National Clinical Research Center for Child Health, The Children's Hospital, Zhejiang University School of Medicine, Hangzhou, China

***Correspondence:**
Yan Jiang
jiangy@zju.edu.cn

† These authors have contributed equally to this work and share first authorship

Carbapenem-resistant *Klebsiella pneumoniae* (CRKP) is an urgent public health problem worldwide, and its rapid evolution in the clinical environment has been a major concern. A total of 99 CRKP isolates spreading in the intensive care unit (ICU) setting were included and subjected to whole-genome sequencing, and their sequence types (STs), serotype loci, and virulence determinants were screened based on genome data. The phylogenetic structure was reconstructed based on the core genome multilocus sequence typing method. Regions of recombination were assessed. Biofilm formation, serum resistance assays, and a *Galleria mellonella* infection model were used to evaluate strain virulence. A novel ST, designated ST4496, emerged in the ICU and spread for 6 months before its disappearance. ST4496 was closely related to ST11, with only a single-allele variant, and ST11 is the most dominant clinical clone in China. Recombination events occurred at capsule biosynthesis loci and divided the strains of ST11 and its derivative ST4496 into three clusters, including ST11-KL47, ST11-KL64, and ST4496-KL47. The phylogenetic structure indicated that ST11-KL47 was probably the origin of ST11-related strain evolution and presented more diversity in terms of both sequence similarity and phenotypes. ST4496-KL47 cluster strains presented less virulence than ST11-KL64, which was probably one of the factors preventing the former from spreading widely. In conclusion, ST4496-KL47 was probably derived from ST11-KL47 via intraspecies shifting but was less competitive than ST11-KL64, which also evolved from ST11-KL47 and developed increased virulence via capsule biosynthesis locus recombination. ST11-KL64 has the potential to be the predominant CRKP clone in China.

**Keywords: virulence, capsule biosynthesis locus, intraspecies shifting, recombination, carbapenem-resistant**

## INTRODUCTION

*Klebsiella pneumoniae* is a common cause of community- and hospital-acquired infections (Paczosa and Mecsas, 2016; Bengoechea and Sa Pessoa, 2019). In recent decades, carbapenem-resistant *K. pneumoniae* (CRKP) has emerged as a major clinical concern worldwide with few treatment options (Munoz-Price et al., 2013; Grundmann et al., 2017). More worrisome is the emergence of hypervirulence-associated genetic determinants in CRKP, which may lead to even higher mortality and morbidity (Gu et al., 2018).

The capsule of *K. pneumoniae* confers resistance to antimicrobial peptides, phagocytosis, and complement-mediated killing and contributes to its ability to thrive in the environment or in a host. More than 77 capsular types (K-types) have been reported in clinical isolates of *K. pneumoniae*, and recombination events involving the capsule biosynthesis (cps) region are frequently observed within several dominant sequence type (ST) clones, such as CG258 (ST258, ST512, ST11, etc.) isolates (Wyres et al., 2015; Chiarelli et al., 2020). In China, ST11 is believed to be the most dominant CRKP clone, with a prevalence greater than 60% (Zhang et al., 2017; Wang et al., 2018). The diversity of K-type capsule polysaccharides is one of the important forces driving the extensive evolution of these bacteria and has been proven to be associated with virulence (Zhao et al., 2020; Zhou et al., 2020). Enhanced virulence may lead to subclonal replacement and thus to great challenges in clinical management and infection control (Zhou et al., 2020).

In this study, we observed an intraspecies shift in CRKP at our center, and we attempted to decipher the underlying mechanisms by determining the genetic and phenotypic diversity of related groups.

## MATERIALS AND METHODS

### CRKP Isolates

A common CRKP surveillance was conducted from January 1, 2017, at Sir Run Run Shaw Hospital, Zhejiang, China, which is a 1,200-bed tertiary medical center. A novel ST closely related to ST11 with a single-locus variant in *mdh* (allele: 1, C59T) was identified. Sixteen isolates with the novel ST (designated ST4496) were collected between January 2017 and May 2017. A rough *mdh* allele polymerase chain reaction analysis and subsequent sequencing screening were then applied to the isolates that were collected 2 months before January 2017 and after May 2017. Only two isolates from late December 2016 were found to harbor the novel *mdh* variant and were later identified as ST4496 by sequencing all seven alleles.

Altogether, 18 non-duplicated ST4496 CRKP isolates were detected, and the clinical data of the corresponding patients were collected from electronic medical records. All of the contemporaneous (from January to May 2017) CRKP isolates from the same intensive care unit (ICU) ward were collected and sequenced, resulting in a total of 99 CRKP isolates.

Species identification was performed by using matrix-assisted laser desorption ionization time-of-flight mass spectrometry (Bruker Daltonics, Bremen, Germany) and verified by genome sequencing. Isolates were considered carbapenem-resistant if the minimal inhibitory concentrations (MICs) of meropenem or imipenem were $\geq$ 4 mg/L or the MIC of ertapenem was $\geq$ 2, in accordance with the Clinical and Laboratory Standards Institute guidelines (2017).

The project was approved by the Ethical Review Committee of Sir Run Run Shaw Hospital (no. 20191231-20).

### Whole-Genome Sequencing

Genomic DNA was extracted using the QIAamp DNA Minikit (Qiagen, Hilden, Germany) according to the manufacturer's recommendations and subsequently sequenced on the Illumina HiSeq X Ten platform (Illumina, San Diego, CA, United States) via a 150-bp paired-end approach. The generated short reads were *de novo* assembled using CLC Genomics Workbench 9.5.1 software, and the draft genome contigs were used for further analysis. One strain was also subjected to long-read sequencing using a MinION Sequencer (Nanopore, Oxford, United Kingdom). The *de novo* hybrid assembly of both short (Illumina) and long (Nanopore) reads was performed using Unicycler v0.4.8 in conservative mode (Wick et al., 2017).

### ST, K-Type, and Virulence Gene Analysis

Multilocus sequence typing (MLST) was performed by using the CGE database,[1] and the novel ST was submitted to Institut Pasteur to obtain the specific ST number. The K-types were identified with Kaptive, and virulence genes were identified using the Institut Pasteur database[2] (Wyres et al., 2016). Virulence genes [i.e., siderophore system yersiniabactin (*ybtAEPQSTUX*), salmochelin (*iroBCDN*), aerobactin (*iucABCDiutA*), and polysaccharide regulator *rmpA*/*rmpA2* genes] were chosen as genotypic biomarkers for virulence evaluation (Russo et al., 2018; Turton et al., 2019; Lan et al., 2020).

### Core Genome MLST and Recombination Analysis

All 99 assembled genomes were imported into Ridom Seqsphere + 4.1.9 (Ridom GmbH, Germany) for core genome MLST (cgMLST) analysis according to the default parameters. *K. pneumoniae* NTUH-K2044 (GenBank accession no. NC_012731.1) was used as a reference with a standard set of 2,358 genes for gene-by-gene comparisons, and the minimum spanning tree was constructed.

ST11-KL64, ST11-KL47, and ST4496 were subjected to further phylogenetic and recombination analyses. Genome alignment was established by using Snippy[3] with the default parameters. Recombination analysis was performed by using Gubbins (Croucher et al., 2015), and the complete genome acquired by long-read sequencing was used as a reference. The region of recombination was extracted and annotated with Prokka (rapid prokaryotic genome annotation) (Seemann, 2014) and PHAST (PHAge Search Tool). Figures illustrating the phylogenetic

[1] http://www.genomicepidemiology.org/

[2] https://bigsdb.pasteur.fr/klebsiella/klebsiella.html

[3] https://github.com/tseemann/snippy

and recombination results were produced with Phandango (Hadfield et al., 2018).

## Biofilm Formation

Microtiter dish biofilm formation assays were used to determine the capacity of biofilm formation, with minor modifications (Naparstek et al., 2014). Briefly, bacteria [$10^7$ colony-forming units (CFU)/mL] were inoculated into Mueller Hinton (MH) medium in polystyrene microtiter 96-well plates (Grenier Bio-One, Frickenhausen, Germany) and incubated at 37°C for 20 h. The biofilm that formed in each well was quantified via crystal violet (Sigma, St. Louis, MO, United States) staining followed by elution with 95% ethanol and optical density (OD) measurements (OD595). Three independent cultures for each strain and quantification in four wells for each culture were performed.

## Serum Resistance Assay

Serum resistance was determined by comparing the lag phase of the growth curve in MH broth or MH broth with 10% pooled normal human serum (1 mL serum mixed with 9 mL MH broth), which was collected from healthy volunteers. Three independent cultures for each strain were grown overnight until saturation and diluted 1:1,000 in MH broth or MH broth with 10% pooled normal human serum. Three replicates of each culture were aliquoted into a flat-bottom 100-well plate (0.2 mL/well). Growth curves were determined by measuring the OD at 600 nm every 5 min for 20 h using a Bioscreen C MBR machine (Oy Growth Curves Ab Ltd., Finland). The lag phase was estimated based on the OD600 curves using an R script defined as previously described (Hua et al., 2017).

## *Galleria mellonella* Infection Model

A *Galleria mellonella* infection model was used to evaluate the virulence level among different CRKP clone groups. For strain assessment, bacteria from a freshly streaked plate were grown overnight and underwent 10-fold serial dilutions in 1 × phosphate-buffered saline (PBS). Prior to inoculation into *G. mellonella* larvae, bacterial cells were washed with PBS and then diluted to an appropriate cell density, as determined by measuring the OD at 600 nm. Groups of 30 larvae (~200 mg; Yuejiayin, Tianjin, China) were stored in the dark at 4°C prior to use. For virulence evaluation, every larva was infected with 10-μL aliquots of $1 \times 10^6$ CFU bacteria ($n = 10$) via the last left proleg by using a 10-μL Hamilton syringe. Survival was monitored every 3 h up to 24 h postinfection at 37°C. Experiments were performed in triplicate.

## Statistical Analysis

A two-tailed Mann–Whitney *U*-test was used to calculate the differences between all pairs of the ST11-KL47, ST11-KL64, and ST4496-KL47 groups regarding the median number of different core genes, biofilm formation, and the lag phase of the growth curve in MH broth or MH broth with 10% human serum. The survival rates of *G. mellonella* were evaluated using Kaplan–Meier survival curves and analyzed with the log-rank (Mantel–Cox) test. The mean numbers of bases involved in recombination were compared among these three clone groups by using one-way analysis of variance. All $p$-values $\leq 0.05$ were considered statistically significant.

# RESULTS

## Clinical Characteristics of Patients Infected With ST4496 Strains

The novel allele and ST were submitted to the administrator of the Pasteur database and assigned as ST4496 with an mdh335 allele (allelic profile of 3-3-335-1-1-1-79 for *gapA*, *infB*, *mdh*, *pgi*, *phoE*, *rpoB*, and *tonB*, respectively).

The clinical characteristics of the patients infected with ST4496 strains are presented in **Table 1**. All 18 isolates were collected from the ICU. Notably, none of the isolates originated from blood or primary abscesses, and the patients tended to show a good prognosis, even though five of them were discharged against medical advice because of uncontrolled underlying conditions. Moreover, the relatively good outcomes of the majority of the patients receiving no effective antimicrobials for CRKP indicated a colonized status of the strains rather than an infectious status. The non-invasive clinical manifestations indicated a hypovirulent character of the ST4496 CRKP.

## cgMLST for Contemporaneous CRKP

Altogether, 99 contemporaneous isolates were included in the cgMLST analysis and the subsequent phylogenetic analysis. K-type was also considered as capsule synthesis loci are recombination hotspots in multidrug-resistant *K. pneumoniae* and are associated with virulence.

The minimum spanning tree based on the cgMLST profiles is presented in **Figure 1**. The results showed that ST11 (70/99) accounted for the majority of CRKP isolates, among which KL64 and KL47 were the overwhelmingly dominant serotypes. ST4496 (18/99) was the second most common ST, and all of the isolates with this ST belonged to the KL47 serotype. There were five ST15 isolates, and the remaining six isolates included five distinct STs. ST4496 and ST11 were closely related to each other but displayed relatively long distances from other STs. ST4496 showed a shorter phylogenetic distance from ST11-KL47 strains than from ST11-KL64 based on the core gene difference. As ST4496 strains have never previously been detected at this center or reported in any other studies, it is logical to believe that they may have originated from ST11-KL47.

ST4496-KL47 ($n = 18$), ST11-KL64 ($n = 58$), and ST11-KL47 ($n = 8$) were selected for further analysis, as these three groups were very closely related to each other according to cgMLST and were the predominant CRKP groups. Notably, ST11-KL47 exhibited greater genetic diversity than the other two clusters; among the clusters, the median number of different core genes between each pair of strains within the group was 25 in ST11-KL47 vs. 5 in ST11-KL64 and 2 in ST4496-KL47, and these differences were significant (both $p < 0.0001$; **Figure 2A**).

**TABLE 1** | Clinical characteristics of the patients infected with ST4496 CRKP.

| Isolates | Time of isolation | Origin | Department | Underlying conditions | Clinical outcome | Antimicrobials |
|---|---|---|---|---|---|---|
| NST-1 | 21/12/2016 | Bile | ICU | Severe acute pancreatitis | Improved | Cefoperazone and sulbactam, tigecycline |
| NST-2 | 26/12/2016 | Ascites | ICU | Pseudomyxoma peritonei | Improved | Imipenem |
| NST-3 | 05/01/2017 | Sputum | ICU | Colon cancer | Improved | Amoxicillin and clavulanic acid |
| NST-4 | 09/01/2017 | Urine | ICU | Bladder cancer | Improved | Cefoperazone and sulbactam |
| NST-5 | 16/01/2017 | Sputum | ICU | Sepsis | Improved | Cefoperazone and sulbactam, tigecycline |
| NST-6 | 26/01/2017 | Ascites | ICU | Hepatic carcinoma | Improved | Imipenem |
| NST-7 | 26/01/2017 | Sputum | ICU | Heart failure | Improved | Moxifloxacin, imipenem |
| NST-8 | 02/02/2017 | Urine | ICU | Deep vein thrombosis, GI bleeding | Improved | Cefoperazone and sulbactam |
| NST-9 | 02/02/2017 | Purulent discharge from surgical site | ICU | Femoral artery embolectomy, atrial fibrillation, heart failure | Against-advice discharge | Amoxicillin and clavulanic acid, cefepime |
| NST-10 | 02/02/2017 | Sputum | ICU | Brain ischemia | Improved | Piperacillin and tazobactam |
| NST-11 | 11/03/2017 | Sputum | ICU | Esophageal cancer, pyothorax, respiratory failure | Against-advice discharge | Tigecycline, meropenem |
| NST-12 | 22/03/2017 | Sputum | ICU | Brain hemorrhage | Improved | Meropenem |
| NST-13 | 22/03/2017 | Sputum | ICU | GI bleeding | Improved | Piperacillin and tazobactam |
| NST-14 | 23/03/2017 | Sputum | ICU | Cerebral infarction, pulmonary infection | Against-advice discharge | Amoxicillin and clavulanic acid, cefepime |
| NST-15 | 02/04/2017 | Sputum | ICU | Brain hemorrhage | Improved | Cefoperazone and sulbactam |
| NST-16 | 05/04/2017 | Ascites | ICU | Acute generalized suppurative peritonitis, exploratory laparotomy | Improved | Imipenem, Tigecycline |
| NST-17 | 10/04/2017 | Purulent discharge from surgical site | ICU | Esophageal perforation from foreign body, mediastinal abscess | Against-advice discharge | Imipenem |
| NST-18 | 02/05/2017 | Urine | ICU | Malignant tumor of the meninges, lymphoma suspected | Against-advice discharge | Cefoperazone and sulbactam |

## Phylogenetic and Recombination Analysis

Further phylogenetic analysis was performed on 84 isolates and revealed three distinct clusters, corresponding to ST11-KL47, ST4496-KL47, and ST11-KL64 (**Figure 3**). The strains in cluster ST11-KL47 had longer branches, continuing to show more genetic diversity than the other two clusters. The mean number of bases involved in recombination in ST11-KL64 was 270,666.7, whereas 56,866.6 and 10,879.2 bases were found in ST11-KL47 and ST4496-KL47, respectively ($p < 0.0001$). The three major regions of recombination were annotated, and the largest region corresponded to the K locus and O locus (149,594 bases), deciphering the K-type and LPS shifts. The other two regions were *fimA*/*oqxAB* (27,879 bases) and the prophage sequence (45,116 bases).

## Virulence Genes

Several key virulence genes were screened, including the capsular polysaccharide regulator *rmpA* or *rmpA2*, and siderophore systems (yersiniabactin, salmochelin, and aerobactin). Yersiniabactin was the most common of these genes and was found in all strains, whereas salmochelin was not found in three lineages, ST11-KL47, ST11-KL64, and ST4496-KL47. However, great differences in other virulence genes were observed among the three lineages. Among ST11-KL64 isolates, not only did the majority (56/58, 96.6%) possess aerobactin/*rmpA2** genes [*rmpA2** indicates a frameshift mutation compared to empirical *rmpA2* gene (Zhou et al., 2020)], but a relatively high proportion (15/58, 25.9%) also carried the *rmpA* gene. Only one isolate of ST11-KL47 contained aerobactin and the empirical *rmpA2* gene. The ST4496 isolates carried no targeted virulence genes beyond the yersiniabactin gene cluster *ybtAEPQSTUX*.

## Phenotypic Assessment

All eight ST11-KL47 isolates were included in the following phenotypic analysis. For biofilm formation and serum resistance assays, eight isolates were randomly chosen as representatives for the phenotypic assessment of ST4496-KL47 and ST11-KL64, respectively. In the biofilm formation assay, the OD measurements indicated that ST4496-KL47 isolates produced the least biofilm, whereas ST11-KL64 isolates produced the most biofilm. The differences between the three groups were significant (median OD595 values in ST11-KL47, ST11-KL64, and ST4496-KL47 of 0.4264, 0.8531, and 0.2340, respectively, **Figure 2B**). Greater diversity in biofilm formation was observed for ST11-KL47 than for ST11-KL64 and ST4496-KL47. In the serum resistance assay, similar lag phases were detected for the three groups in the MH broth (**Figure 2C**). However, a significantly prolonged lag phase was observed for ST4496-KL47 and some

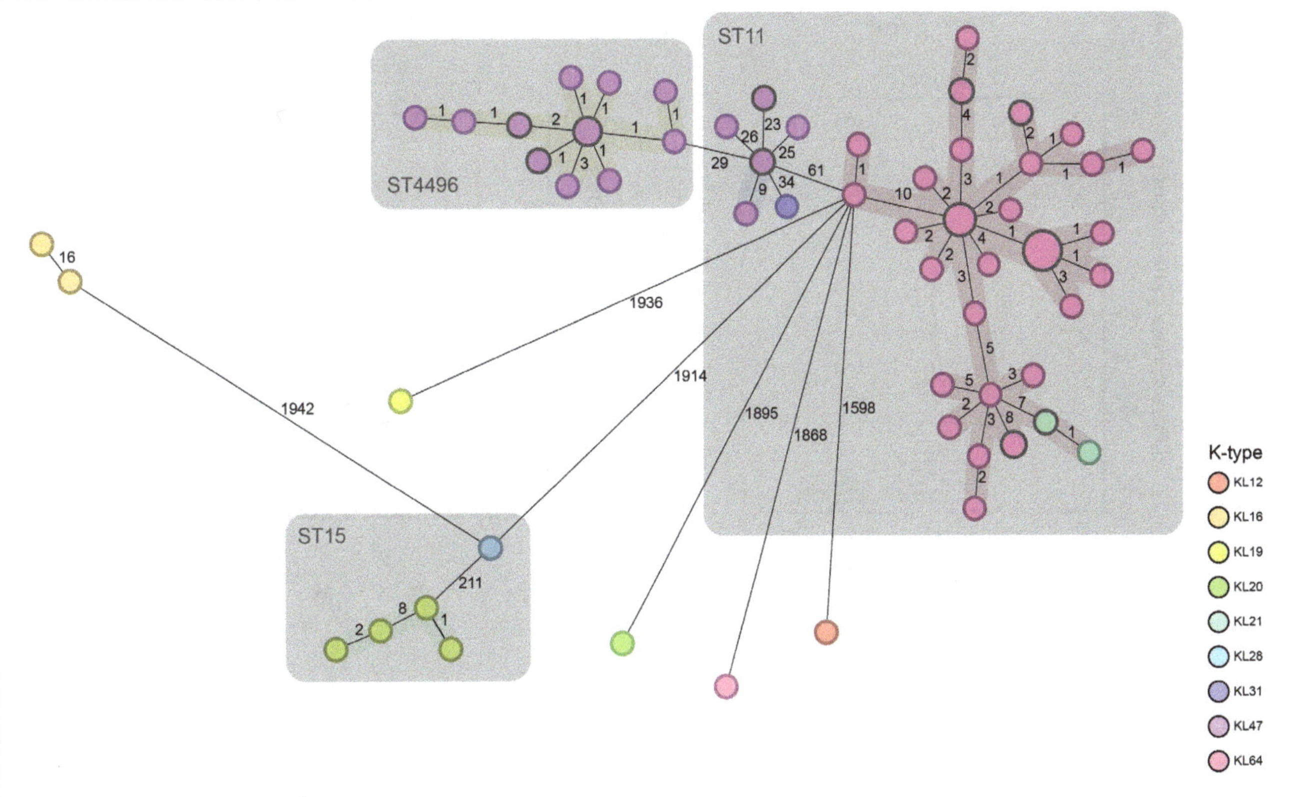


**FIGURE 1 |** Minimum spanning tree based on the cgMLST profiles of contemporaneous CRKP strains. cgMLST profiles are represented by circles, and the size of the circle is proportional to the number of isolates with an identical cgMLST profile. The color of each circle is encoded by the K-type, and the length of lines connecting the cgMLST profiles is proportional to the number of core gene differences between circles. A gray zone surrounds a group of circles that share the same sequence type.

of the ST11-KL47 isolates in MH broth with 10% human serum relative to ST11-KL64. The differences between ST11-KL47 and ST4496-KL47 or between ST11-KL64 and ST4496-KL47 were significant ($p < 0.0001$). Similarly, greater variation in the lag phase in MH broth with 10% pooled normal human serum was observed in ST11-KL47 (**Figure 2D**). Furthermore, we generated a *G. mellonella* infection model to evaluate the virulence among these three groups. The survival percentage of *G. mellonella* larvae in the ST11-KL64 group was significantly lower than that in the ST11-KL47 or ST4496-KL47 group, indicating that the ST11-KL64 isolates had the highest virulence compared to other KL47 serotype isolates (**Figure 4**).

## DISCUSSION

In this study, a novel ST with one single-locus variant in *mdh* emerged in the ST11 CRKP and was assigned ST4496. Unlike other successful descendants (e.g., ST258) of ST11, ST4496 did not show successful persistence or dissemination in the hospital setting. The characteristics of patients infected with ST4496 indicated a hypovirulent nature, as ST4496 strains mostly presented colonization rather than infection, and no bloodstream infection involving ST4496 was detected. We presumed that hypovirulence was mainly responsible for the restriction of the spread of ST4496 after it caused occasional outbreaks in the hospital setting for a couple of months.

There are growing reports of convergent evolution of resistance and virulence in *K. pneumoniae*. Although convergence can result from hypervirulent strains gaining multidrug resistance (MDR) elements or MDR strains gaining virulence elements, MDR clones are more likely to acquire virulence genes than hypervirulent clones are to acquire resistance genes (Wyres et al., 2019). Following sporadic reports of isolates showing the phenomenon of convergence in clinical isolates, there has recently been growing evidence of increasing virulence in the CRKP population, especially in the dominant ST11 clone in China (Shen et al., 2020; Zhao et al., 2020; Zhou et al., 2020). To reveal the genotypic and phenotypic basis of this convergence, novel ST4496 isolates and contemporary CRKP isolates were included in the present study. The K-type was also investigated because it has been proven to be associated with virulence, and recent evidence showed that the previously prevalent ST11-KL47 has been gradually replaced by ST11-KL64, which was derived from an ST11-KL47–like ancestor through recombination (Zhao et al., 2020; Zhou et al., 2020).

From the cgMLST analysis and the derived minimum spanning tree, we can see that ST4496-KL47, ST11-KL64, and ST11-KL47 were closely related to each other and were the predominant CRKP groups. The relationships of the three groups

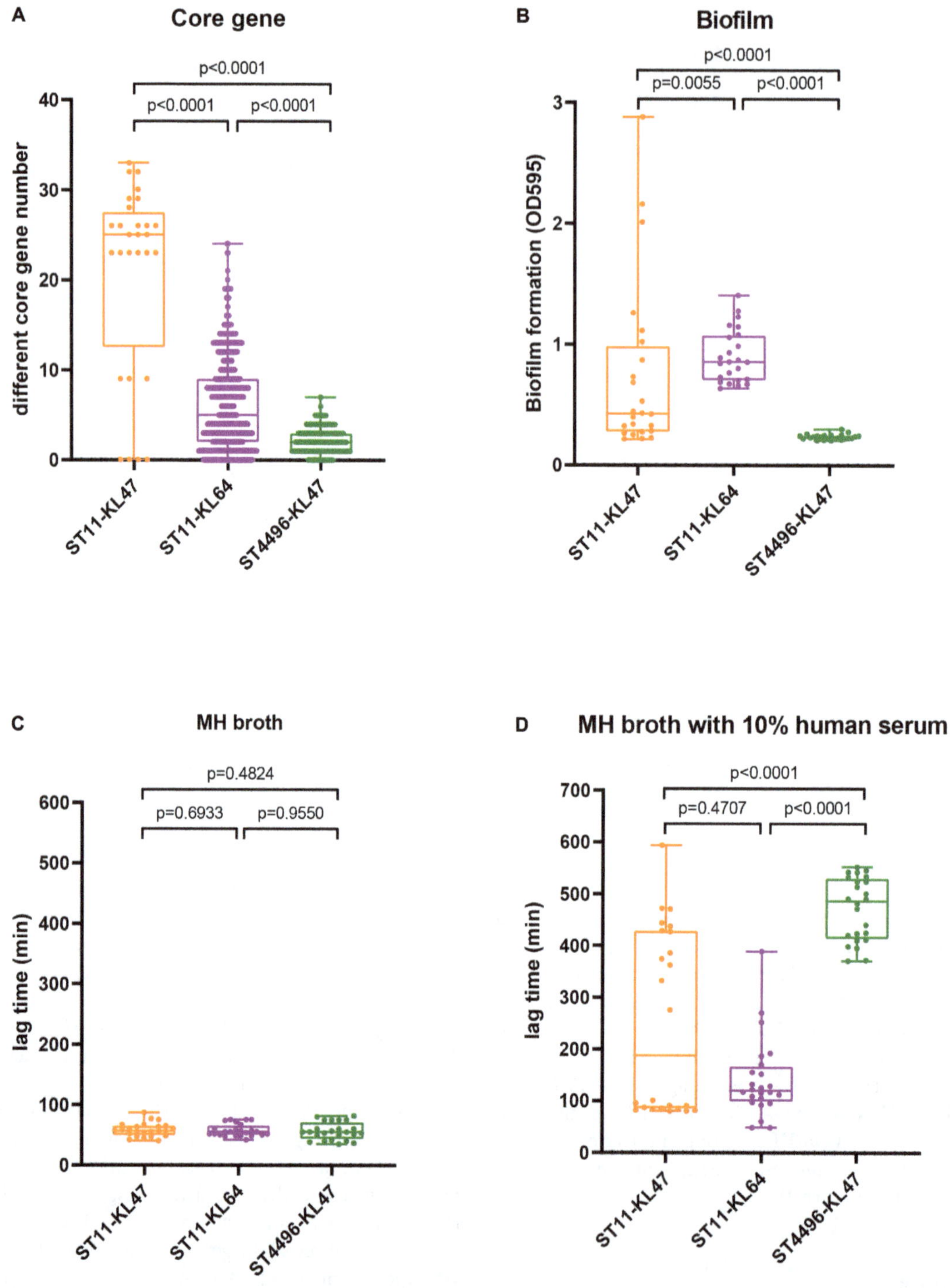


**FIGURE 2 |** Genetic evidence and phenotypic manifestations among the ST11-KL47, ST11-KL64, and ST4496-KL47 groups: **(A)** The distribution of different core gene numbers between each pair of strains within the group; **(B)** biofilm formation (OD595); **(C)** lag phase in MH broth; **(D)** lag phase in MH broth with 10% human serum. The middle lines represent the median value for each group. Error bars indicate the region from the lowest to highest values in each group.

were further confirmed by single-nucleotide polymorphism (SNP)–based phylogenetic and recombination analysis. ST11-KL47 is much more diverse genetically. Since it has been reported that enhanced virulence promotes the replacement of ST11-KL47 by ST11-KL64 (Zhou et al., 2020), it is logical to presume that different levels of virulence may be one of the factors leading to the different fates of the three CRKP groups, that is, the disappearance of ST4496-KL47, the decrease in ST11-KL47, and the proliferation of ST11-KL64, although both ST4496-KL47 and ST11-KL64 may have evolved from ST11-KL47.

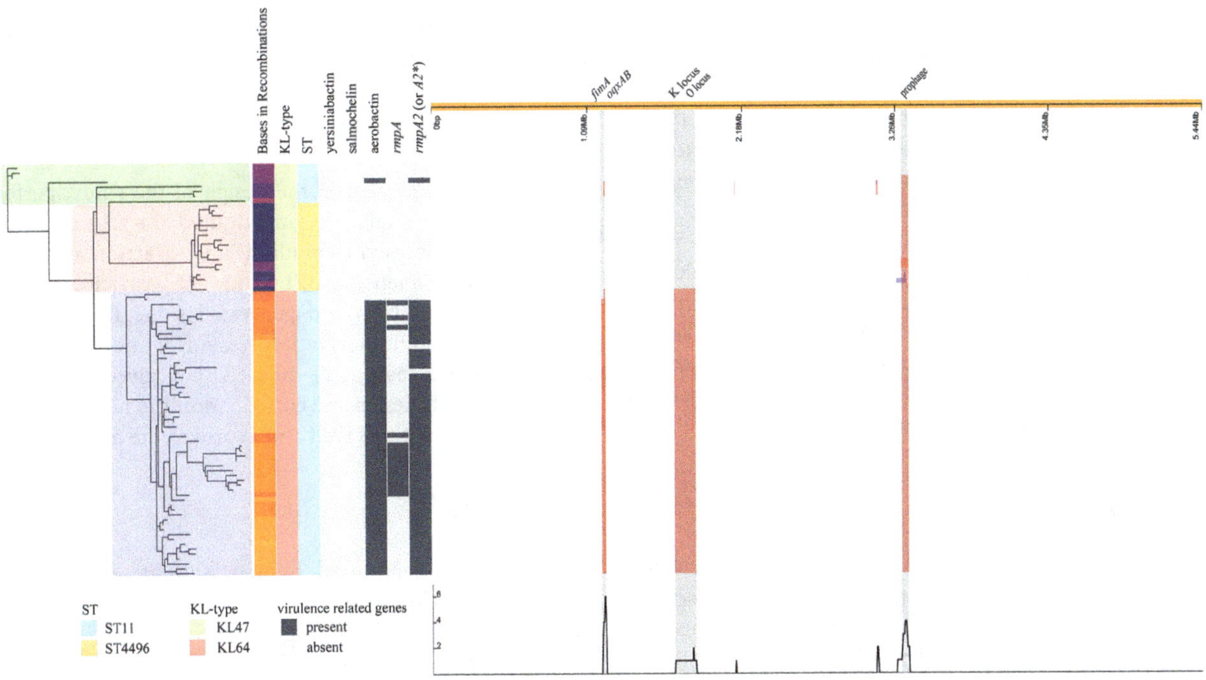


**FIGURE 3 |** Phylogenetic structure combined with the molecular characteristics and the regions of recombination in the ST11-KL47, ST4496-KL47, and ST11-KL64 strains. The SNP-based phylogenetic tree is shown to the left; green zone, ST11-KL47; pink zone, ST4496-KL47; blue zone, ST11-KL64. The distributions of bases in recombinations, KL type, ST type, and some virulence-related genes are shown in the middle. The three major regions of recombination are shown to the right, and the largest region corresponds to the K locus and O locus.

This assumption was supported by the fact that enhanced virulence of ST11-KL64 and weakened virulence of ST4496-KL47 were observed both genetically and phenotypically. Genetically, ST11-KL64 has the most virulence genes, and ST4496-KL47 has the fewest virulence genes. As previously reported, *iuc* (the aerobactin locus) is important for the production of siderophores to promote iron acquisition, and some researchers have even considered aerobactin as an indicator of hypervirulent *K. pneumoniae* (Zhang et al., 2016). The presence of *rmpA/A2*, which encodes regulators of mucoid phenotype genes, is strongly associated with the phenotype of hypermucoviscosity. Positivity for *iuc*, *rmpA*, and *rmpA2* (or *rmpA2**) may indicate the presence of a virulence plasmid (Wyres et al., 2020).

Virulence levels were further determined by phenotypic tests. First, the observation of biofilm formation supported bacterial adhesion to indwell medical devices and potentially better survival in adverse environmental conditions, which may lead to drug ineffectiveness and failure to eradicate infection (O'Toole et al., 2000; Zheng et al., 2018). Previous studies have shown that biofilm formation ability is associated with genetic factors such as *iucA* and *rmpA/rmpA2* in *K. pneumoniae* (Zheng et al., 2018). Second, a significantly prolonged lag phase was observed for ST4496-KL47 and some of the ST11-KL47 isolates in MH broth with 10% human serum. In fact, some ST4496-KL47 and ST11-KL47 isolates failed to grow in MH broth with a higher concentration of human serum (20%) over a 20-h period (data not shown). A shorter lag phase may indicate a relatively high serum resistance ability of ST11-KL64. Finally, the highest virulence level in ST11-KL64 isolates was also observed based on the *G. mellonella* infection model, implying that this clone was more likely to cause pandemic outbreaks than other KL47 serotype isolates.

Relative to ST4496-KL47 and ST11-KL64, diversity is much higher in ST11-KL47 based on both genetic evidence and phenotypic findings. This is consistent with the fact that this group is much more ancient and has therefore had a higher chance to evolve and develop greater diversity.

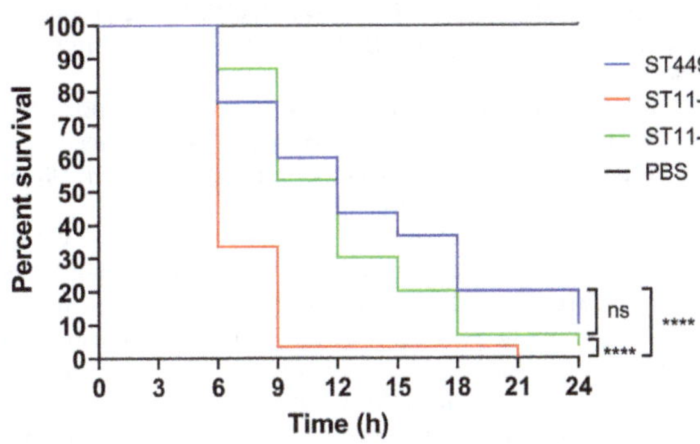


**FIGURE 4 |** Percent survival curve of *G. mellonella* infected with ST11-KL64 isolates (red line), ST11-KL47 isolates (green line), and ST4496-KL47 (blue line). ns, no significant difference; ****$p < 0.0001$.

Our findings are relevant for understanding the risk of carbapenem-resistant hypervirulent *K. pneumoniae* strains as highly virulent MDR strains may be able to persist and be disseminated in hospital settings and may even spread to community settings, leading to public health disasters (Chen and Kreiswirth, 2018). The early detection and containment of spreading through comprehensive infection control measures could be the most feasible solution to this problem.

This work provides a glimpse of intraspecies shifts from one hospital, and a preliminary investigation has been conducted. Certainly, more studies are needed to verify this assumption. To better understand the mechanisms of evolution, we should pay attention to "unsuccessful" evolution as well as successful evolution. Thus, unsuccessful ST4496 could be an excellent reference when studying the evolution of *K. pneumoniae*.

## CONCLUSION

The present study provided further evidence that virulence enhancement in ST11-KL64 was the reason for intraspecies replacement, as further demonstrated by the disappearance of ST4496-KL47, with weakened virulence. The results indicate that ST11-KL64 has the potential to be the predominant CRKP strain in China, and it seems that the convergent evolution of virulence and resistance in *K. pneumoniae* is inevitable under current antimicrobial strategies and infection control policies.

## AUTHOR CONTRIBUTIONS

DZ and QS participated in the design of the study, performed the bioinformatics analysis, and drafted the manuscript. DH, LF, and YM performed Genomic DNA extraction and prepared for illumine sequencing. PL and JQ participated in the bioinformatics analysis and generated some figures. XH and PZ performed biofilm formation assay. HH and YW performed serum resistance assay. YJ and YY conceived of the study, participated in its design and coordination and helped to draft the manuscript. All authors read and approved the final manuscript.

## FUNDING

This work was supported by the National Natural Science Foundation of China (No. 81830069), the China International Medical Foundation for Young Scientists (No. Z-2018-35-2003), and the Key Research and Development Program of Zhejiang (No. 2015C03046).

## REFERENCES

Bengoechea, J. A., and Sa Pessoa, J. (2019). *Klebsiella pneumoniae* infection biology: living to counteract host defences. *FEMS Microbiol. Rev.* 43, 123–144. doi: 10.1093/femsre/fuy043

Chen, L., and Kreiswirth, B. N. (2018). Convergence of carbapenem-resistance and hypervirulence in *Klebsiella pneumoniae*. *Lancet Infect. Dis.* 18, 2–3. doi: 10.1016/S1473-3099(17)30517-0

Chiarelli, A., Cabanel, N., Rosinski-Chupin, I., Zongo, P. D., Naas, T., Bonnin, R. A., et al. (2020). Diversity of mucoid to non-mucoid switch among carbapenemase-producing *Klebsiella pneumoniae*. *BMC Microbiol.* 20:325. doi: 10.1186/s12866-020-02007-y

Croucher, N. J., Page, A. J., Connor, T. R., Delaney, A. J., Keane, J. A., Bentley, S. D., et al. (2015). Rapid phylogenetic analysis of large samples of recombinant bacterial whole genome sequences using Gubbins. *Nucleic Acids Res.* 43:e15. doi: 10.1093/nar/gku1196

Grundmann, H., Glasner, C., Albiger, B., Aanensen, D. M., Tomlinson, C. T., Andrasevic, A. T., et al. (2017). Occurrence of carbapenemase-producing *Klebsiella pneumoniae* and *Escherichia coli* in the European survey of carbapenemase-producing *Enterobacteriaceae* (EuSCAPE): a prospective, multinational study. *Lancet Infect. Dis.* 17, 153–163. doi: 10.1016/S1473-3099(16)30257-2

Gu, D., Dong, N., Zheng, Z., Lin, D., Huang, M., Wang, L., et al. (2018). A fatal outbreak of ST11 carbapenem-resistant hypervirulent *Klebsiella pneumoniae* in a Chinese hospital: a molecular epidemiological study. *Lancet Infect. Dis.* 18, 37–46. doi: 10.1016/S1473-3099(17)30489-9

Hadfield, J., Croucher, N. J., Goater, R. J., Abudahab, K., Aanensen, D. M., and Harris, S. R. (2018). Phandango: an interactive viewer for bacterial population genomics. *Bioinformatics* 34, 292–293. doi: 10.1093/bioinformatics/btx610

Hua, X., Liu, L., Fang, Y., Shi, Q., Li, X., Chen, Q., et al. (2017). Colistin resistance in *Acinetobacter baumannii* MDR-ZJ06 revealed by a multiomics approach. *Front. Cell. Infect. Microbiol.* 7:45. doi: 10.3389/fcimb.2017.00045

Lan, P., Shi, Q., Zhang, P., Chen, Y., Yan, R., Hua, X., et al. (2020). Core genome allelic profiles of clinical *Klebsiella pneumoniae* strains using a random forest algorithm based on multilocus sequence typing scheme for hypervirulence analysis. *J. Infect. Dis.* 221(Suppl. 2), S263–S271. doi: 10.1093/infdis/jiz562

Munoz-Price, L. S., Poirel, L., Bonomo, R. A., Schwaber, M. J., Daikos, G. L., Cormican, M., et al. (2013). Clinical epidemiology of the global expansion of *Klebsiella pneumoniae* carbapenemases. *Lancet Infect. Dis.* 13, 785–796. doi: 10.1016/S1473-3099(13)70190-7

Naparstek, L., Carmeli, Y., Navon-Venezia, S., and Banin, E. (2014). Biofilm formation and susceptibility to gentamicin and colistin of extremely drug-resistant KPC-producing *Klebsiella pneumoniae*. *J. Antimicrob. Chemother.* 69, 1027–1034. doi: 10.1093/jac/dkt487

O'Toole, G., Kaplan, H. B., and Kolter, R. (2000). Biofilm formation as microbial development. *Annu. Rev. Microbiol.* 54, 49–79. doi: 10.1146/annurev.micro.54.1.49

Paczosa, M. K., and Mecsas, J. (2016). *Klebsiella pneumoniae*: going on the offense with a strong defense. *Microbiol. Mol. Biol. Rev.* 80, 629–661. doi: 10.1128/MMBR.00078-15

Russo, T. A., Olson, R., Fang, C. T., Stoesser, N., Miller, M., MacDonald, U., et al. (2018). Identification of biomarkers for differentiation of hypervirulent *Klebsiella pneumoniae* from classical *K. pneumoniae*. *J. Clin. Microbiol.* 56:e00776. doi: 10.1128/JCM.00776-18

Seemann, T. (2014). Prokka: rapid prokaryotic genome annotation. *Bioinformatics* 30, 2068–2069. doi: 10.1093/bioinformatics/btu153

Shen, P., Berglund, B., Chen, Y., Zhou, Y., Xiao, T., Xiao, Y., et al. (2020). Hypervirulence markers among non-ST11 strains of carbapenem- and multidrug-resistant *Klebsiella pneumoniae* isolated from patients with bloodstream infections. *Front. Microbiol.* 11:1199. doi: 10.3389/fmicb.2020.01199

Turton, J., Davies, F., Turton, J., Perry, C., Payne, Z., and Pike, R. (2019). Hybrid resistance and virulence plasmids in "high-risk" clones of *Klebsiella pneumoniae*, including those carrying $bla_{NDM-5}$. *Microorganisms* 7:326. doi: 10.3390/microorganisms7090326

Wang, Q., Wang, X., Wang, J., Ouyang, P., Jin, C., Wang, R., et al. (2018). Phenotypic and genotypic characterization of carbapenem-resistant *Enterobacteriaceae*: data from a longitudinal large-scale CRE study in China (2012-2016). *Clin. Infect. Dis.* 67(suppl. 2), S196–S205. doi: 10.1093/cid/ciy660

Wick, R. R., Judd, L. M., Gorrie, C. L., and Holt, K. E. (2017). Unicycler: resolving bacterial genome assemblies from short and long sequencing reads. *PLoS Comput. Biol.* 13:e1005595. doi: 10.1371/journal.pcbi.1005595

Wyres, K. L., Gorrie, C., Edwards, D. J., Wertheim, H. F., Hsu, L. Y., Van Kinh, N., et al. (2015). Extensive capsule locus variation and large-scale genomic recombination within the *Klebsiella pneumoniae* clonal group 258. *Genome Biol. Evol.* 7, 1267–1279. doi: 10.1093/gbe/evv062

Wyres, K. L., Lam, M. M. C., and Holt, K. E. (2020). Population genomics of *Klebsiella pneumoniae. Nat. Rev. Microbiol.* 18, 344–359. doi: 10.1038/s41579-019-0315-1

Wyres, K. L., Wick, R. R., Gorrie, C., Jenney, A., Follador, R., Thomson, N. R., et al. (2016). Identification of *Klebsiella* capsule synthesis loci from whole genome data. *Microb. Genom.* 2:e000102. doi: 10.1099/mgen.0.000102

Wyres, K. L., Wick, R. R., Judd, L. M., Froumine, R., Tokolyi, A., Gorrie, C. L., et al. (2019). Distinct evolutionary dynamics of horizontal gene transfer in drug resistant and virulent clones of *Klebsiella pneumoniae. PLoS Genet.* 15:e1008114. doi: 10.1371/journal.pgen.1008114

Zhang, R., Liu, L., Zhou, H., Chan, E. W., Li, J., Fang, Y., et al. (2017). Nationwide surveillance of clinical carbapenem-resistant *Enterobacteriaceae* (CRE) strains in China. *EBioMedicine* 19, 98–106. doi: 10.1016/j.ebiom.2017.04.032

Zhang, Y., Zhao, C., Wang, Q., Wang, X., Chen, H., Li, H., et al. (2016). High prevalence of hypervirulent *Klebsiella pneumoniae* infection in China: geographic distribution, clinical characteristics, and antimicrobial resistance. *Antimicrob. Agents Chemother.* 60, 6115–6120. doi: 10.1128/AAC.01127-16

Zhao, J., Liu, C., Liu, Y., Zhang, Y., Xiong, Z., Fan, Y., et al. (2020). Genomic characteristics of clinically important ST11 *Klebsiella pneumoniae* strains worldwide. *J. Glob. Antimicrob. Resist.* 22, 519–526. doi: 10.1016/j.jgar.2020.03.023

Zheng, J. X., Lin, Z. W., Chen, C., Chen, Z., Lin, F. J., Wu, Y., et al. (2018). Biofilm formation in *Klebsiella pneumoniae* bacteremia strains was found to be associated with CC23 and the presence of WCAG. *Front. Cell. Infect. Microbiol.* 8:21. doi: 10.3389/fcimb.2018.00021

Zhou, K., Xiao, T., David, S., Wang, Q., Zhou, Y., Guo, L., et al. (2020). Novel subclone of carbapenem-resistant *Klebsiella pneumoniae* sequence type 11 with enhanced virulence and transmissibility, China. *Emerg. Infect. Dis.* 26, 289–297. doi: 10.3201/eid2602.190594

17

# *Trans*-Cinnamaldehyde and Eugenol Increase *Acinetobacter baumannii* Sensitivity to Beta-Lactam Antibiotics

***Deepti P. Karumathil*[1]*, Meera Surendran Nair*[1]*, James Gaffney*[2]*, Anup Kollanoor-Johny*[3] *and Kumar Venkitanarayanan*[1]****

[1] *Department of Animal Science, University of Connecticut, Storrs, CT, United States,* [2] *College of Veterinary Medicine, Cornell University, Ithaca, NY, United States,* [3] *Department of Animal Science, University of Minnesota, Saint Paul, MN, United States*

***Correspondence:**
*Kumar Venkitanarayanan*
*kumar.venkitanarayanan@uconn.edu*

Multi-drug resistant (MDR) *Acinetobacter baumannii* is a major nosocomial pathogen causing a wide range of clinical conditions with significant mortality rates. *A. baumannii* strains are equipped with a multitude of antibiotic resistance mechanisms, rendering them resistant to most of the currently available antibiotics. Thus, there is a critical need to explore novel strategies for controlling antibiotic resistance in *A. baumannii*. This study investigated the efficacy of two food-grade, plant-derived antimicrobials (PDAs), namely *trans*-cinnamaldehyde (TC) and eugenol (EG) in decreasing *A. baumannii*'s resistance to seven β-lactam antibiotics, including ampicillin, methicillin, meropenem, penicillin, aztreonam, amoxicillin, and piperacillin. Two MDR *A. baumannii* isolates (ATCC 17978 and AB 251847) were separately cultured in tryptic soy broth (~6 log CFU/ml) containing the minimum inhibitory concentration (MIC) of TC or EG with or without the MIC of each antibiotic at 37°C for 18 h. *A. baumannii* strains not exposed to the PDAs or antibiotics served as controls. Following incubation, *A. baumannii* counts were determined by broth dilution assay. In addition, the effect of PDAs on the permeability of outer membrane and efflux pumps in *A. baumannii* was measured. Further, the effect of TC and EG on the expression of *A. baumannii* genes encoding resistance to β-lactam antibiotics (*blaP*), efflux pumps (*adeABC*), and multi-drug resistant protein (*mdrp*) was studied using real-time quantitative PCR (RT-qPCR). The experiment was replicated three times with duplicate samples of each treatment and control. The results from broth dilution assay indicated that both TC and EG in combination with antibiotics increased the sensitivity of *A. baumannii* to all the tested antibiotics ($P < 0.05$). The two PDAs inhibited the function of *A. baumannii* efflux pump, (AdeABC), but did not increase the permeability of its outer membrane. Moreover, RT-qPCR data revealed that TC and EG down-regulated the expression of majority of the genes associated with β-lactam antibiotic resistance, especially *blaP* and *adeABC* ($P < 0.05$). The results suggest that TC and EG could potentially be used along with β-lactam antibiotics for controlling MDR *A. baumannii* infections; however, their clinical significance needs to be determined using *in vivo* studies.

**Keywords: *A. baumannii, trans*-cinnamaldehyde, eugenol, antibiotic resistance**

## INTRODUCTION

*Acinetobacter baumannii* is a multi-drug resistant (MDR) Gram-negative, aerobic bacillus that has emerged as a major cause of nosocomial infections with mortality rates ranging from 34 to 61% (Karageorgopoulos and Falagas, 2008; Wieczorek et al., 2008; Esterly et al., 2011). In humans, MDR *A. baumannii* causes a wide-spectrum of clinical conditions, including pneumonia (Leung et al., 2005), blood-stream infections (Wisplinghoff et al., 2004; Centers for Disease Control and Prevention [CDC], 2004), meningitis (Metan et al., 2007), urinary tract infections (Sunenshine et al., 2007), and wound infections (Scott et al., 2007) In addition, reports of other manifestations such as endocarditis, peritonitis, and osteomyelitis associated with *A. baumannii* have been reported (Olut and Erkek, 2005; Menon et al., 2006) *A. baumannii* is ranked as one of the most common bacteria associated with intensive care units (Garnacho-Montero and Amaya-Villar, 2010; Ulu-Kilic et al., 2013), and is difficult to treat due to its resistance to most of the currently available antibiotics (Maragakis and Perl, 2008; Doi et al., 2009; Neonakis et al., 2011; Al Mobarak et al., 2014; Ellis et al., 2015) For example, carbapenems, which were once the antimicrobials of choice for treating *A. baumannii*, are no longer completely effective due to resistance development by the bacterium (Falagas et al., 2006; Bassetti et al., 2008; Abbott et al., 2013; Fonseca et al., 2013). Similarly, although polymyxins have been successfully used to treat *A. baumannii* infections, strains resistant to these drugs have appeared (Hernan et al., 2009; Lean et al., 2014; Pogue et al., 2015). In light of these reports, the Infectious Diseases Society of America ranked *A. baumannii* as one of the top priority, antibiotic-resistant pathogens to target due to its rapid propensity to develop drug resistance, and a limited choice of antibiotics available to treat infections caused by this bacterium (Talbot et al., 2006; Shlaes et al., 2013).

*A. baumannii* is considered to be multidrug resistant, if it exhibits resistance to more than three classes of antibiotics (Falagas et al., 2006). The resistance of *A. baumannii* to antibiotics has been attributed to multiple mechanisms, including reduced permeability of its outer membrane to antibiotics, constitutive expression of drug efflux pumps, and its ability to acquire and incorporate genetic elements such as plasmids, transposons, and integrons (Giamarellou et al., 2008; Cai et al., 2012). In addition, *A. baumannii* has a significant ability to produce biofilms on various surfaces (Espinal et al., 2012; Longo et al., 2014), which not only increases the potential of *A. baumannii* for nosocomial spread, but also contributes to its resistance to antibiotics and virulence (Lee et al., 2008; Rao et al., 2008). Thus, there is a critical need to explore novel strategies for treating *A. baumannii* infections.

Traditionally, plants have served as a source of novel drugs for treating a variety of diseases in humans (Cowan, 1999). A variety of plant-derived compounds possessing antimicrobial properties against a wide range of microorganisms have been documented (Kon and Rai, 2012; Upadhyay et al., 2014). The antimicrobial effects of four components of ginger against MDR strains of *A. baumannii* has been reported (Wang et al., 2010). Similarly, the essential oil from coriander was found to exert either synergistic or additive effects with antibiotics such as tetracycline, chloramphenicol, ciprofloxacin, gentamicin, piperacillin, and cefoperazone against *A. baumannii* (Duarte et al., 2012). Recently, aqueous extract of kiwi (*Actinidia deliciosa*) and clove (*Syzygium aromaticum*) were found to exert anti-biofilm activity against *A. baumannii* (Tiwari et al., 2017). Similarly, it was shown that plant extract from *Aegle marmelos* and imipenem had synergistic effect against carbapenem resistant strain of *Acinetobacter baumannii* (Tiwari et al., 2016). In another study, the essential oil from *Origanum vulgare* possessed potent antimicrobial activity against MDR *A. baumannii* (Saghi et al., 2015). In addition, previous research from our laboratory indicated that several plant-derived antimicrobials (PDAs), including *trans*-cinnamaldehyde (TC), an ingredient in cinnamon, eugenol (present in clove) and carvacrol and thymol obtained from oregano oil and oil of thyme, respectively, decreased antibiotic resistance in MDR *S.* Typhimurium DT 104 (Johny et al., 2010). These investigators observed that TC reduced DT 104's resistance to five antibiotics, where thymol and carvacrol decreased resistance to three antibiotics.

The β-lactam group of antibiotics are the most commonly prescribed antibiotics for the treatment of bacterial infections worldwide (Pitout et al., 1997; Thakuria and Lahon, 2013). *A. baumannii* is capable of producing β-lactamases that can hydrolyze the β-lactam ring of penicillins, cephalosporins, and carbapenems, thereby conferring resistance to these antibiotics. Therefore, this study investigated the efficacy of TC and eugenol (EG) in increasing the sensitivity of *A. baumannii* to seven β-lactam antibiotics. In addition, the effect of these PDAs on genes conferring resistance to β-lactam antibiotics in *A. baumannii* was determined.

## MATERIALS AND METHODS

### *A. baumannii* Cultures and Growth Conditions

Two clinical isolates of *A. baumannii*, namely 251847 (International Health Management Associates, IL), and 17978 (ATCC; fatal meningitis isolate) were used in the study. All bacteriological media used in the study, except Leeds MDR *Acinetobacter* agar, were purchased from Difco (Becton Dickinson, Sparks, MD, United States). Leeds MDR agar was procured from Hardy Diagnostics (Santa Maria, CA, United States). The bacterial isolates were cultured separately overnight in 10 ml tryptic soy broth (TSB), followed by streaking on Leeds MDR *Acinetobacter* agar plates and incubation at 37°C for 24 h. An individual colony from Leeds MDR *Acinetobacter* agar was sub-cultured twice in 10 ml of TSB at 37°C for 24 h with agitation to reach ~8 $\log_{10}$ CFU/ml. The cultures were sedimented by centrifugation (3,700 × *g*, 15 min, 4°C), and the pellet was washed twice and re-suspended in sterile phosphate buffered saline (PBS; pH 7.2). The cultures were then diluted appropriately in PBS to obtain ~5 to 6 $\log_{10}$ CFU/ml to be used as the inoculum. The bacterial population in the inoculum was confirmed by plating on tryptic soy agar (TSA) with incubation at 37°C for 24 h.

## Plant-Derived Antimicrobials (PDAs) and Chemicals

*Trans*-cinnamaldehyde ($\geq$98%; TC, *trans*-3-phenyl-2-propenal), eugenol ($\geq$98%; EG,4-allyl-2-methoxyphenol), 1-*N*-phenylnaphthylamine (NPN), EDTA, ethidium bromide (EtBr), carbonyl cyanide m-chlorophenylhydrazone (CCP) and pyronin Y were purchased from Sigma-Aldrich (St. Louis, MO, United States).

## Determination of Sub-inhibitory Concentration (SIC) and Minimum Inhibitory Concentration (MIC) of PDAs Against *A. baumannii*

The sub-inhibitory concentration (SIC) and minimum inhibitory concentration (MIC) of TC and EG against *A. baumannii* were determined as previously reported (Johny et al., 2010; Amalaradjou and Venkitanarayanan, 2011) TSB (10 ml) tubes containing 0.75–7.5 μM (TC) and 0.61–6.1 μM (EG) in increments of 0.375 μM (TC) and 0.305 μM (EG were inoculated separately with *A. baumannii* at ~ 6 $\log_{10}$ CFU/ml, and incubated at 37°C for 24 h. Tubes without any added PDAs served as controls. After incubation, the samples were serially diluted (1:10) in PBS, plated on TSA, and incubated at 37°C for 24 h before counting the colonies. The highest concentration of TC or EG that did not inhibit *A. baumannii* growth after 24 h of incubation was selected as the SIC, while the lowest concentration of the antimicrobial that inhibited visible growth of the bacteria after 24 h incubation was taken as the MIC of that treatment. The experiment was done in duplicates and repeated three times.

## Effect of PDAs on Antibiotic Resistance in *A. baumannii*

The β-lactam antibiotics tested in the current study included Ampicillin, Meropenem, Methicillin, Penicillin, Aztreonam, Amoxicillin, and Piperacillin (Sigma-Aldrich). Previously published MIC of each aforementioned antibiotic against *A. baumannii* was used in the study (Vashist et al., 2011; Morfin-Otero and Dowzicky, 2012; Malone and Kwon, 2013) (**Table 1**). To determine the effect of combination of PDAs and antibiotics on *A. baumannii*, the MIC of each antibiotic and that of TC/EG were added to 10 ml TSB containing *A. baumannii* (~ 6 $\log_{10}$ CFU/ml), and incubated at 37°C for 24 h (Johny et al., 2010). The bacterial counts were determined after broth dilution assay and surface plating of appropriate dilutions on TSA. The treatments included only *A. baumannii* (positive control), *A. baumannii* + antibiotic, *A. baumannii* + PDA and *A. baumannii* + antibiotic + PDA. In addition, suitable controls, including *A. baumannii* + diluent (ethanol) and *A. baumannii* + ethanol + antibiotic were also included. Duplicate samples were included for each treatment, and the experiment was replicated three times.

**TABLE 1** | MIC of antibiotics used in testing against *A. baumannii*.

| Antibiotics | MIC (μg/ml) |
|---|---|
| Ampicillin | 64 |
| Meropenem | 32 |
| Methicillin | 256 |
| Penicillin | 256 |
| Aztreonam | 256 |
| Amoxicillin | 64 |
| Piperacillin | 128 |

## Efflux Pump Inhibition Assay

To study the effect of TC and EG on inhibiting the action of efflux pumps in *A. baumannii*, EtBr and pyronin Y efflux assays were performed according to a published protocol (Chusri et al., 2009). Overnight cultures of *A. baumannii* were washed twice and resuspended in PBS containing 0.4% glucose to an $OD_{600}$ of ~0.5. The bacterial suspension was added with the MIC of TC/EG or CCP (positive control, 100 μM), and incubated at 37°C for 5 h. *A. baumannii* suspension in PBS + 0.4% glucose served as control. After incubation, 200 μl of the treatments/control was separately transferred to a 96-well microtiter plate, followed by addition of EtBr (Sigma) to a final concentration of 4 mg/l, and the fluorescence was measured at excitation 530 nm and emission 645 nm. The assay was repeated with pyronin Y (Sigma) at a final concentration of 5 mg/l at 530 nm and emission 645 nm. The experiment was repeated three times with duplicates for *A. baumannii* 17978 and *A. baumannii* 251847.

## Outer Membrane Permeabilization Assay

To study the effect of TC and EG on the outer membrane of *A. baumannii*, NPN uptake assay was performed using a published protocol (Chusri et al., 2009). Overnight *A. baumannii* 17978 and *A. baumannii* 251847 cultures were separately washed and resuspended in 5 mM HEPES buffer to an $OD_{600}$ ~ 0.5. Aliquots of 100 μl of *A. baumannii* suspension were transferred to a microtiter plate along with the MIC of TC/EG or EDTA 1 mM/HEPES buffer. This was followed by addition of 40 μM of NPN to make the total volume to 200 μl, the fluorescence was measured within 3 min at excitation 355 nm and emission 460 nm, and continuously recorded for 3 h every 10 min. The experiment was repeated three times with duplicates in each treatment.

## Effect of PDAs on Antibiotic Resistance Gene Expression in *A. baumannii*

### RNA Extraction and cDNA Synthesis

To study the effect of TC and EG on genes associated with resistance to β-lactam antibiotics in *A. baumannii*, bacterial cultures were grown separately with or without the SIC of TC/EG at 37°C in TSB to mid-log phase. *A. baumannii* grown with either antibiotic alone or PDA alone were also included as controls. After incubation, the cultures were subjected to centrifugation (12,000 × *g*, 15 min, 4°C) and the resultant pellet was added with 0.5 ml of RNAse free, sterile water and 1 ml of RNA protect reagent (Qiagen, Valencia, CA, United States). The total RNA from each sample was extracted using the RNeasy mini kit (Qiagen), and the manufacturer's instructions were followed in estimating the total RNA using Nanodrop (Thermo Fisher Scientific, Waltham, MA, United States). Super-script II reverse transcriptase kit (Invitrogen, Carlsbad, CA, United States) was used for cDNA synthesis, and the resultant cDNA was used as a template for RT-qPCR. The amplified product was detected using SYBR Green reagents.

### Real-Time Quantitative PCR (RT-qPCR)

The antibiotic resistance genes of *A. baumannii* assayed for expression analysis included efflux pump genes, namely *adeA*, *adeB*, *adeC*; β-lactam resistance gene, *blaP*; and the multidrug resistance protein gene, *mdrp*. Primer Express software® (Applied Biosystems, Foster city, CA, United States) was used for designing the primers specific for the genes and for the endogenous control (16S rRNA). The primers were designed from *A. baumannii* AB0057 genome (CP001182.1) published in the NCBI database (Adams et al., 2008) and their sequences are provided in **Table 2**. The custom synthesized primers were obtained from Integrated DNA Technologies (Foster City, CA, United States). RT-qPCR was performed with StepOnePlus™ Real Time PCR system (Applied Biosystems) using the SYBR green assay (Applied Biosystems) under custom thermal cycling conditions with the normalized RNA as the template (Bookout and Mangelsdorf, 2003). Duplicate samples were analyzed and standardized against 16S rRNA gene expression. The relative changes in mRNA expression levels were determined using comparative threshold cycle (CT) method ($2^{-\Delta\Delta C_T}$) between the control and the treatments.

## Statistical Analysis

A completely randomized design with a factorial treatment structure was used. The factors included two *A. baumannii* strains, seven antibiotics, and two PDAs. The data were analyzed using the PROC GENMOD procedure of Statistical Analysis Software (SAS ver. 9.4; SAS Institute Inc., Cary, NC, United States). Least square means were considered significant at $P < 0.05$. The data comparisons for gene expression study were made using Students *t*-test. The difference was considered significant at $P < 0.05$.

**TABLE 2** | List of primers used in detecting *A. baumannii* antibiotic resistance genes.

| Gene | Sequence (5'→3') | Function |
|---|---|---|
| *adeA* (F) | TGACCGACCAATGCACCTT | Efflux pump |
| (R) | GCAACAGTTCGAGCGCCTAT | |
| *adeB* (F) | CCGATGACGTATCGAAGTTAGGA | Efflux pump |
| (R) | CCGATGACGTATCGAAGTTAGGA | |
| *adeC* (F) | ACGGCCCCAGAAGTCTAGTTC | Efflux pump |
| (R) | CGATTAACCCCAATAACCCAGTT | |
| *blaP* (F) | ACACTAGGAGAAGCCATGAAGCTT | Beta-lactam resistance Antibiotics |
| (R) | GCATGAGATCAAGACCGATAC G | |
| *mdrp* (F) | GTACGGCTTCTAGACCCACCATTTT | Multiple drug resistance protein |
| (R) | ACAAAGAGCCGTGCACAGTTT | |
| rRNA-16S (F) | TCGCTAGTAATCGCGGATCA CGCTGGCGGC | Endogenous control |
| (R) | GACGGGCGGTGTGTACAAG | |

*F, forward; R, reverse.*

## RESULTS

The SICs of TC and EG against *A. baumannii* were found to be 1.1 mM (0.015%) and 1.8 mM (0.03%), respectively, while the MIC was 4 mM (0.05% TC and 0.065% EG) for both PDAs. Although a previously reported MIC of each antibiotic against *A. baumannii* was used in the study, both *A. baumannii* isolates grew ~ by 2.0 $\log_{10}$ CFU/ml after 24 h (antibiotic control), as observed in **Figures 1, 2** and Supplementary Figures 1, 2. In the presence of the MIC of TC, the bacterial count after 24 h did not change significantly from the inoculation of level of 6.0 $\log_{10}$ CFU/ml (**Figure 1**) as expected. However, when *A. baumannii* was grown in the presence of each antibiotic and TC, its growth after 24 h was significantly decreased in comparison to that in the positive control, antibiotic control and TC control ($P < 0.05$). In both *A. baumannii* isolates, the greatest sensitivity was observed to methicillin and lowest sensitivity was seen against ampicillin and meropenem (**Figure 1** and Supplementary Figure 1). Similarly, the sensitivity of both *A. baumannii* isolates to all seven antibiotics was significantly increased in the presence of EG, as indicated by the reduced growth after 24 h ($P < 0.05$) (**Figure 2** and Supplementary Figure 2). In *A. baumannii* 17978, the greatest sensitivity was observed against ampicillin (**Figure 2**), whereas *A. baumannii* 251847 was maximally sensitive to amoxicillin (Supplementary Figure 2).

The results of the efflux pump inhibition assay using EtBr and pyronin Y in *A. baumannii* ATCC 17978 and *A. baumannii* 251847 are presented in **Figures 3, 4** and Supplementary Figures 3, 4. EtBr and pyronin Y are known substrates for AdeABC and AdeIJK efflux pumps, respectively (Magnet et al., 2001; Xing et al., 2014). The MIC of TC and EG resulted in an increased accumulation of EtBr inside bacterial cells, as indicated by an increase in fluorescence compared to the PBS control ($P < 0.05$) (**Figures 5A–G**). CCP, an efflux pump inhibitor used as a positive control (Magnet et al., 2001) also resulted in an increase in fluorescence indicating suppression of efflux pump in *A. baumannii*. However, a similar increase in the fluorescence

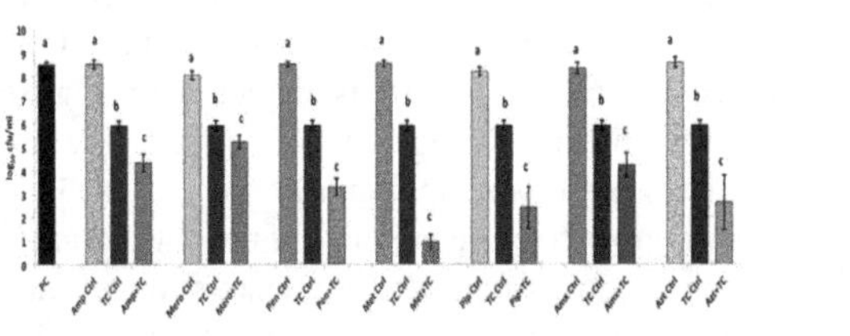

**FIGURE 1** | Effect of TC in combination with β-lactam antibiotics in *A. baumannii* 17978. Bars with different superscripts differ from each other within a cluster ($P < 0.05$). *A. baumannii* 17978 was grown with each β-lactam antibiotic either alone or in combination with TC. Bacteria not exposed to any treatments (PC) and bacteria exposed to only TC (TC Ctrl) served as controls for the experiment.

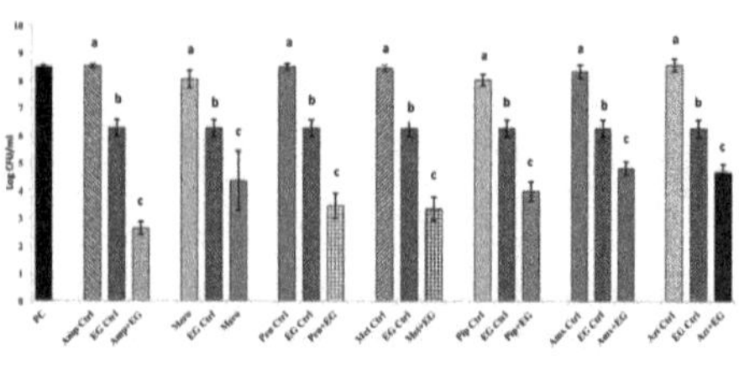

FIGURE 2 | Effect of EG in combination with β-lactam antibiotics in *A. baumannii* 17978. Bars with different superscripts differ from each other within a cluster ($P < 0.05$). *A. baumannii* 17978 was grown with each β-lactam antibiotic either alone or in combination with EG. Bacteria not exposed to any treatments (PC) and bacteria exposed to only EG (EG Ctrl) served as controls for the experiment.

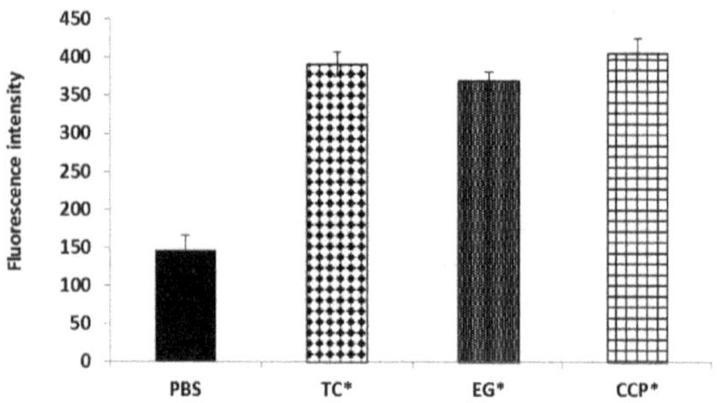


FIGURE 3 | Intracellular accumulation of ethidium bromide (EtBr) in *A. baumannii* ATCC 17978 after treatment with MIC of TC and EG, as measured by fluorescence intensity. *A. baumannii* ATCC 17978 was added with MIC of TC/EG or CCP (100 μM) and incubated for 5 h at 37°C. Fluorescence (excitation 530 nm and emission 645 nm) was measured after addition of EtBr (4 mg/l). Treatments with * are significantly different from PBS (control) ($P < 0.05$).

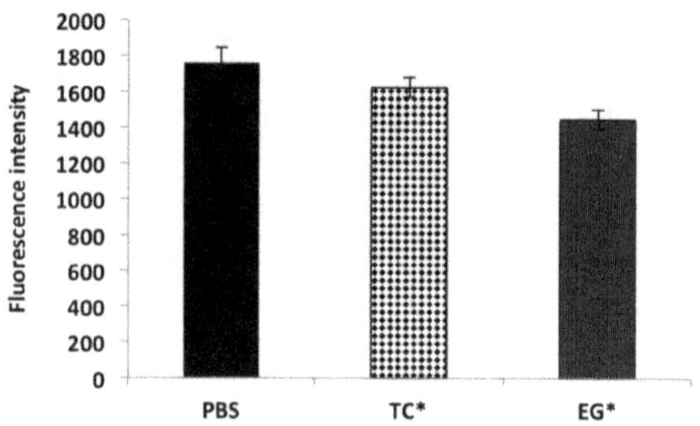


FIGURE 4 | Intracellular accumulation of pyronin Y in *A. baumannii* ATCC 17978 after treatment with MIC of TC and EG, as measured by fluorescence intensity. *A. baumannii* ATCC 17978 was added with MIC of TC/EG and incubated for 5 h at 37°C. Fluorescence (excitation 530 nm and emission 645 nm) was measured after addition of pyronin Y (5 mg/l). Treatments with * are significantly different from PBS (control) ($P < 0.05$).

was not observed for pyronin Y compared to the PBS control (**Figure 4** and Supplementary Figure 4). The results of NPN uptake assay in *A. baumannii* ATCC 17978 and *A. baumannii* 251847 are presented in Supplementary Figures 5, 6, respectively. Neither TC nor EG increased NPN uptake, while the EDTA control did show an increase in fluorescence. Further, the samples treated with TC or EG demonstrated a decrease in fluorescence over time (data not shown).

The effect of seven antibiotics and two PDAs and their combination on the expression of various antibiotic resistance genes in *A. baumannii* 17978 is depicted in **Figures 5A–G.** It was observed that compared to control, the expression of all tested genes was up-regulated ($P < 0.05$) following *A. baumannii* growth in the presence of the antibiotics. However, TC significantly down-regulated the expression of major genes conferring resistance to β-lactam antibiotics compared to control ($P < 0.05$). The genes encoding efflux pump *adeA* and *adeB* were down regulated by ~6- and 9-fold, respectively. Moreover, the expression of genes encoding β-lactamase (*blaP*) and the multiple drug resistance protein (*mdrp*) was decreased by ~3-fold ($P < 0.05$). Similar to the results observed with TC, all antibiotic resistance genes were down-regulated on exposure to EG compared to control ($P < 0.05$). The expression of genes encoding efflux pumps, *adeA* and *adeB* were down-expressed by 3- and 14-fold, respectively. Similarly, *blaP* and *mdrp* were also down-regulated in both strains ($P < 0.05$). The combination of TC or EG with the antibiotics also resulted in a down-regulation of majority of the tested genes ($P < 0.05$). Among the combinations of TC or EG with the seven antibiotics, the combination containing aztreonam resulted in a significant down-regulation of all the tested genes compared to control (**Figure 5D**). The combination of EG with piperacillin (**Figure 5C**) or penicillin (**Figure 5F**) also significantly reduced the expression of all the antibiotic resistance genes ($P < 0.05$).

## DISCUSSION

Rapid emergence of antibiotic resistance in pathogenic microorganisms, especially to multiple antibiotics has ignited research efforts to discover novel antibiotics and develop effective derivatives of currently available antibiotics. However, no promising antibiotics are under development, and the rapidity and complexity of resistance development in pathogens have further exacerbated the situation. In light of this, a potential viable approach was explored to reduce bacterial antibiotic resistance in the development of inhibitors of resistance mechanisms in bacteria (Renau et al., 1999; Walsh and Fanning, 2008). This strategy involves the co-administration of an antibiotic with an "inhibitor," which counteracts bacterial resistance mechanism(s), thereby rendering the resistant pathogen sensitive to the drug. The advantage of this approach is that it makes it possible to continue the use of current antibiotics, for which in-depth pharmacological and toxicological data are already available. In this regard, PDAs represent a potential natural group of "inhibitors" of bacterial antibiotic resistance mechanisms.

Abundant literature exists on the antimicrobial properties of a variety of plant compounds against a wide range of microorganisms (Burt, 2004; Upadhyay et al., 2014). However, only a handful of studies have addressed their effect on bacterial

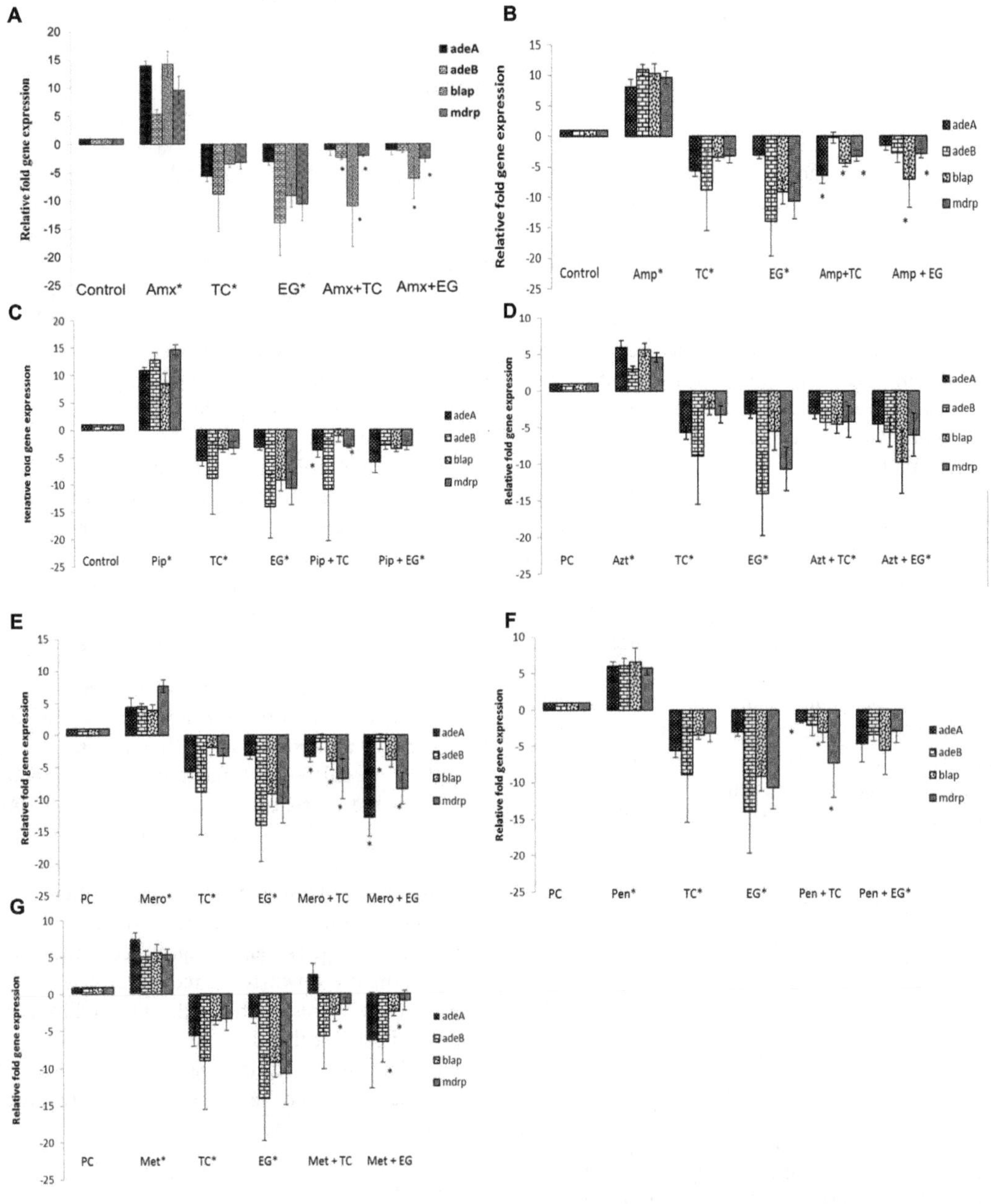


**FIGURE 5 |** Effect of TC and EG on antibiotic resistance genes in *A. baumannii* 17978. **(A)** *A. baumannii* 17978 was grown with the SIC of TC/EG either alone or in combination with amoxicillin, and RT-qPCR was done to test the effect of the treatments on major antibiotic genes in *A. baumannii.* Bacteria exposed to amoxicillin alone and bacteria not exposed to any treatments served as controls. Bars with * are significantly different from control ($P < 0.05$). **(B)** *A. baumannii* 17978 was treated with SICs of TC/EG either alone or in combination with ampicillin and RT-qPCR was done to test the effect of the treatments on major antibiotic genes in *A. baumannii.* Bacteria exposed to ampicillin alone and bacteria not exposed to any treatments served as controls. Bars with * are significantly different from control ($P < 0.05$). **(C)** *A. baumannii* 17978 was treated with SICs of TC/EG either alone or in combination with piperacillin and RT-qPCR was done to test the effect of the treatments on major antibiotic genes in *A. baumannii.* Bacteria exposed to piperacillin alone and bacteria not exposed to any treatments served as controls. Bars with * are significantly different from control ($P < 0.05$). **(D)** *A. baumannii* 17978 was treated with SICs of TC/EG either alone or in combination with aztreonam and RT-qPCR was done to test the effect of the treatments on major antibiotic genes in *A. baumannii.* Bacteria exposed to aztreonam alone and bacteria not exposed to any treatments served as controls. Bars with * are significantly different from control ($P < 0.05$). **(E)** *A. baumannii* 17978 was treated with SICs of TC/EG either alone or in combination with meropenem and RT-qPCR was done to test the effect of the treatments on major antibiotic genes in *A. baumannii.* Bacteria exposed to meropenem alone and bacteria not exposed to any treatments served as controls. Bars with * are significantly different from control ($P < 0.05$). **(F)** *A. baumannii* 17978 was treated with SICs of TC/EG either alone or in combination with penicillin and RT-qPCR was done to test the effect of the treatments on major antibiotic genes in *A. baumannii.* Bacteria exposed to penicillin alone and bacteria not exposed to any treatments served as controls. Bars with * are significantly different from control ($P < 0.05$). **(G)** *A. baumannii* 17978 was treated with SICs of TC/EG either alone or in combination with methicillin and RT-qPCR was done to test the effect of the treatments on major antibiotic genes in *A. baumannii.* Bacteria exposed to methicillin alone and bacteria not exposed to any treatments served as controls. Bars with * are significantly different from control ($P < 0.05$).

antibiotic resistance, especially in Gram negative bacteria (Gallucci et al., 2006; Chusri et al., 2009; Johny et al., 2010; Ilić et al., 2014). In the current study, both TC and EG enhanced the sensitivity of *A. baumannii* to all seven β-lactam antibiotics tested (**Figures 1, 2** and Supplementary Figures 1, 2). This is evident from the significant reductions in bacterial counts observed in the samples containing PDA and antibiotics as compared to that in the treatments containing each PDA or antibiotic alone. A checkerboard assay testing a wide range of concentrations of two antimicrobials is commonly used for determining their combinatorial effects on a bacterium (Jayamani et al., 2017; Tharmalingam et al., 2018). However, since our preliminary studies revealed that concentrations of TC and EG below the MIC were not significantly effective in increasing *A. baumannii* sensitivity to antibiotics, we did not use a checkerboard assay, but instead tested the combinatorial effect of MIC of plant molecules and antibiotics on the pathogen.

A recent study also reported synergistic effect of *Eucalyptus camaldulensis* with polymyxin B against MDR *Acinetobacter baumannii* (Knezevic et al., 2016). In another study, Enrofloxacin and cinnamon were observed to possess synergistic effect against *Salmonella enterica* (Solarte et al., 2017). Further, extracts of medicinal plant *Holarrhena antidysenterica* with Conessine increased susceptibility of extensively drug resistant *A. baumannii* to novobiocin and rifampicin (Siriyong et al., 2016). Additionally, no cytotoxic effects on human epithelial cells at the tested concentrations were reported previously with TC and EG (Amalaradjou et al., 2010; Karumathil et al., 2016). Moreover our previous studies revealed that in-feed supplementation of TC and EG in broiler chicks (Kollanoor-Johny et al., 2012) and TC in mice (Narayanan et al., 2017) for 10 days did not result in any toxicity.

*A. baumannii* has been reported to exhibit resistance to β-lactam antibiotics through several mechanisms, including the production of β-lactamases, changes in penicillin-binding proteins (PBPs), altering the structure and number of porin proteins, decreased membrane permeability, and by use of efflux pumps that exit antibiotics out of the bacterial cell (Vila et al., 2007; Manchanda et al., 2010; Bonnin et al., 2013; Tang et al., 2014). Moreover, the presence of efflux pumps and MDR proteins in *A. baumannii* contribute significantly to both intrinsic and acquired resistance to antibiotics (Lomovskaya and Bostian, 2006). *A. baumannii* genome encodes a wide array of multidrug efflux systems, including AdeABC, a resistance-nodulation-division (RND) family-type pump (Damier-Piolle et al., 2008; Wieczorek et al., 2008; Yoon et al., 2013; Sun et al., 2014). The substrates for this pump include beta-lactams, aminoglycosides, erythromycin, chloramphenicol, tetracycline, fluoroquinolone, trimethoprim, and EtBr (Magnet et al., 2001; Higgins et al., 2004; Heritier et al., 2005; Peleg et al., 2007). The three component structures of AdeABC include the inner membrane fusion protein (AdeA), transmembrane component (AdeB) and an outer membrane protein (AdeC), with the inactivation of *adeB* resulting in the loss of pump function and multidrug resistance (Magnet et al., 2001).

In order to determine if TC or EG exerted an inhibitory effect on the aforementioned efflux pumps in *A. baumannii*, an efflux pump inhibition assay was performed with EtBr and pyronin Y along with CCP, a documented efflux pump inhibitor (Magnet et al., 2001; Chusri et al., 2009). EtBr and pyronin Y are known substrates for AdeABC and AdeIJK efflux pumps, respectively (Magnet et al., 2001; Damier-Piolle et al., 2008; Chusri et al., 2009; Xing et al., 2014). Both TC and EG resulted in the inhibition of AdeABC efflux pump in the two tested *A. baumannii* strains, as evident from the increase in fluorescence in the treated samples compared to PBS control (**Figure 3** and Supplementary Figure 3). However, the PDAs did not exert any inhibitory effect on the action of AdeIJK efflux pump in *A. baumannii*, as evident from the lack of difference in fluorescence units between PDA-treated and PBS control samples (**Figure 4** and Supplementary Figure 4). Similarly, the results from the NPN uptake assay revealed that TC and EG did not increase *A. baumannii*'s outer membrane permeability, as seen from Supplementary Figures 5, 6, where no increase in fluorescence was observed in PDA-treated *A. baumannii* as against the samples treated with EDTA, a known outer membrane permeabilizer in Gram-negative bacteria (Helander and Mattila-Sandholm, 2000; Alakomi et al., 2006). These results indicate that TC and EG increased the sensitivity of *A. baumannii* to the tested antibiotics at least in part by inhibiting the efflux pump, AdeABC.

For ascertaining if TC or EG exerted an inhibitory effect on any of the antibiotic resistance genes conferring resistance to β-lactam antibiotics in *A. baumannii*, we performed a RT-qPCR on mRNA extracted from *A. baumannii* following growth in the presence and absence of the PDAs. The results from the RT-qPCR revealed that TC and EG in combination with or without each antibiotic significantly down-regulated the expression of the majority of genes that confer resistance to β-lactam antibiotics (**Figures 5A–G**). Among the various genes screened, those encoding efflux pumps, *adeA* and *adeB* were maximally down-regulated by both PDAs. These results concur with the results from the EtBr efflux pump inhibition assay, and suggest that TC and EG enhanced the efficacy of the seven β-lactam antibiotics against *A. baumannii* by thwarting the various resistance mechanisms, especially those involving the efflux pumps.

## CONCLUSION

The results of this study suggest the potential use of TC and EG in conjunction with the currently available β-lactam antibiotics for the treatment for MDR *A. baumannii* infections and could lead to development of new treatment options with reduced antibiotic dosage. However, efficacy studies in suitable animal models are warranted before recommending their clinical usage.

## AUTHOR CONTRIBUTIONS

KV is the corresponding author and primary contact during manuscript submission, review, and publication process. The work was done under his supervision as the principal investigator. He significantly contributed to the design, drafting, revisions, and interpretation of data. The manuscript is being submitted with his final approval for publication. MN is the submitting author. DK and AK-J designed the study. DK and JG conducted the experiments. DK and MN prepared the manuscript for submission.

## REFERENCES


Abbott, I., Cerqueira, G. M., Bhuiyan, S., and Peleg, A. Y. (2013). Carbapenem resistance in *Acinetobacter baumannii*: laboratory challenges, mechanistic insights and therapeutic strategies. *Expert Rev. Anti. Infect. Ther.* 11, 395–409. doi: 10.1586/eri.13.21

Adams, M. D., Goglin, K., Molyneaux, N., Hujer, K. M., Lavender, H., Jamison, J. J., et al. (2008). Comparative genome sequence analysis of multidrug-resistant *Acinetobacter baumannii. J. Bacteriol.* 190, 8053–8064. doi: 10.1128/JB.00834-08

Al Mobarak, M. F., Matbuli, R. M., Meir, H., Al Gehani, N., ElToukhy, A. A. M., Al Qureshey, K. F., et al. (2014). Antimicrobial resistance patterns among *Acinetobacter baumannii* isolated from King Abdulaziz Hospital, Jeddah, Saudi Arabia, Four-Year Surveillance Study (2010–2013). *Egypt. J. Med. Microbiol.* 23, 53–60. doi: 10.12816/0025920

Alakomi, H. L., Paananen, A., Suihko, M. L., Helander, I. M., and Saarela, M. (2006). Weakening effect of cell permeabilizers on gram-negative bacteria using biodeterioration. *Appl. Environ. Microbiol.* 72, 4695–4703. doi: 10.1128/AEM.00142-06

Amalaradjou, M. A. R., Narayanan, A., Baskaran, S. A., and Venkitanarayanan, K. (2010). Antibiofilm effect of trans-cinnamaldehyde on uropathogenic *Escherichia coli. J. Urol.* 184, 358–363. doi: 10.1016/j.juro.2010.03.006

Amalaradjou, M. A. R., and Venkitanarayanan, K. (2011). Effect of trans-cinnamaldehyde on reducing resistance to environmental stresses in Cronobacter sakazakii. *Foodborne Pathog. Dis.* 8, 403–409. doi: 10.1089/fpd.2010.0691

Bassetti, M., Righi, E., Esposito, S., Petrosillo, N., and Nicolini, L. (2008). Drug treatment for multidrug-resistant *Acinetobacter baumannii* infections. *Future Microbiol.* 3, 649–660. doi: 10.2217/17460913.3.6.649

Bonnin, R. A., Nordmann, P., and Poirel, L. (2013). Screening and deciphering antibiotic resistance in *Acinetobacter baumannii*: a state of the art. *Expert Rev. Anti. Infect. Ther.* 11, 571–583. doi: 10.1586/eri.13.38

Bookout, A. L., and Mangelsdorf, D. J. (2003). Quantitative real-time PCR protocol for analysis of nuclear receptor signaling pathways. *Nucl. Recept. Signal.* 1, 1–7. doi: 10.1621/nrs.01012

Burt, S. (2004). Essential oils: their antibacterial properties and potential applications in foods—a review. *Int. J. Food Microbiol.* 94, 223–253. doi: 10.1016/j.ijfoodmicro.2004.03.022

Cai, Y., Chai, D., Wang, R., Liang, B., and Bai, N. (2012). Colistin resistance of *Acinetobacter baumannii*: clinical reports, mechanisms and antimicrobial strategies. *J. Antimicrob. Chemother.* 67, 1607–1615. doi: 10.1093/jac/dks084

Centers for Disease Control and Prevention [CDC] (2004). Acinetobacter baumannii infections among patients at military medical facilities treating injured US service members, 2002-2004. *Morb. Mortal Wkly. Rep.* 53, 1063–1066.

Chusri, S., Villanueva, I., Voravuthikunchai, S. P., and Davies, J. (2009). Enhancing antibiotic activity: a strategy to control Acinetobacter infections. *J. Antimicrob. Chemother.* 64, 1203–1211. doi: 10.1093/jac/dkp381

Cowan, M. M. (1999). Plant products as antimicrobial agents. *Clin. Microbiol. Rev.* 12, 564–582.

Damier-Piolle, L., Magnet, S., Bremont, S., Lambert, T., and Courvalin, P. (2008). AdeIJK, a resistance-nodulation-cell division pump effluxing multiple antibiotics in *Acinetobacter baumannii. Antimicrob. Agents Chemother.* 52, 557–562. doi: 10.1128/AAC.00732-07

Doi, Y., Husain, S., Potoski, B. A., McCurry, K. R., and Paterson, D. L. (2009). Extensively drug-resistant *Acinetobacter baumannii. Emerg. Infect. Diseases* 15, 980–982. doi: 10.3201/eid1506.081006

Duarte, A., Ferreira, S., Silva, F., and Domingues, F. C. (2012). Synergistic activity of coriander oil and conventional antibiotics against *Acinetobacter baumannii. Phytomedicine* 19, 236–238. doi: 10.1016/j.phymed.2011.11.010

Ellis, D., Cohen, B., Liu, J., and Larson, E. (2015). Risk factors for hospital-acquired antimicrobial-resistant infection caused by *Acinetobacter baumannii*: antimicrob. *Resist. Infect. Control.* 4, 1–5. doi: 10.1186/s13756-015-0083-2

Espinal, P., Marti, S., and Vila, J. (2012). Effect of biofilm formation on the survival of *Acinetobacter baumannii* on dry surfaces. *J. Hosp. Infect.* 80, 56–60. doi: 10.1016/j.jhin.2011.08.013

Esterly, J. S., Griffith, M., Qi, C., Malczynski, M., Postelnick, M. J., and Scheetz, M. H. (2011). Impact of carbapenem resistance and receipt of active antimicrobial therapy on clinical outcomes of *Acinetobacter baumannii* bloodstream infections. *Antimicrob. Agents Chemother.* 55, 4844–4849. doi: 10.1128/AAC.01728-10

Falagas, M. E., Koletsi, P. K., and Bliziotis, I. A. (2006). The diversity of definitions of multidrug-resistant (MDR) and pandrug-resistant (PDR) *Acinetobacter baumannii* and *Pseudomonas aeruginosa. J. Med. Microbiol.* 55, 1619–1629. doi: 10.1099/jmm.0.46747-0

Fonseca, E. L., Scheidegger, E., Freitas, F. S., Cipriano, R., and Vicente, A. C. (2013). Carbapenem-resistant *Acinetobacter baumannii* from Brazil: role of carO alleles expression and blaOXA-23 gene. *BMC Microbiol.* 13:245. doi: 10.1186/1471-2180-13-245

Gallucci, N., Casero, C., Oliva, M., Zygadlo, J., and Demo, M. (2006). Interaction between terpenes and penicillin on bacterial strains resistant to beta-lactam antibiotics. *Mol. Med. Chem.* 10, 30–32.

Garnacho-Montero, J., and Amaya-Villar, R. (2010). Multiresistant *Acinetobacter baumannii* infections: epidemiology and management. *Curr Opin Infect Dis.* 23, 332–339. doi: 10.1097/QCO.0b013e32833ae38b

Giamarellou, H., Antoniadou, A., and Kanellakopoulou, K. (2008). *Acinetobacter baumannii*: a universal threat to public health? *Int. J. Antimicrob. Agents* 32, 106–119. doi: 10.1016/j.ijantimicag.2008.02.013

Helander, I. M., and Mattila-Sandholm, T. (2000). Fluorometric assessment of gram-negative bacterial permeabilization. *J. Appl. Microbiol.* 88, 213–219. doi: 10.1046/j.1365-2672.2000.00971.x

Heritier, C., Poirel, L., Lambert, T., and Nordmann, P. (2005). Contribution of acquired carbapenem-hydrolyzing oxacillinases to carbapenem resistance in *Acinetobacter baumannii. Antimicrob. Agents Chemother.* 49, 3198–3202. doi: 10.1128/AAC.49.8.3198-3202.2005

Hernan, R. C., Karina, B., Gabriela, G., Marcela, N., Carlos, V., and Angela, F. (2009). Selection of colistin-resistant *Acinetobacter baumannii* isolates in postneurosurgical meningitis in an intensive care unit with high presence of heteroresistance to colistin. *Diagn. Microbiol. Infect. Dis.* 65, 188–191. doi: 10.1016/j.diagmicrobio.2009.05.019

Higgins, P. G., Wisplinghoff, H., Stefanik, D., and Seifert, H. (2004). Selection of topoisomerase mutations and overexpression of adeB mRNA transcripts during an outbreak of *Acinetobacter baumannii. J. Antimicrob. Chemother.* 54, 821–823. doi: 10.1093/jac/dkh427

Ilić, B. S., Kocić, B. D., Ćirić, V. M., Cvetković, O. G., and Miladinović, D. L. (2014). An In Vitro synergistic interaction of combinations of *Thymus glabrescens* essential oil and its main constituents with chloramphenicol. *Sci.World J.* 2014:826219.. doi: 10.1155/2014/826219

Jayamani, E., Tharmalingam, N., Rajamuthiah, R., Coleman, J. J., Kim, W., Okoli, I., et al. (2017). Characterization of a *Francisella tularensis-Caenorhabditis elegans* pathosystem for the evaluation of therapeutic compounds. *Antimicrob. Agents Chemo.* 61, e310–e317. doi: 10.1128/AAC.00310-17

Johny, A. K., Hoagland, T., and Venkitanarayanan, K. (2010). Effect of subinhibitory concentrations of plant-derived molecules in increasing the sensitivity of multidrug-resistant *Salmonella enterica* serovar Typhimurium DT104 to antibiotics. *Foodborne Pathog. Dis.* 7, 1165–1170. doi: 10.1089/fpd.2009.0527

Karageorgopoulos, D. E., and Falagas, M. E. (2008). Current control and treatment of multidrug-resistant *Acinetobacter baumannii* infections. *Lancet Infect. Dis.* 8, 751–762. doi: 10.1016/S1473-3099(08)70279-2

Karumathil, D. P., Surendran-Nair, M., and Venkitanarayanan, K. (2016). Efficacy of trans-cinnamaldehyde and eugenol in reducing *Acinetobacter baumannii* adhesion to and invasion of human keratinocytes and controlling wound infection in vitro. *Phytother. Res.* 30, 2053–2059. doi: 10.1002/ptr.5713

Knezevic, P., Aleksic, V., Simin, N., Svircev, E., Petrovic, A., and Mimica-Dukic, N. (2016). Antimicrobial activity of *Eucalyptus camaldulensis* essential oils and their interactions with conventional antimicrobial agents against multi-drug resistant *Acinetobacter baumannii*. *J. Ethnopharmacol.* 178, 125–136. doi: 10.1016/j.jep.2015.12.008

Kollanoor-Johny, A., Mattson, T., Baskaran, S. A., Amalaradjou, M. A., Babapoor, S., March, B., et al. (2012). Reduction of *Salmonella enterica* serovar Enteritidis colonization in 20-day-old broiler chickens by the plant-derived compounds trans-cinnamaldehyde and eugenol. *Appl. Environ. Microbiol.* 78, 2981–2987. doi: 10.1128/AEM.07643-11

Kon, K. V., and Rai, M. K. (2012). Plant essential oils and their constituents in coping with multidrug-resistant bacteria. *Expert Rev. Anti. Infect. Ther.* 10, 775–790. doi: 10.1586/eri.12.57

Lean, S. S., Suhaili, Z., Ismail, S., Rahman, N. I. A., Othman, N., Abdullah, F. H., et al. (2014). Prevalence and genetic characterization of carbapenem-and polymyxin-resistant *Acinetobacter baumannii* Isolated from a tertiary hospital in Terengganu, Malaysia. *ISRN Microbiol.* 2014:953417. doi: 10.1155/2014/953417

Lee, H. W., Koh, Y. M., Kim, J., Lee, J. C., Lee, Y. C., Seol, S. Y., et al. (2008). Capacity of multidrug-resistant clinical isolates of *Acinetobacter baumannii* to form biofilm and adhere to epithelial cell surfaces. *Clin. Microbiol. Infect.* 14, 49–54. doi: 10.1111/j.1469-0691.2007.01842.x

Leung, W. S., Chu, C. M., Chan, V. L., Lam, J. Y., and Ho, P. L. (2005). Fulminant community acquired *Acinetobacter baumannii* pneumonia as a distinct clinical syndrome. *Chest* 128, 149S–149S. doi: 10.1378/chest.128.4_MeetingAbstracts.149S

Lomovskaya, O., and Bostian, K. A. (2006). Practical applications and feasibility of efflux pump inhibitors in the clinic–a vision for applied use. *Biochem. Pharmacol.* 71, 910–918. doi: 10.1016/j.bcp.2005.12.008

Longo, F., Vuotto, C., and Donelli, G. (2014). Biofilm formation in *Acinetobacter baumannii*. *New Microbiol.* 37, 119–127.

Magnet, S., Courvalin, P., and Lambert, T. (2001). Resistance-nodulation-cell division-type efflux pump involved in aminoglycoside resistance in *Acinetobacter baumannii* strain BM4454. *Antimicrob. Agents Chemother.* 45, 3375–3380. doi: 10.1128/AAC.45.12.3375-3380.2001

Malone, L., and Kwon, D. H. (2013). Carbapenem-associated multidrug-resistant *Acinetobacter baumannii* are sensitised by aztreonam in combination with polyamines. *Int. J. Antimicro. Agents* 41, 70–74. doi: 10.1016/j.ijantimicag.2012.08.009

Manchanda, V., Sanchaita, S., and Singh, N. (2010). Multidrug resistant Acinetobacter. *J. Glob. Infect. Dis.* 2, 291–304. doi: 10.4103/0974-777X.68538

Maragakis, L. L., and Perl, T. M. (2008). *Acinetobacter baumannii*: epidemiology, antimicrobial resistance, and treatment options. *Clin. Infect. Dis.* 46, 1254–1263. doi: 10.1086/529198

Menon, T., Shanmugasundaram, S., Nandhakumar, B., Nalina, K., and Balasubramaniam. (2006). Infective endocarditis due to *Acinetobacter baumannii* complex–a case report. *Indian J. Pathol. Microbiol.* 49, 576–578.

Metan, G., Alp, E., Aygen, B., and Sumerkan, B. (2007). *Acinetobacter baumannii* meningitis in post-neurosurgical patients: clinical outcome and impact of carbapenem resistance. *J. Antimicrob. Chemother.* 60, 197–199. doi: 10.1093/jac/dkm181

Morfin-Otero, R., and Dowzicky, M. J. (2012). Changes in MIC within a global collection of *Acinetobacter baumannii* collected as part of the Tigecycline Evaluation and Surveillance Trial, 2004 to 2009. *Clin. Ther.* 34, 101–112. doi: 10.1016/j.clinthera.2011.11.028

Narayanan, A., Muyyarikkandy, M. S., Mooyottu, S., Venkitanarayanan, K., and Amalaradjou, M. A. R. (2017). Oral supplementation of trans-cinnamaldehyde reduces uropathogenic *Escherichia coli* colonization in a mouse model. *Lett. Appl. Microbiol.* 64, 192–197. doi: 10.1111/lam.12713

Neonakis, I. K., Spandidos, D. A., and Petinaki, E. (2011). Confronting multidrug-resistant *Acinetobacter baumannii*: a review. *Int. J. Antimicro. Agents* 37, 102–109. doi: 10.1016/j.ijantimicag.2010.10.014

Olut, A. I., and Erkek, E. (2005). Early prosthetic valve endocarditis due to *Acinetobacter baumannii*: a case report and brief review of the literature. *Scand. J. Infect. Dis.* 37, 919–921. doi: 10.1080/00365540500262567

Peleg, A. Y., Adams, J., and Paterson, D. L. (2007). Tigecycline efflux as a mechanism for nonsusceptibility in *Acinetobacter baumannii*. *Antimicrob. Agents Chemother.* 51, 2065–2069. doi: 10.1128/AAC.01198-06

Pitout, J. D., Sanders, C. C., and Sanders, W. E. (1997). Antimicrobial resistance with focus on β-lactam resistance in gram-negative bacilli. *Am. J. Med.* 103, 51–59. doi: 10.1016/S0002-9343(97)00044-2

Pogue, J., Kaye, K., Cohen, D., and Marchaim, D. (2015). Appropriate antimicrobial therapy in the era of multidrug-resistant human pathogens. *Clin. Microbiol. Infect.* 21, 302–312. doi: 10.1016/j.cmi.2014.12.025

Rao, R. S., Karthika, R. U., Singh, S. P., Shashikala, P., Kanungo, R., Jayachandran, S., et al. (2008). Correlation between biofilm production and multiple drug resistance in imipenem resistant clinical isolates of *Acinetobacter baumannii*. *Indian J. Med. Microbiol.* 26, 333–337. doi: 10.4103/0255-0857.43566

Renau, T. E., Léger, R., Flamme, E. M., Sangalang, J., She, M. W., Yen, R., et al. (1999). Inhibitors of efflux pumps in *Pseudomonas aeruginosa* potentiate the activity of the fluoroquinolone antibacterial levofloxacin. *J. Med. Chem.* 42, 4928–4931. doi: 10.1021/jm9904598

Saghi, H., Bahador, A., Khaledi, A., Kachoei, R. A., Dastjerdi, F. A., and Esmaeili, D. (2015). Antibacterial effects of origanum vulgare essence against multidrug-resistant *Acinetobacter baumannii* isolated from selected hospitals of Tehran, Iran. *Avicenna J. Clin. Microb. Infect.* 2, 1–5. doi: 10.17795/ajcmi-22982

Scott, P., Deye, G., Srinivasan, A., Murray, C., Moran, K., Hulten, E., et al. (2007). An outbreak of multidrug-resistant *Acinetobacter baumannii*-calcoaceticus complex infection in the US military health care system associated with military operations in Iraq. *Clin. Infect. Dis.* 44, 1577–1584. doi: 10.1086/518170

Shlaes, D. M., Sahm, D., Opiela, C., and Spellberg, B. (2013). The FDA reboot of antibiotic development. *Antimicrob. Agents Chemother.* 57, 4605–4607. doi: 10.1128/AAC.01277-13

Siriyong, T., Chusri, S., Srimanote, P., Tipmanee, V., and Voravuthikunchai, S. P. (2016). Holarrhena antidysenterica extract and its steroidal alkaloid conessine as resistance modifying agents against extensively drug resistant *Acinetobacter baumannii*. *Microb. Drug Resist.* 22, 273–282. doi: 10.1089/mdr.2015.0194

Solarte, A. L., Astorga, R. J., Aguiar, F., Galan-Relano, A., Maldonado, A., and Huerta, B. (2017). Combination of antimicrobials and essential oils as an alternative for the control of *Salmonella enterica* multiresistant strains related to foodborne disesase. *Foodborne Pathog. Dis.*. 14, 558–563. doi: 10.1089/fpd.2017.2295

Sun, J., Deng, Z., and Yan, A. (2014). Bacterial multidrug efflux pumps: Mechanisms, physiology and pharmacological exploitations. *Biochem. Biophys. Res. Commun.* 453, 254–267. doi: 10.1016/j.bbrc.2014.05.090

Sunenshine, R. H., Wright, M. O., Maragakis, L. L., Harris, A. D., Song, X., Hebden, J., et al. (2007). Multidrug-resistant Acinetobacter infection mortality rate and length of hospitalization. *Emerg. Infect. Dis* 13, 97–103. doi: 10.3201/eid1301.060716

Talbot, G. H., Bradley, J., Edwards, J. E. Jr., Gilbert, D., Scheld, M., and Bartlett, J. G. (2006). Antimicrobial availability task force of the infectious diseases society of America, 2006. Bad bugs need drugs: an update on the development pipeline from the antimicrobial availability task force of the infectious diseases society of America. *Clin. Infect. Dis.* 42, 657–668. doi: 10.1086/499819

Tang, S. S., Apisarnthanarak, A., and Hsu, L. Y. (2014). Mechanisms of β-lactam antimicrobial resistance and epidemiology of major community- and healthcare-associated multidrug-resistant bacteria. *Adv. Drug Deliv. Rev.* 78, 3–13. doi: 10.1016/j.addr.2014.08.003

Thakuria, B., and Lahon, K. (2013). The beta lactam antibiotics as an empirical therapy in a developing country: an update on their current status and recommendations to counter the resistance against them. *J. Clin. Diagn. Res.* 7, 1207–1214. doi: 10.7860/JCDR/2013/5239.3052

Tharmalingam, N., Rajmuthiah, R., Kim, W., Fuchs, B. B., Jeyamani, E., Kelso, M. J., et al. (2018). Antibacterial properties of four novel hit compounds from a methicillin-resistant *Staphylococcus aureus–Caenorhabditis elegans* high-throughput screen. *Microb. Drug Resist.* doi: 10.1089/mdr.2017.0250 [Epub ahead of print].

Tiwari, M., Roy, R., and Tiwari, V. (2016). Screening of Herbal based bioactive extract against Carbapenem-resistant strain of *Acinetobacter baumannii*. *Microb. Drug Resist.* 22, 364–371. doi: 10.1089/mdr.2015.0270

Tiwari, V., Tiwari, D., Patel, V., and Tiwari, M. (2017). Effect of secondary metabolite of *Actinidia deliciosa* on the biofilm and extra-cellular matrix components of *Acinetobacter baumannii*. *Microb. Pathog.* 110, 345–351. doi: 10.1016/j.micpath.2017.07.013

Ulu-Kilic, A., Ahmed, S. S., Alp, E., and Doğanay, M. (2013). Challenge of intensive care unit-acquired infections and *Acinetobacter baumannii* in developing countries. *OA Crit. Care* 1:3. doi: 10.13172/2052-9309-1-1-382

Upadhyay, A., Upadhyaya, I., Kollanoor-Johny, A., and Venkitanarayanan, K. (2014). Combating pathogenic microorganisms using plant-derived antimicrobials: a mini review of the mechanistic basis. *Biomed. Res. Int.* 2014:761741. doi: 10.1155/2014/761741

Vashist, J., Tiwari, V., Das, R., Kapil, A., and Rajeswari, M. R. (2011). Analysis of penicillin-binding proteins (PBPs) in carbapenem resistant *Acinetobacter baumannii*. *Indian J. Med. Res.* 133, 332–338.

Vila, J., Martí, S., and Sánchez-Céspedes, J. (2007). Porins, efflux pumps and multidrug resistance in *Acinetobacter baumannii*. *J. Antimicrob. Chemother.* 59, 1210–1215. doi: 10.1093/jac/dkl509

Walsh, C., and Fanning, S. (2008). Antimicrobial resistance in food borne pathogens-A cause for concern? *Curr. Drug Targets.* 9, 808–815. doi: 10.2174/138945008785747761

Wang, H. M., Chen, C. Y., Chen, H. A., Huang, W. C., Lin, W. R., Chen, T. C., et al. (2010). *Zingiber officinale* (ginger) compounds have tetracycline-resistance modifying effects against clinical extensively drug resistant *Acinetobacter baumannii*. *Phytother. Res.* 24, 1825–1830. doi: 10.1002/ptr.3201

Wieczorek, P., Sacha, P., Hauschild, T., Zórawski, M., Krawczyk, M., and Tryniszewska, E. (2008). Multidrug resistant *Acinetobacter baumannii*–the role of AdeABC (RND family) efflux pump in resistance to antibiotics. *Folia Histochem. Cytobiol.* 46, 257–267. doi: 10.2478/v10042-008-0056-x

Wisplinghoff, H., Bischoff, T., Tallent, S. M., Seifert, H., Wenzel, R. P., and Edmond, M. B. (2004). Nosocomial bloodstream infections in US hospitals: analysis of 24,179 cases from a prospective nationwide surveillance study. *Clin. Infect. Dis.* 39, 309–317. doi: 10.1086/421946

Xing, L., Barnie, P., Su, Z., and Xu, H. (2014). Development of efflux pumps and inhibitors (EPIs) in *A. baumanii*. *Clin. Microbial.* 3:135.

Yoon, E. J., Courvalin, P., and Grillot-Courvalin, C. (2013). RND-type efflux pumps in multidrug-resistant clinical isolates of *Acinetobacter baumannii*: major role for AdeABC overexpression and AdeRS mutations. *Antimicrob. Agents Chemother.* 57, 2989–2995. doi: 10.1128/AAC.02556-12

# 18

# Phenotypic Antimicrobial Susceptibility and Genotypic Characterization of Clinical *Ureaplasma* Isolates Circulating in Shanghai, China

***Hongxia Ma[1†], Xuemei Zhang[2†], Xiaoxing Shi[3], Jun Zhang[4*] and Yunheng Zhou[5*]***

*[1]Department of Health Management Medicine, Shanghai East Hospital, Tongji University School of Medicine, Shanghai, China, [2]Department of Oncology, Shanghai East Hospital, Tongji University School of Medicine, Shanghai, China, [3]Department of Clinical Laboratory, Shanghai Provincial Crops Hospital of Chinese People's Armed Police Forces, Shanghai, China, [4]Department of Clinical Laboratory, Sir Run Run Shaw Hospital Zhejiang University School of Medicine, Hangzhou, China, [5]Department of Clinical Laboratory, Zhabei Central Hospital of Jing'an District, Shanghai, China*

***Correspondence:**
*Jun Zhang*
*jameszhang2000@zju.edu.cn*
*Yunheng Zhou*
*hongniwan@aliyun.com*

*[†]These authors have contributed equally to this work*

There is a growing global concern regarding the rise of antimicrobial resistance among *Ureaplasma* spp. isolates. However, studies on the antimicrobial susceptibility profiles, resistance mechanisms, and clonality of *Ureaplasma* spp. clinical isolates are still limited and cover only some geographic regions. Firstly, *Ureaplasma* species from the urogenital tracts of patients in Shanghai, China, were isolated by using the culture medium (A8 and 10B broth), and identified the genotype by polymerase chain reaction (PCR). Secondly, the antimicrobial susceptibility tests were determined by using broth microdilution assay. Then, the resistance genetic determinants to fluoroquinolones (FQs), macrolides, and tetracyclines were investigated through PCR/DNA sequencing. Finally, the molecular epidemiology of *Ureaplasma* species was studied by multilocus sequence typing (MLST). Among 258 isolates, *Ureaplasma parvum* (UPA) and *Ureaplasma urealyticum* (UUR) were found in 226 (87.60%) and 32 (12.40%) isolates, respectively. The minimum inhibitory concentrations (MICs) of 258 *Ureaplasma* spp. strains ranged from 0.015 to 64 μg/ml for all 11 kinds of antimicrobials. Regardless of species, the isolates were most sensitive to AZI (1.94%), JOS (3.49%), and CLA (4.23%). Among them, there were 39 (15.12%) multidrug-resistant (MDR) strains, including 32 UPA isolates. The resistance rates of UPA to CIP (91.59%), and ROX (36.28%) were significantly higher than those of UUR. Twenty six FQ-resistant isolates had amino acid substitutions in *gyrA* and in *parC* (Ser83Leu). Mutations were detected in genes encoding ribosomal proteins L4 (Thr84Ile) and L22 (Ser81Pro) in macrolide-resistant isolates. *Tet*(M) was found in four UPA isolates. These mutations were mainly found in UPA isolates. Sequence type 1 (ST1) was the predominant ST, which contained 18 isolates. In conclusion, this study showed a higher resistance rate (especially to ROX and CIP), higher substitution rate, and higher MDR rate among UPA strains. The most active antimicrobial agents were AZI, JOS, and CLA. Identifying UPA or UUR in clinical isolates could help clinicians to choose appropriate drugs for treatment. The main resistance mechanisms may involve gene substitution of Ser83Leu in *parC* and Ser81Pro in L22. ST1 was the predominant ST of *Ureaplasma* isolates with MDR to FQs and macrolides in Shanghai, China.

**Keywords: *Ureaplasma* spp., drug resistance, urogenital tract samples, multilocus sequence typing, resistance mechanism, multidrug resistance**

## INTRODUCTION

*Ureaplasma* spp. are among the best characterized mycoplasmal bacteria because they are tightly associated with the urogenital tract pathology in humans (Beeton and Spiller, 2017). Owing to their small genome and limited metabolic and biosynthetic capacities, *Ureaplasma* spp. are dependent on an exogenous supply of amino acids and require a close association with host cells for survival. As a result, *Ureaplasma* spp. infections have emerged as a clinical issue in a large group of patients with various diseases, such as nonchlamydial and nongonococcal urethritis (Beeton et al., 2019), prostatitis, cervicitis, as well as pelvic inflammatory disease (Hartmann, 2009). To date, reports have indicated that *Ureaplasma* spp. could be related to adverse neonatal and pregnancy outcomes, including miscarriage and meningitis in newborns (Waites, et al., 2005; Capoccia et al., 2013; Sprong et al., 2020), fatal hyperammonemia in adults (Bharat et al., 2015).

*Ureaplasma* spp. have no cell wall and belong to the class *Mollicutes*; they are characterized by small cell size and genome (Hartmann, 2009). Based on molecular analyses, human *Ureaplasma* spp. are now divided into *Ureaplasma parvum* (UPA) and *Ureaplasma urealyticum* (UUR), which contain at least 14 serovars: UPA (serovars 1, 3, 6, and 14) and UUR (serovars 2, 4, 5, and 7–13; Robertson et al., 2002).

Because *Ureaplasma* spp. lack cell wall and folic acid synthesis capacity, they are naturally insusceptible to β-lactams, sulfonamides, and trimethoprim (Beeton and Spiller, 2017). However, they are generally considered susceptible to tetracyclines, fluoroquinolones (FQs), and macrolides, which interfere with bacterial protein synthesis or DNA replication (Sweeney et al., 2016). In 2011, the Clinical and Laboratory Standards Institute (CLSI) issued the document M43-A: a standard method for performing and validating *in vitro* susceptibility tests for clinical *Ureaplasma* spp. (Clinical and Laboratory Standards Institute, 2011). CLSI M43-A highlights the requirement for standardized media (10B broth or A8 agar). The document lists only five kinds of selected antimicrobials with breakpoints. However, most laboratories lack the capability to cultivate, isolate, and purify fastidious bacteria such as *Ureaplasma* spp. Only a few studies have characterized antimicrobial resistance levels of *Ureaplasma* spp. in China and other countries (Zhang et al., 2014a; Fernández et al., 2016).

We have recently reported the relationship between *Ureaplasma* spp. infection, male infertility, and semen quality, and determined the minimum inhibitory concentrations (MICs) of some antimicrobials for *Ureaplasma* spp. (Zhou et al., 2018b; Wang et al., 2019). Although some studies have evaluated acquired resistance against several of the above-mentioned agents, the detailed mechanisms underlying the resistance and clonality of *Ureaplasma* spp. are still scarce and are limited to several geographic regions (Pereyre et al., 2007; Beeton et al., 2009; Leli et al., 2012; De Francesco et al., 2013; Schneider et al., 2015; Fernández et al., 2016). Therefore, the aim of this study was to study the genotype, the antimicrobial susceptibility; corresponding molecular resistance mechanisms; multidrug resistance (MDR) and sequence type (ST) distribution and clonality of large-scale clinical *Ureaplasma* spp. isolated from the urogenital tracts of patients in Shanghai, China.

## MATERIALS AND METHODS

### Clinical Specimens and Species Identification

The study was approved by the Ethics Committee of Shanghai Crops Hospital of Chinese People's Armed Police (No. 20121206). Clinical specimens were collected from the urogenital tracts of patients (33 men and 225 women; medium age, 28.40 years; age range, 19–54 years) between 2013 and 2014 in three departments (i.e., departments of dermatology, gynecology and obstetrics, and infertility) of the Shanghai Crops Hospital of Chinese People's Armed Police. The specimens were collected by picking up endocervical cells or vaginal secretion using sterile swabs in women and from urethral secretions or semen in men.

The secretions were inoculated directly on the selective solid culture medium (A8) and the liquid culture medium at 37°C in an atmosphere of 5% $CO_2$; the results were observed after 48 and 72 h. Liquefied semen was inoculated in the broth medium (100 µl) and on the selective agar medium in parallel (20 µl). Due to an increase in pH caused by *Ureaplasma* spp. growth, a phenol red indicator was added to media to display a color change. A Leitz Orthoplan microscope was used for direct examination of colonies at 100× magnification. Colonies of *Ureaplasma* spp. were identified presumptively by their characteristic echinus appearance (brown and tiny) on A8 agar in the presence of the Mn indicator (Viscardi, 2010).

### Isolation and Purification

A single *Ureaplasma* spp. colony was placed into 10B broth media under microscope for purification at 37°C. After the color of the liquid medium had changed into light pink or peach after approximately 16–18 h of incubation, the liquid medium was measured and adjusted to pH 7.0; then, the purified strains were identified by PCR and stored in multiple aliquots at −80°C in fetal bovine serum in strains bank of Shanghai Crops Hospital. The selective medium agar (A8) and the liquid medium (10B broth) kits and reference strains (ATCC 33175 and ATCC 15488) were provided by Zhongaisheng Hebei Bioscience Technology Inc. (Xingtai, China).

For *Ureaplasma* spp. samples, genomic DNA extraction was performed using a Takara DNA Minikit (Shiga, Japan). These samples were reconfirmed by amplification of the *Ureaplasma* spp.-specific urease gene (a 430-bp DNA product) using U4 and U5 primers. Detection of 284 *Ureaplasma* spp. isolates was done using DNA sequences of the UM-1 primers (UMS125 and UMA226; Blanchard et al., 1993; Teng et al., 1994; Cunningham et al., 2013) and/or 16S-rRNA gene primers UMS 57-UMA 222 for the detection of UPA (327 bp), as well as UMS 170-UMA 263 for the detection of UUR (476 bp; Kong et al., 2000; Xie et al., 2009).

### Antimicrobial Susceptibility Testing

In this study, 11 antimicrobials were used, including macrolides [erythromycin (ERY), azithromycin (AZI), roxithromycin (ROX), clarithromycin (CLA), josamycin (JOS)], FQs [levofloxacin (LEV), moxifloxacin (MXF), ciprofloxacin (CIP)], and tetracyclines [tetracycline (TET), doxycycline (DOX), and minocycline (MIN)]. All agents (Sigma-Aldrich, St. Louis, MO, United States) were obtained in a powdered form of known purity and were diluted in accordance with their respective manufacturer's instructions. The MICs were determined in duplicate by broth microdilution performed in 96-well microtiter plates in accordance with the Clinical and Laboratory Standards (CLSI) guidelines and previous reports (Kechagia et al., 2008; Clinical and Laboratory Standards Institute, 2011) using a range of antimicrobial concentrations from 0.0625 to 128 μg/ml in 10B broth (Zhong ai sheng). American Type Culture Collection (ATCC) 33,175 (*Ureaplasma urealyticum*) was used as a quality control strain in each broth microdilution assay.

Briefly, we first quantified these organisms for use in MIC determination; then, the frozen culture aliquots were thawed and enriched, where one part was used for colony counting and the rest was stored at 4°C for 48 h for MIC. Next, all the antimicrobials were added to 96-well plates in duplicate. The 96-well plates were placed in a biosafety cabinet, dried at room temperature overnight, and then stored at 4°C for use. Then, the microdilution plates were incubated in ambient air at 37°C until the color change of the positive growth control due to the phenol red pH indicator after approximately 16–24 h of incubation. The MIC was then determined as the lowest concentration of an antimicrobial agent that did not show any color change at the time of the growth control's color change. The $MIC_{50}$ and $MIC_{90}$ values were recorded.

## Analysis of Macrolide, FQ and Tetracycline Resistance Mechanisms

Among FQ-resistant isolates ($n = 31$; MIC ≥ 32 μg/ml), the quinolone resistance-determining regions (QRDRs) of the *gyrA*, *gyrB*, *parC*, and *parE* genes were studied by PCR/DNA sequencing. Primers were designed for amplification, and PCR-amplified DNA was sequenced in both directions to verify the existence by previously described methods (Bébéar et al., 1999, 2000). The *tet*(M) gene was assessed by PCR using Blanchard et al. (1992) primers and cycling conditions described previously in a total of 20 tetracycline-resistant isolates (15 UPA and five UUR isolates) and 59 tetracycline-susceptible isolates (Blanchard et al., 1992). For all macrolide-resistant isolates ($n = 59$, 51 UPA and eight UUR isolates), PCR amplification and sequencing were performed for both 23S rRNA alleles and the genes encoding ribosomal proteins L4 and L22 (Pereyre et al., 2007; Beeton et al., 2009; Fernández et al., 2016).

The acquired sequences were analyzed using DNAStar Lasergene 7.1 and were translated into protein sequences by blastx in NCBI. Nucleotide mutations in the 23S rRNA alleles as well as amino acid substitutions in L4 and L22, *gyrA*, *gyrB*, *parC*, and *parE* were identified by comparison with wild-type sequences, i.e., *Ureaplasma parvum* serovar 3 str. ATCC 700970 (GenBank accession numbers AF222894), UPA ATCC 700970, *Ureaplasma urealyticum* serovar 10 str. ATCC 33699 (GenBank accession numbers CP001184; Pereyre et al., 2007; Schneider et al., 2015; Fernández et al., 2016), and UPA serovar 3 str. SV3F4 (GenBank accession numbers AP 014584; Wu et al., 2014).

## Multilocus Sequence Typing

Multilocus sequence typing (MLST; involving the *ftsH*, *rpl22*, *valS*, and *thrS* genes) was performed on a selection of 59 isolates (51 UPA and eight UUR isolates) that were resistant to FQs and macrolides as well as partially susceptible to tetracyclines (Fernández et al., 2016). Population structures of 59 *Ureaplasma* spp. isolates were predicted by eBURST. All the STs were analyzed.

## Statistical Analysis

Data analysis was performed using SPSS, version 21. The Chi-square test was used for comparison of qualitative variables. $p < 0.05$ was considered statistically significant.

# RESULTS

## Species Identification and Prevalence of Resistance in *Ureaplasma* spp.

Of the 258 tested specimens, 226 (87.60%) were only positive for UPA and 32 (12.40%) were only positive for UUR (**Table 1**). There was no significant difference in the distribution of *Ureaplasma* spp. between the two genders ($p > 0.05$). More than 40% of all the *Ureaplasma* spp. were isolated from patients aged 19–25 years. There was no significant difference in the distribution of UPA and UUR isolates among the age groups ($p > 0.05$; **Table 2**).

The detailed results for the MIC range, $MIC_{50}$ and $MIC_{90}$ values, and the antimicrobial resistance of *Ureaplasma* spp. (UPA and UUR) are shown in **Table 3**. The MICs of 258 *Ureaplasma* spp. strains ranged from 0.015 to 64 μg/ml for all 11 kinds of antimicrobials *in vitro*. Among them, ciprofloxacin had the least effective activity ($MIC_{50}$ of 16 μg/ml and $MIC_{90}$ of 64 μg/ml) against *Ureaplasma* spp. CLA was the most active

**TABLE 1** | Distribution of *Ureaplasma* spp. species isolated from 258 cases between female and male.

| | UPA (N %) | UUR (N %) | Total (N %) |
|---|---|---|---|
| Female | 196 (87.11%) | 29 (12.89%) | 225 (87.21%) |
| male | 30 (90.91%) | 3 (9.09%) | 33 (12.79%) |
| Total | 226 (87.60%) | 32 (12.40%) | 258 (100%) |

*UPA, Ureaplasma parvum; UUR, Ureaplasma urealyticum.*

**TABLE 2** | The distribution of *Ureaplasma* spp. of 258 cases from the urogenital tracts of patients among different age groups.

| Age group (range, years) | UPA (N %) | UUR (N %) | Total (N %) |
|---|---|---|---|
| 19–25 | 98 (88.29%) | 13 (11.71%) | 111 (43.02%) |
| 26–30 | 63 (86.30%) | 10 (13.70%) | 73 (28.29%) |
| 31–35 | 31 (93.94%) | 2 (6.06%) | 33 (14.44%) |
| >35 | 34 (82.93%) | 7 (17.07%) | 41 (16.55%) |
| Total | 226 (87.60%) | 32 (12.40%) | 258 (100%) |

*UPA, Ureaplasma parvum; UUR, Ureaplasma urealyticum.*

**TABLE 3** | Antimicrobial *in vitro* resistance profiles of 258 clinical *Ureaplasma* spp. isolates.

| | ERY N (%) | AZI N (%) | ROX N (%) | CLA N (%) | JOS N (%) | LEV N (%) | MXF N (%) | CIP N (%) | TET N (%) | DOX N (%) | MIN N (%) |
|---|---|---|---|---|---|---|---|---|---|---|---|
| UPA | 39 (17.26) | 4 (1.77) | 82 (36.28) | 9 (3.98) | 6 (2.65) | 167 (73.89) | 61 (27.00) | 207 (91.59) | 39 (17.2) | 22 (9.73) | 18 (7.96) |
| UUR | 6 (18.75) | 1 (3.2) | 3 (9.37) | 3 (9.37) | 3 (9.37) | 21 (65.63) | 11 (34.37) | 25 (78.12) | 6 (18.75) | 7 (21.87) | 6 (18.75) |
| *p* value | 0.806 | - | 0.002 | - | - | 0.395 | 0.403 | 0.027 | 0.806 | 0.042 | - |
| Total | 45 (17.44) | 5 (1.94) | 85 (32.95) | 12 (4.23) | 9 (3.49) | 188 (72.87) | 72 (27.91) | 232 (89.92) | 45 (17.44) | 29 (11.24) | 24 (9.30) |
| MIC range | 0.03–64 | 0.015–16 | 0.03–64 | 0.015–16 | 0.015–16 | 0.03–64 | 0.03–64 | 0.03–64 | 0.015–16 | 0.015–16 | 0.015–16 |
| $MIC_{50}$ | 2 | 1 | 1 | 0.125 | 0.125 | 8 | 1 | 16 | 0.5 | 0.25 | 0.5 |
| $MIC_{90}$ | 16 | 4 | 8 | 0.5 | 1 | 64 | 16 | 64 | 8 | 2 | 4 |

**TABLE 4** | Occurrence of ROX-CIP and MDR among *Ureaplasma* spp.

| ***Ureaplasma* spp. (N %)** | **ROX-CIP** | **MDR** | **Total** |
|---|---|---|---|
| UPA | 67 (29.65%) | 32 (14.16%) | 226 (87.60%) |
| UUR | 10 (31.25%) | 7 (21.87%) | 32 (12.40%) |
| Total | 77 (29.84%) | 39 (15.12%) | 258 (100%) |

*ROX-CIP: both resistant to roxithromycin (ROX) and ciprofloxacin (CIP). MDR, multi-drug resistance: resistant to at least one agent in ≥ 3 antimicrobial categories: macrolides, tetracyclines, and fluoroquinolones. UPA, Ureaplasma parvum; UUR, Ureaplasma urealyticum.*

antimicrobial with an $MIC_{50}$ of 0.125 µg/ml and $MIC_{90}$ of 0.5 µg/ml. ERY was the least effective among macrolides ($MIC_{50}$ of 2 µg/ml and $MIC_{90}$ of 16 µg/ml). DOX was the most active tetracycline, with $MIC_{50}$ of 0.25 µg/ml and $MIC_{90}$ of 2 µg/ml.

According to the CLSI, the top three drug resistance rates of *Ureaplasma* spp. were those to CIP (89.92%), LEV (72.87%), and ROX (32.95%). Among them, the drug resistance rates of UPA were as follows: CIP (91.59%), and ROX (36.28%); they were significantly higher than those of UUR. The most active antimicrobial agents were AZI (1.94%), JOS (3.49%), CLA (4.23%), and MIN (9.30%). Of the 258 *Ureaplasma* spp. strains, there were 77(29.84%) isolates uniformly resistant to ROX and CIP, and 39(15.12%) MDR isolates; both of them were dominated by UPA strains (**Table 4**).

## Molecular Characterization of Antimicrobial Resistance

In the comparison with the relative DNA and protein sequences of reference strains, none of the isolates possessed mutations in 23S rRNA. A Thr84Ile mutation was detected in the ribosomal protein L4 of one roxithromycin-resistant UPA isolate. A Ser81Pro mutation was detected in the ribosomal protein L22 of seven *Ureaplasma* spp. isolates (five roxithromycin-resistant UPA isolates, one erythromycin-resistant UPA isolate, and an UPA isolate resistant to roxithromycin and erythromycin); the latter also had another mutation, Lys91Asn in the protein L22.

The comparison between the QRDR DNA sequences of reference strains and the QRDRs of FQ-resistant isolates ($n = 31$; MIC ≥ 32 µg/ml) revealed no mutations in *gyrB* or *parE* in any of the isolates. However, *gyrA* and *parC* quinolone resistance-associated mutations were found. One FQ-resistant UPA isolate showing a levofloxacin MIC of 32 µg/ml harbored a Val120Phe mutation in *gyrA*, but no QRDR mutations were found in *gyrA* of FQ-resistant UUR isolates. The most frequent mutation was Ser83Leu in *parC*, which was present in 22 (88%) and three (50%) of the FQ-resistant UPA and UUR isolates, respectively. Among 32 MDR UPA isolates, there were 14 cases of mutation in *parC* S83L (Ser83Leu); 2 isolates with Ser83Leu (Ser81Pro) and 1 isolates with *Tet*(M) Screening of the *tet*(M) gene, which is associated with tetracycline resistance, was performed among 79 isolates. Two tetracycline-resistant UPA isolates were positive for this gene, but two tetracycline-susceptible UPA isolates also harbored this gene.

## Multilocus Sequence Typing

Among the 59 *Ureaplasma* spp. isolates resistant to FQs and macrolides, the *ftsH* gene and *thrS* gene, with the highest discriminatory power, had 10 alleles and 8 alleles, respectively, while the *rpL22* gene and *valS* gene had four and three alleles, respectively.

The lineage of the 21 STs in 59 strains was analyzed, and two major clonal complexes (CC1 and CC2) were revealed by the eBURST package. ST2 was the predicted ancestor, highlighted in the blue circle, while the other STs are displayed in the yellow circle. The size of the circle reflects the number of isolates in the relevant ST, and STs are represented as numbers. Twenty one STs appeared among the 59 clinical isolates. ST1 was the predominant ST, which contained 18 UPA isolates. CC1 contained the vast majority of 17 STs in 44 isolates, while the remaining four STs (ST9, ST52, ST101, and ST161) were singletons (**Figure 1**).

## DISCUSSION

In recent years, many questions regarding the role of *Ureaplasma* spp. as human pathogens, therapeutic strategies, and the antimicrobial susceptibility of individual species remain open. In this study, we examined the antimicrobial susceptibility, resistance mechanisms, and ST distribution of contemporary 258 clinical *Ureaplasma* spp. isolated from 2013 to 2014 in Shanghai, China. Few previous studies have focused on the individual UPA and UUR distributions in clinical *Ureaplasma* spp. samples (Kawai et al., 2015; Schneider et al., 2015; Yang et al., 2020). In our study, the positive rate of UPA among clinical *Ureaplasma* spp. isolates of the urogenital tract was 87.60%, similar to a recent estimate obtained by Fernández et al. (2016) in the United States. Studies of the frequencies

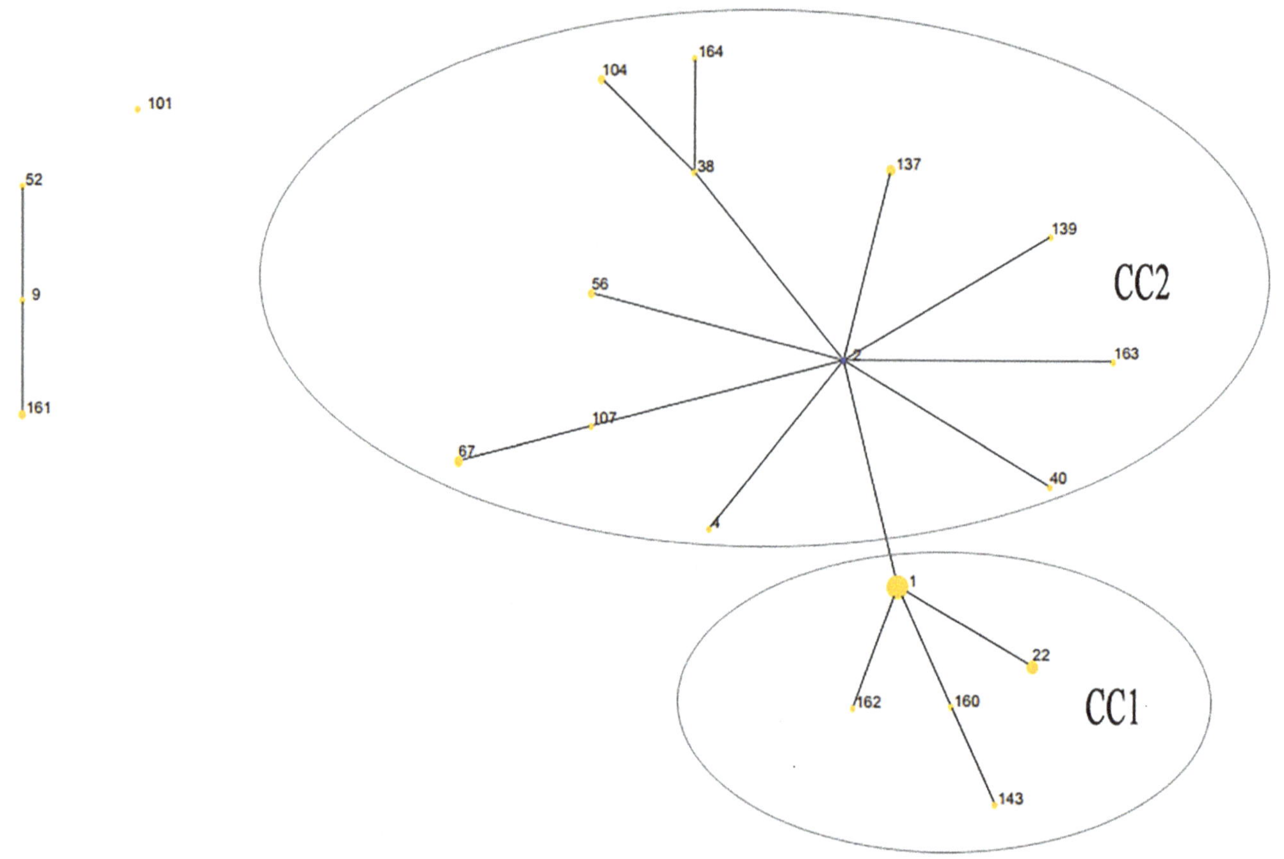


**FIGURE 1** | Population structures of 59 *Ureaplasma* spp. isolates resistant to quinolones and macrolides predicted by eBURST. CC, clonal complex.

of individual species may be useful for further analyses of their clinical characteristics.

The continuous increase in the prevalence of *Ureaplasma* spp. raised questions regarding their antimicrobial resistance (Zeng et al., 2016; Zhou et al., 2018a). Here, we analyzed the susceptibility of *Ureaplasma* spp. to 11 kinds of antimicrobial drugs. As expected, UPA and UUR had low resistance to most macrolides and tetracyclines, while their resistance to LEV (72.87%) was very high. While the resistance to macrolides is less than 5% in most countries, our study showed a higher rate of ERY (17.44%) and ROX (32.95%) resistance among clinical strains from Shanghai. Additionally, our results significantly differed from those of previous reports. For instance, Fernández et al. have reported a lower resistance rate to LEV (6%) and no macrolide resistance among the 250 clinical isolates in the United States (Fernández et al., 2016). Some domestic studies of *Ureaplasma* spp. strains indicated a 20.09% resistance rate to LEV (Zhu et al., 2012), less than 10% to macrolides (Song et al., 2014), and 76.9% to LEV (Song et al., 2015). In addition, *Ureaplasma* spp. exhibited high resistance to CIP (100%) and to ERY (100% in Tunisia and 80% in South Africa; Redelinghuys et al., 2014; Boujemaa et al., 2020).

Higher resistance rates to ERY, ROX, and LEV may be attributed to the following four factors. First, our study population (87.21% women with border age distribution) may have had higher antimicrobial exposure (especially to macrolides and FQs) and higher resistance levels. Kobayashi et al. found that each age group over 30 years had significantly higher odds of receiving FQs for treatment compared with women between 18 and 29 years (Kobayashi et al., 2016). However, in Europe and the United States, the macrolide resistance rates of *M. pneumoniae* are substantially lower than those in Asia (Waites et al., 2017). Second, these overall figures indicate that resistance rates vary significantly among countries; in some instances, there are even dramatic differences within the same country, which may be related to the different strategy or preference of antimicrobials usage in different areas (Yang et al., 2020). Third, another explanation for this variation may be related to the shortcomings of different Mycoplasma testing kits and the reference broth microdilution method currently used to estimate the antimicrobial susceptibility of *Ureaplasma* spp. Schneider et al. reported that there was conflicting results from the IST 2 kit and standard broth microdilution was observed for CIP and AZI (Schneider et al., 2015). Namely, the Mycoplasma IST2 assay identifies a number of false positives and does not conform to the approved CLSI guidelines (Beeton et al., 2009, 2015). The accuracy of some reports is still questionable since there are no standardized methods for *in vitro* susceptibility testing and no MIC interpretive breakpoints were designated before 2011. Of note, acidic pH and incubation time affect erythromycin MICs (Kenny and Cartwright, 1993).

Furthermore, mutations, biofilm formation, and the distribution pattern of species or serovars of *Ureaplasma* spp. can also lead to this phenomenon. The top three drug resistance rates of *Ureaplasma* spp. were those to CIP, LEV, and ROX. Among CIP and ROX, the drug resistance rates of UPA were significantly higher than those of UUR. The drug resistance rates to AZI, CLA, JOS, and MIN were very low (less than 10%) regardless of *Ureaplasma* spp.

The relationship and the molecular mechanism between the antimicrobial susceptibility and genotype of *Ureaplasma* spp. have seldom been reported (Song, 2019). Valentine-King and Brown (2017) reported a trend to higher MIC of UUR compared with UPA. The resistance rates were different for different kinds of antimicrobial between UUR and UPA (Fernández et al., 2016). Therefore, analyses of resistance rates of *Ureaplasma* spp. require more data to properly explain and interpret the observed trends.

In this study, we also studied *Ureaplasma* spp. resistance mechanisms to the above-mentioned drugs. As described previously, FQ resistance has been attributed to mutations in *gyrA*, *gyrB*, S83L, S83W, and S84P mutations in the *parC* genes and *parE* genes (Pereyre et al., 2007; Beeton et al., 2015; Kawai et al., 2015; Schneider et al., 2015; Fernández et al., 2016; Valentine-King and Brown, 2017; Meygret et al., 2018). A sequence analysis of the QRDRs revealed that the resistance mechanism of FQ-resistant isolates involves mutations at position 248 (C-T) of *parC*, which leads to a substitution of Ser83 by Leu, followed by a Val120Phe substitution, which was mostly found in UPA isolates. As in previous studies, Beeton et al. (2009) also found that about 80% of isolates were UUR, and the *ParC* Ser83Leu mutation was largely found in all FQ-resistant *Ureaplasma* spp. We found that three FQ-resistant UPA isolates and three FQ-resistant UUR isolates among 31 *Ureaplasma* spp. isolates with high MICs (≥32 μg/ml) for LEV, MXF and CIP did not harbor QRDR mutations, suggesting the existence of other undescribed resistance mechanisms in these isolates.

Macrolide resistance has been related to mutations in domain V of 23S rRNA, ribosomal proteins L4 and L22, similar to the mechanism underlying *Mycoplasma pneumoniae* resistance (Schneider et al., 2015; Song et al., 2015, 2019). The macrolide resistance of *Ureaplasma* spp. is still a controversial issue. The A2066G (A to G) mutation and C2243N (T or C) mutation in the 23S rRNA may be associated with *Ureaplasma* spp. macrolide resistance in the Chinese population (Meng et al., 2008; Song et al., 2019). We analyzed the aforementioned resistance traits for 59 *Ureaplasma* spp. isolates showing drug resistance to macrolides; while none of the isolates possessed mutations in the 23S rRNA, we found a mutation in the L4 protein gene and two mutations of the L22 protein gene in eight macrolide-resistant UPA isolates. Yang et al. (2020) reported double alterations (A121S and T141I) or a single mutation (D66N) in L22 within five strains, including one sample harboring an S21A substitution in L4 at the same time. In addition, Pereyre et al. detected two mutations (Lys91Asn and Ala94Asp) in the ribosomal protein L22 and three mutations (Thr70Lys, Gly71Val, and Trp65Arg) in the ribosomal protein L4 (Pereyre et al., 2007); the Lys91Asn mutation in L22 of an erythromycin-resistant UPA isolate was also found in one UPA isolate resistant to erythromycin and roxithromycin and harboring another mutation, Ser81Pro, in our study. The most resistance mechanism to macrolides included the gene mutations in L4 and L22 ribosomal proteins.

The presence of *tet*(M) has been reported in both tetracycline-susceptible and -resistant *Ureaplasma* spp. isolates. In this study, the prevalence of *tet*(M) gene (5.1%, 4/79) was lower than in other reports (Kenny and Cartwright, 1993; Teng et al., 1994; Pereyre et al., 2007; Kotrotsiou et al., 2015). We also found that the *tet*(M) gene may not be a specific indicator of tetracycline-resistant *Ureaplasma* spp. isolates.

In this study, uniform resistance to ROX and CIP was the most frequently observed pattern (29.84%) among *Ureaplasma* spp. isolates; an elevated MDR rate among *Ureaplasma* spp. (15.12%) was detected, particularly among UPA isolates. Zhu et al. (2016) reported only 1.08% MDR of *Ureaplasma* spp. in Nanjing, China, while Boujemaa et al. found an elevated MDR rate (37.62%) with 60.71% of UUR strains and 28.76% of UPA being MDR (Boujemaa et al., 2020). To the best of our knowledge, this is the first report of a higher MDR rate of *Ureaplasma* spp. isolates in Shanghai, China.

To study the molecular epidemiology and population structure of *Ureaplasma* spp., an MLST approach based on four housekeeping genes (*ftsH*, *rpL22*, *valS*, and *thrS*) was first developed by Zhang et al. (2014b) who used 14 serovar reference strains and 269 clinical strains. ST1 and ST22 were the predominant STs and contained 68 and 70 isolates, respectively. Zhang et al. (2014a) also found that isolates of CC1 were UPA and those of CC2 were UUR. CC2 was found more often in symptomatic patients with vaginitis, tubal obstruction, and cervicitis. In addition, two recent studies evaluated the molecular epidemiology of clinical *Ureaplasma* spp. isolates in the United States and Switzerland, making reference to the research of Zhang et al.; these studies suggested the association of molecular epidemiology of *Ureaplasma* spp. isolates with pathogenicity or spread of antimicrobial resistance (Schneider et al., 2015; Fernández et al., 2016). We found that ST1 (18 UPA isolates) was the predominant ST among 59 MDR isolates, followed by ST22 (5 UPA isolates). Among 18 ST1 UPA isolates, there was higher MDR rate (8 cases, 44.44%) and the mutations found as the following: *parC* gene (4 cases), GyrA/*parC* (one case), and L22: S81P (one case). ST1 was the main clone both in Hangzhou (Zhang et al., 2014a) and Shanghai, which may hypothesize that ST1 can be associated with spread of the urogenital tracts of different populations or the antimicrobial resistance. MLST is a well-accepted way for illustrating the diversity and population structure of different bacterial species compared to any other molecular subtyping method. As the strain numbers of STs were very limited, it was difficult to draw any decisive conclusions on any possible correlations between STs and pathologies or molecular resistance mechanisms of *Ureaplasma* spp.

In conclusion, using a large number of clinical isolates, which were mainly obtained from women, this study addressed the lack of data in China related to the antimicrobial susceptibility of *Ureaplasma* spp. The prevalence of antimicrobial resistance in *Ureaplasma* spp., especially that to ERY, ROX, and LEV, is markedly higher in China than in European countries. The most active antimicrobial agents were AZI, JOS, and CLA. Identifying UPA or UUR in clinical isolates could help clinicians to choose appropriate drugs for treatment. For UPA in particular, ERY, ROX, and FQs should be used with caution due to the relatively high rate of MDR. ST1 was the predominant ST of *Ureaplasma* isolates with MDR to FQs and macrolides in Shanghai, China. The main resistance mechanisms may involve gene substitution of Ser83Leu in *parC* and Ser81Pro in L22, in addition to other, undescribed mechanisms. One of the limitations of this study is that it did not provide sufficient data to better understand the epidemiology of *Ureaplasma* spp. in China. Future work should extend our investigations to address the resistance mechanisms related to the spread of antimicrobial resistance, particularly MDR strains, and the difference in drug resistance in different *Ureaplasma* spp.

## AUTHOR CONTRIBUTIONS

HM, JZ, and YZ contributed to conception and design of the study. HM, XZ, XS, and YZ performed the experimental studies and analysis. HM, XZ, and YZ wrote the section of the manuscript. All authors contributed to the article and approved the submitted version.

## FUNDING

This work was financially supported by the Key Programs of Science and Technology Commission Foundation of Changning District, Shanghai (CNKW2016Z05), the Jiangxi Provincial Health Technology Project (20202114), the National Natural Science Foundation of China (NSFC81370047), and Natural Science Foundation of Shanghai (13ZR1449700).

## ACKNOWLEDGMENTS

We thank LetPub (www.letpub.com) for its linguistic assistance during the preparation of this manuscript.

## REFERENCES

Bébéar, C. M., Grau, O., Charron, A., Renaudin, H., Gruson, D., and Bébéar, C. (2000). Cloning and nucleotide sequence of the DNA gyrase (gyrA) gene from Mycoplasma hominis and characterization of quinolone-resistant mutants selected in vitro with trovafloxacin. *Antimicrob. Agents Chemother.* 44, 2719–2727. doi: 10.1128/AAC.44.10.2719-2727.2000

Bébéar, C. M., Renaudin, J, Charron, A., Renaudin, H., de Barbeyrac, B., Schaeverbeke, T., et al. (1999). Mutations in the gyrA, parC, and parE genes associated with fluoroquinolone resistance in clinical isolates of Mycoplasma hominis. *Antimicrob. Agents Chemother.* 43, 954–956. doi: 10.1128/AAC.43.4.954

Beeton, M. L., Chalker, V. J., Jones, L. C., Maxwell, N. C., and Spiller, O. B. (2015). Antibiotic resistance among clinical *Ureaplasma* isolates recovered from neonates in England and Wales between 2007 and 2013. *Antimicrob. Agents Chemother.* 60, 52–56. doi: 10.1128/AAC.00889-15

Beeton, M. L., Chalker, V. J., Maxwell, N. C., Kotecha, S., and Spiller, O. B. (2009). Concurrent titration and determination of antibiotic resistance in *Ureaplasma* species with identification of novel point mutations in genes associated with resistance. *Antimicrob. Agents Chemother.* 53, 2020–2027. doi: 10.1128/AAC.01349-08

Beeton, M. L., Payne, M. S., and Jones, L. (2019). The role of *Ureaplasma* spp. in the development of nongonococcal urethritis and infertility among men. *Clin. Microbiol. Rev.* 32:e00137. doi: 10.1128/CMR.00137-18

Beeton, M. L., and Spiller, O. B. (2017). Antibiotic resistance among *Ureaplasma* species isolates: cause for concern? *J. Antimicrob. Chemother.* 72, 330–337. doi: 10.1093/jac/dkw425

Bharat, A., Cunningham, S. A., Scott Budinger, G. R., Kreisel, D., DeWet, C. J., Gelman, A. E., et al. (2015). Disseminated *Ureaplasma* infection as a cause of fatal hyperammonemia in humans. *Sci. Transl. Med.* 7:258.re3. doi: 10.1126/scitranslmed.aaa8419

Blanchard, A., Crabb, D. M., Dybvig, K., Duffy, L. B., and Cassell, G. H. (1992). Rapid detection of tetM in mycoplasma hominis and Ureaplasma urealyticum by PCR: tetM confers resistance to tetracycline but not necessarily to doxycycline. *FEMS Microbiol. Lett.* 95, 277–281. doi: 10.1016/0378-1097(92)90442-q

Blanchard, A., Hentschel, J., Duffy, L., Baldus, K., and Cassell, G. H. (1993). Detection of Ureaplasma urealyticum by polymerase chain reaction in the urogenital tract of adults, in amniotic fluid, and in the respiratory tract of newborns. *Clin. Infect. Dis.* 17(Suppl. 1), S148–S153. doi: 10.1093/clinids/17.supplement_1.s148

Boujemaa, S., Mlik, B., Ben Allaya, A., Mardassi, H., and Ben Abdelmoumen Mardassi, B. (2020). Spread of multidrug resistance among *Ureaplasma serovars*, Tunisia. *Antimicrob. Resist. Infect. Control* 9:19. doi: 10.1186/s13756-020-0681-5

Capoccia, R., Greub, G., and Baud, D. (2013). *Ureaplasma urealyticum, mycoplasma hominis* and adverse pregnancy outcomes. *Curr. Opin. Infect. Dis.* 26, 231–240. doi: 10.1097/QCO.0b013e328360db58

Clinical and Laboratory Standards Institute (2011). *Methods for Antimicrobial Susceptibility Testing for Human Mycoplasmas; Approved Guideline.* CLSI document M43-A. Wayne, PA: Clinical and Laboratory Standards Institute.

Cunningham, S. A., Mandrekar, J. N., Rosenblatt, J. E., and Patel, R. (2013). Rapid PCR detection of *Mycoplasma hominis, Ureaplasma urealyticum,* and *Ureaplasma parvum. Int. J. Bacteriol.* 2013, 1–7. doi: 10.1155/2013/168742

De Francesco, M. A., Caracciolo, S., Bonfanti, C., and Manca, N. (2013). Incidence and antibiotic susceptibility of *Mycoplasma hominis* and *Ureaplasma urealyticum* isolated in Brescia, Italy, over 7 years. *J. Infect. Chemother.* 19, 621–627. doi: 10.1007/s10156-012-0527-z

Fernández, J., Karau, M. J., Cunningham, S. A., Greenwood-Quaintance, K. E., and Patela, R. (2016). Antimicrobial susceptibility and clonality of clinical *Ureaplasma* isolates in the United States. *Antimicrob. Agents Chemother.* 60, 4793–4798. doi: 10.1128/AAC.00671-16

Hartmann, M. (2009). Genital mycoplasmas. *J. Dtsch. Dermatol. Ges.* 7, 371–377. doi: 10.1111/j.1610-0387.2008.06965.x

Kawai, Y., Nakura, Y., Wakimoto, T., Nomiyama, M., Tokuda, T., Takayanagi, T., et al. (2015). In vitro activity of five quinolones and analysis of the quinolone resistance-determining regions of gyrA, gyrB, parC, and parE in Ureaplasma parvum and Ureaplasma urealyticum clinical isolates from perinatal patients in Japan. *Antimicrob. Agents Chemother.* 59, 2358–2364. doi: 10.1128/AAC.04262-14

Kechagia, N., Bersimis, S., and Chatzipanagiotou, S. (2008). Incidence and antimicrobial susceptibilities of genital mycoplasmas in outpatient women with clinical vaginitis in Athens, Greece. *J. Antimicrob. Chemother.* 62, 122–125. doi: 10.1093/jac/dkn158

Kenny, G. E., and Cartwright, F. D. (1993). Effect of pH, inoculum size, and incubation time on the susceptibility of *Ureaplasma urealyticum* to erythromycin *in vitro. Clin. Infect. Dis.* 17(Suppl. 1), S215–S218. doi: 10.1093/clinids/17.supplement_1.s215

Kobayashi, M., Shapiro, D. J., Hersh, A. L., Sanchez, G. V., and Hicks, L. A. (2016). Outpatient antibiotic prescribing practices for uncomplicated urinary tract infection in women in the United States, 2002–2011. *Open. Forum. Infect. Dis.* 3:ofw159. doi: 10.1093/ofifid/ofw159

Kong, F., Ma, Z., James, G., Gordon, S., and Gilbert, G. L. (2000). Species identification and subtyping of Ureaplasma parvum and Ureaplasma urealyticum using PCR-based assays. *J. Clin. Microbiol.* 38, 1175–1179. doi: 10.1128/JCM.38.3.1175-1179.2000

Kotrotsiou, T., Exindari, M., Diza, E., Gioula, G., Melidou, A., and Malisiovas, N. (2015). Detection of the *tetM* resistance determinant among phenotypically sensitive *Ureaplasma* species by a novel real-time PCR method. *Diagn. Microbiol. Infect. Dis.* 81, 85–88. doi: 10.1016/j.diagmicrobio.2014.10.013

Leli, C., Mencacci, A., Bombaci, J. C., D'Alò, F., Farinelli, S., Vitali, M., et al. (2012). Prevalence and antimicrobial susceptibility of *Ureaplasma urealyticum* and *Mycoplasma hominis* in a population of Italian and immigrant outpatients. *Infez. Med.* 20, 82–87.

Meng, D. Y., Xue, W. C., Ma, X. B., and Wang, L. (2008). Transition mutations in 23S rRNA account for acquired resistance to macrolides in *Ureaplasma urealyticum*. *Microb. Drug Resist.* 14, 183–186. doi: 10.1089/mdr.2008.0817

Meygret, A., Le Roy, C., Renaudin, H., Bébéar, C., and Pereyre, S. (2018). Tetracycline and fluoroquinolone resistance in clinical *Ureaplasma* spp. and *Mycoplasma hominis* isolates in France between 2010 and 2015. *J. Antimicrob. Chemother.* 73, 2696–2703. doi: 10.1093/jac/dky238

Pereyre, S., Métifiot, M., Cazanave, C., Renaudin, H., Charron, A., Bébéar, C., et al. (2007). Characterisation of *in vitro*-selected mutants of *Ureaplasma parvum* resistant to macrolides and related antibiotics. *Int. J. Antimicrob. Agents* 29, 207–211. doi: 10.1016/j.ijantimicag.2006.09.008

Redelinghuys, M. J., Ehlers, M. M., Dreyer, A. W., Lombaard, H. A., and Kock, M. M. (2014). Antimicrobial susceptibility patterns of *Ureaplasma* species and mycoplasma hominis in pregnant women. *BMC Infect. Dis.* 14:171. doi: 10.1186/1471-2334-14-171

Robertson, J. A., Stemke, G. W., Davis, J. W. Jr., Harasawa, R., Thirkell, D., Kong, F., et al. (2002). Proposal of *Ureaplasma parvum* sp. nov. and emended description of *Ureaplasma urealyticum* (Shepard et al. 1974). *Int. J. Syst. Evol. Microbiol.* 52, 587–597. doi: 10.1099/00207713-52-2-587

Schneider, S. C., Tinguely, R., Droz, S., Hilty, M., Dona, V., Bodmer, T., et al. (2015). Antibiotic susceptibility and sequence type distribution of *Ureaplasma* species isolated from genital samples in Switzerland. *Antimicrob. Agents Chemother.* 59, 6026–6031. doi: 10.1128/AAC.00895-15

Song, T., Huang, J., Liu, Z., Zhang, Y., Kong, Y., and Ruan, Z. (2019). Antibiotic susceptibilities and genetic variations in macrolide resistance genes of *Ureaplasma* spp. isolated in China. *New Microbiol.* 42, 225–227.

Song, J., Qiao, Y., Kong, Y., Ruan, Z., Huang, J., Song, T., et al. (2015). Frequent topoisomerase IV mutations associated with fluoroquinolone resistance in *Ureaplasma* species. *J. Med. Microbiol.* 64, 1315–1320. doi: 10.1099/jmm.0.000153

Song, T., Ye, A., Xie, X., Huang, J., Ruan, Z., Kong, Y., et al. (2014). Epidemiological investigation and antimicrobial susceptibility analysis of *Ureaplasma* species and *Mycoplasma* hominis in outpatients with genital manifestations. *J. Clin. Pathol.* 67, 817–820. doi: 10.1136/jclinpath-2014-202248

Sprong, K. E., Mabenge, M., Wright, C. A., and Govender, S. (2020). *Ureaplasma* species and preterm birth: current perspectives. *Crit. Rev. Microbiol.* 46, 169–181. doi: 10.1080/1040841X.2020.1736986

Sweeney, E. L., Dando, S. J., Kallapur, S. G., and Knox, C. L. (2016). The human *Ureaplasma* species as causative agents of chorioamnionitis. *Clin. Microbiol. Rev.* 30, 349–379. doi: 10.1128/CMR.00091-16

Teng, L. J., Zheng, X., Glass, J. I., Watson, H. L., Tsai, J., and Cassell, G. H. (1994). *Ureaplasma urealyticum* biovar specificity and diversity are encoded in multiple-banded antigen gene. *J. Clin. Microbiol.* 32, 1464–1469. doi: 10.1128/jcm.32.6.1464-1469.1994

Valentine-King, M. A., and Brown, M. B. (2017). Antibacterial resistance in *Ureaplasma* species and *Mycoplasma hominis* isolates from urine cultures in college-aged females. *Antimicrob. Agents Chemother.* 61, e01104–e01117. doi: 10.1128/AAC.01104-17

Viscardi, R. M. (2010). *Ureaplasma* species: role in diseases of prematurity. *Clin. Perinatol.* 37, 393–409. doi: 10.1016/j.clp.2009.12.003

Waites, K. B., Katz, B., and Schelonka, R. L. (2005). *Mycoplasmas* and *Ureaplasmas* as neonatal pathogens. *Clin. Microbiol. Rev.* 18, 757–789. doi: 10.1128/CMR.18.4.757-789.2005

Waites, K. B., Xiao, L., Liu, Y., Balish, M. F., and Atkinson, T. P. (2017). *Mycoplasma pneumoniae* from the respiratory tract and beyond. *Clin. Microbiol. Rev.* 30, 747–809. doi: 10.1128/CMR.00114-116

Wang, N., Liu, W., Zhou, Y., and Liu, Y. (2019). *In vitro* activities of Nemonoxacin and other antimicrobial agents against human *Mycoplasma* and *Ureaplasmas* isolates and their defined resistance mechanisms. *Front. Microbiol.* 10:1890. doi: 10.3389/fmicb.2019.01890

Wu, H. N., Nakura, Y., Motooka, D., Nakamura, S., Nishiumi, F., Ishino, S., et al. (2014). Complete genome sequence of *Ureaplasma parvum* Serovar 3 strain SV3F4, isolated in Japan. *Genome Announc.* 2, e00256–e00214. doi: 10.1128/genomeA.00256-14

Xie, X. M., Huang, K. S., Li, W. H. (2009). Species identification genotyping of Ureaplasma in urogenital tract of male with secondary infertility and its clinical application. *J. Reprod. Med.* 18, 25–28.

Yang, T., Pan, L., Wu, N., Wang, L., Liu, Z., Kong, Y., et al. (2020). Antimicrobial resistance in clinical *Ureaplasma* spp. and *Mycoplasma hominis* and structural mechanisms underlying quinolone resistance. *Antimicrob. Agents Chemother.* 64:e02560-19. doi: 10.1128/AAC.02560-19

Zeng, X. Y., Xin, N., Tong, X. N., Wang, J. Y., and Liu, Z. W. (2016). Prevalence and antibiotic susceptibility of Ureaplasma urealyticum and mycoplasma hominis in Xi'an, China. *Eur. J. Clin. Microbiol. Infect. Dis.* 35, 1941–1947. doi: 10.1007/s10096-016-2745-2

Zhang, J., Kong, Y., Feng, Y., Huang, J., Song, T., Ruan, Z., et al. (2014a). Development of a multilocus sequence typing scheme for Ureaplasma. *Eur. J. Clin. Microbiol. Infect. Dis.* 33, 537–544. doi: 10.1007/s10096-013-1981-y

Zhang, J., Kong, Y., Ruan, Z., Huang, J., Song, T., Song, J., et al. (2014b). Correlation between Ureaplasma subgroup 2 and genitourinary tract disease outcomes revealed by an expanded multilocus sequence typing (eMLST) scheme. *PLoS One* 9:e104347. doi: 10.1371/journal.pone.0104347

Zhou, Y. H., Ma, H. X., Shi, X. X., and Liu, Y. (2018b). Ureaplasma spp. in male infertility and its relationship with semen quality and seminal plasma components. *J. Microbiol. Immunol. Infect.* 51, 778–783. doi: 10.1016/j.jmii.2016.09.004

Zhou, Y. H., Ma, H. X., Yang, Y., and Gu, W. M. (2018a). Prevalence and antimicrobial resistance of Ureaplasma spp. and mycoplasma hominis isolated from semen samples of infertile men in Shanghai, China from 2011-2016. *Eur. J. Clin. Microbiol. Infect. Dis.* 37, 729–734. doi: 10.1007/s10096-017-3167-5

Zhu, X., Li, M., Cao, H., Yang, X., and Zhang, C. (2016). Epidemiology of *Ureaplasma urealyticum* and *Mycoplasma hominis* in the semen of male outpatients with reproductive disorders. *Exp. Ther. Med.* 12, 1165–1170. doi: 10.3892/etm.2016.3409

Zhu, C. T., Liu, J. M., Ling, Y., Dong, C. L., Wu, T. T., Yu, X. Y., et al. (2012). Prevalence and antimicrobial susceptibility of Ureaplasma urealyticum and *Mycoplasma hominis* in Chinese women with genital infectious diseases. *Indian J. Dermatol. Venereol. Leprol.* 78, 406–407. doi: 10.4103/0378-6323.95480

# 19

# AI-Blue-Carba: A Rapid and Improved Carbapenemase Producer Detection Assay Using Blue-Carba With Deep Learning

*Ling Jia[1,2], Lu Han[1,2], He-Xin Cai[3], Ze-Hua Cui[1,2], Run-Shi Yang[1,2], Rong-Min Zhang[1,2], Shuan-Cheng Bai[1,2], Xu-Wei Liu[1,2], Ran Wei[1,2], Liang Chen[4], Xiao-Ping Liao[1,2], Ya-Hong Liu[1,2,5], Xi-Ming Li[3]* and Jian Sun[1,2]**

*[1] National Risk Assessment Laboratory for Antimicrobial Resistance of Animal Original Bacteria, South China Agricultural University, Guangzhou, China, [2] Guangdong Provincial Key Laboratory of Veterinary Pharmaceutics Development and Safety Evaluation, South China Agricultural University, Guangzhou, China, [3] College of Mathematics and Informatics, South China Agricultural University, Guangzhou, China, [4] Public Health Research Institute Tuberculosis Center, New Jersey Medical School, Rutgers University, Newark, NJ, United States, [5] Jiangsu Co-Innovation Center for Prevention and Control of Important Animal Infectious Diseases and Zoonoses, Yangzhou, China*

***Correspondence:**
*Xi-Ming Li*
*liximing@scau.edu.cn*
*Jian Sun*
*jiansun@scau.edu.cn*

A rapid and accurate detection of carbapenemase-producing Gram-negative bacteria (CPGNB) has an immediate demand in the clinic. Here, we developed and validated a method for rapid detection of CPGNB using Blue-Carba combined with deep learning (designated as AI-Blue-Carba). The optimum bacterial suspension concentration and detection wavelength were determined using a Multimode Plate Reader and integrated with deep learning modeling. We examined 160 carbapenemase-producing and non-carbapenemase-producing bacteria using the Blue-Carba test and a series of time and optical density values were obtained to build and validate the machine models. Subsequently, a simplified model was re-evaluated by descending the dataset from 13 time points to 2 time points. The best suitable bacterial concentration was determined to be 1.5 optical density (OD) and the optimum detection wavelength for AI-Blue-Carba was set as 615 nm. Among the 2 models (LRM and LSTM), the LSTM model generated the higher ROC-AUC value. Moreover, the simplified LSTM model trained by short time points (0–15 min) did not impair the accuracy of LSTM model. Compared with the traditional Blue-Carba, the AI-Blue-Carba method has a sensitivity of 95.3% and a specificity of 95.7% at 15 min, which is a rapid and accurate method to detect CPGNB.

**Keywords: carbapenemase-producing gram-negative bacteria, rapid detection, Blue-Carba, deep learning, OD value**

## INTRODUCTION

Antimicrobial resistance (AMR) poses a serious global threat to human, animal, and environment health, as multidrug resistant bacteria continue to emerge and spread worldwide. Carbapenems are one of the last-resort antibiotics to treat infections caused by multidrug-resistant Gram-negative pathogens. Carbapenem resistance in Gram-negative bacteria is primarily due to the production of various carbapenemases, which leaves the clinicians with limited therapeutic options. Carbapenemase-producers showed broad spectrum enzyme activity for various β-lactam substrates, and were associated with resistance to other antibiotic classes, and demonstrated rapid transmission in healthcare facilities, animals and the environments (Codjoe and Donkor, 2017). Notably, carbapenemase genes are frequently located on mobile genetic elements and plasmids, therefore facilitating the horizontal of resistance to other bacteria (Dortet et al., 2014; Nordmann and Poirel, 2014). It is of paramount importance to develop reliable methods for rapid detection and characterization of carbapenemase-producers.

Different phenotypic and molecular-based methods have been used to identify these carbapenemase producers. For known mechanisms, molecular methods of gene detection are usually fast and accurate. However, molecular detection of carbapenemase genes can be costly and may require substantial expertise, and more importantly they fail to detect unknown or novel carbapenemase genes (Stuart et al., 2012). A solution to this problem is the detection of carbapenem enzymatic degradation, using Matrix Assisted Laser Desorption Ionization-Time of Flight Mass Spectrometry (MALDI-TOF MS) (Yu et al., 2018); or by chromogenic agar or UV spectrophotometry (e.g., Carba NP and Blue Carba) (Bernabeu et al., 2012); or the rapid Carbapenem Inactivation Method (Muntean et al., 2018).

In 2012, Nordmann et al. developed the Carba NP test which is based on visual monitoring of medium acidification of a mixture containing bacterial cells, a carbapenem and the pH indicator phenol red (Dortet et al., 2012). However, some subtle color variations could be hard to differentiate by visual interpretation. This method was then adapted to microtiter plates and spectrophotometric measurement of optical density and interpreted using a pre-programmed Excel spreadsheet (Surre et al., 2018). However, the assay was not comprehensive enough and the data analysis of this assay is still not straightforward.

In this study, a deep learning approach was used to predict carbapenemase production, taking into consideration the similarity in the OD value distributions at different time points, instead of only the best hit. Deep learning has been proven to be the most powerful machine learning approach to date for many applications, including image processing (LeCun et al., 2015), biomedical signaling (Tabar and Halici, 2017), speech recognition (Hinton et al., 2012), and genomic related analysis, such as the predicting antibiotic resistance genes from metagenomic data (Pan and Shen, 2017; Li et al., 2018). Particularly in the case of predicting new genetic markers, the deep learning model surpasses all known binding site for prediction approaches (Drouin et al., 2016).

To the best our knowledge, this is the first time that contact the carbapenemase detection method with Deep learning. Here we describe the AI-Blue-Carba test, an improved variant of Blue-Carba to determine carbapenemase producers using a uniform standard.

## MATERIALS AND METHODS

### Sample Collection and Bacterial Strains

In this study, we mainly collected fecal samples from animals (anal swabs and feces). These fecal samples were randomly collected from pigs, chickens, ducks, and goose, if possible, the soil, dust, sewage and vegetable samples were also collected. These samples were screened from 14 animal farms (pig farms, $n = 5$; chicken houses, $n = 5$; duck farms, $n = 3$; goose farms, $n = 1$) in 6 provinces (Guangxi, Guangdong, Heilongjiang, Jiangsu, Jiangxi, and Zhejiang provinces) in China. In total, 498 strains were collected from June 2016 to Nov 2017 and subjected to selection onto MacConkey (MAC) agars containing meropenem (1 mg l-1). In order to enrich the diversity of carbapenem-resistant strains and genes, we also collected some strains from human and flower sources. Sixty clinical isolates were collected from the hospitals of Guangdong and Shandong provinces. In addition, 273 strains were isolated from flowers including carnations, roses and lilies which were collected from Mar 2018 to Apr 2018 in Guangzhou Flower Market and selected on MAC plates without any antibiotics.

We utilized 130 among the 831 collected strains from different sources above, including 49 isolates from animal anal swabs and feces samples which were characterized, 60 clinical isolates collected from two hospitals in Guangdong and Shandong provinces, and then 21 isolates from flowers. Carbapenemase genes were characterized by PCR and Sanger sequencing (Rahman et al., 2013). Strains from different Enterobacteriaceae species (*E. coli, Klebsiella pneumoniae, Citrobacter freundii, Enterobacter cloacae*, etc.) as well as *Pseudomonas spp.* were included. We identified 107 carbapenem-resistant strains able to produce at least one carbapenem-hydrolyzing β-lactamase, whereas the remaining 23 carbapenem-susceptible strains were carbapenemase negative (**Table 1**). The MICs for ertapenem, meropenem, and imipenem were determined by agar dilution and interpreted according to the Clinical and Laboratory Standards Institute guidelines (CLSI, 2018).

### Blue-Carba Test

The Blue-Carba test was performed and interpreted as previously described (Pires et al., 2013). Briefly, 5 μL loopfuls of bacteria cultured on Mueller-Hinton agar (HuanKai, Guangzhou, China) were suspended in 0.04% bromothymol blue (Macklin, Shanghai, China) solution containing (test) or lacking (control) 3 mg/mL imipenem (MedChemExpress, New Jersey, United States) and 0.1 mM $ZnSO_4$ (Damao, Tianjin, China). Color changes were registered after incubation at 37°C for 2 h. The result was considered positive when the solution containing imipenem became green or yellow and differed from the negative control. The result was negative if the solution lacking antibiotic presented the same or a stronger color change as the solution containing imipenem. A previously characterized NDM-5 producer (CQ02-121) was used as positive control (Sun et al., 2016) and a test tube containing only bacterial inoculum (*E. coli* ATCC 25922) and Blue-Carba solution was used as negative control for each isolate tested.

**TABLE 1** | Results of carbapenemase and non-carbapenemase producers' PCR and MIC.

| Species | MIC(μg/ml) | | | | No. of isolates with a positive test/no. of isolates tested for 2 h | |
|---|---|---|---|---|---|---|
| | **Carbapenemase content** | **MEM** | **IPM** | **ERT** | **AI-Blue-Carba** | **Blue-Carba** |
| **Carbapenemase producers *E. coli* (47)** | NDM-5(43) | 1–64 | 1- >64 | >64 | 41/43 | 41/43 |
| | NDM-1(4) | 4–8 | 8–16 | 16–64 | 4/4 | 4/4 |
| ***Pseudomonas putida*(7)** | VIM-2(6) | ≥64 | 8-≥64 | >64 | 6/6 | 6/6 |
| | IMP-4(1) | >64 | 8 | >64 | 1/1 | 1/1 |
| ***Klebsiella pneumoniae* (44)** | NDM-1(15) | 2–32 | 2–32 | 8- >64 | 13/15 | 13/15 |
| | NDM-5(4) | 2–64 | 4- >64 | 16–64 | 4/4 | 4/4 |
| | NDM-1 + IMP-4(2) | 32 | 8- ≥64 | >64 | 1/1 | 1/1 |
| | KPC-2(23) | 32 | >64 | >64 | 23/23 | 23/23 |
| ***Citrobacter freundii* (1)** | NDM-1(1) | 16 | 8 | 64 | 1/1 | 1/1 |
| ***Enterobacter cloacae* (5)** | IMP-4(1) | 8 | 16 | 64 | 1/1 | 1/1 |
| | NDM-1(3) | 16 | 16–32 | 32- >64 | 3/3 | 3/3 |
| | VIM-1(1) | 1 | 2 | 2 | 1/1 | 1/1 |
| ***Providencia rettgeri* (4)** | NDM-1(4) | 2- ≥64 | 4 | 8 | 4/4 | 4/4 |
| ***Enterobacter mucus* (2)** | NDM-1(2) | 32 | 32 | >64 | 2/2 | 2/2 |
| ***Pseudomonas aeruginosa* (1)** | NDM-5(1) | 64 | >64 | >64 | 1/1 | 1/1 |
| **Non-carbapenemase producers** | | | | | | |
| ***E. coli (10)*** | CTX-M | <0.0625 | <0.0625–4 | <0.0625–2 | 0/10 | 0/10 |
| ***Citrobacter freundii (8)*** | CTX-M | <0.0625 | <0.0625–4 | <0.0625–2 | 0/8 | 0/8 |
| ***Enterobacter cloacae (4)*** | CTX-M | <0.0625 | <0.0625–4 | <0.0625–2 | 0/4 | 0/4 |
| ***Providencia rettgeri (1)*** | CTX-M | <0.0625 | <0.0625–4 | <0.0625–2 | 0/1 | 0/1 |

*MEM, meropenem; IPM, imipenem; ERT, ertapenem.*

## Experiment Condition of AI-Blue-Carba

In order to overcome the limitation of lower the sensitivity with visual interpretation, we used the OD values to indicate the color's change of the Blue-Carba result. To obtain a stable OD value, the optimum wavelength for detection of CPGNB was determined using a wavelength scan of test solutions generated using known carbapenemase producers up to 2 h in a Multimode Plate Reader (PerkinElmer, Hamburg, Germany) to obtain the absorbance maxima corresponding to yellow and blue (negative control).

Bacteria were diluted in 500 μL phosphate buffered saline (PBS, pH 7.4) and distilled water, respectively, the OD600 nm was adjusted to 1.0, 1.5, and 2.0 and the 100 μL of the bacteria suspension was used for testing. The wells were scanned and the OD was recorded every 5 min for 2 h at 37°C in the plate reader.

## Deep Learning

The problem of distinguishing carbapenemase and non-carbapenemase producers based on the OD values and the results of the Blue-Carba test can be formalized as a machine learning or supervised learning question. It is assumed that a data sample $S$ that contains $m$ machine learning examples were given at the beginning. These examples are pairs $(x, y)$, where $x$ represents OD values detected over time and y is a label that corresponds to one of the two possible results (positive or negative). In addition, we assume that $x \in \{a_1, a_2 \ldots a_{13}\}$ which corresponds to the set of all 13 OD values and that $y \in \{0, 1\}$. Label $y = 1$ is assigned to the carbapenemase producers group and $y = 0$ is assigned to the non-carbapenemase producers group. We assumed the examples in $S$ are drawn independently from an unknown and fixed data generating distribution $D$, resulting in the equation of $S \overset{\text{def}}{=} \{(x_1, y_1), \ldots (x_m, y_m)\} \sim D^m$.

Usually, learning algorithms are designed to learn from a vector representation of the data. In order to learn from detected OD values, a function $\emptyset : \{x_1, x_2, \ldots x_m\}^* \to R^d$ is defined, which takes time as input and maps it to some $d$ dimensional vector space. Then a learning algorithm can be applied to the set $S' \overset{\text{def}}{=} \{\emptyset(x_1), y_1, \ldots \emptyset(x_m, y_m)\}$ to obtain a model $h : R^d \to \{0, 1\}$. The model is a function which maps the feature representation of OD values over time to the associated results of the carbapenemase producers. Our objective is to achieve a model $h$ that has a good generalization performance, i.e., that minimizes the probability, $R(h)$, of making a prediction error for any example drawn according to the distribution $D$, where

$$R(h) \overset{\text{def}}{=} Pr^R_{(x,y)\sim D}\left[h(\emptyset(x)) \neq y\right] \quad (1)$$

## Construct Models

The LSTM (Long Short-Time Memory) cells store and access information over long periods of time using multiplicative gates (Hochreiter and Schmidhuber, 1997). It retains useful long-term information through the threshold mechanism and removes useless short-term information to realize the mining of timing information. In this work, the rules were individual units that detect the carbapenemase-producer using OD values over time. These rules are Boolean-valued, i.e., the output is either positive or negative. The models learned by the LSTM are logical combinations of such rules, which can be conjunctions (logical-AND) or disjunctions (logical-OR). To predict the results of detection of carbapenemase producers using OD values over time, each rule in the model was evaluated and the results were aggregated to obtain the prediction.

Real-time prediction of data traffic requires continuous data input and learning. The dataset was therefore split into a training set (80% of the OD values) to construct the LSTM model that can output a $y$ value randomly (0 or 1 which represent the positive or negative results of carbapenemase producer) if input a group of OD values. In addition, a separate testing set (20% of the data) were used with the results of Blue-Carba to validate and evaluate LSTM's prediction accuracy. In this study, we used a 10-fold cross validation to test the prediction model and select the best hyperparameter (Webb et al., 2019).

In order to display data characteristics to more accurately predict the carbapenemase-producing strains, we compared the LSTM with LRM (Linear Regression model). The LRM is a linear approach to find the relationship between a scalar response and one or more explanatory variables (Kumaresan and Riyazuddin, 2007). In this paper, LRM modeled the relation between OD values and Blue-Carba test.

## Evaluation Metrics

We evaluated the performance of the two models using the confusion matrix assessment method. The prediction quality was evaluated by the following evaluation metrics: The ROC curve describes the classifier's True Positive Rate (TPR, the ratio of the number of positive samples correctly classified by the classifier to the total number of positive samples) and False Positive Rate (FPR, the number of negative samples that the classifier misclassified accounts for the total negative samples) Ratio of the number). Recall [Equation 2] shows the number of correct positive results divided by the number of all relevant samples that were identified as positive. Precision [Equation 3] expresses the number of correct positive results divided by the number of positive results predicted by the classifier. F1 Score [Equation 4] indicates the Harmonic Mean between Precision and Recall that tells you how precise your models is. The possible outcomes of a classification model include: true positive, TP; false positive, FP; true negative, TN; false negative, FN.

$$\text{Recall} = \frac{\text{TP}}{\text{TP} + \text{FN}} \tag{2}$$

$$\text{Precision} = \frac{\text{TP}}{\text{TP} + \text{FP}} \tag{3}$$

$$\text{F1} - \text{score} = \frac{2\text{TP}}{2\text{TP} + \text{FP} + \text{FN}} \tag{4}$$

## Model Simplification

To achieve the purpose for rapid detection of a carbapenemase producer, we choose the OD values at 12 time points groups: 2 time points,3 time points, and so on 13 time points (**Figure 1B**) to optimize the best model from the above LSTM. We then evaluated the performance of the 12 models on the basis of the 12 sets of time points (OD value data set) using the above evaluation metrics to get the optimal detection time.

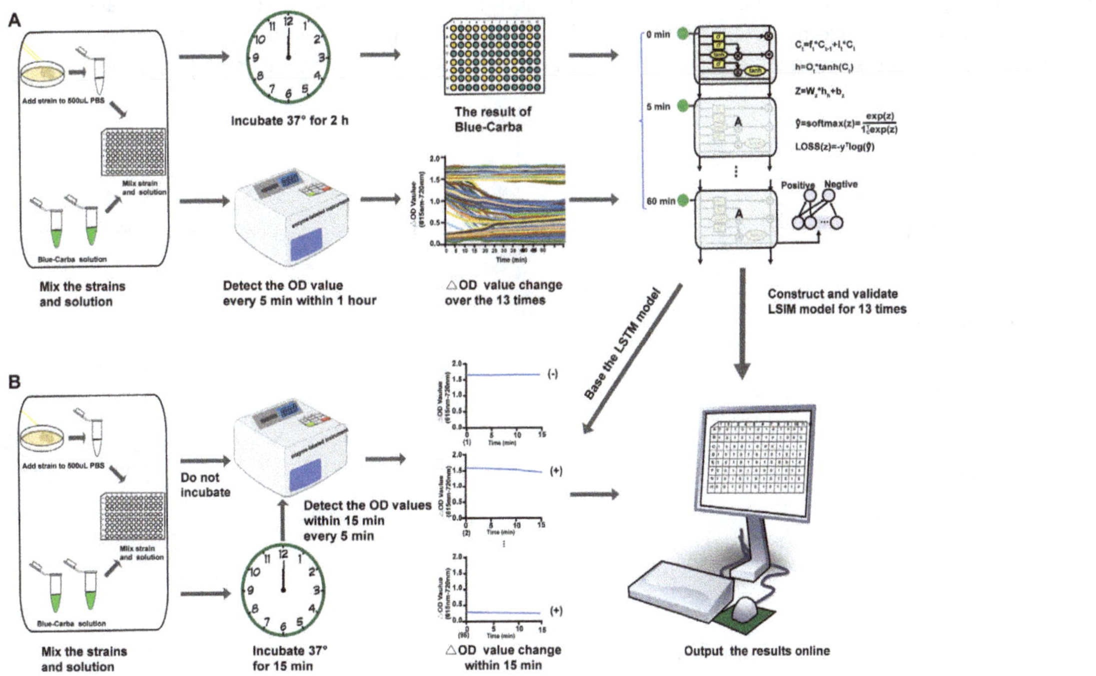


**FIGURE 1 |** Rapid detection of carbapenemase producers by AI-Blue-Carba. **(A)**. Process to construct and validate the AI model; **(B)** Process to optimize the AI-Blue-Carba.

# RESULTS

## Optimum Conditions for AI-Blue-Carba Test

The scanning results of positive and negative carbapenemase producers indicated a maximum absorption peak at 615 nm and this was chosen as the detection wavelength in following experiments (**Supplementary Figure S1A**). At the same time, we chose 720 nm as the detection wavelength of negative carbapenemase producers due to its stable absorption after 700 nm (**Supplementary Figure S1B**) to stabilize the OD values. Finally, the experimental data was the difference in OD ($\Delta$OD) values between 615 and 720 nm.

We next examined differing bacterial concentrations and diluents at these wavelengths and found that the $\Delta$OD values varied. The general trend in $\Delta$OD values over time showed a more rapid decrease using the PBS diluent vs. ultrapure water at different bacterial concentrations (**Supplementary Figures S2A–F**). The weak carbapenemase producers showed a more rapid decrease in OD values as the bacterial concentration increased. However, when the bacterial concentration was set at 2.0 OD (at 600 nm), the strong carbapenemase producers generated with an ascending pattern over time (**Supplementary Figures S2C,F**). As such, we choose 1.5 OD (at 600 nm) for the bacterial concentration in PBS as the most appropriate testing condition for the AI-Blue-Carba test, due to more reliable stable OD values were acquired for both strong and weak carbapenemase producers.

We measured the OD values every 5 min up to 1 h (13 time points) using our 160 isolates (**Table 1**) to obtain the data characteristics. In brief, the trend in the $\Delta$OD values of non-carbapenemase producers over time demonstrated a smooth linear pattern and ranged from 1.5 OD to 2.0 OD. The strong carbapenemase-producers generated a trend of $\Delta$OD values over time that were also smooth lines, but the range was 0.2 OD – 0.4 OD while for weak carbapenemase producers, the trend of $\Delta$OD values decreased gradually over time (**Figure 1A**).

**TABLE 2 |** Prediction results for the majority prediction rule of four models.

| Model | ACC | F1 | REC | PRE |
|---|---|---|---|---|
| LRM | 0. 93 | 0.93 | 0.62 | 0.94 |
| LSTM | 0.98 | 0.98 | 0.98 | 0.98 |

*ACC, Accuracy; PRE, Precision; REC, Recall; F1, F1-score.*

## Construction and Evaluation of Deep Learning Model

In the following, we discuss the results of a 10-fold cross-validation study on the entire data set of 2 models. Across all cross-validation folds, predictor performance generalizes well to independent data. The degree of certainty of a read prediction can be measured by the prediction probability (see Methods). As **Table 2** shows, the REC of LSTM is bigger (0.98) than LRM (0.62), other parameter values (ACC, REC, F1) of LSTM still higher than LRM. The model receiver operating characteristic (ROC) curves with the performances of LRM and LSTM (**Figure 2A**). The ROC-AUC of LSTM (0.99) was also better than LRM (0.94). Considering these factors, the LSTM model is the optimal model to detect the carbarpenemase producers.

## The Simplified Model

In order to determine the earliest time required to accurately detect carbapenemase producers, we used OD values with lesser time points and constructed and evaluated the models in a manner similar to that described above. To find a suitable model for specific application, we get the corresponding ACC, PRE, REC, and F1 values, sensitivity, specificity to adjust the threshold

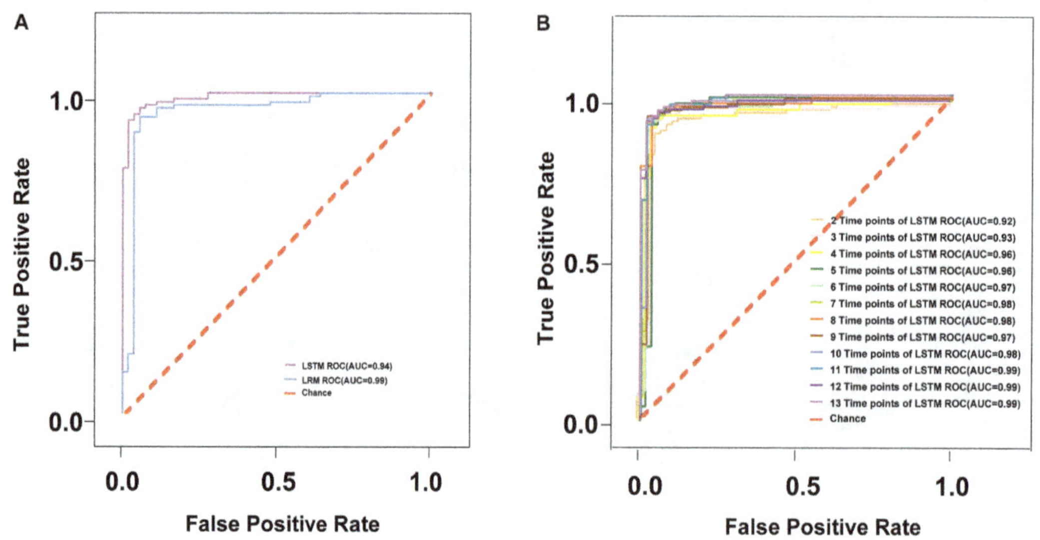


**FIGURE 2 |** The ROC curves of different models. **(A)** The ROC curves are shown for the models trained with the multispecies data sets of Linear Regression model and LSTM model; **(B)** The ROC curves of different time points of LSTM.

of the model, the ACC, PRE, REC, and F1 values of 12 optimized LSTM models were all >96% after 20 min in **Table 3**. In addition, the ROC-AUC values of the 12 time points group was >96% after 15 min (**Figure 2B**). Additionally, the 95.3% specificity and 95.7% sensitivity of AI-Blue-Carba were higher than Blue-Carba at 0–15 min. Consequently, we used the 0–15 min internal for rapid detecting the carbapenemase producers.

We examined some weak (*Klebsiella pneumonia* E-3F3 and *Citrobacter freundii* 2N3001), strong (*E. coli* FS89) and non-carbapenemase producers (*E. coli* ATCC 25922) using the Blue-Carba test. Isolates FS89 and ATCC 25922 could be detected in 0 min, while E-3F3 and 2N3001 could be accurately judged after 30 min but the confirmation of the final results took 2 h by Blue-Carba. The ΔOD values for FS89 and 25922 from 0–15 min, 0–30 min and 0–60 min were consistent with the trend of the 13-time points taken over 1 h. This indicated that the strong carbapenemase and the non-carbapenemase producers can be rapidly detected within 15 min. For E-3F3 and 2N3001, the ΔOD values for the 13-time points was relatively slow for the 0–15 min, 0–30 min, and 0–60 min intervals (**Figure 3A**). The colors change of Blue-Carba (**Figure 3B**) and the results of AI-Blue-Carba (**Figure 3C**) were consistent with the PCR results.

**TABLE 3** | Prediction results for the different time groups by LSTM model.

| Time Group | ACC | F1 | REC | PRE |
|---|---|---|---|---|
| 0–5 min | 0.87 | 0.87 | 0.88 | 0.89 |
| 0–10 min | 0.90 | 0.92 | 0.92 | 0.92 |
| 0–15 min | 0.93 | 0.93 | 0.94 | 0.94 |
| 0–20 min | 0.96 | 0.96 | 0.96 | 0.96 |
| 0–25 min | 0.97 | 0.97 | 0.97 | 0.97 |
| 0–30 min | 0.98 | 0.98 | 0.98 | 0.98 |
| 0–35 min | 0.97 | 0.97 | 0.97 | 0.97 |
| 0–40 min | 0.97 | 0.97 | 0.97 | 0.97 |
| 0–45 min | 0.97 | 0.97 | 0.97 | 0.97 |
| 0–50 min | 0.97 | 0.97 | 0.96 | 0.97 |
| 0–55 min | 0.97 | 0.97 | 0.97 | 0.97 |
| 0–60 min | 0.98 | 0.98 | 0.98 | 0.98 |

## DISCUSSION

The rapid increase of carbapenem resistance in Gram-negative bacilli is of great concern worldwide (Zhang et al., 2018). Public health surveillance for a disease is traditionally viewed as the first step in disease prevention and data obtained from surveillance help to enforce public health action. Therefore, rapid and user-friendly assays are crucial.

To rapidly and efficiently detect carbapenemase producers, the Carba NP test was modified according to CLSI guidelines by measuring the *in vitro* hydrolysis of imipenem to produce a color change within 2 h (Dortet et al., 2012). The RAPID ECCARBA NP test could be useful for screening carbapenemase producers from colonized patients (Poirel and Nordmann, 2015). The commercially available β CARBA test is based on the change of color of an undisclosed chromogenic substrate in the presence of carbapenem-hydrolyzing activity. The test is simple to perform and interpret by non-specialized staff members (Mancini et al., 2017). In addition, the CarbAcineto NP test, which is rapid and reproducible, detects all types of carbapenemases including *Acinetobacter spp.* with a sensitivity of 94.7% and a specificity of 100%. Its use will facilitate its recognition and prevent its spread.

All these modified Carba NP tests have an obvious shortcoming that the color intensity is somewhat low, so we choose the LSTM model to correct this deficiency. Carbapenemase detection by spectrophotometric assays is a more accurate approach for the detection of carbapenemases and has

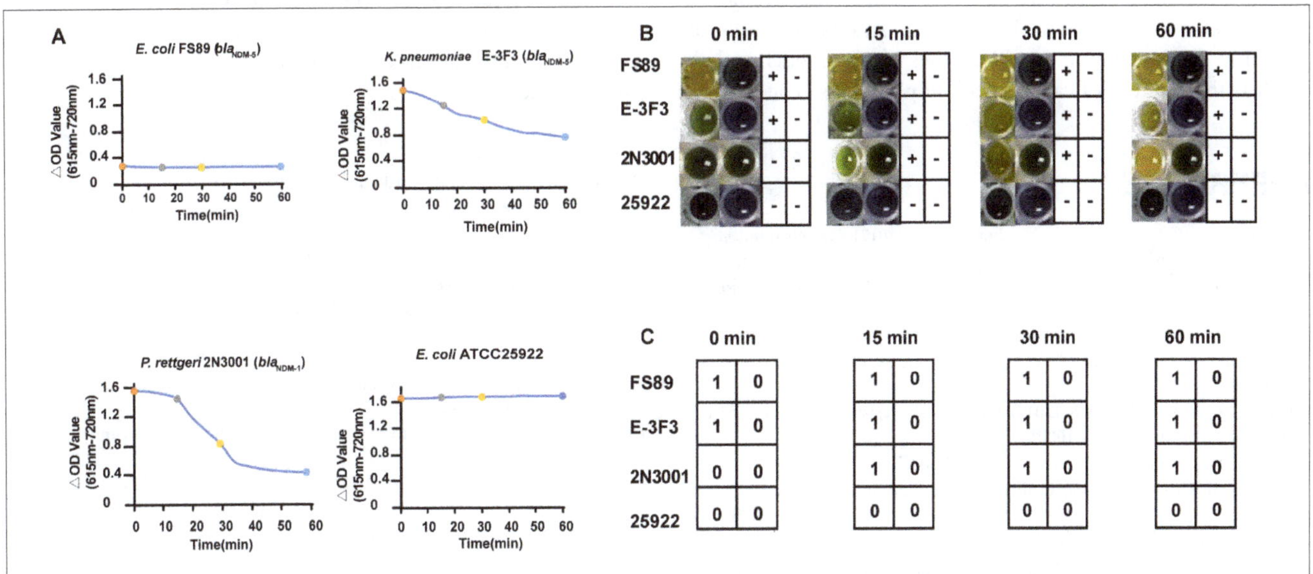


**FIGURE 3** | Comparison of the result of AI-Blue-Carba and Blue-Carba. **(A)** shows the ΔOD values' change of different time points (within in 0 min, 0–15 min, 0–30 min, 0–60 min); **(B)** shows the results of carbapenamase producer by Blue-Carba; **(C)** shows the results of carbapenamase producer by AI -Blue-Carba within.

excellent sensitivity and specificity for the Enterobacteriaceae. The results are usually comparable between different labs and were suggested to be implemented in national reference laboratories (Nordmann et al., 2012). Moreover, all the above methods can use these tools (OD values and the LSTM model) to improve their sensitivity and specificity.

A pioneering study illustrated the huge potential of using Big Data for epidemiology in which the epidemics can be detected early by tracking online queries on disease symptoms using social media such as Google Search and Twitter (Deiner et al., 2016). We introduce a "deep learning" approach to improve the objectivity and efficiency of detecting carbapenemase producers. The deep learning model can be applied to new data to make decisions after training, and decision making can involve detection, discrimination, and classification. Therefore, we trained the LRM and LSTM models using OD values generated by the Blue Carba test and compared the evaluation metrics of the four models. The results presented below could not be notably improved by further parameter tuning or feature selection efforts. An auxiliary assessment further shows that our classifiers are very robust. We chose LSTM to construct the website because it was optimized by the evaluation metrics independent of the values of the F1-scores. As we expected, its advantages are most pronounced for problems requiring the use of long-range contextual information. Consequently, LSTM has also been applied to various real-world problems, such as protein secondary structure prediction, music generation, reinforcement learning, speech recognition, and handwriting recognition. Furthermore, similar to any software systems, updating this classification system or model can be conducted at regular intervals whenever new dataset/information/evidence is available.

To achieve the aim of the rapid detection of the carbapenemase producers, we simplified the LSTM model by reducing detection times and chose 15 min as test interval. The deep learning analysis platform illustrates that $\Delta$OD values change over time intuitively and then judges the strength of carbapenemase production by the test strains. In addition, you only need to input the OD values to the model and the result is the number of carbapenemase producers. The data can be output directly to reduce the time for manual entry and analysis of data. Lastly, the model gives a standard procedure for reading experimental results of carbapenemase producers and climates reading errors. In the next step, we will create a website platform that co-networking with hospitals and research laboratories, the results of carbapenemase producers in different areas can be compared to effectively monitor the prevalence of carbapenemases in the region. By providing actionable data directly to governments, a website that could analyze those areas containing CPGNB could forewarn healthcare facilities to take the appropriate infection control measures.

We evaluated a deep learning method (AI-Blue-Carba) which allows detection of CPGNB in less than 15 min. This test can be used as the first step in detecting the carbapenemase activity of candidate isolates. In addition, it is also useful for checking carbapenemase activity as part of the infection control process for outbreaks caused by carbapenemase producers. AI-Blue-Carba is a robust assay which user-friendly (no need for trained staff), high in performance (sensitive and specific), and low in cost.

## AUTHOR CONTRIBUTIONS

JS and X-ML conceived of the study. LJ, LH, and S-CB performed the experiments. LJ and H-XC constructed models. LJ, Z-HC, R-SY, and R-MZ analyzed the data. LJ, X-WL, and RW made the figures. LJ wrote the manuscript. JS, LC, X-ML, and X-PL edited and revised the manuscript. Y-HL coordinated the whole project. All authors have read and approved the final manuscript.

## FUNDING

This work was jointly supported by the National Key Research and Development Program of China (2016YFD0501300), the National Natural Science Foundation of China (31972735), the Program for Innovative Research Team in the University of Ministry of Education of China (IRT_17R39), and the 111 Project (D20008).

## REFERENCES

Bernabeu, S., Poirel, L., and Nordmann, P. (2012). Spectrophotometry-based detection of carbapenemase producers among *Enterobacteriaceae*. *Diagn. Microbiol. Infect. Dis.* 74, 88–90. doi: 10.1016/j.diagmicrobio.2012.05.021

CLSI (2018). *Performance Standards for Antimicrobial Susceptibility Testing*, 28th Edn. ClSI Supplement. M100. Wayne, PA: Clinical and Laboratory Standards Institute. .

Codjoe, F. S., and Donkor, E. S. (2017). Carbapenem resistance: a review. *Med Sci* 6:1. doi: 10.3390/medsci6010001

Deiner, M. S., Lietman, T. M., Mcleod, S. D., Chodosh, J., and Porco, T. C. (2016). Surveillance tools emerging from search engines and social media data for determining eye disease patterns. *JAMA Ophthalmol.* 134, 1024–1030. doi: 10.1001/jamaophthalmol.2016.2267

Dortet, L., Poirel, L., and Nordmann, P. (2012). Rapid identification of carbapenemase types in *Enterobacteriaceae* and *Pseudomonas* spp. by using a biochemical test. *Antimicrob. Agents Chemother.* 56, 6437–6440. doi: 10.1128/aac.01395-12

Dortet, L., Poirel, L., and Nordmann, P. (2014). Worldwide dissemination of the NDM-type carbapenemases in Gram-negative bacteria. *Biomed. Res. Int.* 2014:249856.

Drouin, A., Giguere, S., Deraspe, M., Marchand, M., Tyers, M., Loo, V. G., et al. (2016). Predictive computational phenotyping and biomarker discovery using reference-free genome comparisons. *BMC Genomics* 17:754. doi: 10.1186/s12864-016-2889-6

Hinton, G., Deng, L., Yu, D., Dahl, G. E., Mohamed, A. R., Jaitly, N., et al. (2012). Deep neural networks for acoustic modeling in speech recognition. *IEEE Signal Process. Mag.* 29, 82–97.

Hochreiter, S., and Schmidhuber, J. (1997). Long short-term memory. *Neural Comput.* 9, 1735–1780.

Kumaresan, M., and Riyazuddin, P. (2007). Factor analysis and linear regression model (LRM) of metal speciation and physico-chemical characters of groundwater samples. *Environ. Monit. Assess.* 138, 65–79. doi: 10.1007/s10661-007-9761-8

LeCun, Y., Bengio, Y., and Hinton, G. (2015). Deep learning. *Nature* 521, 436–444.

Li, L. G., Yin, X., and Zhang, T. (2018). Tracking antibiotic resistance gene pollution from different sources using machine-learning classification. *Microbiome* 6:93.

Mancini, S., Kieffer, N., Poirel, L., and Nordmann, P. (2017). Evaluation of the RAPIDEC(R) CARBA NP and beta-CARBA(R) tests for rapid detection of Carbapenemase-producing *Enterobacteriaceae*. *Diagn. Microbiol. Infect. Dis.* 88, 293–297. doi: 10.1016/j.diagmicrobio.2017.05.006

Muntean, M. M., Muntean, A. A., Gauthier, L., Creton, E., Cotellon, G., Popa, M. I., et al. (2018). Evaluation of the rapid carbapenem inactivation method (rCIM): a phenotypic screening test for carbapenemase-producing *Enterobacteriaceae*. *J. Antimicrob. Chemother.* 73, 900–908. doi: 10.1093/jac/dkx519

Nordmann, P., Gniadkowski, M., Giske, C. G., Poirel, L., Woodford, N., Miriagou, V., et al. (2012). Identification and screening of carbapenemase-producing *Enterobacteriaceae*. *Clin. Microbiol. Infect.* 18, 432–438. doi: 10.1111/j.1469-0691.2012.03815.x

Nordmann, P., and Poirel, L. (2014). The difficult-to-control spread of carbapenemase producers among *Enterobacteriaceae* worldwide. *Clin. Microbiol. Infect.* 20, 821–830. doi: 10.1111/1469-0691.12719

Pan, X., and Shen, H. B. (2017). RNA-protein binding motifs mining with a new hybrid deep learning based cross-domain knowledge integration approach. *BMC Bioinformatics* 18:136. doi: 10.1186/s12859-017-1561-8

Pires, J., Novais, A., and Peixe, L. (2013). Blue-carba, an easy biochemical test for detection of diverse carbapenemase producers directly from bacterial cultures. *J. Clin. Microbiol.* 51, 4281–4283. doi: 10.1128/jcm.01634-13

Poirel, L., and Nordmann, P. (2015). RAPIDEC(R) CARBA NP test for rapid detection of carbapenemase producers. *J. Clin. Microbiol.* 53, 3003–3008. doi: 10.1128/jcm.00977-15

Rahman, M., Uddin, M., Sultana, R., Moue, A., and Setu, M. (2013). Polymerase chain reaction (PCR): a short review. *Anwer Khan Mod. Med. Coll. J.* 4, 30–36.

Stuart, J. C., Voets, G., Scharringa, J., Fluit, A. C., and Leverstein-Van Hall, M. A. (2012). Detection of carbapenemase-producing *Enterobacteriaceae* with a commercial DNA microarray. *J. Med. Microbiol.* 61, 809–812. doi: 10.1099/jmm.0.041673-0

Sun, J., Yang, R. S., Zhang, Q., Feng, Y., Fang, L. X., Xia, J., et al. (2016). Co-transfer of blaNDM-5 and mcr-1 by an IncX3-X4 hybrid plasmid in *Escherichia coli*. *Nat. Microbiol.* 1:16176.

Surre, J., Canard, I., Bourne-Branchu, P., Courbiere, E., Franceschi, C., Chatellier, S., et al. (2018). Enhanced detection of carbapenemase-producing *Enterobacteriaceae* by an optimized phenol red assay. *Diagn. Microbiol. Infect. Dis.* 90, 11–17. doi: 10.1016/j.diagmicrobio.2017.09.005

Tabar, Y. R., and Halici, U. (2017). A novel deep learning approach for classification of EEG motor imagery signals. *J. Neural Eng.* 14:016003. doi: 10.1088/1741-2560/14/1/016003

Webb, C. A., Trivedi, M. H., Cohen, Z. D., Dillon, D. G., Fournier, J. C., Goer, F., et al. (2019). Personalized prediction of antidepressant *v.* placebo response: evidence from the EMBARC study. *Psychol. Med.* 49, 1118–1127. doi: 10.1017/S0033291718001708

Yu, J., Liu, J., Li, Y., Yu, J., Zhu, W., Liu, Y., et al. (2018). Rapid detection of carbapenemase activity of *Enterobacteriaceae* isolated from positive blood cultures by MALDI-TOF MS. *Ann. Clin. Microbiol. Antimicrob.* 17:22.

Zhang, H., Ma, G., Zhu, Y., Zeng, L., Ahmad, A., Wang, C., et al. (2018). Active-Site Conformational Fluctuations Promote the Enzymatic Activity of NDM-1. *Antimicrob. Agents Chemother.* 62:e1579-18.

20

# Harnessing the mTOR Pathway for Tuberculosis Treatment

*Pooja Singh and Selvakumar Subbian**

*Public Health Research Institute at New Jersey Medical School, Rutgers Biomedical and Health Sciences Rutgers, The State University of New Jersey, Newark, NJ, United States*

***Correspondence:**
*Selvakumar Subbian*
*subbiase@njms.rutgers.edu*

Tuberculosis (TB) remains as one of the leading killer infectious diseases of humans. At present, the standard therapeutic regimen to treat TB comprised of multiple antibiotics administered for a minimum of six months. Although these drugs are useful in controlling TB burden globally, they have not eliminated the disease. In addition, the lengthy duration of treatment with multiple drugs contributes to patient non-compliance that can result in the development of drug resistant strains (MDR and XDR) of Mycobacterium tuberculosis (Mtb), the causative agent of TB. Therefore, new and improved therapeutic strategies are urgently needed for effective control of TB worldwide. The intracellular survival of Mtb is regarded as a cumulative effect of the host immune response and the bacterial ability to resist or subvert this response. When the host innate defensive system is manipulated by Mtb for its survival and dissemination, the host develops disease conditions that are hard to overcome. The host intrinsic factors also contributes to the poor efficacy of anti-mycobacterial drugs and to the emergence of drug resistance. Hence, strengthening the immune repertoire involved in combating Mtb through host-directed therapeutics (HDT) can be one of the approaches for effective bacterial killing and clearance of infection/disease. Recently, more scientific research has been focused toward HDT strategies that empowers host cells for effective killing of Mtb, reduce the duration of treatment and/or alleviates the development of MDR/XDR, since Mtb cannot develop resistance against a drug that targets the host cell function. Autophagy is a conserved cellular process critical for maintaining cellular integrity and function. Autophagy is regulated by multiple pathways that are either dependent or independent of mTOR (mechanistic target of rapamycin; a.k.a. mammalian target of rapamycin), a master regulatory molecules that impacts several cellular functions. In this review, we summarize the role of autophagy in Mtb pathogenesis, the mTOR pathway and, modulating the mTOR pathway with inhibitors as potential adjunctive HDT, in combination with standard anti-TB antibiotics, to improve the outcome of current TB treatment.

**Keywords: mTOR, autophagy, everolimus, host directed therapy, tuberculosis, drug resistance, adjunct therapy, phagocytosis**

## INTRODUCTION

Tuberculosis (TB) is one of the leading killer among infectious diseases of humans, accounting for about 10.4 million new cases and 1.8 million deaths in 2015 (World Health Organization, 2016). The global burden of TB has also been exacerbated by other co-morbid conditions, including diabetes and HIV-infection, and TB is a leading cause of mortality among HIV infected individuals with nearly 400,000 deaths reported in 2015. The standard therapeutic regimen recommended by the WHO for treating drug-sensitive pulmonary TB, known as DOTS (Directly Observed Treatment, Short course), is comprised of four antibiotics: isoniazid (INH), rifampicin (RIF), pyrazinamide (PZA) and ethambutol (ETH) for 2 months (initial phase) followed by INH, and RIF for 4 months (continuation phase). This multi-drug regimen is essential and necessary to ensure successful bacteriological cure in patients with TB. Although these drugs are useful in controlling the overall disease burden at the level of individual patients as well as global TB control measures, they have not eliminated the disease at both these levels (Ryan, 1992). This is in part due to the lengthy duration of treatment with multiple drugs, which promotes the fear of drug dependency and doubts of not getting cured and contributes to drug-induced tissue toxicity issues. Adverse effects, ranging from serious ones, like hepatitis and pneumonia, to minor ones, like vomiting, acne and nausea, have been reported to be associated with DOTs therapy (Michael et al., 2016). Thus, high drop-out rate of TB patients from treatment regimens (a.k.a. patient non-compliance) is a serious issue contributing directly to the development of drug resistance in *Mycobacterium tuberculosis* (Mtb), the causative agent of TB.

Development of drug resistance in a single bacterium has been suggested to be sufficient to create an outbreak of drug resistant bacteria (Borrell and Gagneux, 2009). In 2015, nearly 4.8 million cases of isoniazid- and rifampicin-resistant [a.k.a. multidrug-resistant TB (MDR-TB)] cases were reported. In addition to INH and RIF (the first line drugs), Mtb can develop resistance to PZA and ETH (second line drugs) and other injectable aminoglycosides, leading to extensively drug-resistant TB (XDR-TB) cases. Nearly 9.5 % of all MDR-TB cases in 2015 were estimated to be XDR-TB. A recent study aimed at predicting the future burden of TB suggests an increased prevalence of MDR and XDR cases due mainly to person-to-person transmission of drug-resistant Mtb, rather than the pathogen acquiring drug resistance within the infected host (Sharma et al., 2017). Hence, current treatment strategies demand intense patient monitoring during and after drug treatment, which poses major strategical and economical challenges for the global TB control programs conducted by various health agencies. Therefore, it is imperative that new anti-TB therapies are developed and implemented to shorten the number of antibiotics taken and/or duration of treatment, to lower the drug- induced toxicities, and to improve the drug efficacy among TB patients with co-morbid conditions, such as HIV-infection and/or patients with MDR/XDR-TB.

Development of drug resistance among infecting Mtb is also dependent on host intrinsic factors, such as genetic make-up, health, and well-being, all of which impact the immune response against the bacteria. A key component of the host innate defense system are macrophages, phagocytic cells that engulf and destroy infecting microorganisms. However, Mtb can "invade" macrophages (and other host cells), where it is able to survive, proliferate and cause infection/disease. Invasion of macrophages by Mtb brings changes to the normal phagocytosis events, such as calcium ion homeostasis, membrane protein distribution and phagosome-lysosome fusion. If/when Mtb survives, it continues to multiply intracellularly and induce a pro-inflammatory response, leading to the onset of cell mediated/adaptive immunity and granuloma formation, which is generally thought of as a region of equilibrium between the host and the bacterium. For Mtb, the granuloma serves as an environment where the bacteria can exist in a dormant, semi- and/or non-replicating state. For the host, the granulomas restrict the spread of Mtb to other tissues/organs because the diseased area is cordoned-off by the activated immune cells (Guirado et al., 2013). The host-pathogen interactions in the granuloma are highly complex, where the bacteria may get killed or able to survive and persist (Flynn and Chan, 2003). Taken together, the intracellular survival of Mtb is regarded as a cumulative effect of the host immune response and the bacterial ability to resist or subvert this response. Hence, strengthening the immune repertoire involved in combating Mtb through host-directed therapeutics (HDT) can be one of the approaches for effective bacterial killing and clearance of infection/disease.

Host directed therapy (HDT) aims at manipulating the metabolism and/or immune cell function to optimize the pro-inflammatory response or to modify the tissue physiology (Subbian et al., 2011a,b; Tobin et al., 2012). Recently, research on HDT as potential therapeutic strategy for infectious diseases has gained significant momentum due to the possibility of re-purposing drugs that have been already approved to treat chronic ailments and the advantage that pathogenic bacteria, such as Mtb, cannot develop resistance against a HDT, which targets host cell functions (Zumla et al., 2015). Autophagy is a homeostatic cellular process that removes intracellular debris derived from endo-and exo-genous sources, thus ensuring efficient functioning of cells. It is also a key innate immune response of the host cells to protect against invading pathogens. Therefore, targeting the autophagy machinery using small molecules and drugs to improve the host cell effector functions is an emerging concept in the treatment of several chronic diseases (Rubinsztein et al., 2012). Autophagy is regulated by multiple, complex networks and pathways that are either dependent or independent of mTOR (mechanistic target of rapamycin; a.k.a. mammalian target of rapamycin), a master regulatory molecule that impacts several cellular functions (**Figure 1**). In this review, we focus mainly on the role of autophagy in Mtb pathogenesis and modulating the mTOR pathway as potential adjunctive HDT to improve current, antibiotic-based treatment for pulmonary TB.

## MODULATION OF PHAGOCYTE FUNCTION BY *MYCOBACTERIUM TUBERCULOSIS*

Successful intracellular pathogens inhibit host cell antimicrobial processes involved in restricting their survival (Flynn and Chan, 2003; Kim et al., 2012). In that context, Mtb is known to inhibit killing within the phagolysosome of macrophages and other antigen presenting cells (APC) by modulating phagosome maturation and its fusion with the lysosome. In the infected APC, pathogenic Mtb inhibits actin assembly around the phagosome, thereby inhibiting host lipid molecules from interacting with

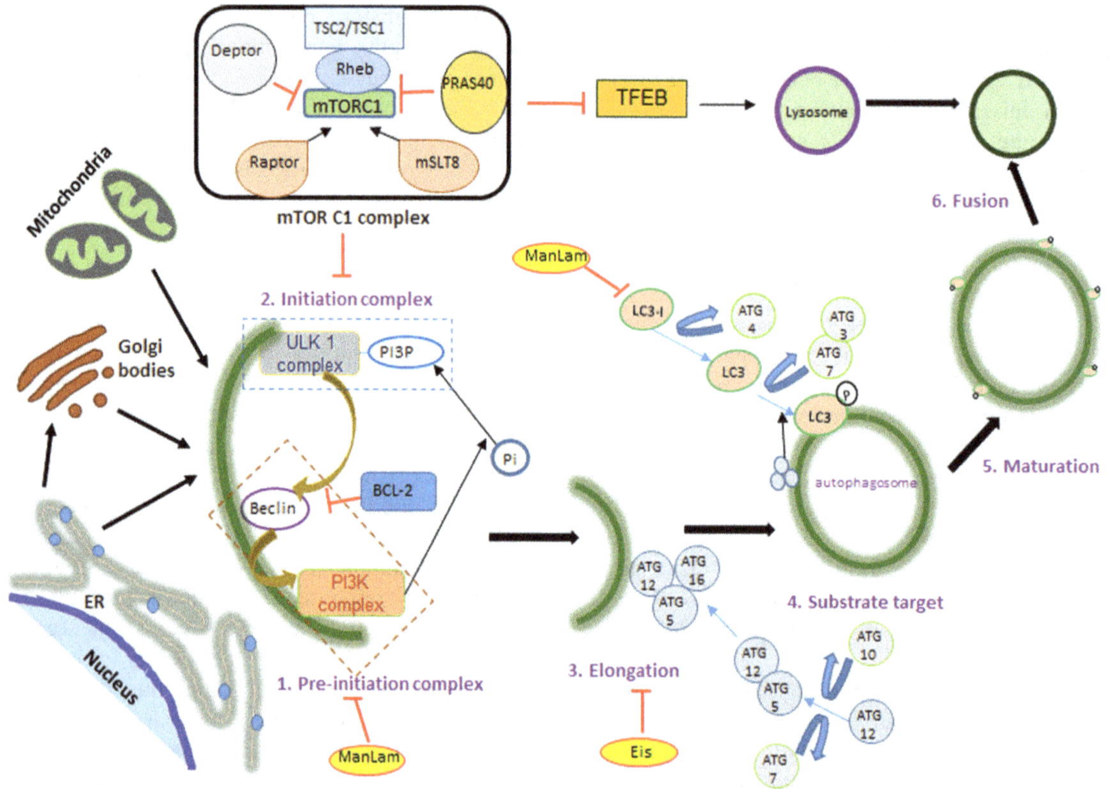


**FIGURE 1** | mTOR signaling during autophagy. mTOR has two complexes: mTORC1 and mTORC2, differentiated according to their activator proteins Raptor and Rictor. When activated, mTOR blocks ULK complex formation by phosphorylating it. ULK and PI3K complex formation marks the initiation of autophagy, followed by ATG-5, 12, and 16 binding on the phagophore membrane. This leads to LC3 translocation on the autophagosome membrane, which is required for fusion with lysosome and ultimately bacterial killing. Autophagy activating factors and pathways are denoted in black color and autophagy inhibitors are in red color letters and lines; mTOR activation leads to protein synthesis, nucleotide synthesis, cytoskeletal regulation and ion transport. These are denoted in blue color. Yellow color highlight denotes mycobacterial factors influencing autophagy.

phagosomal proteins necessary for further maturation and fusion with the lysosome (Vergne et al., 2003; Rohde et al., 2007; Ehrt and Schnappinger, 2009; Shui et al., 2011; Seto et al., 2012). When bacteria are phagocytosed by APC, the phagosome acquires early endosomal protein markers, such as EEA1 (early endosomal antigen 1) and Rab5, which are gradually replaced with Rab7 during the maturation of the phagosome (Chandra et al., 2015); ultimately, LAMP1 (lysosome-associated membrane protein 1) and acid hydrolases mark the late phagosome for fusion with lysosome (Huynh et al., 2007). It has been reported that phagosomes containing live Mtb do not acquire Rab5 due to the presence of tryptophan aspartate coat protein (TACO). Phagosomal association with TACO is also reported in macrophages that can engulf other pathogenic mycobacteria, which also result in the inhibition of phagosomal maturation (Pieters and Gatfield, 2002). Proper maturation of phagosomes is the key to its fusion with lysosomes, which can kill the bacteria by delivering toxic molecules. However, due to the absence of proton-ATPase molecules in Mtb-containing phagosomes, the phagosome-lysosome fusion does not take place and the bacteria survive intracellularly (Vergne et al., 2005).

Another mechanism used by Mtb to manipulate APC involves perturbation of intracellular calcium ion ($Ca^{2+}$) levels (Kusner and Barton, 2001). Several studies have demonstrated fluctuations in intracellular $Ca^{2+}$ levels in Mtb-infected macrophages (Vergne et al., 2003; Jayachandran et al., 2007). During phagocytosis of opsonized or heat-killed Mtb, intracellular $Ca^{2+}$ concentrations increase, while macrophages infected with live pathogenic Mtb have reduced calcium ion level, which in turn significantly reduce the levels of $Ca^{2+}$ associated-calmodulin and the phosphorylated $Ca^{2+}$/calmodulin-dependent protein kinase II (CaMKII) (Jayachandran et al., 2007). Reduction in CaKMII level also blocks the delivery of lysosomal components to phagosome. Mtb reportedly prevents intracellular $Ca^{2+}$ increase through its cell wall glycolipid, ManLAM (mannose-capped lipoarabinomannan), and by inhibiting host sphingosine kinase (SK). ManLAM also inhibits ionophore-induced increase in $Ca^{2+}$ levels in macrophages. Reduced $Ca^{2+}$/Calmodulin association impairs PI3K signaling, which inhibits recruitment of EEA1 to phagosomes (Rojas et al., 2000). Inhibition of SK abrogates phosphorylation of sphingosine, which is required for G-protein coupled receptor (GPCR) signaling that regulates $Ca^{2+}$ homeostasis. Thus, ManLAM triggers a sequence of events leading to $Ca^{2+}$ signaling disruption and phagosomal maturation arrest, which facilitate successful intracellular survival of infecting Mtb (Chan et al., 1991; Rojas et al., 2000).

Apart from its function in maintaining cellular homeostasis, autophagy is also known to sense and destroy intracellular bacteria in innate immune cells, such as macrophages. Although intracellular Mtb can efficiently modulate the bactericidal mechanisms of phagocytes, autophagy has been shown to be effective in killing Mtb (Gutierrez et al., 2004; Maiuri et al., 2007). Xenophagy, a type of autophagy whereby microorganisms can be sequestered and subject to lysosomal degradation, has been proposed to play an important role in elimination of bacteria (Gutierrez et al., 2004; Rubinsztein et al., 2012; Songane et al., 2012). In Mtb-infected host cells, the autophagosome collects ubiquitin while maturing, which then ultimately fuses with lysosome, thereby enhancing the lysosome-mediated bacterial killing. Survival of Mtb in macrophages has been reported to be dependent on the autophagosome delivery to the lysosome. However, *in vivo* and *in vitro* results have shown disparity in Mtb survival following inhibition of autophagy markers (**Table 1**) (Levine and Deretic, 2007; Lerena et al., 2008; Levine et al., 2011). Mutation or knockdown of autophagy associated host genes, such as Unc-51-like kinase 1 (Ulk1), Beclin1, Atg5, Atg7 or p62, has been reported to increase the survival of intracellular bacteria (Kim et al., 2011; Mizushima et al., 2011; Shang et al., 2011; Alers et al., 2012). However, although xenophagy is reported to restrict the survival of Mtb and BCG (bacille Calmette-Guerin) within macrophages, there are studies suggesting that intracellular pathogens such as *Shigella flexneri, Listeria monocytogenes, Burkholderia pseudomallei, Orientia tsutsugamushi, Porphyromonas gingivalis, Staphylococcus, Brucella abortus,* and *Salmonella typhimurium* are capable of blocking induction of autophagy by downregulating the co-localization of LC3 (microtubule-associated protein 1A/1B-light chain 3), restoring activation of mTOR, and utilizing nutrients for their growth and survival (Thurston et al., 2009; Yoshikawa et al., 2009; Zheng et al., 2009; Choy et al., 2012; Fraunholz and Sinha, 2012; Asrat et al., 2014; Yu et al., 2014).

Pathogenic Mtb also inhibits phagosome function in infected macrophages by releasing vesicle-bound lipids and glycolipids, which accumulate in lysosomes and interfere with the phagosome-lysosome fusion (Beatty et al., 2000). Taken together, pathogenic intracellular Mtb uses multiple strategies to manipulate the host defense machinery of APC for its own survival. Manipulation of APC function by Mtb impacts subsequent downstream events, including autophagy, antigen presentation, apoptosis, and activation of various signaling pathways involved in the production of cytokines, chemokines and other effector molecules that are crucial for controlling bacterial growth and replication (Briken et al., 2004; Cooper, 2009; Guenin et al., 2009; Rajaram et al., 2010).

## AUTOPHAGY AND mTOR SIGNALING

Autophagy, a Greek word meaning "eating of self," is a conserved cellular process critical for maintaining cellular integrity and function. This catabolic process is activated in cells due to lack of nutrient availability or cellular damage or stress, and involves degradation of damaged organelles and misfolded or abnormal proteins. During starvation, cytosolic components of cells are sequestered by autophagy to release nutrients for de novo biosynthesis of molecules (Laplante and Sabatini, 2012). Autophagy can also be activated by pathological factors, such as infections and other diseases. In these cases, normal cellular functions are facilitated by the elimination of pathogens through autophagy-dependent mechanisms, such as surface antigen presentation (Rubinsztein et al., 2012; Songane et al., 2012). Moreover, autophagy is one of the macrophage defense mechanisms against Mtb infection.

Autophagy is characterized by phagophore formation, elongation and maturation of the autophagosome, which ultimately fuse with the lysosome for the degradation of its contents. Formation of the autophagosome begins with a double membranous structure derived from the lipid bilayers of the endoplasmic reticulum (ER) or Golgi apparatus and conjugated with autophagy related (ATG) proteins (Maiuri et al., 2007; Alers et al., 2012). The three main components of autophagosome generation are: PI3KC3 (class III phosphoinositide 3-kinase

**TABLE 1** | Major differences and similarities between mTOR complexes- mTORC1 and mTORC2.

| Similarities | Differences | |
|---|---|---|
| | **mTOR C1** | **mTOR C2** |
| • Both belong to mTOR signaling cascade.<br>• Member of PI3K related kinase family.<br>• mLST8 is a common positive regulator protein.<br>• Cellular stress, such as low level of growth factors, generation of reactive oxygen species and energy depletion inhibits mTOR signaling. | Five components: mTOR, RAPTOR, mLST8, PRAS40, and DEPTOR. | Six components: mTOR, RICTOR, DEPTOR, mSIN-1, mLST8, and PROCTOR. |
| | Positive regulators: RAPTOR and mLST8. | Positive regulators: RICTOR and mSIN-1. |
| | Negative regulators; PRAS40 and DEPTOR. | Negative regulators: DEPTOR. |
| | Rapamycin sensitive. | Rapamycin insensitive. |
| | Inhibits autophagy by directly interacting with pre initiation complex (ULK complex). | Inhibits autophagy indirectly by regulating mTORC1. |
| | Regulates p70-S6K and 4E-BP-1 to influence cellular metabolism. | Regulates AKT to influence cellular growth. |
| | Activating signaling: Growth factors, energy molecules, amino acids level. | Not known. |

complex 3), ULK1 (unc-51-like kinase 1) complex and ATG complex (**Figure 1**). This process is negatively regulated by mTOR kinase, which, when activated, blocks the ULK1 complex (Kim et al., 2011; Shang et al., 2011). Under stress conditions, such as nutrient deprivation or bacterial invasion, mTOR gets inactivated, enabling the ULK1 complex to recruit and activate PI3KC3 (Dibble and Cantley, 2015). This initiation complex, formed on the ER, leads to the nucleation of cell membrane, which is followed by recruitment of an ubiquitin-like molecule, LC3. In the final step, LC3 conjugates with phosphotidylethanolamine, resulting in self-fusion of the double membrane to form the autophagosome, which subsequently fuses with lysosome to degrade the engulfed contents.

Apart from mTOR signaling pathway (Lipinski et al., 2010), autophagy is also regulated by the inositol signaling pathway (Sarkar et al., 2005), $Ca^{2+}$ /Calpain signaling pathway (Gordon et al., 1993) and cAMP (cyclic adenosine monophosphate) (Noda and Ohsumi, 1998). Inhibition of these mTOR-independent pathways for promoting autophagy has been studied under different disease conditions (Floto et al., 2007; Grumati et al., 2010; Hidvegi et al., 2010). Promising outcomes of autophagy induction via mTOR-independent pathway have been observed only with a combination therapy strategy, where the small molecules enhancers (SMERs) or inhibitors (SMIRs) of mTOR-independent pathway are used in combination with an mTOR inhibitor. For example, lithium, an inositol (1,4,5)-triphosphate inhibitor, when administered with rapamycin results in a stronger induction of autophagy (Sarkar et al., 2008). On the other hand, rapamycin alone can induce autophagy even at high intracellular inositol (1,4,5)-triphosphate levels, which has autophagy inhibitory effects. Since targeting ULK complex formation or ATG complex, rather than affecting the upstream pathways, seems to have a specific and stronger impact on autophagy, mTOR has been the target of interest for promoting autophagy upon infection with *Mycobacteria* (Gutierrez et al., 2004).

## THE mTOR COMPLEX

In addition to its role in autophagy, mTOR is also a master regulator of cell metabolism, growth, proliferation, translation initiation, and cytoskeletal organization. It belongs to the family of phosphoinoside 3-kinase- (PI3K-) related kinase and is a highly conserved serine/threonine protein kinase, which exists in host cells as part of two protein complexes—mTORC1 and mTORC2 (Laplante and Sabatini, 2012; Singh and Cuervo, 2012) (**Figure 2**). Theses complexes differ in their structure and activity, in part due to the difference in mTOR regulatory proteins such as RAPTOR (regulatory associated protein of mTOR; rapamycin sensitive) in mTORC1 and RICTOR (rapamycin-insensitive companion of mTOR) in mTORC2, as well as other accessory proteins (Laplante and Sabatini, 2009). The proteins that are common to both mTORC1 and C2 complexes are the mammalian lethal with Sec13 protein 8 (mLST8) and DEP domain containing mTOR interacting protein (DEPTOR). While mLST8 acts as a positive regulator, DEPTOR functions as a negative regulator of mTOR signaling. The mTORC1 is activated by RAPTOR, PRAS40 (proline-rich AKT substrate 40 kDa) and by phosphorylation of tuberous sclerosis protein 2 (TSC2) (Huang et al., 2008). The PI3K/AKT pathway is a positive regulator of mTOR signaling (Kim et al., 2011; Ng et al., 2011; Pan et al., 2012). Apart from PI3K/AKT, arginine, DNA damage, AMPK (AMP-activated protein kinase) and ERK1/2 (extracellular signal-regulated protein kinases 1 and 2) signaling were also reported to regulate mTORC1 activation (Kim et al., 2002; Inoki et al., 2003; Fingar and Blenis, 2004; Laplante and Sabatini, 2009). Importantly, mTORC1 activation inhibits autophagy (Jung et al., 2010). Deactivation of mTORC1 in cells under nutrition depletion or treatment with rapamycin leads to initiation of autophagy. (Seto et al., 2013). Similarly, dephosphorylating ULK1 by inactivation of mTORC1 induces autophagy (Egan et al., 2011; Kim et al., 2011; Shang et al., 2011).

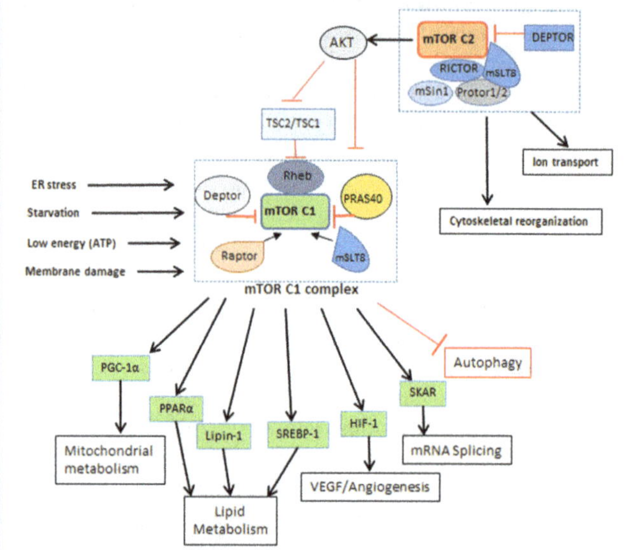


**FIGURE 2 |** mTORC1 and mTORC2 complexes. mTORC1: Is a five component complex with DEPTOR and PRAS40 as negative regulators and RAPTOR and mSLT8 as positive regulators. It regulates different cellular processes like lipid metabolism and protein metabolism other than autophagy as seen in **Figure 1**. It is influenced by the nutrient and energy level in cell and gets shut down or inhibited when cell encounters reducing nutrient level and decrease in energy. Inhibition of mTORC1 leads to inhibition of cellular metabolic processes. mTORC2; A six component complex has DEPTOR as its negative regulator and RICTOR and mSLT8 as positive regulators. This complex influences activation of mTORC1 by phosphorylation of AKT. How nutrient level influences mTORC2 is not known yet.

The binding of mTORC2 with RICTOR facilitates the interaction of these proteins with TSC2 and mammalian stress-activated protein kinase interacting protein (mSIN-1); another protein found in association with RICTOR is PROTOR-1, which promotes activation of serum and glucorticoid-induced kinase 1 (SGK1). Interaction of all these proteins ultimately promotes mTORC2 complex formation and phosphorylation of AKT. Therefore, mTORC2 activation also regulates mTORC1 activation via AKT phosphorylation. Similarly, while mTORC1 activation is mediated by PI3K-AKT/PKB pathway in response to nutrient availability and mitogenic stimulation of the cell, phosphorylation of growth factors by autophosphorylation of their receptor tyrosine kinases activates mTORC2 complex, which also activates class I PI3K-AKT/PKB pathway (Dibble and Cantley, 2015). mTOR complexes also differ in the nature of their stimulant, for example, mTORC1 is activated by low levels of amino acids and growth factors, energy molecules and stress, while mTORC2 remains unaffected by the changing levels of these mTORC1 stimulants. However, role of mTORC2 is important for the regulation of AKT, which in turn governs mTORC1 functions. With use of TSC deficient cells importance of autophagy for cell survival was validated. In conditions like TSC (tuberous sclerosis complex), mTOR inhibition by rapamycin and pro-survival due to autophagy may have beneficial effects (Parkhitko et al., 2011).

In addition to regulating autophagy, activation of mTORC1 also promotes cellular metabolic pathways, such as glucose metabolism, protein and lipid synthesis, all of which contributes to cell growth and proliferation. S6Ks (p70 ribosomal protein S6 kinase 1/2) and 4E-BPs (eukaryotic initiation factor4 binding protein) are the two major proteins interacting with mTORC1 and play a major role in protein synthesis. mTORC1 phosphorylates 4E-BP1 thereby inhibiting its interaction with elF4E, which is then able to promote cap-dependent translation. Similarly, mTORC1 interaction with S6K1 stimulates cap-dependent translation of ribosomal proteins. Phosphorylation of S6K by mTORC1 also activates glucose transporter protein (Glut1) which activates glycolysis, lipogenesis and increases glucose uptake (Zeng et al., 2016). This increased glycolysis due to Glut1 is also reported to elevate T cell function and proliferation (Macintyre et al., 2014). Likewise, lipid synthesis is influenced by positive regulation of SREBP1 (sterol regulatory element binding protein 1) and PPARγ (peroxisome proliferator-activated receptor-γ) (Kim and Chen, 2004), which are regulated by mTORC1. The mTOR inhibitor, rapamycin, reduced phosphatidic acid phosphatase (lipin-1) phosphorylation, which is essential for glycerolipid synthesis; lipin-1 also activates PPARγ and other proteins associated with lipid synthesis (Huffman et al., 2002). Oxidative metabolism is also influenced by mTOR signaling. In a mouse model, inhibition of mTORC1 reduced the muscle mass and oxidative metabolism, leading to early death. It has been shown that PGC1-α is associated with the oxidative metabolism and that mTOR directly interacts with this regulatory protein (Laplante and Sabatini, 2012). Other proteins interacting with mTORC1 are HIF-1α (hypoxia-inducible factor 1-alpha) and STAT3 (signal transducer and activator of transcription 3), which are involved in a plethora of cellular functions, ranging from angiogenesis to inflammation and cytokine response (Laughner et al., 2001).

## mTOR INHIBITORS AS POTENTIAL HDT FOR TB

Since mTOR signaling pathway regulates several cellular processes, including autophagy, that are linked to the host immune response to pathogens, it is an attractive target for developing/testing small molecules to modulate host immunity for better protection against infectious agents. Moreover, the peripheral blood mononuclear cells (PBMCs) and $CD^{4+}CD^{25+}FoxP^{3+}$Treg cells isolated from active tuberculosis patients demonstrated mTOR inhibition during infection (Zhang et al., 2017). In contrast, mTOR activation, by deletion of *Tsc1* in hematopoietic stem cells, induces accumulation CDK (cyclin-dependent kinase) inhibitors $p16^{ink4a}$, $p19^{Arf}$, $p21^{Cip1}$ leading to impaired hematopoietic system and decreased lymphopoiesis (Chen et al., 2009). These observations establish that mTOR inhibition improves cell survival and the understanding that mTOR inhibition may be promoting host cell defense mechanisms against invading pathogens (Harrison et al., 2009).

The following are some of the key mTOR inhibitors in use to treat chronic conditions in humans.

### Rapamycin

Rapamycin, specifically known for its mTOR inhibitory activity, was first isolated from *Streptomyces hygroscopicus*. Despite of its antifungal and antibacterial properties, Rapamycin is well-known for its immunosuppressant activity, which led to its use in organ transplant cases to reduce graft rejection. Similar to temsirolimus, rapamycin, which is also known as sirolimus, targets FKBP12 (FK506-binding protein 1A, 12 kDa) and inhibits the formation of active mTOR complex. Thus all of the currently known sirolimus derivatives target FKBP12 and inhibit mTOR complex.

In a zebrafish model of *M. marinum* infection, mTOR was shown to be associated with the host resistance to infection. In this model, mTOR mutants were hyper-susceptible to *M. marinum* at higher infection dose; however, when the inoculum size was decreased, the mTOR-deficient zebrafish cleared infection early (Pagan et al., 2016). Inhibition of mTOR in mice by rapamycin treatment at early age did not significantly affect the life expectancy or susceptibility to disease, but administration at an old age improved the survival expectancy (Harrison et al., 2009). In another study, administration of rapamycin to BCG-vaccinated mice has been shown to elicit better vaccination efficacy against Mtb infection, which is associated with induced autophagy, increased antigen presentation on dendritic cells and elevated Th1-type immune response (Gutierrez et al., 2004; Jagannath et al., 2009). Results from a low dose Mtb infection (MOI = 1) of human monocyte-derived-macrophages pre-infected with HIV, showed elevated bacterial load upon administration of rapamycin (1 $\mu$M) (Andersson et al., 2016). This study described mTOR inhibition as an advantage for the intracellular survival of Mtb; however, in an already immunocompromised cell (due to HIV infection), it is difficult to assess the impact of mTOR inhibition on Mtb growth. Although rapamycin used to be the popular drug of interest to achieve cellular mTOR inhibition, poor solubility and long intracellular half-life complicates the consideration of this molecule as potential HDT for TB therapy.

### Temsirolimus

Temsirolimus, commercially known as CCI-779 or Torisel, is currently approved by the US-FDA for use in renal cell carcinoma

(RCC) treatment. This prodrug can transform to sirolimus when dihydroxymethyl propionic acid ester group at C40 position is removed. Temsirolimus is metabolized by the enzyme CYP3A4 (cytochrome P450 3A4) and has a half-life of 9–27 h (MacKeigan and Krueger, 2015). Intravenous administration of temsirolimus increases its bioavailability and dose intensity (Boni et al., 2009). Mechanistically, temsirolimus targets host FKBP-12 protein. The drug-FKBP-12 interaction inhibits the formation of mTOR-FKBP-12 complex, leading to the inactivation of mTOR complex and inhibition of p70S6k and S6 phosphorylation. These effects cumulatively results in arrested cell growth, proliferation and survival in RCC patients. Nonspecific pneumonitis and gastrointestinal disorders are major side effects in RCC patients treated with this drug. In addition, metabolic diseases such as hyperglycemia, and hypercholesterolemia are associated with temsirolimus administration in these patients (Malizzia and Hsu, 2008). Importantly, temsirolimus treatment has been widely associated with reactivation of latent Mtb infection among RCC patients. Also, progression of tumor was noted in these patients when temsirolimus was administered in combination with rifampicin, a first-line anti-TB drug (Bossé et al., 2016).

## Ridaforolimus

Ridaforolimus (AP23573 or MK-8669) is an analog of sirolimus with improved bioavailability, solubility and half-life (30–75 h) (Rivera et al., 2011). It is administered orally or intravenously for the treatment of solid tumors of soft tissues, bone and other hematologic malignancies (Huang et al., 2015). In a phase I clinical trial with 87 $ER^+$/high-proliferative breast cancer cases, majority of patients treated with ridaforolimus demonstrated reduced tumor activity (Di Cosimo et al., 2015). Similarly, a phase II clinical trial showed promising results for ridaforolimus to treat patients with endometrial, soft tissue and bone cancers (Palavra et al., 2017). The effect of ridaforolimus on cell metabolism and growth is largely dependent on the dose of drug used for treatment. This is due to its varying effect on mTOR inhibition with variation in dosage (Rivera et al., 2011). However, no reactivation of latent Mtb infection has been reported in these studies (Huang et al., 2015; Palavra et al., 2017).

## Everolimus

Everolimus (40-O-(2-Hydroxy)-ethyl-rapamycin), commercially known as SDZ-RAD, RAD001, Certican and Afinitor, is a derivative of rapamycin bearing a stable 2-hydroxy ethyl chain substitution at position 40. This agent has a better solubility, oral availability, and decreased mean elimination half-life (~18–30 h), leading to early removal of drug from the body compared to the parent compound (rapamycin). Because of the better absorption, it has higher bio-availability (30–60%) and a $T_{max}$ of 1–2 h. Everolimus is an immunosuppressive, anti-inflammatory drug that inhibits host cell proliferation by arresting the progression of cell cycle from G1 to S phase; the immune suppressive function is exerted by inhibiting IL-2 and IL-15 mediated lymphocyte proliferation (Kovarik et al., 2002; Lingaraju et al., 2010; Ahya et al., 2011). In addition, everolimus promotes autophagy by inhibiting mTORC1 (Saran et al., 2015).

Inhibition of mTOR pathway by everolimus treatment has been reported to improve cellular immune response in both animal models and human studies. In a study performed with 218 healthy volunteers of >65 years of age, everolimus treatment had beneficial effects over aging-related issues (Mannick et al., 2014). Specifically, these elderly volunteers treated with a low dose of everolimus showed about 20% improvement in their protective response after influenza vaccination. This improvement was associated with reduced expression of programmed death-1 receptor, which is otherwise highly expressed in aging individuals, on CD4 and CD8 T cells, thus increasing T cell antigen processing and expression. This low dose administration (0.5 mg daily or 5 mg weekly) of eveolimus demonstrated minimum number of adverse events, (35 adverse events) compared to a higher dose administration (20 mg weekly), which resulted in 109 adverse events amongst 53 elderly individuals (Mannick et al., 2014). This study clearly highlights the importance of optimizing the dose of mTOR inhibitors, such as everolimus in this case, for better efficacy with minimal adverse effects. In contrast, case studies with organ transplant patients have mentioned a higher risk of Mtb infection and reactivation of LTBI as possible side-effects of everolimus administration (Kovarik et al., 2002; Fijałkowska-Morawska et al., 2011). Although patients in this study were treated with a higher dose of everolimus, than the influenza vaccine study mentioned above, the mechanism underlying the connection between dose of everolimus and reactivation of LTBI is not clearly understood. However, the negative consequences of high dose administration of everolimus can be overcome by co-administration with CYP3A4 enzyme inducers, such as rifampicin, which are used to treat opportunistic TB infections in organ transplant patients (Eisen et al., 2003). Thus, it is important to understand the dose-response of everolimus in the context of host cellular functions and how the drug influences phagocytosis and autophagy-mediated elimination of Mtb during infection.

All the mTOR inhibitors described above are also frequently used in the treatment of various forms of cancer, including breast cancer, renal cell carcinoma and tuberous sclerosis complex, due to their ability to inhibit host cell proliferation and growth (Pohanka, 2006; Koh et al., 2013). However, the idea of using these mTOR inhibitors as potential adjunct HDT for TB therapy needs to be substantiated through experimental evidences related to dosage, pharmacokinetics and pharmacodynamics (PK/PD) parameters and, cost vs. benefit effects on the host immunity. Such evidences need to be reinforced by series of studies on reliable and relevant pre-clinical animal models of Mtb infection. In addition, metabolic dysfunctions, such as hyperglycemia is a common side effect in cancer patients treated with mTOR inhibitors, including everolimus (Porta et al., 2011). Although the impact of such inhibitors in the context of TB treatment remains to be determined, serious side effects of HDT drugs preclude their potential use in any treatment. Moreover, as immune-suppressing agents, the application of mTOR inhibitors as a stand-alone HDT therapy for TB holds a significant risk of reactivation of latent Mtb infection, similar to the situation observed in rheumatoid arthritis patients treated with anti-TNF-α antibody (Kovarik et al., 2002). However, when used at an immune modulating-, as opposed to immune suppressing-dose, these mTOR inhibitors can be potential candidates to serve as an adjunct therapeutic molecule, along with standard anti-TB drugs, in improving the treatment outcome. Thus, fine-tuning the dose of mTOR inhibitors is an important and necessary step toward application of these HDT compounds for TB treatment. Importantly, since Mtb cannot develop resistance to a drug that targets host signaling pathway, such as mTOR or cellular processes, such as autophagy, HDT drugs has the potential to alleviate the development of MDR- and XDR-Mtb strains and their transmission in the community. Analogous to the trend in cancer treatment that have shifted from chemotherapeutic and radiologic regimens to more-host targeted treatment approaches, Mtb infection and/or disease can benefit from specific HDT drugs that targets, for example, the mTOR pathway and/or autophagy.

## SUMMARY AND CONCLUSION

Pathogenic Mtb possess several virulent determinants, such as the unusually lipid-rich cell wall, that serve as permeability barriers and protects the bacteria from the harsh intracellular environment within phagocytes, and from the bactericidal activities of anti-TB drugs. Additionally, these mycobacteria-derived molecules interact with the host immune cells and modulates their function, promoting bacterial survival/persistence, causing disease within the host and enabling the development of bacterial drug resistance. Thus, when the innate defensive mechanisms of phagocytes are manipulated by the pathogen to promote its survival, the host develops active disease, which is hard to overcome. This can be one of the reasons for the inefficiency of current anti-mycobacterial drugs to eliminate TB, and for the emergence of drug-resistant Mtb strains. Perturbing host cell functions through HDT molecules has the potential to enhance the effector functions of these cells, which are the ultimate arsenals in combating bacterial infection. Moreover, these immune modulating drugs do not contribute to the emergence of drug resistance by the infecting bacteria. This criterion is crucial when considering therapy, particularly for patients with MDR, XDR-TB, as well as those patients with co-existing chronic conditions, such as diabetes or HIV infection, in which conventional antibiotics therapy has been shown to be complex, complicated, toxic and insufficient in achieving a bacteriological cure. Host cell autophagy, regulated by mTOR pathway, plays an important role in cellular homeostasis as well as in antibacterial defense mechanism. Therefore, targeting mTOR pathway with small molecules, such as everolimus, has the potential to develop novel and better combination drug therapy, along with standard anti-TB drugs to combat various forms of TB in patients with/without other co-morbid conditions. This approach can also enhance bacterial killing, reduce treatment duration, and/or improve clinical outcome. Clearly, more research and experimental evidence is warranted on these and other HDT molecules, for their efficacy, toxicity and other properties, through extensive pre-clinical studies using appropriate animal models of TB, before they are tried as therapeutic intervention for TB in human clinical trial.

## AUTHOR CONTRIBUTIONS

SS: conceived the concept; PS and SS: wrote/edited the manuscript and agreed for submission.

## FUNDING

This study was supported by a grant from the Bill and Melinda Gates Foundation (OPP1157210) to SS.

## REFERENCES

Ahya, V. N., McShane, P. J., Baz, M. A., Valentine, V. G., Arcasoy, S. M., Love, R. B., et al. (2011). Increased risk of venous thromboembolism with a sirolimus-based immunosuppression regimen in lung transplanta-tion. *J. Heart Lung Transplant.* 30, 175–181. doi: 10.1016/j.healun.2010.08.010

Alers, S., Löffler, A. S., Wesselborg, S., and Stork, B. (2012). Role of AMPK-mTOR-Ulk1/2 in the regulation of autophagy: cross talk, shortcuts, and feedbacks. *Mol. Cell. Biol.* 32, 2–11. doi: 10.1128/MCB.06159-11

Andersson, A. M., Andersson, B., Lorell, C., Raffetseder, J., Larsson, M., and Blomgran, R. (2016). Autophagy induction targeting mTORC1 enhances *Mycobacterium tuberculosis* replication in HIV co-infected human macrophages. *Sci. Rep.* 6:28171. doi: 10.1038/srep28171

Asrat, S., de Jesús, D. A., Hempstead, A. D., Ramabhadran, V., and Isberg, R. R. (2014). Bacterial pathogen manipulation of host membrane trafficking. *Ann. Rev. Cell Dev. Biol.* 30, 79–109. doi: 10.1146/annurev-cellbio-100913-013439

Beatty, W. L., Rhoades, E. R., Ullrich, H. J., Chatterjee, D., Heuser, J. E., and Russell, D. G. (2000). Trafficking and release of mycobacterial lipids from infected macrophages. *Traffic* 1, 235–247. doi: 10.1034/j.1600-0854.2000.010306.x

Boni, J. P., Hug, B., Leister, C., and Sonnichsen, D. (2009). Intravenous temsirolimus in cancer patients: clinical pharmacology and dosing considerations. *Semin. Oncol.* 36(Suppl. 3), S18–S25. doi: 10.1053/j.seminoncol.2009.10.009

Borrell, S., and Gagneux, S. (2009). Infectiousness, reproductive fitness and evolution of drug-resistant *Mycobacterium tuberculosis*. *Int. J. Tuberc. Lung Dis.* 13, 1456–1466.

Bossé, D., Ng, T., Ahmad, C., Alfakeeh, A., Alruzug, I., Biagi, J., et al. (2016). Eastern Canadian gastrointestinal cancer consensus conference 2016. *Curr. Oncol.* 23, e605–e614. doi: 10.3747/co.23.3394

Briken, V., Porcelli, S. A., Besra, G. S., and Kremer, L. (2004). Mycobacterial lipoarabinomannan and related lipoglycans: from biogenesis to modulation of the immune response. *Mol. Microbiol.* 53, 391–403. doi: 10.1111/j.1365-2958.2004.04183.x

Chan, J., Fan, X. D., Hunter, S. W., Brennan., P. J., and Bloom, B. R. (1991). Lipoarabinomannan, a possible virulence factor involved in persistence of *Mycobacterium tuberculosis* within macrophages. *Infect. Immun.* 59, 1755–1761.

Chandra, P., Ghanwat, S., Matta, S. K., Yadav, S. S., et al. (2015). *Mycobacterium tuberculosis* inhibits RAB7 recruitment to selectively modulate autophagy flux in macrophages. *Sci. Rep.* 5:16320. doi: 10.1038/srep16320

Chen, C., Liu, Y., Liu, Y., and Zheng, P. (2009). mTOR regulation and therapeutic rejuvenation of aging hematopoietic stem cells. *Sci. Signal.* 2:ra75. doi: 10.1126/scisignal.2000559

Choy, A., Dancourt, J., Mugo, B., O'Connor, T. J., Isberg, R. R., Melia, T. J., et al. (2012). The Legionella effector RavZ inhibits host autophagy through irreversible Atg8 deconjugation. *Science* 338, 1072–1076. doi: 10.1126/science.1227026

Cooper, A. M. (2009). Cell-mediated immune responses in tuberculosis. *Annu. Rev. Immunol.* 27, 393–422. doi: 10.1146/annurev.immunol.021908.132703

Di Cosimo, S., Sathyanarayanan, S., Bendell, J. C., Cervantes, A., Stein, M. N., Braña, I., et al. (2015). Combination of the mTOR inhibitor ridaforolimus and the anti-IGF1R monoclonal antibody dalotuzumab: preclinical characterization and phase I clinical trial. *Clin. Cancer Res.* 21, 49–59. doi: 10.1158/1078-0432.CCR-14-0940

Dibble, C. C., and Cantley, L. C. (2015). Regulation of mTORC1 by PI3K signaling. *Trends Cell Biol.* 25, 545–555. doi: 10.1016/j.tcb.2015.06.002

Egan, D. F., Shackelford, D. B., Mihaylova, M. M., Gelino, S., Kohnz, R. A., Mair, W., et al. (2011). Phosphorylation of ULK1 (hATG1) by AMP-activated protein kinase connects energy sensing to mitophagy. *Science* 331, 456–461. doi: 10.1126/science.1196371

Ehrt, S., and Schnappinger, D. (2009). Mycobacterial survival strategies in the phagosome: defence against stresses. *Cell. Microbiol.* 11, 1170–1178. doi: 10.1111/j.1462-5822.2009.01335.x

Eisen, H. J., Tuzcu, E. M., Dorent, R., Kobashigawa, J., Mancini, D., Valantine-von Kaeppler, H. A., et al. (2003). Everolimus for the prevention of allograft rejection and vasculopathy in cardiac-transplant recipients. *N. Engl. J. Med.* 349, 847–858. doi: 10.1056/NEJMoa022171

Fijałkowska-Morawska, J. B., Jagodzinska, M., and Nowicki, M. (2011). Pulmonary embolism and reactivation of tuberculosis during everolimus therapy in a kidney transplant recipient. *Ann. Transplant.* 16, 107–110. doi: 10.12659/AOT.882226

Fingar, D. C., and Blenis, J. (2004). Target of rapamycin (TOR): an integrator of nutrient and growth factor signals and coordinator of cell growth and cell cycle progression. *Oncogene* 23, 3151–3171. doi: 10.1038/sj.onc.1207542

Floto, R. A., Sarkar, S., Perlstein, E. O., Kampmann, B., Schreiber, S. L., and Rubinsztein, D. C. (2007). Small molecule enhancers of rapamycin-induced TOR inhibition promote autophagy, reduce toxicity in Huntington's disease models and enhance killing of mycobacteria by macrophages. *Autophagy* 3, 620–622. doi: 10.4161/auto.4898

Flynn, J. L., and Chan, J. (2003). Immune evasion by *Mycobacterium tuberculosis*: living with the enemy. *Curr. Opin. Immunol.* 15, 450–455. doi: 10.1016/S0952-7915(03)00075-X

Fraunholz, M., and Sinha, B. (2012). Intracellular staphylococcus aureus: Live-in and let die. *Front. Cell. Inf. Microbiol.* 2:43. doi: 10.3389/fcimb.2012.00043

Gordon, P. B., Holen, I., Fosse, M., Røtnes, J. S., and Seglen, P. O. (1993). Dependence of hepatocytic autophagy on intracellularly sequestered calcium. *J. Biol. Chem.* 268, 26107–26112.

Grumati, P., Coletto, L., Sabatelli, P., Cescon, M., Angelin, A., Bertaggia, E., et al. (2010). Autophagy is defective in collagen VI muscular dystrophies, and its reactivation rescues myofiber degeneration. *Nat. Med.*. 16, 1313–1320. doi: 10.1038/nm.2247

Guenin-Macé, L., Siméone, R., and Demangel, C. (2009). Lipids of pathogenic Mycobacteria: contributions to virulence and host immune suppression. *Trans. Emerg. Dis.* 56, 255–268. doi: 10.1111/j.1865-1682.2009.01072.x

Guirado, E., Schlesinger, L. S., and Kaplan, G. (2013). Macrophages in tuberculosis: friend or foe. *Semin. Immunopathol.* 35, 563–583. doi: 10.1007/s00281-013-0388-2

Gutierrez, M. G., Master, S. S., Singh, S. B., Taylor, G. A., Colombo, M. I., and Deretic, V. (2004). Autophagy is a defense mechanism inhibiting BCG and *Mycobacterium tuberculosis* survival in infected macrophages. *Cell* 119, 753–766. doi: 10.1016/j.cell.2004.11.038

Harrison, D. E., Strong, R., Sharp, Z. D., et al. (2009). Rapamycin fed late in life extends lifespan in genetically heterogeneous mice. *Nature* 460, 392–395. doi: 10.1038/nature08221

Hidvegi, T., Ewing, M., Hale, P., Dippold, C., Beckett, C., Kemp, C., et al. (2010). An autophagy-enhancing drug promotes degradation of mutant α1-antitrypsin Z and reduces hepatic fibrosis. *Science* 329, 229–232. doi: 10.1126/science.1190354

Huang, J., Dibble, C. C., Matsuzaki, M., and Manning, B. D. (2008). The TSC1-TSC2 complex is required for proper activation of mTOR complex 2. *Mol. Cell. Biol.* 28, 4104–4115. doi: 10.1128/MCB.00289-08

Huang, Z., Wu, Y., Zhou, X., Qian, J., Zhu, W., Shu, Y., et al. (2015). Clinical efficacy of mTOR inhibitors in solid tumors: a systematic review. *Future Oncol.* 11, 1687–1699. doi: 10.2217/fon.15.70

Huffman, T. A., Mothe-Satney, I., and Lawrence, J. C. Jr. (2002). Insulin-stimulated phosphorylation of lipin mediated by the mammalian target of rapamycin. *Proc. Natl. Acad. Sci. U.S.A.* 99, 1047–1052. doi: 10.1073/pnas.022634399

Huynh, K. K., Eskelinen, E.-L., Scott, C. C., Malevanets, A., Saftig, P., and Grinstein, S. (2007). LAMP proteins are required for fusion of lysosomes with phagosomes. *EMBO J.* 26, 313–324. doi: 10.1038/sj.emboj.7601511

Inoki, K., Zhu, T., and Guan, K. L. (2003). TSC2 mediates cellular energy response to control cell growth and survival. *Cell* 115, 577–590. doi: 10.1016/S0092-8674(03)00929-2

Jagannath, C., Lindsey, D. R., Dhandayuthapani, S., Xu, Y., Hunter, R. L. Jr., and Eissa, N. T. (2009). Autophagy enhances the efficacy of BCG vaccine by increasing peptide presentation in mouse dendritic cells. *Nat. Med.* 15, 267–276. doi: 10.1038/nm.1928

Jayachandran, R., Sundaramurthy, V., Combaluzier, B., Mueller, P., Korf, H., Huygen, K., et al. (2007). Survival of mycobacteria in macrophages is mediated by coronin-1 dependent activation of calcineurin. *Cell* 130, 37–50. doi: 10.1016/j.cell.2007.04.043

Jung, C. H., Ro, S. H., Cao, J., Otto, N. M., and Kim, D. H. (2010). mTOR regulation of autophagy. *FEBS Lett.* 584, 1287–1295. doi: 10.1016/j.febslet.2010.01.017

Kim, D. H., Sarbassov, D. D., Ali, S. M., King, J. E., Latek, R. R., Erdjument-Bromage, H., et al. (2002). mTOR interacts with raptor to form a nutrient sensitive complex that signals to the cell growth machinery. *Cell* 110, 163–175. doi: 10.1016/S0092-8674(02)00808-5

Kim, J. E., and Chen, J. (2004). Regulation of peroxisome proliferator-activated receptor-gamma activity by mammalian target of rapamycin and amino acids in adipogenesis. *Diabetes* 53, 2748–2756. doi: 10.2337/diabetes.53.11.2748

Kim, J. J., Lee, H. M., Shin, D. M., Kim, W., Yuk, J. M., Jin, H. S., et al. (2012). Host cell autophagy activated by antibiotics is required for their effective antimycobacterial drug action. *Cell Host Microbe.* 11, 457–468. doi: 10.1016/j.chom.2012.03.008

Kim, J., Kundu, M., Viollet, B., and Guan, K. L. (2011). AMPK and mTOR regulate autophagy through direct phosphorylation of Ulk1. *Nat. Cell Biol.* 13, 132–141. doi: 10.1038/ncb2152

Koh, Y., Lim, H. Y., Ahn, J. M., Lee, J. L., Rha, S. Y., Kim, Y. J., et al. (2013). Phase II trial of everolimus for the treatment of nonclear-cell renal cell carcinoma. *Ann. Oncol.* 24, 1026–1031. doi: 10.1093/annonc/mds582

Kovarik, J. M., Hartmann, S., Figueiredo, J., Rouilly, M., Port, A., and Rordorf, C. (2002). Effect of rifampin on apparent clearance of everolimus. *Ann. Pharmacother.* 36, 981–985. doi: 10.1345/aph.1A384

Kusner, D. J., and Barton, J. A. (2001). ATP stimulates human macrophages to kill intracellular virulent *Mycobacterium tuberculosis* via calcium dependent phagosome-lysosome fusion. *J. Immunol.* 167, 3308–3315. doi: 10.4049/jimmunol.167.6.3308

Laplante, M., and Sabatini, D. M. (2009). mTOR signaling at a glance. *J. Cell. Sci.* 122(Pt 20), 3589–3594. doi: 10.1242/jcs.051011

Laplante, M., and Sabatini, D. M. (2012). mTOR signaling in growth control and disease. *Cell* 149, 274–293. doi: 10.1016/j.cell.2012.03.017

Laughner, E., Taghavi, P., Chiles, K., Mahon, P. C., and Semenza, G. L. (2001). HER2 (neu) signaling increases the rate of hypoxia-inducible factor 1α (HIF-1α) synthesis: novel mechanism for HIF-1-mediated vascular endothelial growth factor expression. *Mol. Cell. Biol.* 21, 3995–4004. doi: 10.1128/MCB.21.12.3995-4004.2001

Lerena, C., Calligaris, S. D., and Colombo, M. I. (2008). Autophagy: for better or for worse, in good times or in bad times. *Curr. Mol. Med.* 8, 92–101. doi: 10.2174/156652408783769634

Levine, B., and Deretic, V. (2007). Unveiling the roles of autophagy in innate and adaptive immunity. *Nat. Rev. Immunol.* 7, 767–777. doi: 10.1038/nri2161

Levine, B., Mizushima, N., and Virgin, H. W. (2011). Autophagy in immunity and inflammation. *Nature* 469, 323–335. doi: 10.1038/nature09782

Lingaraju, R., Blumenthal, N. P., Mendez, J., Hadjiliadis, O., Lee, J. C., Ahya, V. N., et al. (2010). Venous thromboembolic disease after lung transplantation: special focus on sirolimus. *Open. Transplant. J.* 4, 1–4. doi: 10.2174/1874418401004010001

Lipinski, M. M., Hoffman, G., Ng, A., Zhou, W., Py, B. F., Hsu, E., et al. (2010). A genome-wide siRNA screen reveals multiple mTORC1 independent signaling pathways regulating autophagy under normal nutritional conditions. *Dev. Cell* 18, 1041–1052. doi: 10.1016/j.devcel.2010.05.005

Macintyre, A. N., Gerriets, V. A., Nichols, A. G., Michalek, R. D., Rudolph, M. C., Deoliveira, D., et al. (2014). The glucose transporter Glut1 is selectively essential for CD4 T cell activation and effector function. *Cell Metab.* 20, 61–72. doi: 10.1016/j.cmet.2014.05.004

MacKeigan, J. P., and Krueger, D. A. (2015). Differentiating the mTOR inhibitors everolimus and sirolimus in the treatment of tuberous sclerosis complex. *Neuro-Oncology* 17, 1550–1559. doi: 10.1093/neuonc/nov152

Maiuri, M. C., Zalckvar, E., Kimchi, A., and Kroemer, G. (2007). Self-eating and self-killing: crosstalk between autophagy and apoptosis. *Nat. Rev. Mol. Cell Biol.* 8, 741–752. doi: 10.1038/nrm2239

Malizzia, L. J., and Hsu, A. (2008). Temsirolimus, an mTOR inhibitor for treatment of patients with advanced renal cell carcinoma. *Clin. J. Oncol. Nurs.* 12, 639–646. doi: 10.1188/08.CJON.639-646

Mannick, J. B., Del Giudice, D., Lattanzi, M., Valiante, N. M., Praestgaard, J., Huang, B., et al. (2014). mTOR inhibition improves immune function in the elderly. *Sci. Transl. Med.* 6:68ra179. doi: 10.1126/scitranslmed.3009892

Michael, O. S., Sogaolu, O. M., Fehintola, F. A., Ige, O. M., and Falade, C. O. (2016). Adverse events to first line anti-tuberculosis drugs in patients co-infected with HIV and tuberculosis. *Ann. Ib. Postgrad. Med.* 14, 21–29.

Mizushima, N., Yoshimori, T., Ohsumi, Y. (2011). The role of Atg proteins in autopha-gosome formation. *Annu. Rev. Cell Dev. Biol.* 27, 107–132. doi: 10.1146/annurev-cellbio-092910-154005

Ng, S., Wu, Y. T., Chen, B., Zhou, J., and Shen, H. M. (2011). Impaired autophagy due to constitutive mTOR activation sensitizes TSC2-null cells to cell death under stress. *Autophagy* 7, 1173–1186. doi: 10.4161/auto.7.10.16681

Noda, T., and Ohsumi, Y. (1998). Tor, a phosphatidylinositol kinase homologue, controls autophagy in yeast. *J. Biol. Chem.* 273, 3963–3966. doi: 10.1074/jbc.273.7.3963

Pagan, A. J., Levitte, S., Berg, R. D., Hernandez, L., Zimmerman, J., Tobin, D., et al. (2016). mTOR deficiency reveals an immunological trade-off in innate resistance to mycobacterial infection *in vivo*. *J. Immunol.* 196(1 Suppl.) 200.6.

Palavra, F., Robalo, C., and Reis, F. (2017). Recent advances and challenges of mTOR inhibitors use in the treatment of patients with tuberous sclerosis complex. *Oxid. Med. Cell. Longev.* 2017:9820181. doi: 10.1155/2017/9820181

Pan, H., O'Brien, T. F., Zhang, P., and Zhong, X. P. (2012). The role of tuberous sclerosis complex 1 in regulating innate immunity. *J. Immunol.* 188, 3658–3666. doi: 10.4049/jimmunol.1102187

Parkhitko, A., Myachina, F., Morrison, T. A., Hindi, K. M., Auricchio, N., Karbowniczek, M., et al. (2011). Tumorigenesis in tuberous sclerosis complex is autophagy and p62/sequestosome 1 (SQSTM1)-dependent. *Proc. Natl. Acad. Sci. U.S.A.* 108, 12455–12460. doi: 10.1073/pnas.1104361108

Pieters, J., and Gatfield, J. (2002). Hijacking the host: survival of pathogenic mycobacteria inside macrophages. *Trends Microbiol.* 10, 142–146. doi: 10.1016/S0966-842X(02)02305-3

Pohanka, E. (2006). Conversion to everolimus in maintenance patients - current clinical strategies. *Nephrol. Dial. Transplant.* 21(Suppl. 3), iii24–iii29. doi: 10.1093/ndt/gfl301

Porta, C., Osanto, S., Ravaud, A., Climent, M. A., Vaishampayan, U., White, D. A., et al. (2011). Management of adverse events associated with the use of everolimus in patients with advanced renal cell carcinoma. *Eur. J. Cancer* 47, 1287–1298. doi: 10.1016/j.ejca.2011.02.014

Rajaram, M. V., Brooks, M. N., Morris, J. D., Torrelles, J. B., Azad, A. K., and Schlesinger, L. S. (2010). *Mycobacterium tuberculosis* activates human macrophage peroxisome proliferator-activated receptor gamma linking mannose receptor recognition to regulation of immune responses. *J. Immunol.* 185, 929–942. doi: 10.4049/jimmunol.1000866

Rivera, V. M., Miller, S. D., Berk, L., Wardwell, S. D., Ning, Y., Pollock, R., et al. (2011). Ridaforolimus (AP23573; MK-8669), a potent mTOR inhibitor, has broad antitumor activity and can be optimally administered using intermittent dosing regimens. *Mol. Cancer Ther.* 10, 1059–1071. doi: 10.1158/1535-7163.MCT-10-0792

Rohde, K., Yates, R. M., Purdy, G. E., and Russell, D. G. (2007). *Mycobacterium tuberculosis* and the environment within the phagosome. *Immunol. Rev.* 219, 37–54. doi: 10.1111/j.1600-065X.2007.00547.x

Rojas, M., García, L. F., Nigou, J., Puzo, G., and Olivier, M. (2000). Mannosylated lipoarabinomannan antagonizes *Mycobacterium tuberculosis* induced macrophage apoptosis by altering $Ca^{2+}$-dependent cell signaling. *J. Infect. Dis.* 182, 240–251. doi: 10.1086/315676

Rubinsztein, D. C., Codogno, P., and Levine, B. (2012). Autophagy modulation as a potential therapeutic target for diverse diseases. *Nat. Rev. Drug Discov.* 11, 709–730. doi: 10.1038/nrd3802

Ryan, F. (1992). *The Forgotten Plague: How the Battle against Tuberculosis was Won and Lost.* Boston, MA: Little Brown.

Saran, U., Foti, M., and Dufour, J. F. (2015). Cellular and molecular effects of the mTOR inhibitor everolimus. *Clin. Sci.* 129, 895–914. doi: 10.1042/CS20150149

Sarkar, S., Floto, R. A., Berger, Z., Imarisio, S., Cordenier, A., Pasco, M., et al. (2005). Lithium induces autophagy by inhibiting inositol monophosphatase. *J. Cell Biol.* 170, 1101–1111. doi: 10.1083/jcb.200504035

Sarkar, S., Krishna, G., Imarisio, S., Saiki, S., O'Kane, C. J., and Rubinsztein, D. C. (2008). A rational mechanism for combination treatment of Huntington's disease using lithium and rapamycin. *Hum. Mol. Genet.* 17, 170–178. doi: 10.1093/hmg/ddm294

Seto, S., Tsujimura, K., Horii, T., and Koide, Y. (2013). Autophagy adaptor protein p62/SQSTM1 and autophagy-related gene Atg5 mediate autophagosome formation in response to *Mycobacterium tuberculosis* infection in dendritic cells. *PLoS ONE* 8:e86017. doi: 10.1371/journal.pone.0086017

Seto, S., Tsujimura, K., and Koideet, Y. (2012). Coronin-1a inhibits autophagosome formation around *Mycobacterium tuberculosis*-containing phago-somes and assists mycobacterial survival in macrophages. *Cell. Microbiol.* 14, 710–727. doi: 10.1111/j.1462-5822.2012.01754.x

Shang, L., Chen, S., Du, F., Li, S., Zhao, L., and Wang, X. (2011). Nutrient starvation elicits an acute autophagic response mediated by Ulk1 dephosphorylation and its subsequent dissociation from AMPK. *Proc. Natl. Acad. Sci. U.S.A.* 108, 4788–4793. doi: 10.1073/pnas.1100844108

Sharma, A., Hill, A., Kurbatova, E., van der Walt, M., Kvasnovsky, C., Tupasi, T. E., et al. (2017). Estimating the future burden of multidrug-resistant and extensively drug-resistant tuberculosis in India, the Philippines, Russia, and South Africa: a mathematical modelling study. *Lancet Infect. Dis.* 17, 707–715. doi: 10.1016/S1473-3099(17)30247-5

Shui, W., Petzold, C. J., Redding, A., Liu, J., Pitcher, A., Sheu, L., et al. (2011). Organelle membrane proteomics reveals differential influence of mycobacterial lipoglycans on macro-phage phagosome maturation and autophagosome accumulation. *J. Proteome Res.* 10, 339–348. doi: 10.1021/pr100688h

Singh, R., and Cuervo, A. M. (2012). Lipophagy: connecting autophagy and lipid metabolism. *Int. J. Cell Biol.* 2012:282041. doi: 10.1155/2012/282041

Songane, M., Kleinnijenhuis, J., Nete, M. G., and van Crevel, R. (2012). The role of autophagy in host defense against *Mycobacterium tuberculosis* infection. *Tuberculosis (Edinb.)* 92, 388–396. doi: 10.1016/j.tube.2012.05.004

Subbian, S., Tsenova, L., O'Brien, P., Yang, G., Koo, M. S., Peixoto, B., et al. (2011a). Phosphodiesterase-4 inhibition alters gene expression and improves isoniazid-mediated clearance of *Mycobacterium tuberculosis* in rabbit lungs. *PLoS Pathog.* 7:e1002262. doi: 10.1371/journal.ppat.1002262

Subbian, S., Tsenova, L., O'Brien, P., Yang, G., Koo, M. S., Peixoto, B., et al. (2011b). Phosphodiesterase-4 inhibition combined with isoniazid treatment of rabbits with pulmonary tuberculosis reduces macrophage activation and lung pathology. *Am. J. Pathol.* 179, 289–301. doi: 10.1016/j.ajpath.2011.03.039

Thurston, T. L. M., Ryzhakov, G., Bloor, S., von Muhlinen, N., and Randow, F. (2009). The TBK1 adaptor and autophagy receptor NDP52 restricts the proliferation of ubiquitin-coated bacteria. *Nat. Immunol.* 10, 1215–1221. doi: 10.1038/ni.1800

Tobin, D. M., Roca, F. J., Oh, S. F., McFarland, R., Vickery, T. W., Ray, J. P., et al. (2012). Host genotype-specific therapies can optimize the inflammatory response to mycobacterial infections. *Cell* 148, 434–446. doi: 10.1016/j.cell.2011.12.023

Vergne, I., Chua, J., and Deretic, V. (2003). Tuberculosis toxin blocking phagosome maturation inhibits a novel $Ca^{2+}$/calmodulin–PI3K hVPS34 cascade. *J. Exp. Med.* 198, 653–659. doi: 10.1084/jem.20030527

Vergne, I., Chua, J., Lee, H. H., Lucas, M., Belisle, J., and Deretic, V. (2005). Mechanism of phagolysosome biogenesis block by viable *Mycobacterium tuberculosis*. *Proc. Natl. Acad. Sci. U.S.A.* 102, 4033–4038. doi: 10.1073/pnas.0409716102

World Health Organization (2016). *Global Tuberculosis Report.* Geneva: World Health Organization.

Yoshikawa, Y., Ogawa, M., Hain, T., Yoshida, M., Fukumatsu, M., Kim, M., et al. (2009). *Listeria monocytogenes* ActA-mediated escape from autophagic recognition. *Nat. Cell Biol.* 11, 1233–1240. doi: 10.1038/ncb1967

Yu, H. B., Croxen, M. A., Marchiando, A. M., Ferreira, R. B., Cadwell, K., Foster, L. J., et al. (2014). Autophagy facilitates Salmonella replication in HeLa cells. *MBio* 5:e00865-14. doi: 10.1128/mBio.00865-14

Zeng, H., Cohen, S., Guy, C., Shrestha, S., Neale, G., Brown, S. A., et al. (2016). mTORC1 and mTORC2 kinase signaling and glucose metabolism drive follicular helper T cell differentiation. *Immunity* 45, 540–554. doi: 10.1016/j.immuni.2016.08.017

Zhang, X. X., Huang, T. Y., Wu, Y., Peng, W. G., Xie, H. B., et al. (2017). Inhibition of the PI3K-Akt-mTOR signaling pathway in T lymphocytes in patients with active tuberculosis. *Int. J. Infect. Dis.* 59, 110–117. doi: 10.1016/j.ijid.2017.04.004

Zheng, Y. T., Shahnazari, S., Brech, A., Lamark, T., Johansen, T., and Brumell, J. H. (2009). The adaptor protein p62/SQSTM1 targets invading bacteria to the autophagy pathway. *J. Immunol.* 183, 5909–5916. doi: 10.4049/jimmunol.0900441

Zumla, A., Maeurer, M., Chakaya, J., Hoelscher, M., Ntoumi, F., Rustomjee, R. et al. (2015). Towards host-directed therapies for tuberculosis. *Nat. Rev. Drug Discov.* 14, 511–512. doi: 10.1038/nrd4696

# 21

# Global Expansion of Linezolid-Resistant Coagulase-Negative Staphylococci

*Vladimir Gostev[1,2], Semen Leyn[3], Alexander Kruglov[4†], Daria Likholetova[1,5], Olga Kalinogorskaya[1], Marina Baykina[4], Natalia Dmitrieva[6], Zlata Grigorievskaya[6], Tatiana Priputnevich[7], Lyudmila Lyubasovskaya[7], Alexey Gordeev[7] and Sergey Sidorenko[1,2*]*

*[1] Department of Medical Microbiology and Molecular Epidemiology, Pediatric Research and Clinical Center for Infectious Diseases, Saint Petersburg, Russia, [2] Department of Medical Microbiology, North-Western State Medical University Named After I. I. Mechnikov, Saint Petersburg, Russia, [3] Infectious and Inflammatory Disease Center, Sanford Burnham Prebys Medical Discovery Institute, La Jolla, CA, United States, [4] Laboratory of Clinical Microbiology, National Agency for Clinical Pharmacology and Pharmacy, Moscow, Russia, [5] Saint Petersburg State University, Saint Petersburg, Russia, [6] Department of Microbiology, N. N. Blokhin Russian Cancer Research Center, Moscow, Russia, [7] Department of Microbiology, Clinical Pharmacology and Epidemiology, National Medical Research Center for Obstetrics, Gynecology and Perinatology, Moscow, Russia*

***Correspondence:**
*Sergey Sidorenko*
*sidorserg@gmail.com*

**†Present address:**
*Alexander Kruglov,*
*City Hospital No 40, Moscow Department of Health, Moscow, Russia*

Coagulase-negative staphylococci (CoNS) for a long time were considered avirulent constituents of the human and warm-blooded animal microbiota. However, at present, *S. epidermidis*, *S. haemolyticus*, and *S. hominis* are recognized as opportunistic pathogens. Although linezolid is not registered for the treatment of CoNS infections, it is widely used off-label, promoting emergence of resistance. Bioinformatic analysis based on maximum-likelihood phylogeny and Bayesian clustering of the CoNS genomes obtained in the current study and downloaded from public databases revealed the existence of international linezolid-resistant lineages, each of which probably had a common predecessor. Linezolid-resistant *S. epidermidis* sequence-type (ST) 2 from Russia, France, and Germany formed a compact group of closely related genomes with a median pairwise single nucleotide polymorphism (SNP) difference of fewer than 53 SNPs, and a common ancestor of this lineage appeared in 1998 (1986–2006) before introduction of linezolid in practice. Another compact group of linezolid-resistant *S. epidermidis* was represented by ST22 isolates from France and Russia with a median pairwise SNP difference of 40; a common ancestor of this lineage appeared in 2011 (2008–2013). Linezolid-resistant *S. hominis* ST2 from Russia, Germany, and Brazil also formed a group with a high-level genome identity with median 25.5 core-SNP differences; the appearance of the common progenitor dates to 2003 (1996–2012). Linezolid-resistant *S. hominis* isolates from Russia demonstrated associated resistance to teicoplanin. Analysis of a midpoint-rooted phylogenetic tree of the group confirmed the genetic proximity of Russian and German isolates; Brazilian isolates were phylogenetically distant. *repUS5*-like plasmids harboring *cfr* were detected in *S. hominis* and *S. haemolyticus*.

**Keywords: coagulase-negative staphylococci, linezolid, resistance, genome epidemiology, tedizolid**

## INTRODUCTION

Coagulase production was introduced as a criterion for the differentiation of members of genus *Staphylococcus* members in 1940 (Fairbrother, 1940). In contrast to the main representative of coagulase-positive staphylococci (*Staphylococcus aureus*), coagulase-negative staphylococci (CoNS) initially were considered avirulent constituents of the human and warm-blooded animal microbiota. However, at present, many CoNS species are recognized as opportunistic pathogens (Coates et al., 2014; Heilmann et al., 2019). The most frequent colonizers of human skin *S. epidermidis, S. haemolyticus,* and *S. hominis* are the main cause of local and bloodstream foreign body–related infections; prosthetic valve endocarditis (Otto, 2012; Becker et al., 2014); and neonatal infections, including bacteremia (Dong and Speer, 2014).

Treatment of CoNS is becoming increasingly complex due to the emergence and rapid spread of methicillin resistance (MR)—a marker of resistance to most beta-lactams (except for ceftaroline and ceftobiprol), mediated by an additional penicillin-binding protein (PBP), designated PBP2a, that has reduced affinity to beta-lactams. After its first description (Kjellander et al., 1963), prevalence of MR among CoNS causing hospital-acquired infections has continuously increased. Publications from the late 2010s confirm high percentages of MR isolates among CoNS causing bacteremia worldwide: 64.2% in the United Kingdom (Henriksen et al., 2018), 64.7% in the United States (Pfaller et al., 2019), and 91% in Iran (Pourakbari et al., 2018).

Methicillin resistance in CoNS is frequently associated with resistance to other antibiotics except for glycopeptides, which for many years were the drugs of choice in the treatment of staphylococcal infections. Over the past decades, treatment options for Gram-positive infections have expanded significantly with new glycopeptides, beta-lactams, lipopetides, glycylcyclins, and oxazolidinones (linezolid and tedizolid). Although linezolid is not registered for the treatment of CoNS infections, it was used off-label for the treatment of meningitis (Krueger et al., 2004; Kruse et al., 2006; Watanabe et al., 2013), ventriculitis (Boak et al., 2006), osteomyelitis (Nam et al., 2008) and prosthetic-joint infections (Ferry et al., 2018) caused by CoNS. However, high rates of oxazolidinone consumption or the use of long courses of therapy promotes resistance (Dortet et al., 2018; Bai et al., 2019). There are four mechanisms of oxazolidinone resistance in CoNS: methylation of 23S rRNA [plasmid-born chloramphenicol–florfenicol resistance (*cfr*) gene], mutations in 23S rRNA and ribosomal proteins (*rpl* genes), and efflux (plasmid-born *optr*A gene) (Long and Vester, 2012; Wang et al., 2015). Resistance due to ribosomal protection (plasmid-born *poxt*A gene) was recently described in enterococci (Antonelli et al., 2018). Isolates harboring the *cfr* gene are resistant to linezolid but susceptible to tedizolid; all other resistance mechanisms confer cross-resistance between both oxazolidinones. Oxazolidinone-resistant CoNS infections and particularly bloodstream infections are associated with poor clinical outcome: high mortality and prolonged hospital stay (Russo et al., 2015).

Recently, several outbreaks of hospital-acquired infections due to oxazolidinone-resistant CoNS were reported from the United States (Tewhey et al., 2014), Brazil (de Almeida et al., 2013), Greece (Karavasilis et al., 2015), Italy (Mendes et al., 2010), France (Dortet et al., 2018), Germany (Layer et al., 2018), China (Cai et al., 2012), and Spain (Seral et al., 2011; Rodríguez-Lucas et al., 2020).

Revealing the genetic structure of bacterial populations is necessary for the identification of their evolution and distribution. Clustering in large databases is most often done using both non-spatial and spatial Bayesian analysis of population structure (BAPS) algorithms developed by Corander et al. (2008). Bayesian evolutionary analysis by sampling trees (BEAST) is used for the estimation of the time of clade formation (or divergence times). It is used to build rooted, time-measured phylogenies inferred using strict or relaxed molecular clock models. Using the combination of BEAST and BAPS (Castillo-Ramirez et al., 2012) several genetically isolated lineages within the MRSA sequence type (ST) 239 clone and chronology of the introduction of these lineages into the specific geographical regions were identified.

In the present study, we describe linezolid-resistant *S. epidermidis* (LRSE), *S. haemolyticus*, and *S. hominis* recovered in several tertiary hospitals in Moscow. Methods of comparative genomics were initially used for the investigation of recovered isolates and followed by comparison with publicly available genomes of oxazolidinone-resistant CoNS. BAPS and chronogram reconstruction using BEAST were implemented to determine clusters and the time of linezolid-resistant CoNS lineage emergence. The possibilities of two scenarios of oxazolidinone resistance dissemination were evaluated: either clonal spread of resistant genetic lineages or emergence of resistance *de novo*.

## MATERIALS AND METHODS

### Bacterial Strains and Antibiotic Susceptibility

*Staphylococcus epidermidis*, *S. hominis*, and *S. haemolyticus* isolates ($n$ = 47) demonstrating reduced susceptibility to linezolid were collected in 2014–2018 in six Moscow hospital laboratories and transferred to the central laboratory Pediatric Research and Clinical Centre for Infectious Diseases (PRCCID) together with record forms. Personal data of patients were not included in record forms; ethical approval for the study was not required. Control of CoNS identification was performed in the central laboratory by MALDI-TOF mass spectrometry (Microflex LT, Bruker Daltonics, Germany) following the manufacturer's instructions. Antimicrobial susceptibilities to 22 antibiotics (Molekula, United Kingdom), including linezolid (Sigma-Aldrich, United States), tedizolid (Bayer, Germany), teicoplanin, oritavancin, telavancin, and dalbavancin (Biosynth Carbosynth, United Kingdom) were tested by broth microdilution in cation-adjusted Mueller–Hinton broth (Bio-Rad, Marnes-la-Coquette, France) and interpreted according to The European Committee on Antimicrobial Susceptibility Testing (EUCAST) (2020) recommendations

(Breakpoint tables for interpretation of MICs and zone diameters, Version 10.0, 2020.[1]).

## Population Analysis Profile

A population analysis profile (PAP) was performed according to the microdilution modification proposed in a previous study (Pfeltz et al., 2001). Four dilutions ($10^{-1}$, $10^{-3}$, $10^{-5}$, and $10^{-7}$) of the initial suspension ($10^{8}$ CFU/mL) of each strain were prepared. Three 10-μL droplets of each dilution were plated on vancomycin-containing brain-heart infusion agar plates (0.5, 1, 1.5, 2.0, 3.0, 4.0, 6.0, 4.0, 8.0, 12.0, and 16.0 mg/mL). The inoculated plates were incubated for 48 h at 37°C. Plated droplets containing 5–50 CFU were selected for counting, and the average number of colonies per vancomycin concentration was determined. Plots showing the log10 CFU in the presence of each concentration of vancomycin were constructed. Area under curve (AUC) was calculated using the R 3.6.3 base package with trapezoidal rule. The ratio of AUC for CoNS to AUC of control hetero-resistant strain *Staphylococcus aureus* Mu50 under the study was calculated ($AUC_{CoNS}/AUC_{Mu50}$). Isolates demonstrating $AUC_{CoNS}/AUC_{Mu50} \geq 0.9$ were considered to be hetero-resistant.

## Whole Genome Sequencing

Genomic DNA was extracted using a PureLink™ Genomic DNA Mini Kit (Invitrogen™, CA, United States) with preliminary lysis of the cells being done with 1 mg/mL lysostaphin (Sigma-Aldrich, United States). The Nextera XT Kit (Illumina, San Diego, CA, United States) was used for DNA library preparation followed by sample indexing and amplification according to the manufacturer's protocol. DNA libraries were sequenced on a MiSeq instrument (Illumina, San Diego, CA, United States). Quality check data on sequencing reads is presented in **Supplementary Table 1**.

## Genome Assembling and Annotation

Sequence reads were filtered and trimmed using the trimmomatic 0.32 (Bolger et al., 2014) under default settings for Illumina raw data. Read quality and length distribution were analyzed with FastQC 0.11.9 (Brown et al., 2017). *De novo* contigs were assembled with SPAdes 3.14.0 (Bankevich et al., 2012). Bowtie 2 2.3.5 (Langmead and Salzberg, 2012) and SAMtools 1.10 (Li et al., 2009) software were used for detection of SNP's conferred antibiotic resistance, including oxazolidinones resistance. Prediction of single nucleotide polymorphism (SNP) effects was done with SNPeff 4.3t (Cingolani et al., 2012) using filtered (minimum SNP coverage 10 and quality Phred per base > 20) and deduplicated reads after SAMtools processing. The following genomes were used as reference: *S. epidermidis* ATCC 12228 (NC_004461.1), *S. hominis* FDAARGOS_746 (NZ_CP046306.1), and *S. haemolyticus* ATCC 29970 (NZ_CP035291.1). Genomes were annotated with PROKKA 1.14.5 (Seemann, 2014), MLST typing, resistance, and virulence gene typing were done using MLST 2.18.0[2] and abricate 0.9.8[3] scripts, respectively.

## Inclusion of Genome Data From Previous Studies

For phylogenetic reconstruction in addition to Moscow genomes, data from previous studies—outbreaks in France (Dortet et al., 2018) and the United States (Tewhey et al., 2014)—were included in the study. These data were downloaded from the NCBI Sequence Read Archive (SRA) (BioProjects PRJEB22222 and PRJNA239883, respectively), assembled, and annotated using methods listed in the previous section. Additionally, 460 genomes of *S. epidermidis*, 60 genomes of *S. hominis*, and 205 genomes of *S. haemolyticus* were downloaded from the NCBI GenBank using the list of genomes from the PATRIC database (update July 2019) (Wattam et al., 2017). The genomes included for phylogenetic analysis are listed in the data set (**Supplementary Table 2**).

## Phylogenetic and Pan-Genome Analysis

Pan-genomic analysis was done with Roary 3.13.0 (Page et al., 2015), and gene content comparison was done with scoary 1.6.16 (Brynildsrud et al., 2016). Genomes of the CoNS were *in silico* genotyped against the PubMLST database update July 2020 (Jolley and Maiden, 2010) using MLST script 2.18.0 (see text footnote 2).

To produce a core genome alignment for phylogenetic tree reconstruction, we developed a nucmer aligner wrapper named panmap (available on[4]). Panmap uses nucmer 3.9.4 (Kurtz et al., 2004) to create a pairwise alignment for every genome against a reference contigs [in our case, we used the complete chromosome of *S. epidermidis* BPH0662 (NZ_LT571449.1), of *S. hominis* FDAARGOS_136 (NZ_CP014107.1), and *S. haemolyticus* JCSC1435 (NC_007168.1)]. Then, it uses reference contig annotations for every region—gene or intergenic—to produce counts of gapped positions. A gapped position is defined as a position in which the proportion of gaps is above some threshold. If the proportions of gapped positions in a region are higher than a second threshold, then the whole region is dropped. Otherwise, the whole region is kept. Both thresholds were set to 1%. We implemented this annotation-based region-to-region approach to keep as much information about distance between SNPs as possible as Gubbins 2.4.1 (Croucher et al., 2015)—the program that identifies potential recombination regions—uses SNP density information. Using Gubbins 2.4.1, we removed potential regions of recombination from the core genome alignment. The resulting alignment was used for phylogenetic tree reconstruction by IQ-tree 1.6.12 software with ModelFinder and ultrafast bootstraps (Nguyen et al., 2015; Kalyaanamoorthy et al., 2017; Hoang et al., 2018). The substitution model chosen by ModelFinder was TVMe + ASC + R4. The substitution model was chosen based on the ModelFinder results under default parameters. Long branches that did not contain genomes of interest were removed from the trees. The core genome

[1]http://www.eucast.org

[2]https://github.com/tseemann/mlst

[3]https://github.com/tseemann/abricate

[4]https://github.com/sleyn/panmap

alignment was clustered using BAPS with the rhierBAPS R package 1.0.1 (Cheng et al., 2013; Tonkin-Hill et al., 2018) with the expected number of populations set as 20 and maximum depth of clustering set as two. Intra- and inter-group pairwise comparison of the number of SNPs was carried out using R script pairwise_snp_differences[5] (**Supplementary Table 3**).

## Timed Phylogeny Analysis

Timed phylogeny calculation was used for the genetically closest groups of CoNS. Several genome groups were chosen: LRSE belonging to ST2 ($n$ = 76), all (susceptible and resistance to linezolid) ST22 isolates ($n$ = 27), and *S. hominis* ST2 ($n$ = 20). BEAST 2.6.4 was used to generate a timed phylogeny (chronogram) assuming a relaxed lognormal clock and, with coalescent constant tree prior, 10 million iterations of a gamma site model with an HKY substitution model. Tree convergence was confirmed using BEAST's Tracer 1.7.1 program (Suchard et al., 2018) using the recommended criterion (ESS > 200). TreeAnnotator was then used to identify the maximum clade credibility (MCC) tree using a 10% burn-in. The resulting tree was visualized using FigTree 1.4.4.

## Annotation and Mapping of Resistance Data

Analysis of resistance-related SNPs was done for SNPs known to cause linezolid resistance: 23S rRNA (G2576T, C2534T, T2504A *Escherichia coli* numbering), ribosomal proteins L3 (Ala157Arg, Asp159Tyr, Met156Thr, Gly152Asp, His146Arg, Gly137Val, Leu101Val), L4 (Asn158Ser), and L2 (Val112Ile, Ile75Thr) with a potential role of oxazolidinone-resistant. *mecA*, *cfr* genes, and mutations in *rpoB* that conferred multidrug resistance were also mapped. The sequence of 23S rRNA was extracted using barrnap tool 0.9[6]. Other genes were extracted with designed in the study Riddikulus script[7]. Genes were aligned by MAFFT 7.407 (Katoh and Standley, 2013). SNPs were extracted using Unipro UGENE software 37.0 (Okonechnikov et al., 2012).

[5]https://github.com/MDU-PHL/pairwise_snp_differences
[6]https://github.com/tseemann/barrnap
[7]https://github.com/dariader/Riddikulus

Calculation of the total number of acquired resistance genes for each genome was done with abricate 0.9.8 (see text footnote 3).

Seventeen proteins associated with decreased glycopeptide susceptibility in *S. aureus* (MprF, Pbp123, WalKR, GraSR, VraSRT, RpoBC, YycIH, Cmk, and MsrR) were selected for analysis, and homology proteins were extracted from *S. epidermidis* and *S. hominis* genomes. Frequency of amino acids substitution (AAS) was compared across the all-genome data set in linezolid-resistant genomes and linezolid-susceptible genomes. AAS with frequency below the threshold of 5 and 1% for *S. epidermidis* and *S. hominis*, respectively, were excluded. For possible associations between mutations and linezolid-resistance phenotype multiple correspondence analysis (MCA) was applied using factoextra R package 1.0.7.

Visualization and annotations of phylogenetic trees were done using ITOL 6.1.1 (Letunic and Bork, 2016). Plasmid structural comparison was done with Mauve 2.4.0 (Darling et al., 2004).

## Accession Numbers

Genomic data have been deposited in NCBI Sequence Read Archive (SRA) and all reads are available from BioProject PRJNA384130 (SRA id: SRR5482186—SRR5482205 and SRR8427123—SRR8427149).

# RESULTS

## Linezolid-Resistant CoNS in Moscow Hospitals

The first two LRSE isolates were recovered at site A in 2014 and 2015 from patients with catheter-associated bloodstream infections in the intensive care unit. These isolates belonged to genetic lineage ST23. Emergence and dissemination of LRSE (ST2, *ST22*), linezolid-resistant *S. hominis* (ST2), and *S. haemolyticus* (ST1) were observed in several Moscow hospitals (A to F), in 2016–2018.

Different combinations of mutations in 23S rRNA and *rlp3* genes and acquisition of the *cfr* gene mediated resistance to oxazolidinones (**Table 1**). To estimate the number of modified copies of 23S rRNA, we aligned sequence reads on the target

**TABLE 1** | Characterization of Oxazolidinone-resistant CoNS isolated in Moscow hospitals.

| Species | MLST | N | Sites | Source | MIC, mg/L | | *cfr* | SNPs | |
|---|---|---|---|---|---|---|---|---|---|
| | | | | | LNZ | TDZ | | *23S rRNA** | *rpl3* |
| *S. epidermidis* | ST2 | 6 | E | Blood, sputum, intubation tube | >32 | 2–4 | – | G2576T, (G2602T) | – |
| | | 2 | F | Intubation tube, feces | >32 | 16 | – | G2576T, (G2602T) | Gly137Val, His146Arg, Met156Thr |
| | ST23 | 2 | A | Blood | 32 | 2 | – | G2576T, (G2602T) | – |
| | ST22 | 20 | A, B, D, E | Blood | >32 | >32 | – | C2534T, (C2560T), T2504A, (T2530A) | Asp159Tyr, Gly152Asp |
| *S. hominis* | ST2 | 10 | A,C,D,E | Blood | >32 | 4–8 | – | G2576T, (G2603T) | Met156Thr, Val154Leu |
| | | 6 | A,F | Blood, feces, sputum | >32 | 4–8 | + | G2576T, (G2603T) | Met156Thr, Val154Leu |
| *S. haemolyticus* | ST1 | 1 | A | Blood | >32 | 0.25 | + | – | – |

**Mutation in 23S rRNA according to E. coli numbering, in brackets mutation according to Staphylococcus numbering (NC_004461.1, NZ_CP046306.1, and NZ_CP035291.1).*

fragment of the reference sequence, and in all isolates, the specific SNPs were detected in 99% of the reads without mixed alleles. These data suggest that mutations are present in all copies of 23S rRNA.

All CoNS isolates demonstrated a high level of linezolid resistance (MIC $\geq$ 32 mg/L). The majority of isolates demonstrated tedizolid MIC $\leq$ 16.0 mg/L. A high level of tedizolid resistance (MIC $\geq$ 32 mg/L) was detected in ST22 isolates carrying double substitution in 23S rRNA. Only one *S. haemolyticus* isolate carrying the *cfr* gene as a single mechanism of resistance demonstrated susceptibility to tedizolid (MIC = 0.25 mg/L).

LRSE, belonging to ST2 and ST22, harbored *mec*–cassette of *SCCmec* III–like type with intact recombinase genes *ccrA3*, *ccrB3*, *mec*-complex class A, and *psm-mecA* regions. ST23 isolates carried *SCCmec* V–like type without the *psm-mecA* region. All *S. hominis* harbored intact SCC*mec* III with *psm-mecA* region. The *S. haemolyticus* isolate lacked SCC*mec* elements with only the *mecA* gene.

CoNS isolates under the study demonstrated high levels of associated resistance to aminoglycosides, fluoroquinolones, macrolides/lincosamides, tetracycline, co-trimoxazole, fusidic acid, rifampicin, and mupirocin but retained susceptibility to ceftaroline, tigecycline, and daptomycin. Resistance phenotypes were confirmed by the detection of corresponding genotypes (**Supplementary Table 4**). Isolates belonging to ST22 demonstrated susceptibility to erythromycin (despite the presence of intact macrolide resistance genes *msrA* and *mphC*) and resistance to clindamycin (L-phenotype). The phenotype is associated with T2504A point mutation (Liakopoulos et al., 2009).

## Molecular Epidemiology of LRSE

Analysis of the *S. epidermidis* population identified a pan-genome consisting of 31,036 genes and 731 core ortholog gene clusters. Phylogenetic analysis of genomes was based on extraction of a 74,628 nt long core genome after alignment.

Bayesian analysis of population structure divided the *S. epidermidis* population into eight clusters (**Figure 1** and **Supplementary Figure 1**), but LRSE genomes were found only in two of them: BAPS clusters 2 and 3 consisting mainly of *mecA*-positive isolates of human origin (from infected persons and carriers). *S. epidermidis* belonging to other clusters (1 and 4–8) were isolated from different sources: environmental samples, animals, and humans and were characterized by maximum diversity and represented by different STs.

## BAPS Cluster 2

Bayesian analysis of population structure cluster 2 consisted mostly of ST2 ($n$ = 260) and a minor number of other STs. Part of LRSE in the cluster forms a compact group of closely related ST2 genomes from Russia, France, and Germany, all of them harbored a mutation in the 23S rRNA gene (G2576T) and *rpoB* gene (Asp471Glu and Ile527Met). LRSE from France carried an additional mutation in *rpl3* (Met156Thr). Part of LRSE from France and Germany harbored the *cfr* gene. Other LRSE were represented by distantly related ST2 and ST23 genomes from the United States, Brazil, and Germany. A pairwise SNP difference between LRSE and linezolid-susceptible ST2 isolates revealed a low level of identity with a median of 191 SNPs with lower and upper interquartile range (IQR): 181–545. LRSE of ST2 demonstrated high genomic identity with a median pairwise SNP difference of 43 SNPs with lower and upper IQR: 16–53 SNPs. A subgroup of isolates from France, Germany, and Russia demonstrated an even higher level of similarity (**Supplementary Table 3**). Intragroup SNP differences between genomes from the same country varied from 2 to 27 and intergroup from 44 to 52. BAPS cluster 2 also includes a group of seven highly similar ST23 isolates from the United States with a median pairwise SNP difference of 35 SNPs (IQR: 29–39).

The timed phylogeny analysis of all LRSE ST2 isolates showed that they could have emerged in the 1960s with a large confidence interval: 1915–1994 (**Figure 2**). A common ancestor of LRSE isolates from Russia, France, and Germany appeared in 1998 (1986–2006) before introduction of linezolid in practice. We can assume two scenarios for the appearance of LRSE in Russia: independent formation (site E) and importation (site F) from Germany. At the same time, the progenitor of the Russian isolates appeared in 2002 (1996–2008). In Brazil and the United States, LRSE isolates emerged independently in 1960–1970.

## BAPS Cluster 3

Bayesian analysis of population structure cluster 3 included ST5, ST2, ST22, ST23, ST186, ST7, ST16, and ST35. Two groups of LRSE were detected within this cluster. The first group included LRSE of ST22 and its single-locus variant ST186 from Russia, France, and the United States. ST22 from Russia and France carried two mutations in 23S rRNA (C2534T and T2504A), and two mutations in *rpl3* (Asp159Tyr and Gly152Asp). Part of the Russian isolates carried a mutation of the *rpoB* gene (His481Asn). ST186 from the United States carried C2534T mutations and harbored the *cfr* gene. The pairwise SNP difference between LRSE and linezolid-susceptible ST22 isolates demonstrated a low level of identity with a median pairwise SNP difference of 214.5 (IQR: 204–233). LRSE from Russia and France were highly similar with a median pairwise SNP difference of 40 (IQR: 35.75–48.25). LRSE of ST186 from the United States were genetically distant from Russian and French isolates with a median pairwise SNP difference of more than 1,000 (**Supplementary Table 3**).

All ST22 isolates were included in BEAST analysis (**Figure 3**), a majority of them were LRSE, and a few were susceptible to linezolid. ST22 has a common time of origin in 1992 (1975–2000), but the LRSE sublineage widespread in France and Russia emerged in 2011 (2008–2013), and further divergence continued. Russian isolates from center A, B, and D are descended from a common ancestor with isolates from France, whose time of origin was 2011 (2009–2013). All isolates are compactly localized and have a short spreading period (which is also reflected in short branches on the chronogram), which indicates a clonal spread. Russian isolates from site E formed a separate cluster and were susceptible to rifampicin due to a wild type of *rpoB*.

The second group of LRSE within BAPS cluster 3 consisted of ST5 isolates from France ($n$ = 23), and the United States ($n$ = 2), and ST23 isolates from the United States ($n$ = 2) and

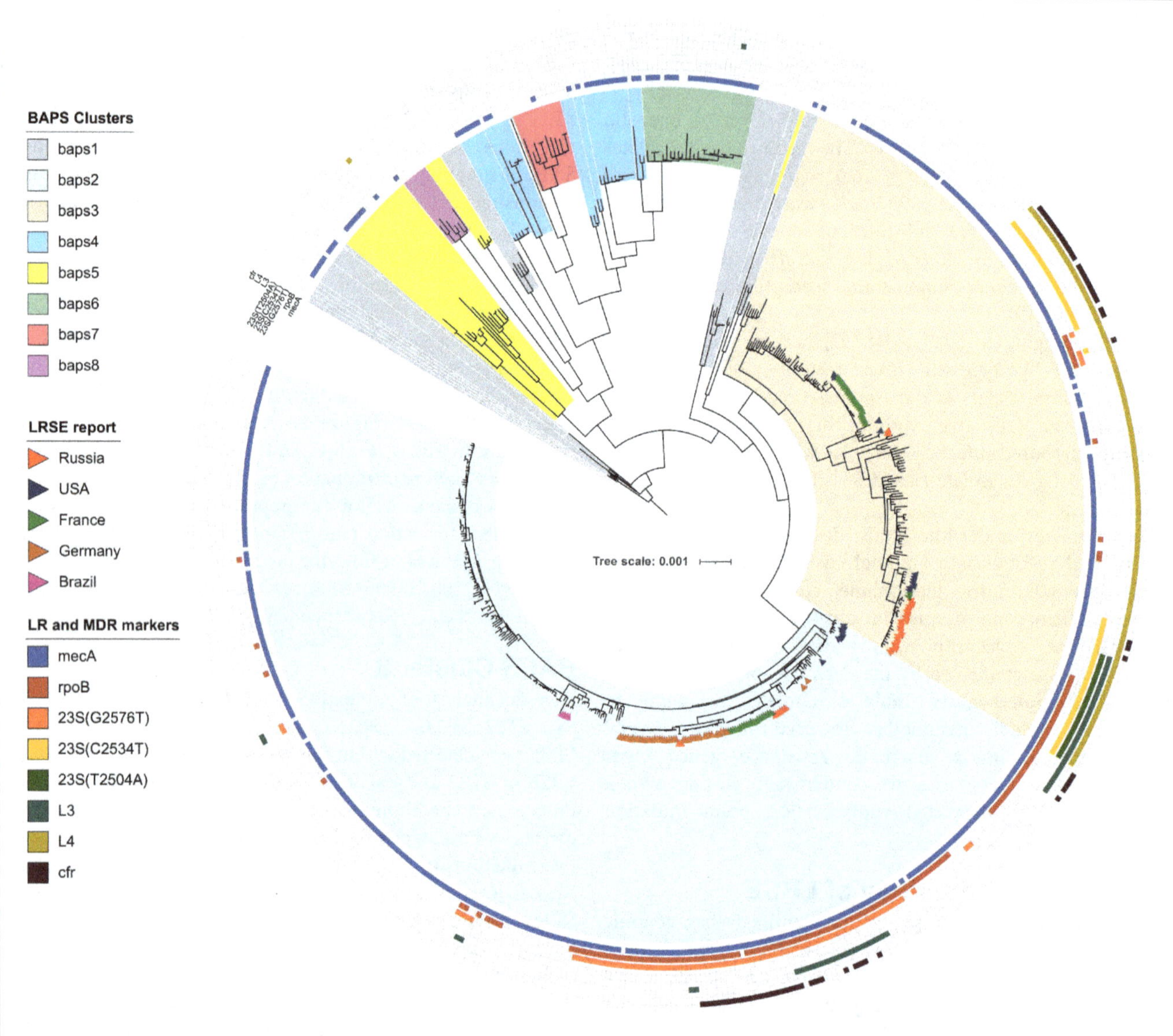


**FIGURE 1 |** Maximum-likelihood phylogeny of *S. epidermidis* population (*n* = 554) with mapped data of linezolid resistance and multidrug resistance data. Background color fill is matched to BAPS clustering. LRSE isolate is marked triangles: from Russia (current study), the United States (Tewhey et al., 2014), France (Dortet et al., 2018), Germany (unpublished data, only metadata is available BioProject PRJNA314440), and Brazil (unpublished data, only metadata is available from BioProjects PRJNA419710, PRJNA419705, PRJNA419706, and PRJNA419711). Annotation from inner to outer circle: presence *mecA*, mutations in *rpoB* (rifampin resistance), linezolid resistance (mutations in 23S rRNA, *rpl3*, *rpl4* genes and presence of *cfr*). Full zoom scalable view of phylogenetic tree with additional data and names of strains and description of calculated acquired resistance genes are available in **Supplementary Figure 1**.

Russia (*n* = 2). LRSE of ST23 harbored mutations in 23S RNA (G2576T or C2534T) and *rpoB* (Asp471Glu and Ile527Met), and one isolate carried the *cfr* gene. LRSE of ST5 carried a C2534T mutation and harbored the *cfr* gene. LRSE of ST23 were characterized by significant heterogeneity between BAPS clusters and between all LRSE of ST23 with median pairwise SNP difference of 4,204 (IQR: 4,167–4,252) SNPs and 4,196 (IQR: 37–4,245), respectively. LRSE of ST5 from France were highly similar with a median pairwise SNP difference of 5 (IQR: 2–7) SNP. Two isolates from Russia were also similar, but four isolates from the United States of ST23 and ST5, belonging to BAPS 3 and located close to the Russian isolates, revealed a high level of heterogeneity with a median pairwise SNP difference of 7,165 (IQR: 1,955.5–7,167.5).

In two genomes from Russia (CNS243, CNS244 from site F) and one from the United States (strain DAR4891, BioProject PRJNA308322) belonging to the ST2 rare mutation in *rpl3*, Gly137Val was detected together with a G2576T mutation in 23S rRNA. The role of this SNP in linezolid resistance development is unknown. Mutations in *rpl2* (Val112Ile and Ile75Thr) and *rpl4* (Asn158Ser) were detected in LRSE and linezolid-susceptible isolates from epidemic sequence types from BAPS cluster 3.

Analysis of distribution of acquired resistance genes in the population shows that the highest mean count of determinants

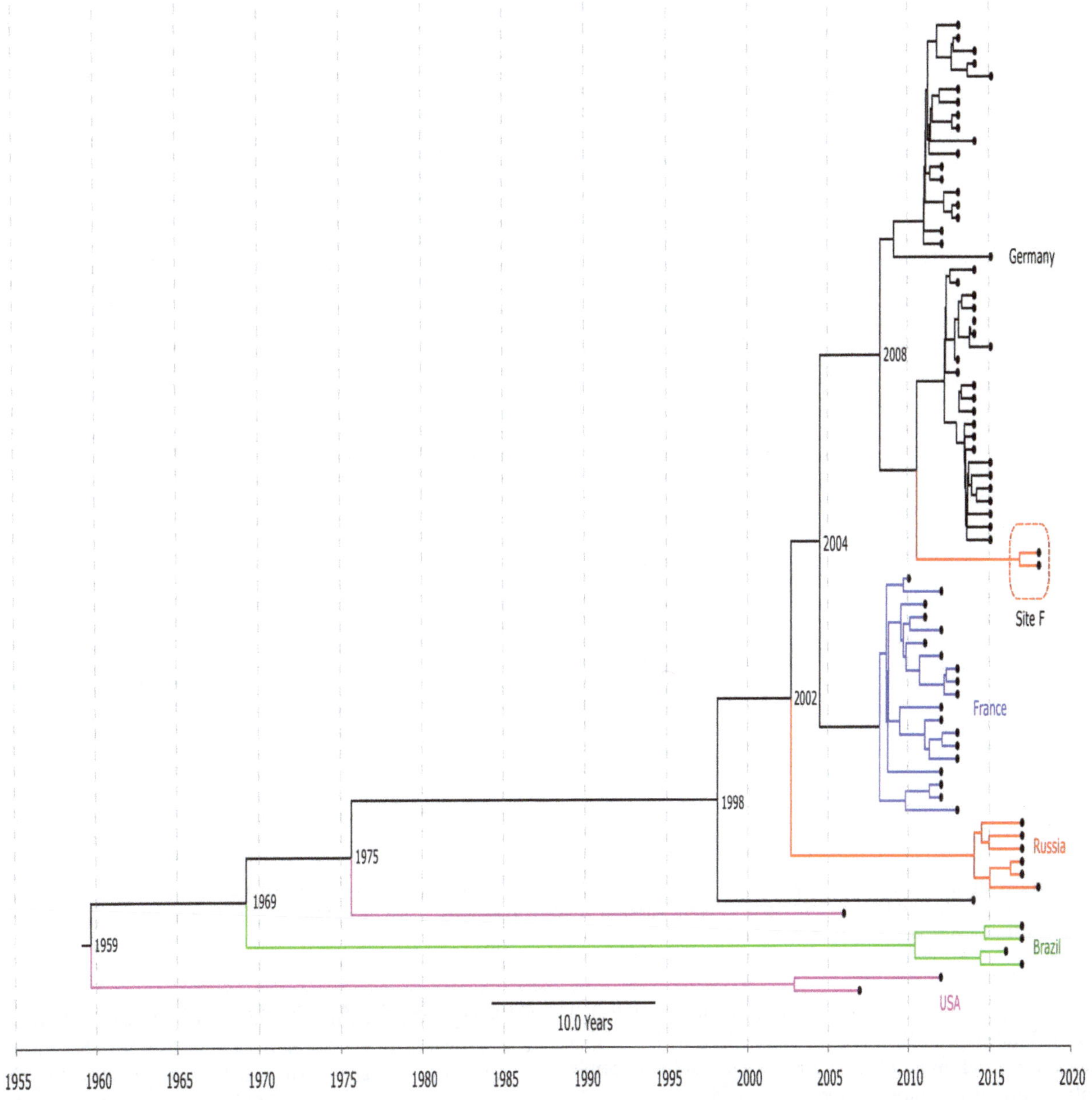


**FIGURE 2 |** Chronogram of LRSE ST2 ($n$ = 76) based on core-SNP alignment and BEAST. Color of branches is matched to country of origin of LRSE: black, Germany; blue, France; green, Brazil, violet, United States; and red, Russia (sites E and F). The time of divergence is given near nodes.

per genome was in genomes of BAPS clusters 2 (6.1) and 3 (5.9). The mean count of resistance genes in the LRSE subpopulation was 6.9.

## Phylogenetic Analysis of *S. hominis*

The pan-genome of *S. hominis* consisted of 7,798 genes, and the core genome included 1,185 genes. Phylogenetic analysis of genomes was based on extraction of 50,332 nt long core genome after alignment. The *S. hominis* population formed six BAPS clusters (**Figure 4**). The 1–3 BAPS clusters were localized closely to the root; they included *mecA*-negative isolates from healthy humans, animals, insects, and environmental specimens with different new unregistered MLST allelic profiles. Comparative analysis of genomes of these clusters showed a high number of core SNPs: for the BAPS 1 cluster, the pairwise median SNP difference was 4,197 (IQR: 3,538.5–4,915), and for BAPS 3, 2,860 SNPs (IQR: 348–7,694). The pairwise median SNP difference of all BAPS clusters is presented in **Supplementary Table 3**.

BAPS clusters 4–6 consisted of ST1, ST2, ST18, ST29, and ST47. Isolates of BAPS cluster 6 belonged to ST2, and they demonstrated high level genome identity with median 25.5 core SNP differences (IQR: 15–92); the cluster included linezolid-resistant isolates: 16 from Russia (current study), one from Lübeck, Germany (LRKNS031 unpublished, data from

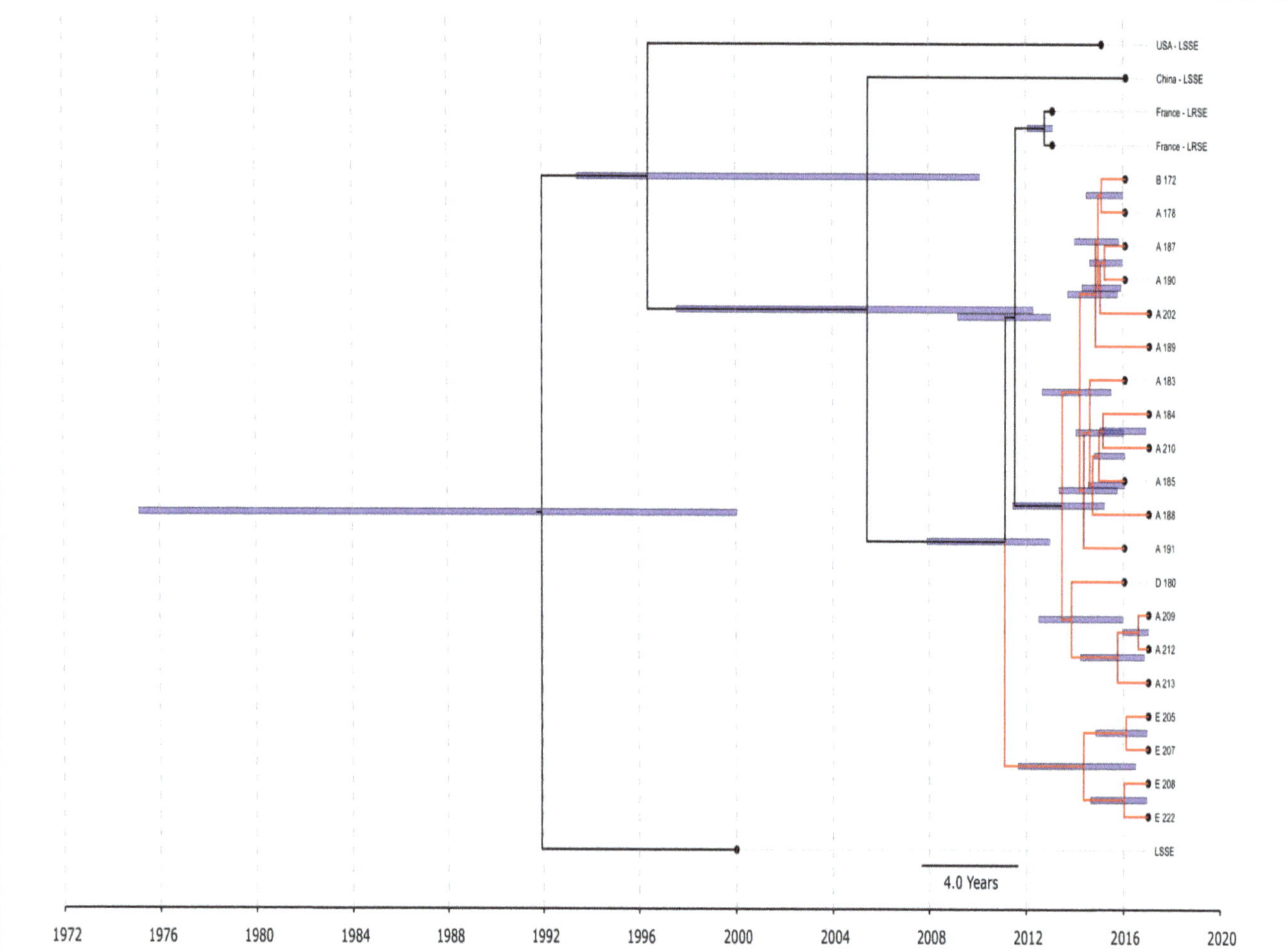


**FIGURE 3 |** Chronogram of *S. epidermidis* ST22 (*n* = 25) based on core-SNP alignment and BEAST. Three linezolid-susceptible *S. epidermidis* from different countries were included in the analysis. LRSE ST22 from Russia (red branches) and France were included in the analysis. Title of Russian isolates is matched of site isolation. 95% CI of time appearance (blue bars) shown near the nodes.

BioProject PRJNA314440), and two from Brazil (unpublished, data from BioProjects PRJNA419707 and PRJNA419709). One isolate from Sweden in BAPS cluster 6 was linezolid susceptible. All isolates carried a mutation in *rpoB* (Asn481His). Phylogenetic analysis of a midpoint rooted tree of BAPS cluster 6 (**Figure 5**) revealed the genetic proximity of the Russian and German isolates; they carried identical mutations in *23S rRNA* (G2603T) and *rpl3* (Met156Thr, Val154Leu). Six Russian isolates carried *cfr* also; most of them were isolated from site F. Isolates with double mechanism resistance and isolates with only mutation in 23S rRNA shared the same core genetic background with a minimum SNP difference. Brazilian isolates were phylogenetically distant; they carried identical mutations in *23S rRNA* but different mutations in *rpl3* (Met156Thr, Phe147Leu). The timed phylogeny analysis (**Figure 5**) showed that the BAPS 6 cluster of the *S. hominis* ST2 appeared in 1993 (95% CI: 1982–1998). The appearance of the common progenitor of linezolid-resistant *S. hominis* dates to 2003 (1996–2012) soon after introduction of linezolid into clinical practice in 2001, emergence of resistance *de novo* looks more probable.

## Phylogenetic Analysis of *S. haemolyticus*

The pan-genome of *S. haemolyticus* consists of 13,524 genes. The population of *S. haemolyticus* was divided into four BAPS clusters based on the extraction of 45,692 core SNPs after alignment of 1,032 core genes (**Figure 6**). BAPS cluster 1 included 82.6% of available *S. haemolyticus* isolates that were recovered at different times from different sources and belonged to 15 different STs, the cluster demonstrated a relatively low-level genome identity with median core-SNP differences of 651 SNPs (IQR: 481–806). A majority (77%) of isolates were *mecA*-positive and carried an average of 6.7 resistant genes per genome. Oxazolidinone-resistant *S. haemolyticus* isolates from Moscow (ST1) and the United States (ST4) (Tewhey et al., 2014) belonged to BAPS cluster 1 and were genetically distant.

## *Staphylococcus haemolyticus* and *S. hominis* Plasmids Carrying *cfr* Genes

One *S. haemolyticus* and six *S. hominis* isolates carried *cfr*-harboring plasmids of approximately 38,000 bp size (only

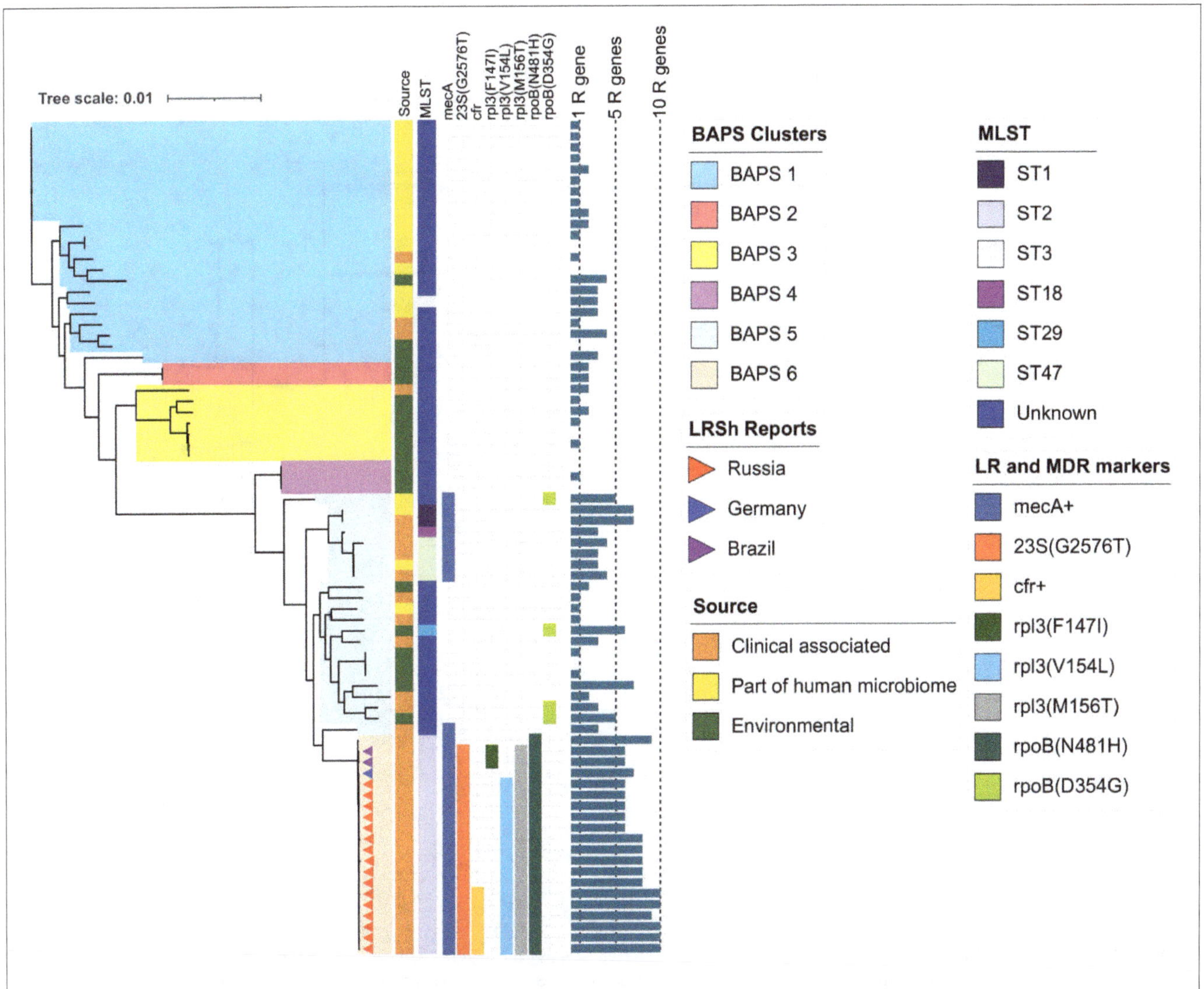


**FIGURE 4 |** Maximum-likelihood phylogeny of *S. hominis* population (76 genomes) based on core-SNP alignment. Background color fill is matched to BAPS clustering (BAPS 1 to BAPS 6). Linezolid-resistant *S. hominis* isolates (LRSh reports) marked as triangles on the tree. Annotation included source of genomes, MLST, linezolid resistance markers (LR): 23S rRNA mutation G2576T, rpl3 (Phe147Ile, Val154Leu, and Met156Thr), *cfr*; and multidrug-resistance markers (MDR): *mecA* and mutations in *rpoB* (Asn481His, Asp354Gly); bar chart is matched to the number of acquired resistance genes from 0 to 10 genes per genome (1R gene to 10R genes). The following genes were screened (mutations were not included): *aac(6')-aph(2''), aadD, ant(6)-Ia, ant(9)-Ia, aph(3')-III, blaZ, cat, ermC, fexA, cfr, fosB, fosD, fusB, fusC, lnu(A), lsa(B), mecA, mph(C), msr(A), str, tetK, tetL, vgaA, and vgaB.*

*de novo* assembled contigs were studied). BLAST analysis of the plasmid sequence revealed in GenBank several similar plasmids, which formed two clusters (**Supplementary Figure 2**). The first cluster included plasmids from *S. haemolyticus* (current study, Moscow), MRSA from the United States (Mendes et al., 2008) and Ireland (Shore et al., 2016), *S. cohnii* from China (Chen et al., 2013), and *S. epidermidis* from France (Dortet et al., 2018). The analysis of core genes of these plasmids revealed differences in no more than five SNPs. The second cluster included similar plasmids from *S. hominis*. They differed from the first cluster in no more than 408 SNPs. Plasmids from both clusters share 90% nucleotide identity and harbored replication gene *repUS5*, which was included in incompatibility group 18 (Inc18). The *Cfr*-gene in all considered plasmids was colocated together with the *fexA* gene coding phenicol resistance.

## Decreased Susceptibility to Glycopeptide in Linezolid-Resistant CoNS

Eight *S. hominis* ST2 and one *S. epidermidis* ST23 isolates demonstrated teicoplanin resistance with MIC = 16 mg/L. At the same time, the MIC of vancomycin was in range 1–4 mg/L (**Table 2**). However, the median parameter of $AUC_{MU50}/AUC_{CoNS}$ with vancomycin across all isolates was 0.74 (0.38–0.98). Nine isolates demonstrated a hetero-resistant phenotype with $AUC_{MU50}/AUC_{CoNS}$ range from 0.90 to 0.99

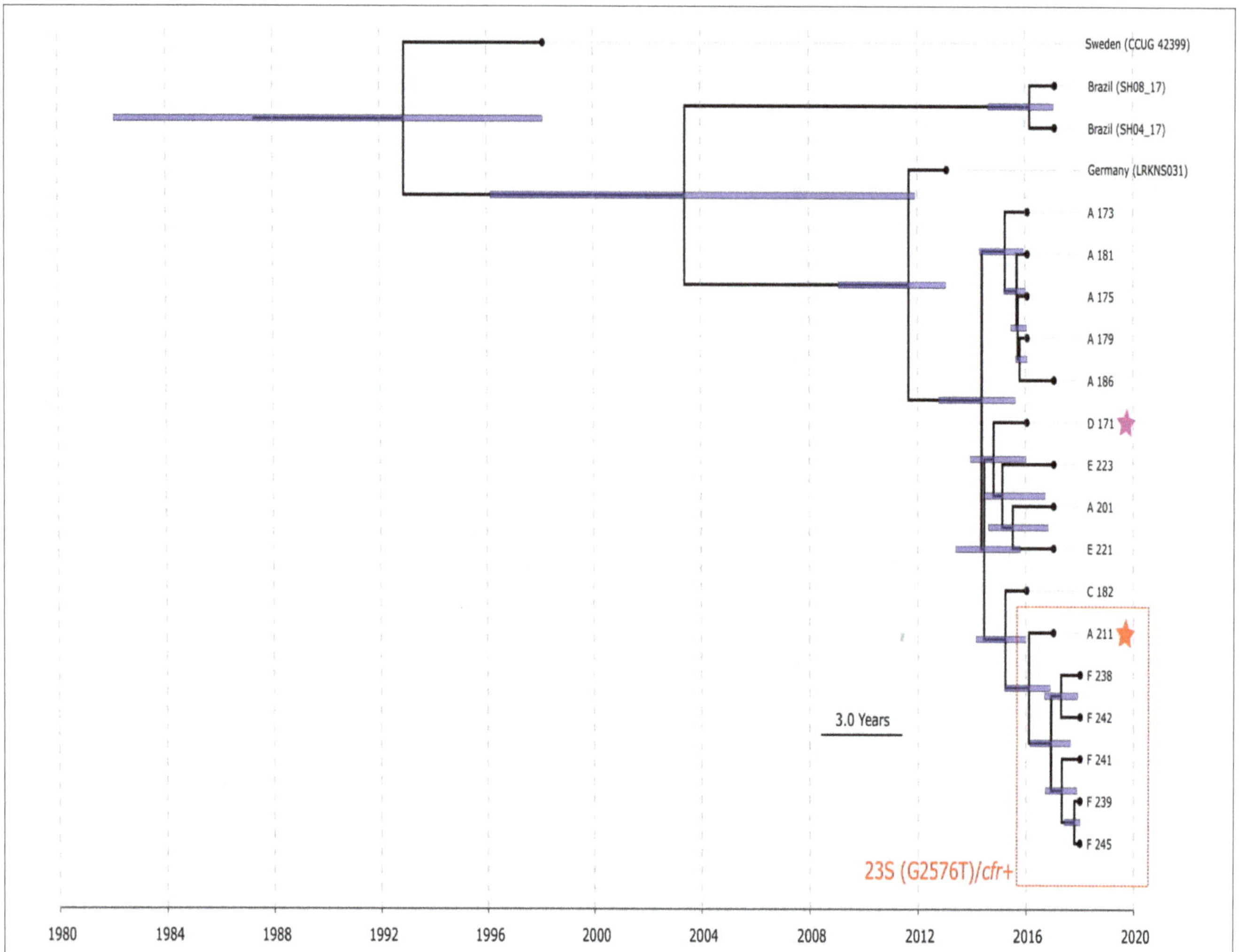


**FIGURE 5 |** Chronogram of *S. hominis* ST2 (BAPS cluster 6, $n = 20$) based on core-SNP alignment and BEAST. The violet star marks first time isolated oxazolidinone-resistant *S. hominis* in Russia, red star—first isolated cfr-positive *S. hominis*. Sites of appearance oxazolidinone-resistant *S. hominis* is shown on the figure (A, C–F). In addition to Russian isolates, this cluster included (blue names of strains): isolate LRKNS031 (linezolid-resistant *S. hominis* from Germany, BioProject PRJNA314440), two isolates from Brazil (BioProject PRJNA419707 and BioProject PRJNA419709) and linezolid-susceptible isolate CCUG 42399 from Sweden. 95% CI of time appearance (blue bars) shown near the nodes.

(**Supplementary Table 4**). Correlation between susceptibility to rifampicin (including mutations in *rpoB*) and PAP/AUC as well as correlation between teicoplanin and vancomycin levels of susceptibility were not found (**Supplementary Figure 3C**). However, a moderate positive correlation ($R = 0.27$, $p < 0.05$) was found between two parameters: $AUC_{MU50}/AUC_{CoNS}$ and teicoplanin susceptibility (**Figure 7**). The new lipoglycopeptides (oritavancin, dalbavancin, and telavancin) demonstrated high potency with an MIC range from 0.03 to 0.125 mg/L (**Table 2** and **Supplementary Table 4**). For *S. hominis* isolates, possible genetic markers associated with teicoplanin resistance were identified. These include the plasmid homolog of teicoplanin resistance-related proteins (*tcaA*), localized together with the *cfr* and *fexA*. However, in the *cfr*-positive isolate of *S. haemolyticus* (CNS200), this gene is also present on the plasmid, but the teicoplanin MIC level was 2 mg/L. Other mutations were also identified only in teicoplanin-resistant isolates. In particular, the Tyr75Asn mutation in the protein with unknown function with the Duf420 domain; mutation of Gly95Glu in the protein containing the DedA family protein domain; mutation (G → T) in the upstream region of DNA polymerase III subunit beta.

Using genomic data of all isolates included in the study, we analyzed the possible association of linezolid-resistance in *S. epidermidis* and *S. hominis* isolates with a decrease susceptibility to glycopeptides. For this purpose, 17 amino acid sequences of homologous proteins involved in the decreased susceptibility to glycopeptides in *S. aureus* were analyzed. A total of 45 mutation variants were identified, including missense and frameshift mutations. Using MCA analysis, the distribution of these mutations in the proteins was not associated with the LRSE genomes (**Supplementary Figure 3B**). However, it was found that the following mutations: YycH (Ser379Ala), RpoB (Ser486Tyr), GraS (Asn2Asp), and GraR (Glu224Gly) are most common in LRSE ($p < 0.01$), then in the other groups (heat

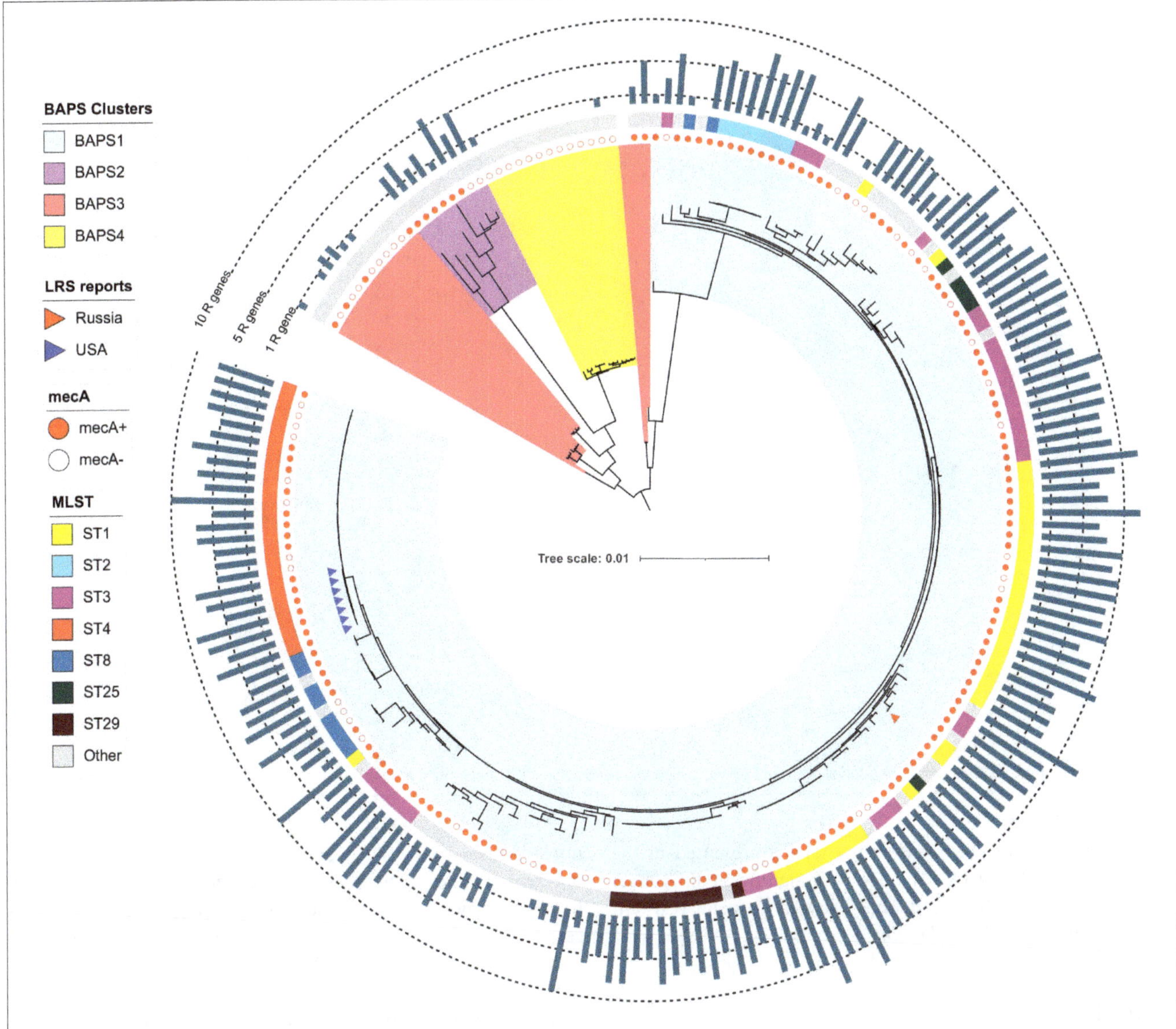


**FIGURE 6 |** Maximum-likelihood phylogeny of *S. haemolyticus* population (*n* = 207) based on core-SNP alignment. Background color fill is matched to BAPS clustering (BAPS 1 to BAPS 4). Linezolid-restant isolates (LRS reports) isolates is marked triangles: from Russia (one isolate in current study) and the United States (Tewhey et al., 2014). Annotation from inner to outer circle: presence *mecA*; MLST data; outer bar chart is matched to the number of acquired resistance genes (from 0 to 13 genes, specific chromosomal mutations were not included). The following genes were screened: *aac(6')-aph(2''), aadD, ant(6)-Ia, ant(9)-Ia, aph(3')-III, blaZ, cat, dfrG, ermA, ermC, cfr, fexA, fosB, fosD, fusB, fusC, lnu(A), lsa(B), mecA, mph(C), msr(A), str, tetC, tetK, tetL, tetM, vgaA, and vgaB.*

**TABLE 2 |** Glycopeptide and lipoglycopeptides susceptibility and PAP analysis in linezolid-resistant coagulase-negative staphylococci.

| | MLST | *n* | Range MIC, mg/L | | | | | | | PAP/AUC | | AAS* in RpoB | | |
|---|---|---|---|---|---|---|---|---|---|---|---|---|---|---|
| | | | **VAN** | **TEC** | **DLB** | **TLV** | **ORI** | **DAP** | **RIF** | **Range** | **M**** | **D471E** | **H481N** | **I527M** |
| LRSE | ST2 | 8 | 1–4 | 0.25–4 | 0.03–0.06 | 0.06–0.125 | <0.06 | 0.25–0.5 | >4 | 0.38–0.9 | 0.59 | + | − | + |
| | ST22 | 16 | 1–2 | 0.125–4 | <0.03 | 0.03–0.125 | <0.06 | 0.125–0.5 | 0.25–1 | 0.37–0.99 | 0.76 | − | + | − |
| | ST22 | 4 | 2–4 | 4 | <0.03 | 0.06–0.125 | <0.06 | 0.25–0.5 | <0.03 | 0.75–0.98 | 0.85 | − | − | − |
| | ST23 | 2 | 2–4 | 2 and 16 | 0.06 | 0.125 | 0.125 | 0.5 | >4 | 0.67–0.85 | NA | + | − | + |
| LRSH | ST2 | 16 | 1–2 | 4–16 | 0.03–0.125 | 0.06–0.125 | 0.03–0.125 | 0.125–0.5 | 0.5–2 | 0.40–0.9 | 0.75 | − | + | − |

*NA, not applicable; VAN, vancomycin; TEC, teicoplanin; DLB, dalbavancin; TLV, telavancin; ORI, oritavancin; DAP, daptomycin; RIF, rifampicin. *amino acid substitution, **median.*

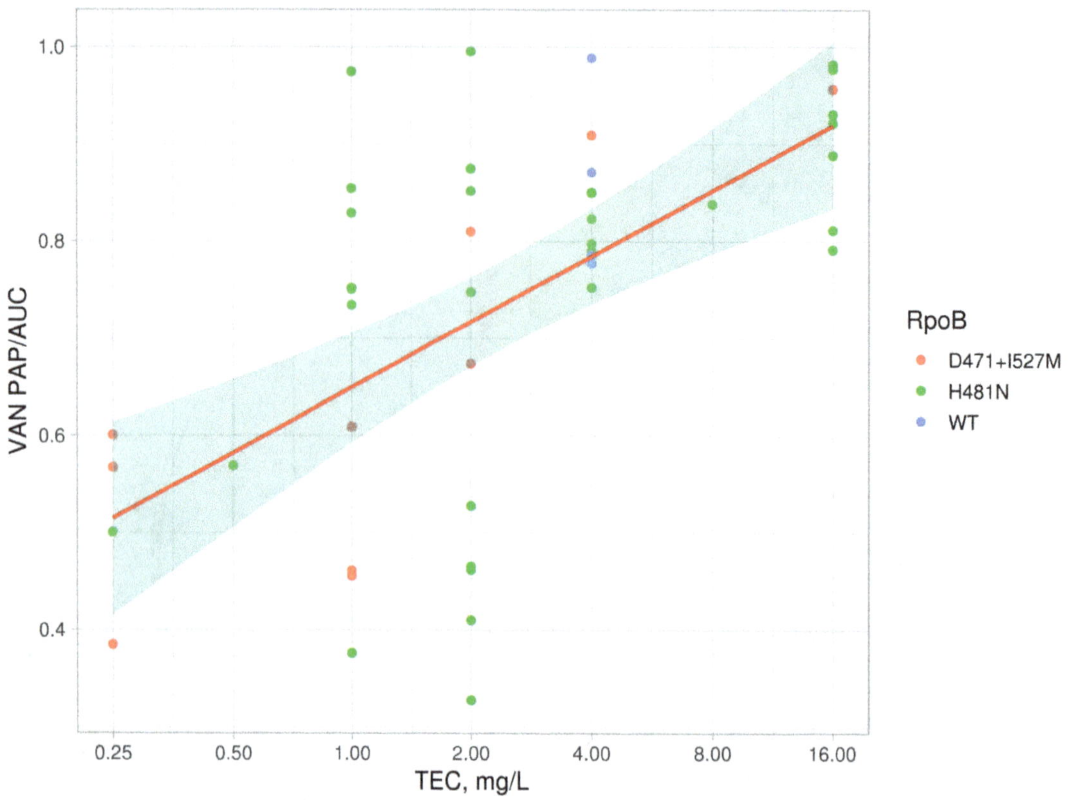


**FIGURE 7 |** Linear model and confidence interval plot with PAP/AUC data and teicoplanin MICs. Each point represented by AAS in RpoB (WT—wild type).

map of frequency of occurrence mutations is presented in the **Supplementary Figure 3A**). There were no significant differences in the prevalence of these mutations between linezolid-resistant and linezolid-susceptible *S. hominis*.

## DISCUSSION

In 2018, the main representative of CoNS group *S. epidermidis* was recognized by the European Centre for Disease Prevention and Control (2018) as a public health threat. The decision was based on the results of a study (Lee et al., 2018). The authors described the international spread of three hospital-adapted, multidrug-resistant lineages of *S. epidermidis*. Among the multidrug-resistant *S. epidermidis* isolates included in the study, the 18 isolates from Germany, France, and Ireland demonstrated resistance to linezolid, 14 of them belonged to ST2, three to ST5, and one to ST23. In the current study, we examined the international spread of LRSE in more detail. We also analyzed the dissemination of linezolid-resistant lineages of other common human skin colonizers: *S. hominis* and *S. haemolyticus*.

Evaluation of pairwise core-SNP differences between isolates of the same group (intragroup comparison) or between isolates of different groups (intergroup comparison) is a powerful tool for the assessment of the level of similarity between bacteria. However, criteria for different levels of similarity or identity are not established, making it difficult to interpret the results and differentiate lineages that have independently acquired resistance to oxazolidinones from lineages originating from a common resistant precursor. In this case, additional approaches could be used, such as BAPS and BEAST, for more detailed analysis of *Staphylococcus* phylogenomic.

In the current study using several approaches, we uncovered the existence of three international LRSE lineages, which largely coincides with the clustering of the *S. epidermidis* obtained in the study (Lee et al., 2018). The first lineage was represented by ST2 BAPS cluster 2 with highly similar isolates from France, Germany, and Russia harboring identical mutations in 23S rRNA and *rpoB*. The SNP difference between genomes from the same country (intragroup) was less than between genomes from different countries (intergroup). The time-scaled tree analysis showed that a common ancestor for LRSE ST2 from European countries and Russia appeared in 1998 (1986–2006) before introduction of linezolid in clinical practice, which indicates a greater likelihood of independent formation of LRSE in various countries. However, possible import of isolates can be observed for isolates from site F, which are in the same clade with LRSE from Germany. After dissemination to different regions, the lineage probably continues to evolve, thus the sublineage in France acquired additional a mutation in *rpl3*-Met156Thr, and some isolates in Germany and France acquired *cfr* genes.

The second LRSE lineage included ST22 isolates from France and Russia and its single-locus variant ST186 from the United States. Two ST22 isolates from France (Dortet et al., 2018) and 20 from Russia demonstrated high levels of intra- and intergroup similarity; they have identical mutations in 23S rRNA and *rpl3*, which suggests the existence of a common resistant precursor that appeared in 2011 (2008–2013). Isolates of this lineage harbored a maximal number of acquired resistance genes between all studied genomes. This genetic lineage may be common not only in Russia and France. ST22 LRSE carrying the same mutations in 23S and *rpl3* were reported from Greece and Turkey (Karavasilis et al., 2015; Freitas et al., 2018; Papadimitriou-Olivgeris et al., 2020). The whole genome sequencing (WGS) data in the mentioned publication are lacking, and it is impossible to evaluate the level of similarity between ST22 isolates from different sources. Seven ST186 isolates from the United States were genetically distant from the ST22 subgroup.

The third LRSE lineage included highly similar ST5 isolates from France ($n = 23$) and the United States ($n = 2$), *cfr* genes, and the 23S rRNA SNP at position 2,534 mediated oxazolidinone resistance in this subgroup. In this case, neither the international spread of LRSE nor the independent acquisition of the plasmid by representatives of closely related genetic lineages can be ruled out.

*S. hominis* is a poorly studied species among CoNS, and it is an uncommon causative agent of different opportunistic infections, including life-threatening nosocomial (d'Azevedo et al., 2008) and neonatal bacteremia's (Chaves et al., 2005). ST16, ST23, and ST2 are major lineages associated with human infections (Zhang et al., 2013). In this study, we found emergence and spread of linezolid-resistant ST2 lineage in Russia, Germany, and Brazil. BEAST analysis revealed that time of divergence of linezolid-resistant *S. hominis* was 2003 (1996–2012). The greatest genetic relationship with isolates from Russia demonstrated a single isolate from Germany. Linezolid-resistant *S. hominis* were previously reported from Europe (Musumeci et al., 2016; Drăgulescu et al., 2018) and Brazil (de Almeida et al., 2013; Chamon et al., 2014); however, data on MLST typing and/or WGS of these isolates are lacking. Six isolates from Russia carried simultaneous mutations in genes 23S rRNA and plasmid-born *cfr*. This combination of resistance mechanisms was previously described only in Romania (Drăgulescu et al., 2018). It cannot be ruled out that the spread of linezolid-resistant *S. hominis* ST2 is underestimated.

Several linezolid-resistant *S. hominis* from Russia demonstrated resistance to teicoplanin while maintaining susceptibility to vancomycin. To our knowledge, only a few reports dealing with teicoplanin-resistant *S. hominis* are published (Cercenado et al., 1996; d'Azevedo et al., 2008). We propose that resistance is caused by mutations in hypothetical proteins with Duf420 and DedA domains. The DedA family membrane proteins are widely represented in Gram-negative and Gram-positive bacteria; however, their biological functions are unknown. In one study, it was shown that DedA protein is associated with colistin resistance in *Burkholderia* (Panta et al., 2019). Further studies are needed for understanding of glycopeptide-resistance mechanisms in CoNS.

*Staphylococcus haemolyticus* is also an opportunistic pathogen and the second most frequent CoNS isolated from human blood cultures. In the study of Cavanagh et al. (2014), the population structure based on analysis of the core-genomes of a large collection of clinical European *S. haemolyticus* isolates showed predominance of one single cluster of genomes. All genomes from Cavanagh's study were included in the current work, and a majority of them were in BAPS cluster 1. This cluster included highly similar linezolid-resistant isolates from the United States (Tewhey et al., 2014) and genetically distant isolate from Russia. Linezolid-resistant *S. haemolyticus* were previously reported from Europe (Rodriguez-Aranda et al., 2009), China (Jian et al., 2018), and India (Brijwal et al., 2016; Mittal et al., 2019); however, data on MLST typing and\or WGS of these isolates are lacking.

A limitation of the study is the impossibility to characterize mobilomes from the short reads of the studied genomes. We were able to demonstrate that *cfr* harboring plasmids from *S. hominis* and *S. haemolyticus* belonged to different clusters of *repUS5*-like plasmids widely disseminated in the *S. aureus* population (Mendes et al., 2008; Chen et al., 2013; Dortet et al., 2018). Lack of epidemiological data supporting this assumption is another limitation of the study. We also have no information about the level of consumption of antibiotics, including linezolid in participating hospitals, which may indicate in favor of the local formation of resistance.

Noteworthy is the small number of available complete genomes of linezolid-resistant strains of CoNS that are not associated with the main genetic lineages. Many linezolid-resistant clones may be quickly eliminated from circulation, and only evolutionarily successful ones remain. However, likely, isolates obtained from local outbreaks were mainly included in the studies with genome-wide sequencing. Larger studies using whole genome sequencing are needed to better understand the molecular epidemiology of linezolid-resistant CoNS.

## CONCLUSION

CoNS are part of the human microbiome and are frequent contaminants of implants and medical devices. The importance of CoNS in the future is likely to increase as the use of invasive technologies in medicine increases, which will require new approaches to antibiotic therapy and, possibly, wider use of oxazolidinones. At present, the global population of linezolid-resistant CoNS is represented by a limited number of homogeneous genetic lineages and a small number of unrelated isolates. The leading mechanisms of resistance are mutations in the 23S rRNA and ribosomal protein genes; resistance due to *cfr* production is relatively rare. The geographic dissemination of resistance to linezolid is mediated by both the spread of resistant clones (LRSE ST22) and the formation of resistance *de novo* in closely related lineages of (LRSE ST2 and *S. hominis* ST2). The rate of further dissemination of resistance in the future is likely to depend on the consumption of oxazolidinones; however, it is almost impossible to predict which of the resistance mechanisms will dominate. Whole genome sequencing should become the main tool in the surveillance of the spread of linezolid-resistant CoNS.

## AUTHOR CONTRIBUTIONS

SS, VG, and AK conceived and designed the study. SL and DL analyzed the data. OK, MB, ND, ZG, TP, LL, and AG performed the experiments. All authors have read and agreed to the published version of the manuscript.

## FUNDING

This study was supported by the Institutional grant 001-05, Pediatric Research and Clinical Center for Infectious Diseases.

## SUPPLEMENTARY MATERIAL

**Supplementary Figure 1 |** Maximum-likelihood phylogeny of *S. epidermidis* population based on core-SNP alignment with additional data and names of strains and description of calculated acquired resistance genes.

**Supplementary Figure 2 |** Structure alignment of *cfr*-harboring plasmids.

**Supplementary Figure 3 | (A)** Heat map of the distribution of AAS in proteins associated with decreased susceptibility to glycopeptides in *S. epidermidis*; **(B)** Results of MCA analysis; **(C)** Distribution of isolates with PAP data, genotypes, and variants of mutations in RpoB.

**Supplementary Table 1 |** Quality of sequence data.

**Supplementary Table 2 |** Genomes included in the study.

**Supplementary Table 3 |** Pairwise SNP differences between genomes of CoNS.

**Supplementary Table 4 |** Description of resistance phenotypes and genotypes of Russian linezolid resistant isolates including MICs and PAP data.

## REFERENCES


Antonelli, A., D'andrea, M. M., Brenciani, A., Galeotti, C. L., Morroni, G., Pollini, S., et al. (2018). Characterization of poxtA, a novel phenicol-oxazolidinone-tetracycline resistance gene from an MRSA of clinical origin. *J. Antimicrob. Chemother.* 73, 1763–1769. doi: 10.1093/jac/dky088

Bai, B., Hu, K., Zeng, J., Yao, W., Li, D., Pu, Z., et al. (2019). Linezolid consumption facilitates the development of linezolid resistance in *Enterococcus faecalis* in a tertiary-care hospital: a 5-year surveillance study. *Microb. Drug Resist.* 25, 791–798. doi: 10.1089/mdr.2018.0005

Bankevich, A., Nurk, S., Antipov, D., Gurevich, A. A., Dvorkin, M., Kulikov, A. S., et al. (2012). SPAdes: a new genome assembly algorithm and its applications to single-cell sequencing. *J. Comput. Biol.* 19, 455–477. doi: 10.1089/cmb.2012.0021

Becker, K., Heilmann, C., and Peters, G. (2014). Coagulase-negative *Staphylococci*. *Clin. Microbiol. Rev.* 27, 870–926.

Boak, L. M., Li, J., Spelman, D., Du Cros, P., Nation, R. L., and Rayner, C. R. (2006). Successful treatment and cerebrospinal fluid penetration of oral linezolid in a patient with coagulase-negative *Staphylococcus ventriculitis*. *Ann. Pharmacother.* 40, 1451–1455. doi: 10.1345/aph.1h029

Bolger, A. M., Lohse, M., and Usadel, B. (2014). Trimmomatic: a flexible trimmer for illumina sequence data. *Bioinformatics* 30, 2114–2120. doi: 10.1093/bioinformatics/btu170

Brijwal, M., Dhawan, B., Rawre, J., Sebastian, S., and Kapil, A. (2016). Clonal dissemination of linezolid-resistant *Staphylococcus haemolyticus* harbouring a G2576T mutation and the cfr gene in an Indian hospital. *J. Med. Microbiol.* 65, 698–700. doi: 10.1099/jmm.0.000279

Brown, J., Pirrung, M., and Mccue, L. A. (2017). FQC dashboard: integrates FastQC results into a web-based, interactive, and extensible FASTQ quality control tool. *Bioinformatics* 33, 3137–3139. doi: 10.1093/bioinformatics/btx373

Brynildsrud, O., Bohlin, J., Scheffer, L., and Eldholm, V. (2016). Rapid scoring of genes in microbial pan-genome-wide association studies with Scoary. *Genome Biol.* 17:238.

Cai, J. C., Hu, Y. Y., Zhang, R., Zhou, H. W., and Chen, G. X. (2012). Linezolid-resistant clinical isolates of meticillin-resistant coagulase-negative staphylococci and *Enterococcus faecium* from China. *J. Med. Microbiol.* 61, 1568–1573. doi: 10.1099/jmm.0.043729-0

Castillo-Ramirez, S., Corander, J., Marttinen, P., Aldeljawi, M., Hanage, W. P., Westh, H., et al. (2012). Phylogeographic variation in recombination rates within a global clone of methicillin-resistant *Staphylococcus aureus*. *Genome Biol.* 13:R126.

Cavanagh, J. P., Hjerde, E., Holden, M. T., Kahlke, T., Klingenberg, C., Flægstad, T., et al. (2014). Whole-genome sequencing reveals clonal expansion of multiresistant *Staphylococcus haemolyticus* in European hospitals. *J. Antimicrob. Chemother.* 69, 2920–2927. doi: 10.1093/jac/dku271

Cercenado, E., Garcia-Leoni, M. E., Diaz, M. D., Sanchez-Carrillo, C., Catalan, P., De Quiros, J. C., et al. (1996). Emergence of teicoplanin-resistant coagulase-negative staphylococci. *J. Clin. Microbiol.* 34, 1765–1768.

Chamon, R. C., Iorio, N. L., Cavalcante, F. S., Teodoro, C. R., De Oliveira, A. P., Maia, F., et al. (2014). Linezolid-resistant *Staphylococcus haemolyticus* and *Staphylococcus hominis*: single and double mutations at the domain V of 23S rRNA among isolates from a Rio de Janeiro hospital. *Diagn. Microbiol. Infect. Dis.* 80, 307–310. doi: 10.1016/j.diagmicrobio.2014.09.011

Chaves, F., Garcia-Alvarez, M., Sanz, F., Alba, C., and Otero, J. R. (2005). Nosocomial spread of a *Staphylococcus hominis* subsp. novobiosepticus strain causing sepsis in a neonatal intensive care unit. *J. Clin. Microbiol.* 43, 4877–4879. doi: 10.1128/jcm.43.9.4877-4879.2005

Chen, H., Wu, W., Ni, M., Liu, Y., Zhang, J., Xia, F., et al. (2013). Linezolid-resistant clinical isolates of enterococci and *Staphylococcus cohnii* from a multicentre study in China: molecular epidemiology and resistance mechanisms. *Int. J. Antimicrob. Agents* 42, 317–321. doi: 10.1016/j.ijantimicag.2013.06.008

Cheng, L., Connor, T. R., Siren, J., Aanensen, D. M., and Corander, J. (2013). Hierarchical and spatially explicit clustering of DNA sequences with BAPS software. *Mol. Biol. Evol.* 30, 1224–1228. doi: 10.1093/molbev/mst028

Cingolani, P., Platts, A., Wang Le, L., Coon, M., Nguyen, T., Wang, L., et al. (2012). A program for annotating and predicting the effects of single nucleotide polymorphisms, SnpEff: SNPs in the genome of *Drosophila melanogaster* strain w1118; iso-2; iso-3. *Fly* 6, 80–92. doi: 10.4161/fly.19695

Coates, R., Moran, J., and Horsburgh, M. J. (2014). Staphylococci: colonizers and pathogens of human skin. *Future Microbiol.* 9, 75–91. doi: 10.2217/fmb.13.145

Corander, J., Marttinen, P., Siren, J., and Tang, J. (2008). Enhanced Bayesian modelling in BAPS software for learning genetic structures of populations. *BMC Bioinformatics* 9:539. doi: 10.1186/1471-2105-9-539

Croucher, N. J., Page, A. J., Connor, T. R., Delaney, A. J., Keane, J. A., Bentley, S. D., et al. (2015). Rapid phylogenetic analysis of large samples of recombinant bacterial whole genome sequences using Gubbins. *Nucleic Acids Res.* 43:e15.

Darling, A. C., Mau, B., Blattner, F. R., and Perna, N. T. (2004). Mauve: multiple alignment of conserved genomic sequence with rearrangements. *Genome Res.* 14, 1394–1403. doi: 10.1101/gr.2289704

d'Azevedo, P. A., Trancesi, R., Sales, T., Monteiro, J., Gales, A. C., and Pignatari, A. C. (2008). Outbreak of *Staphylococcus hominis* subsp. novobiosepticus bloodstream infections in Sao Paulo city, Brazil. *J. Med. Microbiol.* 57, 256–257. doi: 10.1099/jmm.0.47345-0

de Almeida, L. M., De Araujo, M. R., Sacramento, A. G., Pavez, M., De Souza, A. G., Rodrigues, F., et al. (2013). Linezolid resistance in Brazilian *Staphylococcus hominis* strains is associated with L3 and 23S rRNA ribosomal mutations. *Antimicrob. Agents Chemother.* 57, 4082–4083. doi: 10.1128/aac.00437-13

Dong, Y., and Speer, C. P. (2014). The role of *Staphylococcus epidermidis* in neonatal sepsis: guarding angel or pathogenic devil? *Int. J. Med. Microbiol.* 304, 513–520. doi: 10.1016/j.ijmm.2014.04.013

Dortet, L., Glaser, P., Kassis-Chikhani, N., Girlich, D., Ichai, P., Boudon, M., et al. (2018). Long-lasting successful dissemination of resistance to oxazolidinones in MDR *Staphylococcus epidermidis* clinical isolates in a tertiary care hospital in France. *J. Antimicrob. Chemother.* 73, 41–51. doi: 10.1093/jac/dkx370

Drăgulescu, E.-C., Codiţă, I., Nistor, I., Coldea, I. L., and Şerban, R. (2018).

Linezolid resistant *Staphylococcus hominis* isolated in a paediatric Romanian hospital. *Rom. Biotechnol. Lett.* 23, 13255–13263.

European Centre for Disease Prevention and Control (2018). *Multidrug-Resistant Staphylococcus Epidermidis - 8 November 2018.* Stockholm: ECDC.

Fairbrother, R. W. (1940). Coagulase production as a criterion for the classification of the staphylococci. *J. Pathol. Bacteriol.* 50, 83–88. doi: 10.1002/path.1700500112

Ferry, T., Batailler, C., Conrad, A., Triffault-Fillit, C., Laurent, F., Valour, F., et al. (2018). Correction of linezolid-induced myelotoxicity after switch to tedizolid in a patient requiring suppressive antimicrobial therapy for multidrug-resistant *Staphylococcus epidermidis* prosthetic-joint infection. *Open Forum Infect. Dis.* 5:ofy246.

Freitas, A. R., Dilek, A. R., Peixe, L., and Novais, C. (2018). Dissemination of *Staphylococcus epidermidis* ST22 with stable, high-level resistance to linezolid and tedizolid in the Greek-Turkish region (2008-2016). *Infect. Control Hosp. Epidemiol.* 39, 492–494. doi: 10.1017/ice.2018.5

Heilmann, C., Ziebuhr, W., and Becker, K. (2019). Are coagulase-negative staphylococci virulent? *Clin. Microbiol. Infect.* 25, 1071–1080. doi: 10.1016/j.cmi.2018.11.012

Henriksen, A. S., Smart, J., and Hamed, K. (2018). Comparative activity of ceftobiprole against coagulase-negative staphylococci from the BSAC bacteraemia surveillance programme, 2013–2015. *Eur. J. Clin. Microbiol. Infect. Dis.* 37, 1653–1659. doi: 10.1007/s10096-018-3295-6

Hoang, D. T., Chernomor, O., Von Haeseler, A., Minh, B. Q., and Vinh, L. S. (2018). UFBoot2: improving the ultrafast bootstrap approximation. *Mol. Biol. Evol.* 35, 518–522. doi: 10.1093/molbev/msx281

Jian, J., Chen, L., Xie, Z., and Zhang, M. (2018). Dissemination of cfr-mediated linezolid resistance among *Staphylococcus* species isolated from a teaching hospital in Beijing, China. *J. Int. Med. Res.* 46, 3884–3889. doi: 10.1177/0300060518781636

Jolley, K. A., and Maiden, M. C. (2010). BIGSdb: scalable analysis of bacterial genome variation at the population level. *BMC Bioinformatics* 11:595. doi: 10.1186/1471-2105-11-595

Kalyaanamoorthy, S., Minh, B. Q., Wong, T. K. F., Von Haeseler, A., and Jermiin, L. S. (2017). ModelFinder: fast model selection for accurate phylogenetic estimates. *Nat. Methods* 14, 587–589. doi: 10.1038/nmeth.4285

Karavasilis, V., Zarkotou, O., Panopoulou, M., Kachrimanidou, M., Themeli-Digalaki, K., Stylianakis, A., et al. (2015). Wide dissemination of linezolid-resistant *Staphylococcus epidermidis* in Greece is associated with a linezolid-dependent ST22 clone. *J. Antimicrob. Chemother.* 70, 1625–1629.

Katoh, K., and Standley, D. M. (2013). MAFFT multiple sequence alignment software version 7: improvements in performance and usability. *Mol. Biol. Evol.* 30, 772–780. doi: 10.1093/molbev/mst010

Kjellander, J. O., Klein, J. O., and Finland, M. (1963). *In vitro* activity of penicillins against *Staphylococcus Albus*. *Proc. Soc. Exp. Biol. Med.* 113, 1023–1031. doi: 10.3181/00379727-113-28563

Krueger, W. A., Kottler, B., Will, B. E., Heininger, A., Guggenberger, H., and Unertl, K. E. (2004). Treatment of meningitis due to methicillin-resistant *Staphylococcus epidermidis* with linezolid. *J. Clin. Microbiol.* 42, 929–932. doi: 10.1128/jcm.42.2.929-932.2004

Kruse, A. J., Peerdeman, S. M., Bet, P. M., and Debets-Ossenkopp, Y. J. (2006). Successful treatment with linezolid and rifampicin of meningitis due to methicillin-resistant *Staphylococcus epidermidis* refractory to vancomycin treatment. *Eur. J. Clin. Microbiol. Infect. Dis.* 25, 135–137. doi: 10.1007/s10096-006-0097-z

Kurtz, S., Phillippy, A., Delcher, A. L., Smoot, M., Shumway, M., Antonescu, C., et al. (2004). Versatile and open software for comparing large genomes. *Genome Biol.* 5:R12.

Langmead, B., and Salzberg, S. L. (2012). Fast gapped-read alignment with Bowtie 2. *Nat. Methods* 9, 357–359. doi: 10.1038/nmeth.1923

Layer, F., Vourli, S., Karavasilis, V., Strommenger, B., Dafopoulou, K., Tsakris, A., et al. (2018). Dissemination of linezolid-dependent, linezolid-resistant *Staphylococcus epidermidis* clinical isolates belonging to CC5 in German hospitals. *J. Antimicrob. Chemother.* 73, 1181–1184. doi: 10.1093/jac/dkx524

Lee, J. Y. H., Monk, I. R., Goncalves Da Silva, A., Seemann, T., Chua, K. Y. L., Kearns, A., et al. (2018). Global spread of three multidrug-resistant lineages of *Staphylococcus epidermidis*. *Nat. Microbiol.* 3, 1175–1185. doi: 10.1038/s41564-018-0230-7

Letunic, I., and Bork, P. (2016). Interactive tree of life (iTOL) v3: an online tool for the display and annotation of phylogenetic and other trees. *Nucleic Acids Res.* 44, W242–W245.

Li, H., Handsaker, B., Wysoker, A., Fennell, T., Ruan, J., Homer, N., et al. (2009). The sequence alignment/map format and SAMtools. *Bioinformatics* 25, 2078–2079. doi: 10.1093/bioinformatics/btp352

Liakopoulos, A., Neocleous, C., Klapsa, D., Kanellopoulou, M., Spiliopoulou, I., Mathiopoulos, K. D., et al. (2009). A T2504A mutation in the 23S rRNA gene responsible for high-level resistance to linezolid of *Staphylococcus epidermidis*. *J. Antimicrob. Chemother.* 64, 206–207. doi: 10.1093/jac/dkp167

Long, K. S., and Vester, B. (2012). Resistance to linezolid caused by modifications at its binding site on the ribosome. *Antimicrob. Agents Chemother.* 56, 603–612. doi: 10.1128/aac.05702-11

Mendes, R. E., Deshpande, L. M., Castanheira, M., Dipersio, J., Saubolle, M. A., and Jones, R. N. (2008). First report of cfr-mediated resistance to linezolid in human staphylococcal clinical isolates recovered in the United States. *Antimicrob. Agents Chemother.* 52, 2244–2246. doi: 10.1128/aac.00231-08

Mendes, R. E., Deshpande, L. M., Farrell, D. J., Spanu, T., Fadda, G., and Jones, R. N. (2010). Assessment of linezolid resistance mechanisms among *Staphylococcus epidermidis* causing bacteraemia in Rome, Italy. *J. Antimicrob. Chemother.* 65, 2329–2335. doi: 10.1093/jac/dkq331

Mittal, G., Bhandari, V., Gaind, R., Rani, V., Chopra, S., Dawar, R., et al. (2019). Linezolid resistant coagulase negative staphylococci (LRCoNS) with novel mutations causing blood stream infections (BSI) in India. *BMC Infect. Dis.* 19:717. doi: 10.1186/s12879-019-4368-6

Musumeci, R., Calaresu, E., Gerosa, J., Oggioni, D., Bramati, S., Morelli, P., et al. (2016). Resistance to linezolid in *Staphylococcus* spp. clinical isolates associated with ribosomal binding site modifications: novel mutation in domain V of 23S rRNA. *New Microbiol.* 39, 269–273.

Nam, J. R., Kim, M. S., Lee, C. H., and Whang, D. H. (2008). Linezolid treatment for osteomyelitis due to *Staphylococcus epidermidis* with reduced vancomycin susceptibility. *J. Korean Neurosurg. Soc.* 43, 307–310. doi: 10.3340/jkns.2008.43.6.307

Nguyen, L. T., Schmidt, H. A., Von Haeseler, A., and Minh, B. Q. (2015). IQ-TREE: a fast and effective stochastic algorithm for estimating maximum-likelihood phylogenies. *Mol. Biol. Evol.* 32, 268–274. doi: 10.1093/molbev/msu300

Okonechnikov, K., Fursov, M., Golosova, O., and Team, T. U. (2012). Unipro UGENE: a unified bioinformatics toolkit. *Bioinformatics* 28, 1166–1167. doi: 10.1093/bioinformatics/bts091

Otto, M. (2012). Molecular basis of *Staphylococcus epidermidis* infections. *Semin. Immunopathol.* 34, 201–214. doi: 10.1007/s00281-011-0296-2

Page, A. J., Cummins, C. A., Hunt, M., Wong, V. K., Reuter, S., Holden, M. T., et al. (2015). Roary: rapid large-scale prokaryote pan genome analysis. *Bioinformatics* 31, 3691–3693. doi: 10.1093/bioinformatics/btv421

Panta, P. R., Kumar, S., Stafford, C. F., Billiot, C. E., Douglass, M. V., Herrera, C. M., et al. (2019). A DedA family membrane protein is required for *Burkholderia thailandensis* colistin resistance. *Front. Microbiol.* 10:2532. doi: 10.3389/fmicb.2019.02532

Papadimitriou-Olivgeris, M., Kolonitsiou, F., Karamouzos, V., Tsilipounidaki, K., Nikolopoulou, A., Fligou, F., et al. (2020). Molecular characteristics and predictors of mortality among Gram-positive bacteria isolated from bloodstream infections in critically ill patients during a 5-year period (2012–2016). *Eur. J. Clin. Microbiol. Infect. Dis.* 39, 863–869. doi: 10.1007/s10096-019-03803-9

Pfaller, M. A., Flamm, R. K., Duncan, L. R., Shortridge, D., Smart, J. I., Hamed, K. A., et al. (2019). Ceftobiprole activity when tested against contemporary bacteria causing bloodstream infections in the United States (2016–2017). *Diagn. Microbiol. Infect. Dis.* 94, 304–313. doi: 10.1016/j.diagmicrobio.2019.01.015

Pfeltz, R. F., Schmidt, J. L., and Wilkinson, B. J. (2001). A microdilution plating method for population analysis of antibiotic-resistant staphylococci. *Microb. Drug Resist.* 7, 289–295. doi: 10.1089/10766290152652846

Pourakbari, B., Mahmoudi, S., Moradzadeh, M., Mahzari, M., Ashtiani, M. T. H., Tanzifi, P., et al. (2018). Antimicrobial resistance patterns of the gram-positive bacteria isolated from children with bloodstream infection in an Iranian referral hospital: a 6-year study. *Infect. Disord. Drug Targets* 18, 136–144. doi: 10.2174/1871526517666170821164343

Rodriguez-Aranda, A., Daskalaki, M., Villar, J., Sanz, F., Otero, J. R., and Chaves, F. (2009). Nosocomial spread of linezolid-resistant *Staphylococcus haemolyticus* infections in an intensive care unit. *Diagn. Microbiol. Infect. Dis.* 63, 398–402. doi: 10.1016/j.diagmicrobio.2008.12.008

Rodríguez-Lucas, C., Rodicio, M. R., Càmara, J., Domínguez, M. Á, Alaguero, M., and Fernández, J. (2020). Long-term endemic situation caused by a linezolid- and meticillin-resistant clone of *Staphylococcus epidermidis* in a tertiary hospital. *J. Hosp. Infect.* 105, 64–69.

Russo, A., Campanile, F., Falcone, M., Tascini, C., Bassetti, M., Goldoni, P., et al. (2015). Linezolid-resistant staphylococcal bacteraemia: a multicentre case-case-control study in Italy. *Int. J. Antimicrob. Agents* 45, 255–261. doi: 10.1016/j.ijantimicag.2014.12.008

Seemann, T. (2014). Prokka: rapid prokaryotic genome annotation. *Bioinformatics* 30, 2068–2069. doi: 10.1093/bioinformatics/btu153

Seral, C., Saenz, Y., Algarate, S., Duran, E., Luque, P., Torres, C., et al. (2011). Nosocomial outbreak of methicillin- and linezolid-resistant *Staphylococcus epidermidis* associated with catheter-related infections in intensive care unit patients. *Int. J. Med. Microbiol.* 301, 354–358. doi: 10.1016/j.ijmm.2010.11.001

Shore, A. C., Lazaris, A., Kinnevey, P. M., Brennan, O. M., Brennan, G. I., O'connell, B., et al. (2016). First report of cfr-carrying plasmids in the pandemic sequence type 22 methicillin-resistant *Staphylococcus aureus* staphylococcal cassette chromosome mec type IV clone. *Antimicrob. Agents Chemother.* 60, 3007–3015. doi: 10.1128/AAC.02949-15

Suchard, M. A., Lemey, P., Baele, G., Ayres, D. L., Drummond, A. J., and Rambaut, A. (2018). Bayesian phylogenetic and phylodynamic data integration using BEAST 1.10. *Virus Evol.* 4:vey016. doi: 10.1093/ve/vey016

Tewhey, R., Gu, B., Kelesidis, T., Charlton, C., Bobenchik, A., Hindler, J., et al. (2014). Mechanisms of linezolid resistance among coagulase-negative staphylococci determined by whole-genome sequencing. *MBio* 5:e00894-14.

The European Committee on Antimicrobial Susceptibility Testing (EUCAST) (2020). *Breakpoint Tables for Interpretation of MICs and Zone Diameters.* Version 10.0, 2020. Växjö: The European Committee on Antimicrobial Susceptibility Testing.

Tonkin-Hill, G., Lees, J. A., Bentley, S. D., Frost, S. D. W., and Corander, J. (2018). RhierBAPS: an R implementation of the population clustering algorithm hierBAPS. *Wellcome Open Res.* 3:93. doi: 10.12688/wellcomeopenres.14694.1

Wang, Y., Lv, Y., Cai, J., Schwarz, S., Cui, L., Hu, Z., et al. (2015). A novel gene, optrA, that confers transferable resistance to oxazolidinones and phenicols and its presence in *Enterococcus faecalis* and *Enterococcus faecium* of human and animal origin. *J. Antimicrob. Chemother.* 70, 2182–2190. doi: 10.1093/jac/dkv116

Watanabe, S., Tanaka, A., Ono, T., Ohta, M., Miyamoto, H., Tauchi, H., et al. (2013). Treatment with linezolid in a neonate with meningitis caused by methicillin-resistant *Staphylococcus epidermidis. Eur. J. Pediatr.* 172, 1419–1421. doi: 10.1007/s00431-013-1978-7

Wattam, A. R., Davis, J. J., Assaf, R., Boisvert, S., Brettin, T., Bun, C., et al. (2017). Improvements to PATRIC, the all-bacterial bioinformatics database and analysis resource center. *Nucleic Acids Res.* 45, D535–D542.

Zhang, L., Thomas, J. C., Miragaia, M., Bouchami, O., Chaves, F., D'azevedo, P. A., et al. (2013). Multilocus sequence typing and further genetic characterization of the enigmatic pathogen, *Staphylococcus hominis. PLoS One* 8:e66496. doi: 10.1371/journal.pone.0066496

22

# *In vitro* Activity of Lefamulin Against the Common Respiratory Pathogens Isolated From Mainland China During 2017–2019


*Shi Wu[1,2], Yonggui Zheng[1,2], Yan Guo[1,2], Dandan Yin[1,2], Demei Zhu[1,2] and Fupin Hu[1,2]**

[1] *Institute of Antibiotics, Huashan Hospital, Fudan University, Shanghai, China,*

[2] *Key Laboratory of Clinical Pharmacology of Antibiotics, Ministry of Health, Shanghai, China*

***Correspondence:***
*Fupin Hu*
*hufupin@fudan.edu.cn*



**Purpose:** Lefamulin is a novel antibiotic approved by the U.S. Food and Drug Administration in 2019 for the treatment of community-acquired bacterial pneumonia (CABP). In this study we evaluated the *in vitro* antimicrobial activity of lefamulin in order to better understand its antibiogram.

**Methods:** The test strains were isolated from patients across China during the period from 2017 to 2019, including 634 strains of respiratory pathogens. The minimum inhibitory concentrations (MICs) of lefamulin and comparators were determined by broth microdilution method.

**Results:** Lefamulin showed potent activity against *Streptococcus pneumoniae* and *Staphylococcus* evidenced by 100% inhibition at 0.25 mg/L, and favorable $MIC_{50/90}$ (0.125/0.125 mg/L) against *S. pneumoniae* (penicillin MIC $\geq$ 2 mg/L), $MIC_{50/90}$ ($\leq$0.015/0.125 mg/L) against methicillin-resistant *S. aureus*, and $MIC_{50/90}$ ($\leq$0.015/0.06 mg/L) against methicillin-resistant *S. epidermidis*. Lefamulin also had good activity against *Streptococcus pyogenes* and *Streptococcus agalactia* ($MIC_{50/90}$: $\leq$0.015/$\leq$0.015 mg/L), β-lactamase-producing *Haemophilus influenzae* ($MIC_{50/90}$: 0.5/1 mg/L), β-lactamase-negative *H. influenzae* ($MIC_{50/90}$: 1/1 mg/L), *Moraxella catarrhalis* ($MIC_{50/90}$: 0.25/0.25 mg/L), and *Mycoplasma pneumoniae* ($MIC_{50/90}$: 0.03/0.03 mg/L) regardless of resistance to azithromycin. Lefamulin was generally more active than the comparators against the test strains.

**Conclusion:** In summary, lefamulin has good and broad-spectrum coverage of respiratory pathogens (methicillin-sensitive and -resistant *Staphylococcus*, *S. pneumoniae*, β-hemolytic *Streptococcus*, *H. influenzae*, *M. catarrhalis* and *M. pneumoniae*). *In vitro* activity supports the use of lefamulin in the treatment of CABP in China.



**Keywords: lefamulin, antimicrobial susceptibility test, minimum inhibitory concentration, community-acquired bacterial pneumonia, *Mycoplasma pneumoniae***

## INTRODUCTION

Pleuromutilin is a natural antimicrobial substance first found in 1950s. It can be obtained from *Clitopilus scyphoides*, *Clitopilus passeckerianus*, or other *Clitopilus* species in basidiomycota. Lefamulin is the first-in-class semi-synthetic pleuromutilin antibiotic for systemic use. Its molecular formula is $C_{28}H_{45}NO_5S$ (molecular weight 567.79 g). Lefamulin inhibits bacterial protein synthesis by binding to "A" and "P" sites of the peptidyl transferase center (PTC) of the 23s rRNA of the 50S ribosomal subunit of bacterial cell. The binding is through the mutilin core and C-14 side chain in the forms of hydrogen bonds, hydrophobic interactions, and conformational change to prevent correct orientation of tRNA's 3'-CCA ends for peptide transfer (Veve and Wagner, 2018; Rodvold, 2019). The resistance to lefamulin may be related to the mutations in *rplC* gene and *cfr* gene of *Staphylococcus aureus*, Vga (AV) coded by the transposon Tn5406 and *vga(A)* carried by plasmids (encoding ABC transporter) (Mendes et al., 2019; Rodvold, 2019). So far, it is known that lefamulin has no cross resistance to the antimicrobial agents in clinical use.

Studies have shown that lefamulin has good coverage of the pathogens of community-acquired respiratory tract infections, including antibiotic-resistant strains, such as penicillin-resistant *Streptococcus pneumoniae* (PRSP), macrolide-resistant *Mycoplasma pneumoniae*, and methicillin-resistant *S. aureus* (MRSA) (Veve and Wagner, 2018; Rodvold, 2019). In August 2019, lefamulin was approved by the U.S. Food and Drug Administration (FDA) for the treatment of community-acquired bacterial pneumonia (CABP) patients based on its good pharmacodynamic results, pharmacokinetic, and safety profiles in clinical trials.

The antibacterial spectrum and activity of lefamulin have been studied in the United States and Europe (Paukner et al., 2013, 2019), but it is not clear about its antimicrobial activity against the clinical isolates in China. For better understanding the antimicrobial activity of lefamulin against the common respiratory pathogens recently isolated in China, we studied the *in vitro* activity of lefamulin against a broad range of respiratory pathogens.

## MATERIALS AND METHODS

A total of 634 non-duplicate strains of respiratory pathogens were tested, including 580 strains of bacteria and 54 strains of *Mycoplasma pneumoniae*. These strains were isolated from 29 hospitals across China, representing 23 provinces and municipalities, during the period from October 2017 to July 2019. Specifically, the test strains included *S. aureus* ($n$ = 121), *S. epidermidis* ($n$ = 30), β-lactamase-producing *Haemophilus influenzae* ($n$ = 48), β-lactamase-negative *H. influenzae* ($n$ = 48), *Haemophilus parainfluenzae* ($n$ = 10), *Moraxella catarrhalis* ($n$ = 54), *S. pneumoniae* ($n$ = 172), *Streptococcus pyogenes* ($n$ = 30), and *Streptococcus agalactiae* ($n$ = 13). All the strains were re-identified before susceptibility testing. Species identification was confirmed by MALDI-TOF/MS system (bioMérieux, France), and antimicrobial susceptibility testing were controlled with reference strains *S. aureus* ATCC29213, *S. pneumoniae* ATCC49619, *H. influenzae* ATCC49247, and *M. pneumoniae* ATCC 29342.

The minimum inhibitory concentrations (MICs) of lefamulin and the comparators were determined by broth microdilution method according to the Clinical and Laboratory Standards Institute (CLSI) (2018) M07-11th Edition (CLSI, 2018). The MICs against *M. pneumoniae* were measured according to the methods for antimicrobial susceptibility testing for human mycoplasmas described in CLSI document M43-A (2011) (CLSI, 2011). The antimicrobial comparators included tigecycline, moxifloxacin, linezolid, penicillin, ampicillin, oxacillin, ceftriaxone, levofloxacin, vancomycin, trimethoprim-sulfamethoxazole, erythromycin, and azithromycin. The concentrations of the test antimicrobial agents ranged from 32 mg/L to 0.015 mg/L.

WHONET 5.6 software and the breakpoints of CLSI M100-29$^{th}$ Edition (CLSI, 2019) were used to interpret and analyze the results of antimicrobial susceptibility test. Lefamulin and tigecycline were analyzed according to the breakpoints recommended by FDA[1]. The breakpoints of lefamulin was ≤0.25 mg/L active against methicillin-sensitive *S. aureus*, ≤0.5 mg/L against *S. pneumoniae*, and ≤2 mg/L against *H. influenzae*. The breakpoint of tigecycline was ≤0.5 mg/L active against *S. aureus*, and ≤0.25 mg/L against *H. influenzae*.

### Ethics Statement

The study protocol was approved by the Ethics Committee of Huashan Hospital, Fudan University (Number: 2019-319).

## RESULTS

Lefamulin at 0.25 mg/L inhibited the growth of all *Staphylococcus* strains (**Table 1** and **Figure 1**). The $MIC_{90}$ value of lefamulin was 0.125 mg/L against MRSA, 0.06 mg/L against methicillin-resistant *S. epidermidis* (MRSE), 0.06 mg/L against methicillin-sensitive *S. aureus* (MSSA), and 0.03 mg/L against methicillin-sensitive *S. epidermidis* (MSSE). Lefamulin displayed MIC values ranging from ≤0.015 mg/L to 0.25 mg/L ($MIC_{90}$: ≤0.25 mg/L) against 172 strains of *S. pneumoniae*, including penicillin-susceptible (PSSP) strains (penicillin MIC ≤0.06 mg/L), penicillin-intermediate (PISP) strains (penicillin MIC: 0.125 mg/L–1 mg/L), and penicillin-resistant (PRSP) strains (penicillin MIC ≥ 2 mg/L). Lefamulin inhibited the growth of all PSSP strains at ≤0.015 mg/L and all PISP and PRSP strains at 0.25 mg/L. The $MIC_{50/90}$ values of lefamulin were ≤0.015/≤0.015 mg/L against *S. pyogenes* and ≤0.015/0.06 mg/L against *S. agalactiae*. Lefamulin inhibited the growth of all the *S. pyogenes* and *S. agalactiae* strains at 0.06 mg/L (**Table 2** and **Figure 1**).

[1]www.fda.gov/drugs/development-resources/antibacterial-susceptibility-test-interpretive-criteria

**TABLE 1** | *In vitro* activity of lefamulin and comparators against *Staphylococcus*.

| Organism (No. of strains) | Antimicrobial agent | MIC (mg/L) | | | R% | S% |
|---|---|---|---|---|---|---|
| | | MIC Range | $MIC_{50}$ | $MIC_{90}$ | | |
| MRSA (*n* = 60) | Lefamulin | ≤0.015–0.25 | ≤0.015 | 0.125 | – | – |
| | Oxacillin | 32 – >32 | >32 | >32 | 100 | 0 |
| | Levofloxacin | 0.125–>32 | 8 | >32 | 53.3 | 45 |
| | Moxifloxacin | 0.03–16 | 1 | 8 | 48.3 | 48.3 |
| | Erythromycin | 0.25–>32 | >32 | >32 | 85.0 | 11.7 |
| | Azithromycin | 0.5–>32 | >32 | >32 | 85.0 | 15.0 |
| | Vancomycin | 0.5–2 | 1 | 1 | 0 | 100 |
| | Linezolid | 0.5–4 | 2 | 2 | 0 | 100 |
| | Tigecycline | 0.06–0.5 | 0.125 | 0.25 | – | 100 |
| MSSA (*n* = 61) | Lefamulin | ≤0.015–0.125 | 0.06 | 0.06 | - | 100 |
| | Oxacillin | 0.25–2 | 1 | 2 | 0 | 100 |
| | Levofloxacin | 0.125–8 | 0.25 | 0.5 | 3.3 | 96.7 |
| | Moxifloxacin | ≤0.015–2 | 0.06 | 0.25 | 3.3 | 96.7 |
| | Erythromycin | 0.25–>32 | >32 | >32 | 55.7 | 44.3 |
| | Azithromycin | 0.5–>32 | >32 | >32 | 55.7 | 44.3 |
| | Vancomycin | 0.5–1 | 1 | 1 | 0 | 100 |
| | Linezolid | 1–4 | 2 | 4 | 0 | 100 |
| | Tigecycline | 0.06–0.25 | 0.125 | 0.25 | - | 100 |
| MRSE (*n* = 15) | Lefamulin | ≤0.015–0.125 | ≤0.015 | 0.06 | - | - |
| | Oxacillin | 1–>32 | 4 | 32 | 100 | 0 |
| | Levofloxacin | 0.125–>32 | 8 | >32 | 73.3 | 20 |
| | Moxifloxacin | 0.03–32 | 2 | 32 | 53.3 | 20 |
| | Erythromycin | 0.25–>32 | >32 | >32 | 86.7 | 13.3 |
| | Azithromycin | 0.25–>32 | >32 | >32 | 80.0 | 20.0 |
| | Vancomycin | 1–2 | 1 | 2 | 0 | 100 |
| | Linezolid | 0.25–1 | 1 | 1 | 0 | 100 |
| | Tigecycline | 0.06–0.25 | 0.06 | 0.25 | - | - |
| MSSE (*n* = 15) | Lefamulin | ≤0.015–0.06 | ≤0.015 | 0.03 | - | - |
| | Oxacillin | 0.06–0.125 | 0.125 | 0.125 | 0 | 100 |
| | Levofloxacin | 0.125–4 | 0.25 | 4 | 13.3 | 80 |
| | Moxifloxacin | 0.03–1 | 0.06 | 0.5 | 0 | 93.3 |
| | Erythromycin | 0.125–>32 | 32 | >32 | 60.0 | 40.0 |
| | Azithromycin | 0.125–>32 | 32 | >32 | 60.0 | 40.0 |
| | Vancomycin | 1–2 | 1 | 2 | 0 | 100 |
| | Linezolid | 0.5–2 | 1 | 1 | 0 | 100 |
| | Tigecycline | 0.06–0.25 | 0.125 | 0.25 | - | – |

*MIC, minimum inhibitory concentration; $MIC_{50}$, MIC for inhibiting 50% of the isolates; $MIC_{90}$, MIC for inhibiting 90% of the isolates; R, resistant; S, susceptible; MRSA, methicillin-resistant S. aureus; NA, not available; MSSA, methicillin-susceptible S. aureus; MRSE, methicillin-resistant S. epidermidis; MSSE, methicillin-susceptible S. epidermidis.*

The $MIC_{50/90}$ values of lefamulin ≤ 1/ ≤ 1 mg/L against *H. influenzae* and *H. parainfluenzae*, regardless of β-lactamase production. Lefamulin inhibited the growth of all the *Haemophilus* strains at 2 mg/L (**Table 3** and **Figure 1**). Lefamulin showed $MIC_{50/90}$ of 0.25/0.25mg/L against *M. catarrhalis*. Lefamulin inhibited the growth of all *M. catarrhalis* strains at 0.5 mg/L (**Table 3** and **Figure 1**).

Lefamulin inhibited the growth of all *M. pneumoniae* strains at 0.03 mg/L. The MIC ranged from ≤0.015 to 0.03 mg/L ($MIC_{50/90}$: 0.03/0.03 mg/L). Its activity was comparable to moxifloxacin and significantly superior to erythromycin and azithromycin (**Table 4** and **Figure 1**).

## DISCUSSION

In the present study, lefamulin displayed excellent antimicrobial activity against all the respiratory pathogens, including MRSA, MSSA, MRSE, MSSE, *S. pneumoniae*, β-hemolytic *Streptococcus*, *Haemophilus*, *M. catarrhalis*, and *M. pneumoniae*. Our results are consistent with the reports of Susanne Paukner et al. on the antimicrobial activity of lefamulin against 1,473 and 2,661 strains of *S. pneumoniae*, 3,923 and 2,919 strains of *S. aureus* in the SENTRY Antimicrobial Surveillance Program 2010 and 2015–2016 (Paukner et al., 2013, 2019). The $MIC_{90}$ of lefamulin was 0.25 mg/L and 0.12 mg/L against *S. pneumoniae*, regardless

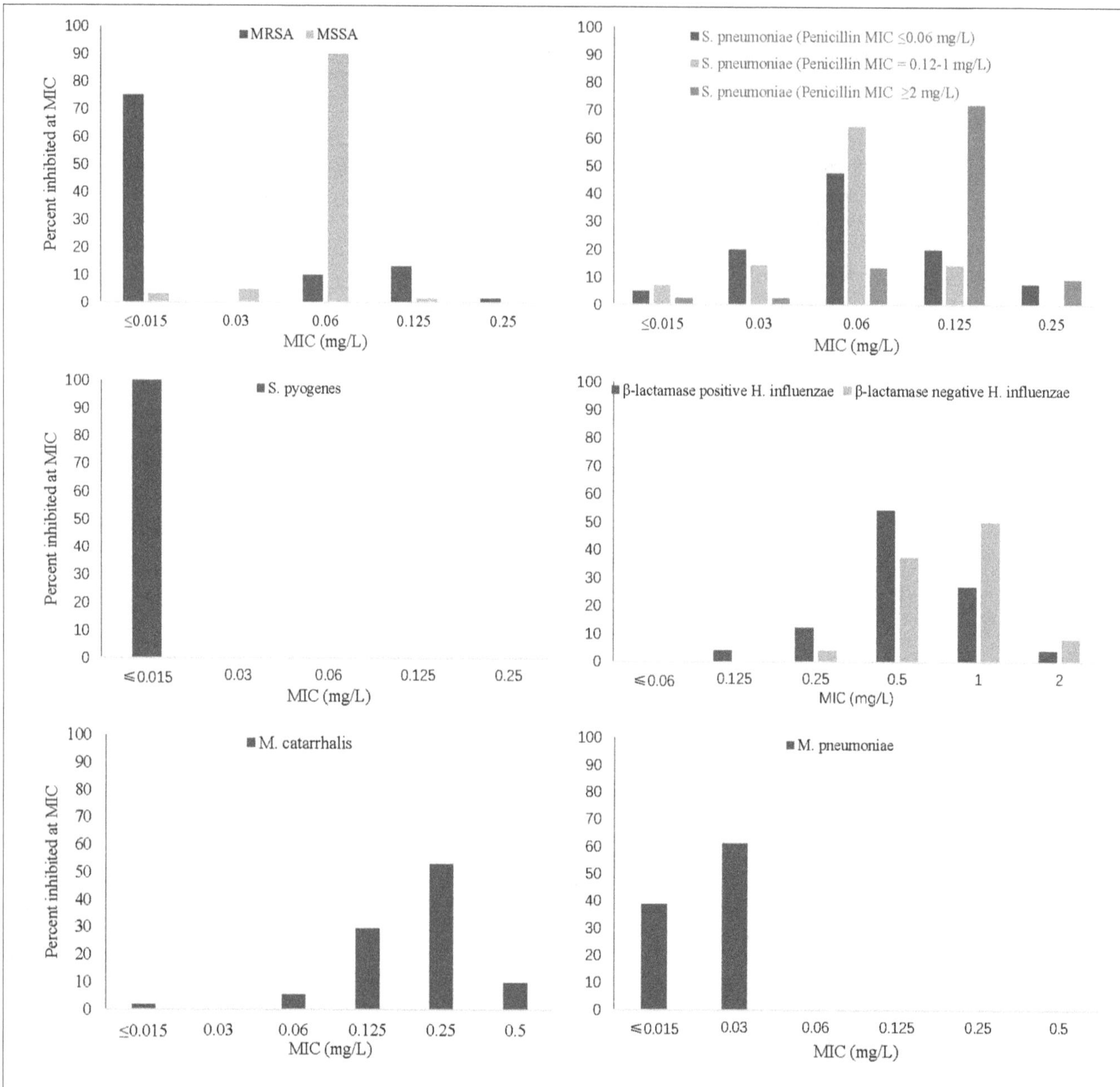


**FIGURE 1 |** MIC frequency distribution of lefamulin against respiratory pathogens. MRSA ($n$ = 60), MSSA ($n$ = 61), *S. pneumoniae* strains (penicillin MIC ≤ 0.06 mg/L, $n$ = 40; penicillin MIC = 0.12–1 mg/L, $n$ = 40; penicillin MIC ≥ 2 mg/L, $n$ = 118), *S. pyogenes* ($n$ = 30), *H. influenzae* (β-lactamase-positive strains, $n$ = 48; β-lactamase-negative strains, $n$ = 48), *M. catarrhalis* ($n$ = 54), and *M. pneumoniae* ($n$ = 54). MIC, minimum inhibitory concentration; MRSA, methicillin-resistant *S. aureus*; MSSA, methicillin-susceptible *S. aureus*.

of resistance to penicillin, ceftriaxone and/or levofloxacin. The $MIC_{50/90}$ was 0.12/0.12 mg/L against MRSA and MSSA. They also reported that the MIC value of lefamulin was 2–>16 mg/L against two MRSA isolates and 5 MSSA isolates in 2010, whereas the MIC value of lefamulin against 11 *S. aureus* isolates in 2015–2016 was higher than its epidemiological cutoff value. However, all the *Staphylococcus* strains tested in the present study were sensitive to lefamulin. All the *Staphylococcus* strains were also susceptible to tigecycline, vancomycin, and linezolid. However, lefamulin inhibited the growth of all *Staphylococcus* strains at concentration of ≤0.25 mg/L, which is far lower than the concentration of 1–2, 1–4, and 0.25–0.5 mg/L required by the above three comparators for 100% inhibition of bacterial growth. Lefamulin was also superior to quinolones (only inhibited 80–96.7% of the strains) in this respect.

Lefamulin also displayed high antimicrobial activity against *Haemophilus* and *M. catarrhalis*. Lefamulin was comparable to ceftriaxone in activity against *S. pneumoniae* strains (PSSP, PISP) and β-hemolytic *Streptococcus*, but better than ceftriaxone against PRSP, better than penicillin against PISP and PRSP, and similar to penicillin against β-hemolytic *Streptococcus*. Lefamulin had similar activity as moxifloxacin, vancomycin,

**TABLE 2** | *In vitro* activity of lefamulin and comparators against *Streptococcus* species.

| Organism (No. of strains) | Antimicrobial agent | MIC (mg/L) | | | R% | S% |
|---|---|---|---|---|---|---|
| | | MIC Range | $MIC_{50}$ | $MIC_{90}$ | | |
| *Streptococcus pneumoniae* (penicillin MIC ≤ 0.06 mg/L) (*n* = 40) | Lefamulin | ≤0.015–≤0.015 | ≤0.015 | ≤0.015 | – | 100 |
| | Ceftriaxone | ≤0.015–0.03 | ≤0.015 | ≤0.015 | 0 | 100 |
| | Penicillin | ≤0.015–≤0.015 | ≤0.015 | ≤0.015 | 0 | 100 |
| | Levofloxacin | 0.125–0.25 | 0.25 | 2 | 3.3 | 97.5 |
| | Moxifloxacin | 0.03–0.25 | 0.06 | 0.125 | 0 | 97.5 |
| | Erythromycin | 0.03–>32 | >32 | >32 | 97.5 | 2.5 |
| | Azithromycin | 0.06–>32 | >32 | >32 | 97.5 | 2.5 |
| | Vancomycin | ≤0.015–0.5 | 0.25 | 0.5 | 0 | 100 |
| | Linezolid | 0.125–1 | 1 | 1 | 0 | 100 |
| *Streptococcus pneumoniae* (penicillin MIC = 0.12–1 mg/L) (*n* = 40) | Lefamulin | 0.03–0.25 | 0.125 | 0.25 | – | 100 |
| | Ceftriaxone | 0.03–1 | 0.125 | 0.5 | 0 | 100 |
| | Penicillin | 0.125–1 | 0.5 | 1 | – | – |
| | Levofloxacin | 0.5–2 | 1 | 1 | 0 | 100 |
| | Moxifloxacin | 0.125–0.25 | 0.125 | 0.25 | 0 | 100 |
| | Erythromycin | 2–>32 | >32 | >32 | 100 | 0 |
| | Azithromycin | 2–>32 | >32 | >32 | 100 | 0 |
| | Vancomycin | 0.06–0.5 | 0.25 | 0.5 | – | 100 |
| | Linezolid | 0.25–1 | 1 | 1 | – | 100 |
| *Streptococcus pneumoniae* (penicillin MIC ≥ 2 mg/L) (*n* = 118) | Lefamulin | ≤0.015–0.25 | 0.125 | 0.125 | – | 100 |
| | Ceftriaxone | 0.5–>32 | 2 | 4 | 45.8 | 47.5 |
| | Penicillin | 2–32 | 8 | 8 | 100 | 0 |
| | Levofloxacin | 0.125–32 | 1 | 1 | 1.7 | 98.3 |
| | Moxifloxacin | 0.06–8 | 0.125 | 0.25 | 0.8 | 98.3 |
| | Erythromycin | 2–>32 | > 32 | >32 | 100 | 0 |
| | Azithromycin | 2–>32 | >32 | >32 | 100 | 0 |
| | Vancomycin | 0.125–1 | 0.25 | 0.5 | – | 100 |
| | Linezolid | 0.25–2 | 1 | 1 | – | 100 |
| *Streptococcus pyogenes* (*n* = 30) | Lefamulin | ≤0.015–≤0.015 | ≤0.015 | ≤0.015 | – | – |
| | Ceftriaxone | ≤0.015–0.03 | ≤0.015 | ≤0.015 | 0 | 100 |
| | Penicillin | ≤0.015–≤0.015 | ≤0.015 | ≤0.015 | 0 | 100 |
| | Levofloxacin | 0.125–0.25 | 0.25 | 2 | 3.3 | 96.7 |
| | Moxifloxacin | 0.03–0.25 | 0.06 | 0.125 | – | – |
| | Erythromycin | 0.03–>32 | >32 | >32 | 93.3 | 6.7 |
| | Azithromycin | 0.06–>32 | >32 | >32 | 93.3 | 6.7 |
| | Vancomycin | 0.25–0.5 | 0.25 | 0.5 | 0 | 100 |
| | Linezolid | 0.5–2 | 1 | 1 | 0 | 100 |
| *Streptococcus agalactiae* (*n* = 13) | Lefamulin | ≤0.015–0.03 | ≤0.015 | 0.03 | – | – |
| | Ceftriaxone | ≤0.015–0.06 | ≤0.015 | 0.06 | 0 | 100 |
| | Penicillin | 0.06–0.125 | 0.06 | 0.06 | 0 | 100 |
| | Levofloxacin | 0.5–1 | 1 | 1 | 0 | 100 |
| | Moxifloxacin | 0.125–0.25 | 0.125 | 0.25 | – | – |
| | Erythromycin | 0.06–>32 | 2 | >32 | 69.2 | 30.8 |
| | Azithromycin | 0.06 –>32 | 16 | >32 | 69.2 | 30.8 |
| | Vancomycin | 0.5–0.5 | 0.5 | 0.5 | – | 100 |
| | Linezolid | 1–2 | 1 | 2 | – | 100 |

*MIC, minimum inhibitory concentration; $MIC_{50}$, MIC for inhibiting 50% of the isolates; $MIC_{90}$, MIC for inhibiting 90% of the isolates; R, resistant; S, susceptible.*

and linezolid against *Streptococcus*. It inhibited the growth of all *Streptococcus* species at 0.125 mg/L, which was lower than the above mentioned three agents. Lefamulin was significantly better than erythromycin and azithromycin in the activity against *S. pneumoniae* and β-hemolytic *Streptococcus*.

In this study, lefamulin also had good antimicrobial effect on the gram-negative bacilli commonly found in CABP. Lefamulin was similar to ceftriaxone, tigecycline, levofloxacin, and moxifloxacin, and better than ampicillin, azithromycin, and trimethoprim-sulfamethoxazole in the activity against

**TABLE 3 |** *In vitro* activity of lefamulin and comparators against *Haemophilus influenzae* and *Moraxella catarrhalis.*

| Organism (No. of strains) | Antimicrobial agent | MIC (mg/L) | | | R% | S% |
|---|---|---|---|---|---|---|
| | | MIC Range | $MIC_{50}$ | $MIC_{90}$ | | |
| *Haemophilus influenzae* (β-lactamase positive) (*n* = 48) | Lefamulin | 0.125–2 | 0.5 | 1 | – | 100 |
| | Ceftriaxone | ≤0.015–1 | 0.03 | 0.125 | – | 100 |
| | Ampicillin | 8–>32 | >32 | >32 | 100 | 0 |
| | Levofloxacin | ≤0.015–1 | ≤0.015 | 0.5 | – | 100 |
| | Moxifloxacin | ≤0.015–1 | ≤0.015 | 0.5 | – | 100 |
| | Erythromycin | 4–>32 | >32 | >32 | – | NA |
| | Azithromycin | 1–>32 | >32 | >32 | – | 27.1 |
| | Tigecycline | 0.06–0.25 | 0.125 | 0.25 | – | 100 |
| | Trimethoprim-sulfamethoxazole | 0.06/1.14–32/608 | 8/152 | 16/304 | 77.1 | 16.7 |
| *Haemophilus influenzae* (β-lactamase negative) (*n* = 48) | Lefamulin | 0.25–2 | 1 | 1 | – | 100 |
| | Ceftriaxone | ≤0.015–0.25 | ≤0.015 | 0.06 | – | 100 |
| | Ampicillin | ≤0.015–1 | 0.5 | 1 | 0 | 100 |
| | Levofloxacin | ≤0.015–1 | ≤0.015 | 0.5 | – | 100 |
| | Moxifloxacin | ≤0.015–1 | ≤0.015 | 0.5 | – | 100 |
| | Erythromycin | 2–>32 | 8 | 8 | – | NA |
| | Azithromycin | 0.5–>32 | 2 | 2 | – | 97.9 |
| | Tigecycline | 0.125–0.25 | 0.25 | 0.25 | – | 100 |
| | Trimethoprim-sulfamethoxazole | 0.03/0.57–16/304 | 4/76 | 16/304 | 56.2 | 37.5 |
| *Haemophilus parainfluenzae* (*n* = 10) | Lefamulin | 0.015–2 | 0.5 | 1 | – | – |
| | Ceftriaxone | 0.015–0.25 | 0.03 | 0.125 | 0 | 100 |
| | Ampicillin | ≤0.015–8 | 0.125 | 4 | 30.0 | 70.0 |
| | Levofloxacin | 0.03–8 | 0.125 | 4 | 0 | 80.0 |
| | Moxifloxacin | 0.125–16 | 0.25 | 4 | 0 | 60.0 |
| | Erythromycin | 2 –>32 | 2 | 8 | – | – |
| | Azithromycin | 0.25–16 | 1 | 2 | 0 | 90 |
| | Tigecycline | 0.125–1 | 0.5 | 0.5 | – | – |
| | Trimethoprim-sulfamethoxazole | 0.015/0.285–16/304 | 0.125/2.375 | 2/38 | 10 | 70 |
| *Moraxella catarrhalis* (*n* = 54) | Lefamulin | ≤0.015–0.5 | 0.25 | 0.25 | – | – |
| | Ceftriaxone | ≤0.015–2 | 0.5 | 1 | 0 | 100 |
| | Ampicillin | ≤0.015–>32 | 1 | 4 | – | – |
| | Levofloxacin | ≤0.015–1 | 0.06 | 0.06 | 0 | 100 |
| | Moxifloxacin | ≤0.015–0.5 | 0.06 | 0.06 | – | – |
| | Erythromycin | 0.125–>32 | 1 | >32 | – | – |
| | Azithromycin | 0.03–>32 | 0.25 | >32 | 0 | 66.7 |
| | Tigecycline | 0.03–2 | 0.06 | 0.125 | – | – |
| | Trimethoprim-sulfamethoxazole | 0.03/0.57 –>32/608 | 0.5/9.5 | 4/76 | 11.1 | 64.8 |

*MIC, minimum inhibitory concentration; $MIC_{50}$, MIC for inhibiting 50% of the isolates; $MIC_{90}$, MIC for inhibiting 90% of the isolates; R, resistant; S, susceptible; NA, not available.*

**TABLE 4 |** *In vitro* activity of lefamulin and comparators against *M. pneumoniae.*

| Organism (no. of strains) | Antimicrobial agent | MIC (mg/L) | | | R% | S% |
|---|---|---|---|---|---|---|
| | | MIC Range | $MIC_{50}$ | $MIC_{90}$ | | |
| *Mycoplasma pneumoniae* (*n* = 54) | Lefamulin | ≤0.015 –0.03 | 0.03 | 0.03 | – | – |
| | Erythromycin | ≤0.015–>32 | 32 | >32 | 94.4 | 5.6 |
| | Azithromycin | ≤0.015–32 | 8 | 16 | 94.4 | 5.6 |
| | Moxifloxacin | 0.06–0.125 | 0.06 | 0.125 | – | 100 |

*MIC, minimum inhibitory concentration; $MIC_{50}$, MIC for inhibiting 50% of the isolates; $MIC_{90}$, MIC for inhibiting 90% of the isolates; R, resistant; S, susceptible; NA, not available.*

β-lactamase-producing *H. influenzae* and *M. catarrhalis*. As for the β-lactamase-negative strains, lefamulin provided significantly better activity than azithromycin. Lefamulin was comparable to tigecycline, ceftriaxone, and levofloxacin, and significantly superior to azithromycin and trimethoprim-sulfamethoxazole in the activity against *M. catarrhalis*. These results are consistent with those reports from other countries (Paukner et al., 2013, 2019).

It has been reported that the *M. pneumoniae* strains isolated from China are highly resistant to macrolides. Our results also confirmed the previous reports. About 94.4% of the 54 *M. pneumoniae* strains were resistant to erythromycin and azithromycin in this study. However, lefamulin still showed MIC range from $\leq$0.015 to 0.03 mg/L, which was not affected by resistance to macrolides. This MIC range is consistent with that from other countries ($MIC_{90}$: 0.002 mg/L) (Waites et al., 2017).

Lefamulin is the first semi-synthetic pleuromutilin antimicrobial agent approved for the treatment of CABP patients. Clinical trials have proved the excellent therapeutic effect of lefamulin. The $MIC_{90}$ value of lefamulin was 0.5 μg/mL against the 50 strains of *S. pneumoniae* isolated from the patients in phase III clinical trial LEAP 1 (File et al., 2019) and 0.25 μg/mL against the 123 strains of *S. pneumoniae* isolated from the patients in clinical trial LEAP 2 (Alexander et al., 2019). The $MIC_{90}$ against *S. aureus* isolates (10 and 13 strains) was 0.12–0.25 μg/mL. The post-treatment bacterial clearance rate was up to 100%. Research results at home and abroad have shown that lefamulin had similar antimicrobial activity against *S. epidermidis* and *S. aureus* (Paukner et al., 2013, 2019).

The above results support the excellent antimicrobial activity of lefamulin against CABP pathogens, especially antibiotic-resistant pathogens, such as PRSP, macrolide-resistant *M. pneumoniae* and MRSA. The major parameter driving efficacy for both *S. aureus* and *S. pneumoniae* is the 24h area under the drug concentration–time curve (AUC) over the MIC (24 h AUC/MIC). Lefamulin achieves rapid and predictable penetration into human tissues, with a mean 5.7-fold higher concentration in the pulmonary epithelial lining fluid compared with plasma. Percent probabilities of attaining the median AUCELF/MIC ratio targets associated with a 1-log10 CFU reduction from baseline by MIC were 97.0% at a MIC of 0.5 μg/mL for *S. pneumoniae* and 99.4% at a MIC of 0.25 μg/mL for *S. aureus* (Falcó et al., 2020). The unique mechanism of action, lack of cross resistance, good and broad coverage of respiratory pathogens regardless of resistance to other antimicrobial agent (Abbas et al., 2017; Lee and Jacobs, 2019) will surely make lefamulin a promising alternative treatment option in Chinese patients with CABP, especially those caused by PRSP, MRSA, or macrolide-resistant *M. pneumoniae*.

## AUTHOR CONTRIBUTIONS

DZ and FH designed the study. SW, YZ, YG, and DY performed the experimental work. SW and YZ collected the data. FH analyzed the data. All authors read and approved the final manuscript, contributed to the article, and approved the submitted version.

## FUNDING

This work was supported by Sinovant Sciences, Major Research and Development Project of Innovative Antibiotics, Ministry of Science and Technology of China (No. 2017ZX09304005), National Mega-project for Innovative Drugs (2019ZX09721001-006-004), and CHINET Antimicrobial Surveillance Network (grant number WI207259).

## REFERENCES

Abbas, M., Paul, M., and Huttner, A. (2017). New and improved? a review of novel antibiotics for Gram-positive bacteria. *Clin. Microbiol. Infect* 23, 697–703. doi: 10.1016/j.cmi.2017.06.010

Alexander, E., Goldberg, L., Das, A. F., Moran, G. J., Sandrock, C., Gasink, L. B., et al. (2019). Oral lefamulin vs moxifloxacin for early clinical response among adults with community-acquired bacterial pneumonia: the LEAP 2 randomized clinical trial. *JAMA* 2019 322, 1661–1671. doi: 10.1001/jama.2019.15468

CLSI (2011). *Methods for Antimicrobial Susceptibility Testing for Human Mycoplasmas; Approved Guideline (M43-A).* Wayne, PA: Clinical and Laboratory Standards Institute.

CLSI (2018). *Methods for Dilution Antimicrobial Susceptibility Tests for Bacteria That Grow Aerobically (M07).* Wayne, PA: Clinical and Laboratory Standards Institute.

CLSI (2019). *Performance standards for antimicrobial susceptibility testing (M100-S29).* Wayne, PA: Clinical and Laboratory Standards Institute.

Falcó, V., Burgos, J., and Almirante, B. (2020). An overview of lefamulin for the treatment of community acquired bacterial pneumonia. *Expert Opin. Pharmacother.* 21, 629–636. doi: 10.1080/14656566.2020.1714592

File, T. M., Goldberg, L., Das, A., Sweeney, C., Saviski, J., Gelone, S. P., et al. (2019). Efficacy and safety of intravenous-to-oral lefamulin, a pleuromutilin antibiotic, for the treatment of community-acquired bacterial pneumonia: the phase III Lefamulin Evaluation Against Pneumonia (LEAP 1) trial. *Clin. Infect. Dis.* 69, 1856–1867. doi: 10.1093/cid/ciz090

Lee, Y. R., and Jacobs, K. L. (2019). Leave it to lefamulin: a Pleuromutilin treatment option in community-acquired bacterial pneumonia. *Drugs* 79, 1867–1876. doi: 10.1007/s40265-019-01219-5

Mendes, R. E., Paukner, S., Doyle, T. B., Gelone, S. P., Flamm, R. K., and Sader, H. S. (2019). Low prevalence of gram-positive isolates showing elevated lefamulin MIC results during the SENTRY surveillance program for 2015-2016 and characterization of resistance mechanisms. *Antimicrob. Agents Chemother* 63:e02158-18. doi: 10.1128/AAC.02158-18

Paukner, S., Gelone, S. P., Arends, S. J. R., Flamm, R. K., and Sader, H. S. (2019). Antibacterial activity of lefamulin against pathogens most commonly causing community-acquired bacterial pneumonia: SENTRY antimicrobial surveillance program (2015–2016). *Antimicrob. Agents Chemother* 63:e02161-18. doi: 10.1128/AAC.02161-18

Paukner, S., Sader, H. S., Ivezic-Schoenfeld, Z., and Jones, R. N. (2013). Antimicrobial activity of the pleuromutilin antibiotic BC-3781 against bacterial pathogens isolated in the SENTRY antimicrobial surveillance program in 2010. *Antimicrob. Agents Chemother* 57, 4489–4495. doi: 10.1128/aac.00358-13

Rodvold, K. A. (2019). Introduction: lefamulin and pharmacokinetic/pharmacodynamics rationale to support the dose selection of lefamulin. *J. Antimicrob. Chemother* 74(Suppl. 3), i2–i4.

Veve, M. P., and Wagner, J. L. (2018). Lefamulin: review of a promising novel pleuromutilin antibiotic. *Pharmacotherapy* 38, 935–946. doi: 10.1002/phar.2166

Waites, K. B., Crabb, D. M., Duffy, L. B., Jensen, J. S., Liu, Y., and Paukner, S. (2017). In vitro activities of lefamulin and other antimicrobial agents against macrolide-susceptible and macrolide-resistant mycoplasma pneumoniae from the United States, Europe, and China. *Antimicrob Agents Chemother* 61:e02008-16. doi: 10.1128/AAC.02008-16

23

# Antibacterial Efficacy of Polysaccharide Capped Silver Nanoparticles is not Compromised by AcrAB-TolC Efflux Pump

*Mitali Mishra[1], Satish Kumar[2], Rakesh K. Majhi[1], Luna Goswami[2], Chandan Goswami[1] and Harapriya Mohapatra[1]**

[1] *School of Biological Sciences, National Institute of Science Education and Research, Homi Bhabha National Institute, Bhubaneswar, India,*

[2] *School of Biotechnology, Kalinga Institute of Industrial Technology, Bhubaneswar, India*

***Correspondence:***
*Harapriya Mohapatra*
*hm@niser.ac.in;*
*hmsbsniser@gmail.com*

Antibacterial therapy is of paramount importance in treatment of several acute and chronic infectious diseases caused by pathogens. Over the years extensive use and misuse of antimicrobial agents has led to emergence of multidrug resistant (MDR) and extensive drug resistant (XDR) pathogens. This drastic escalation in resistant phenotype has limited the efficacy of available therapeutic options. Thus, the need of the hour is to look for alternative therapeutic approaches to mitigate healthcare concerns caused due to MDR bacterial infections. Nanoparticles have gathered much attention as potential candidates for antibacterial therapy. Equipped with advantages of, wide spectrum bactericidal activity at very low dosage, inhibitor of biofilm formation and ease of permeability, nanoparticles have been considered as leading therapeutic candidates to curtail infections resulting from MDR bacteria. However, substrate non-specificity of efflux pumps, particularly those belonging to resistance nodulation division super family, have been reported to reduce efficacy of many potent antibacterial therapeutic drugs. Previously, we had reported antibacterial activity of polysaccharide-capped silver nanoparticles (AgNPs) toward MDR bacteria. We showed that AgNPs inhibits biofilm formation and alters expression of cytoskeletal proteins FtsZ and FtsA, with minimal cytotoxicity toward mammalian cells. In the present study, we report no reduction in antibacterial efficacy of silver nanoparticles in presence of AcrAB-TolC efflux pump proteins. Antibacterial tests were performed according to CLSI macrobroth dilution method, which revealed that both silver nanoparticles exhibited bactericidal activity at very low concentrations. Further, immunoblotting results indicated that both the nanoparticles modulate the transporter AcrB protein expression. However, expression of the membrane fusion protein AcrA did show a significant increase after exposure to AgNPs. Our results indicate that both silver nanoparticles are effective in eliminating MDR *Enterobacter cloacae* isolates and their action was not inhibited by AcrAB-TolC efflux protein expression. As such, the above nanoparticles have strong potential to be used as effective and alternate therapeutic candidates to combat MDR gram-negative Enterobacterial pathogens.

**Keywords: nanoparticles, efflux pump, AcrAB-TolC, *Enterobacter cloacae*, antibiotic resistance**

## INTRODUCTION

The drastic escalation in the proportion of multiple antibiotic resistant bacteria is recognized as a serious health care concern globally (WHO, 2014). The evolution of drug resistant microbes has challenged the success of antimicrobial agents for combating infectious diseases. The group of opportunistic pathogens, belonging to genera *Enterococcus*, *Staphylococcus*, *Klebsiella*, *Acinetobacter*, *Pseudomonas*, and *Enterobacter* (acronymed as ESKAPE) are exhibiting resistance to virtually all available antimicrobial agents (Boucher et al., 2009). Indeed, the acronym 'ESKAPE' is perfect choice to reflect these 'bad bugs.' To complicate the scenario, many of the above-mentioned bacteria are increasingly becoming responsible for spread of multidrug resistant (MDR) community acquired infections (Pendleton et al., 2013).

The *Enterobacter* spp., particularly *E. aerogenes* and *E. cloacae* are often associated with nosocomial infections like urinary tract infection (specifically catheter related), abdominal cavity/intestinal infections, wound infections, pneumonia, and septicemia (Sanders and Sanders, 1997; Fraser and Arnett, 2010). These two clinically predominant species display one or more resistance mechanisms toward antimicrobials like β-lactams, cephalosporins, aminoglycosides. Ironically, *E. aerogenes* and *E. cloacae* are also exhibiting trends of increased resistance toward the last resort antimicrobial agents - carbapenems and colistin (Davin-Regli and Pagès, 2015). Well-equipped with armory of antibiotic resistance strategies such as, outer membrane permeability barrier, efflux pumps and antibiotic degrading enzymes, *Enterobacter* spp. form an interesting infectious model to explore (Grimont and Grimont, 2006; Mezzatesta et al., 2012; Davin-Regli and Pagès, 2015).

The rise in antimicrobial resistance coupled with diminishing available options has necessitated searching for alternative therapeutic options (Martins and McCusker, 2016). One such lucrative direction was use of combinatorial therapy for treatment of infections caused by gram-negative pathogens, such as *Pseudomonas aeruginosa*. Typically, the combinatorial therapies for gram-negative pathogens included a β-lactam with aminoglycoside or fluoroquinolone (Tamma et al., 2012). The strategy was to extract their synergistic potential and broader spectrum of activity. But, in many clinical trials, it developed adverse effects leading to nephrotoxicity and even greater multiple antibiotic resistance (Kerantzas and Jacobs, 2017). The limitations faced by combinatorial therapies led to further improvisation and antimicrobial peptides were the more sought after. These host-defense peptides were investigated due to their antimicrobial properties against both gram-positive and gram-negative pathogens and immunomodulatory roles. However, low metabolic stability and discrepancies between *in vivo* and *in vitro* antimicrobial effectiveness limited the scope of antimicrobial peptides (Mahlapuu et al., 2016). Other interesting alternatives were more conceptual driven, such as bacteriophage therapy (Yang et al., 2014) and/or repurposing the existing drugs for better antibacterial and anti-virulence features (Rangel-Vega et al., 2015). Although both of them appeared as promising candidates, but development of such therapy at large scale remains challenging and yet to be explored.

All of the above-developed strategies faced severe obstacles in getting translated for sustainable, practical and large-scale usage, as demanded by the present situation. Much of the aforementioned limitations were circumvented by development of nanoparticle as drugs (Salata, 2004; Singh and Lillard, 2009). Over the years, nanoparticle-based approaches have gathered much reputation due to their fast and effective antibacterial properties for various pathogens (Gelperina et al., 2005; Tran and Webster, 2011). Nanoparticles endowed with wide bactericidal spectrum, ability to inhibit biofilm, increased permeability and efficacy at low dose, form a powerful weapon to combat MDR bacteria (Kim et al., 2007; Pelgrift and Friedman, 2013; Chen et al., 2014; Sanyasi et al., 2016). Review of the literature reveals that presence of efflux pumps [particularly those belonging to resistance nodulation division (RND) super family, e.g., tripartite efflux pump AcrAB-TolC] in gram-negative bacteria compromises the antibacterial efficacy of the drugs by extruding them out of the cytoplasm (Zgurskaya, 2009). Efflux of drugs reduces their intracellular concentration, leading to increased resistance in pathogens toward the drug. Further, it has been reported that substrates to be effluxed (antibacterial drugs) induce overexpression of the efflux proteins (Rosenberg et al., 2003).

Previously we had reported antibacterial activity of polysaccharide-capped silver nanoparticles (AgNPs) toward several MDR bacteria *viz. E. coli*, *Klebsiella* spp., *Enterobacter* spp., and *S. aureus* (Sanyasi et al., 2016). We had demonstrated AgNPs to inhibit biofilm formation and alter expression of cytoskeletal proteins FtsZ and FtsA, with minimal cytotoxicity toward mammalian cells. In the present study, we have further investigated antibacterial effects of the aforementioned AgNPs and that of a newly developed silver-metal-carbohydrate nanoparticle (Ag-MCNP) particularly on MDR *E. cloacae* isolates. Further, with the objective to consolidate our findings, we also investigated the effect of these silver nanoparticles on expression of AcrAB-TolC efflux pump proteins in MDR *E. cloacae* isolates.

## MATERIALS AND METHODS

### Bacterial Strains and Media

A wild type *E. cloacae* (EspIMS6) urinary tract infection isolate from a tertiary care hospital at Bhubaneswar, India, and *E. cloacae* subsp. *cloacae* ATCC-13047 type strain were used in the present study. The bacterial isolates were identified by biochemical tests followed by 16S rRNA gene sequencing. As prescribed for Enterobacteriaceae (CLSI, 2016), *E. coli* strain ATCC 25922 was used as control during antibiotic susceptibility testing. Unless otherwise mentioned, bacterial cultures were grown on nutrient agar/broth (Hi-Media, India) and incubated at 37°C in a controlled environment shaker (New Brunswick, NJ, United States). Muller Hinton broth (MHB)/agar (MHA) medium (Hi-Media, India) was used for antibiotic susceptibility test. Following sub-culture, the strains were preserved at −80°C in 20% glycerol for further use. All experiments were performed in triplicate and repeated at least three times.

## Resistance Profiling

Antibiotic disks used in resistance profiling were obtained from Himedia, India. Each strain was tested for susceptibility to different antibiotics by disk diffusion method (Bauer et al., 1966). The diameter of the inhibition zones was interpreted following CLSI standard as proposed for Enterobacteriaceae (CLSI, 2016).

## Characterization of Silver Nanoparticles Used

### Physical Characterization of the Nanoparticles Used

Particle size and zeta potential (ζ) of the polysaccharide capped silver nanoparticles were measured by Zetasizer Nano ZS instrument (Malvern Instruments, United Kingdom) at a constant temperature of 25 ± 1°C. The samples (0.1 mg/ml) were suspended in Milli-Q water and sonicated for 1 min. The mean hydrodynamic diameter and zeta potential for each sample was measured in triplicate and the results were measured as mean size ± SD. The surface plasmon resonance (SPR) was recorded at different time points (10–150 min) for polysaccharide-capped silver nanoparticles (AgNP) against the only carboxyl methyl tamarind (CMT) polysaccharide solution as blank.

### Determining Hemocompatibility of Silver Nanoparticle

Hemocompatibility of polysaccharide capped silver nanoparticle was determined in terms of percent hemolysis using sheep blood (Mangalaraj and Devi, 2017). The diluted suspension of extracted RBCs (0.2 ml) was mixed with varied concentrations (1, 3, 6, 9, and 12 μg/ml) of AgNPs in PBS (0.8 ml). Diluted suspension of RBCs mixed with 0.8 ml PBS and 0.8 ml double distilled water were used as negative and positive control, respectively. The mixture was gently vortexed and incubated at room temperature for 3 h. After centrifugation (1600 rpm, 5 min) of the incubated mixture, absorbance of the supernatant was recorded at 541 nm by UV-Vis spectrophotometer (Agilent Cary 100 UV-Vis, Germany). Finally, hemocompatibility was evaluated in terms of percent hemolysis using the formula: $(A_S - A_N)/(A_P - A_N) \times 100$; where "$A_S$" is the sample absorbance, "$A_N$" is the absorbance of negative control and "$A_P$" is the absorbance of positive control (Jana et al., 2016).

### Determining Effect of CMT-Capped Ag-MCNP on Mammalian Cells

The cytotoxic effect of polysaccharide capped nanoparticles against Mouse macrophage (RAW 264.7) cells were evaluated by MTT [3-(4,5-Dimethylthiazol-2-Yl)-2,5-Diphenyltetrazolium Bromide] assay. Approximately, $1 \times 10^4$ cells were seeded in 96-well plates (Tarsons, India) and were incubated for 24 h at 37°C in a 5% $CO_2$ incubator with different concentration of Ag-MCNP's (1, 2, 3, 4, and 6 μg/ml, respectively). Raw cells seeded without nanoparticles were used as control. To determine the cell viability, MTT dye (100 μl from 0.1 mg/ml stock) was added to each well and incubated for 4 h at 37°C, 5% $CO_2$ in dark. In this assay, metabolically active cells reduce the MTT salt into water insoluble purple MTT formazan crystal by mitochondrial dehydrogenase. The formazan crystals formed as a result of cellular reduction of MTT were dissolved in buffer solution (4 g NP-40 detergent in 50 ml 0.02 M HCl and 50 ml isopropanol) and incubated for 1 h at 37°C and absorbance was measured at 570 nm in an ELISA reader (BioTek, Germany). The percentage of cell viability at different doses of Ag-MCNPs was obtained by the following formula: % cell viability = [OD sample - OD control] - 100/OD control.

## Determination of Minimum Inhibitory Concentration (MIC) Breakpoints for Nanoparticles

Minimum inhibitory concentration (MIC) values were determined for both the nanoparticles *viz.* silver nanoparticle (AgNP) and silver-metal-carbohydrate nanoparticles (Ag-MCNP's) by macrobroth double dilution method based on the guidelines of Clinical Laboratory Standard Institute (CLSI) for Enterobacteriaceae (CLSI, 2016). Ten microliters of mid log bacterial cultures ($OD_{600\ nm}$: 0.6–0.8) were inoculated into MHB with different concentration (μg/ml) of nanoparticles. Inoculated tubes were incubated at 37°C, 220 rpm in bacteriological incubator shaker (New Brunswick, NJ, United States). MIC break point values (in μg/ml) were noted after overnight incubation at the above-mentioned conditions. Further, we checked survival of the bacteria by dilution plating onto MHA plates to enumerate viable colonies.

## Determining Effect of Silver Nanoparticles on AcrAB-TolC Efflux Pump Protein Expression

The bacterial cells of ($OD_{600\ nm}$: 0.6–0.8), were treated with sub-MIC concentration of nanoparticles, i.e., AgNPs (6 μg/ml) and Ag-MCNPs (0.75 μg/ml), and incubated for specified time points (e.g., 0, 30, 60, 120, 180 min). Both the treated and control bacterial cells were pelleted down, washed once with 1X PBS (pH 7.4), dissolved in 1X PBS and kept on ice. The protein samples were preserved by adding proteinase-K, lysed by treating with 5X Lamelli buffer and heat denatured at 95°C for 5 min. Extracted protein samples were then loaded onto 12% polyacrylamide gels, transferred to polyvinylidene fluoride (PVDF) membrane (Millipore, United States) for 1 h at 17 V, blocked by 5% skimmed milk in Tris buffered Saline with 0.05% Tween-20 (1X TBST). Blots were incubated with custom synthesized anti-rabbit polyclonal anti-AcrA, anti-AcrB, and anti-TolC primary antibodies (GenScript, United States) at 1:1000 dilutions overnight at 4°C. After incubation, blots were washed thrice with 1X TBST. Further blots were incubated with goat anti-rabbit immunoglobulin secondary antibodies (1:10,000) conjugated to horseradish peroxidase. Specific bands were visualized by Chemiluminescence method using SuperSignal$^{TM}$ West Femto maximum sensitivity substrate kit (Thermo Scientific, United States). The images were acquired using ChemiDoc and analyzed using Quantity-one software (Bio-Rad, United States).

## RESULTS

### Resistance Profile of *Enterobacter* Isolates

The wild type *E. cloacae* clinical isolate (EspIMS6) exhibited extreme drug resistant (XDR) phenotype with resistance to β-lactams, cephalosporins belonging to second and third-generation, imipenem, fluoroquinolones (**Table 1**). The type strain, *E. cloacae* ATCC 13047 displayed MDR phenotype. Both of these isolates harbor multidrug efflux system AcrAB-TolC belonging to RND superfamily (data not shown).

### Characterization of Silver Nanoparticles Used

#### Physical Characterization of the Nanoparticles Used

The size of nanoparticles has direct relevance with the stability, surface charge, bio distribution, cellular uptake, and drug release of nanomedicine (Lamprecht et al., 2001). The average size measured from photon correlation spectroscopy was found to be 140 d.nm in terms of number percent distribution (**Figures 1A,B**). The poly-dispersity index (PDI) of 0.208 indicated the monodispersed pattern of nanoparticles (Chandni et al., 2013). The surface charge of nanoparticles is another vital physical characteristic affecting its stability. The surface characteristics of polysaccharide capped AgNPs was measured upon immediate synthesis and 6 months post-synthesis. The mean zeta potential of AgNP was measured to be $-34.5 \pm 2.2$ mV (**Figures 1C,D**). Nanoparticles with zeta potential values outside the range of +30 to −30 mV are considered stable for a longer period in suspended state (Yue et al., 2008). To validate long-term stability of suspended AgNPs, hydrodynamic diameter, PDI and surface charge were measured 6 months post-synthesis by photon correlation spectroscopy and results compared with those obtained for initially synthesized AgNPs. Our data suggest that there is slight increase in hydrodynamic diameter (161 d.nm), with PDI (0.426) and surface charge (−28.6) (**Figures 1A,B**). However, PDI smaller than 0.5 suggested that there is no agglomeration of nanoparticles and thus these particles are stable at room temperature for longer period of time (Yue et al., 2008). Further CMT-capped AgNP was characterized by SPR observed from UV-Vis spectral analysis. The occurrence of single maximum peak at wavelength 420 nm corresponded to the SPR of AgNPs (**Figure 1E**), and reflected about the size of AgNPs to be around 30–40 nm (Oldenburg, 2012). Further characterization of this AgNP such as size, dispersion, crystallinity and presence of silver has been performed by TEM, FE-SEM, XRD and EDAX methods, which was reported in our previous article (Sanyasi et al., 2016).

**TABLE 1** | Antibiotic susceptibility profile of clinical *Enterobacter cloacae* isolates.

| Strains | Resistant (R) | Susceptible (S) | Intermediate (I) |
|---|---|---|---|
| EspIMS6 | CZX, CX, LE, CTR, TCC, PIT, GAT, A/S, CTX, AMC, OF, CIP, AMP, CXM, IPM, CPM, COT, CAZ, CAC, AT | GEN, AK | MRP |
| ATCC 13047 | AMC, CXM, AMP, CAZ, CX, CAC, A/S | COT, CPM, IPM, CIP, GEN, GAT, AT, OF, AK, MRP, PIT, CZX, LE | CTR, CTX |

*Antibiotic resistance profile of EspIMS6 and E. cloacae type strain ATCC 13047 control using DoDeca Enterobacteriaceae disks 1 and 2 (Himedia, India). Disk 1: Ampicillin-AMP (10 mcg), Gentamicin-GEN (10 mcg), Amikacin-AK (30 mcg), Ciprofloxacin-CIP (5 mcg), Ofloxacin-OF (5 mcg), Co-Trimoxazole-COT (25 mcg), Amoxyclav-AMC (30 mcg), Cefuroxime-CXM (30 mcg), Ceftazidime-CAZ (30 mcg), Ceftazidime/Clavulanic acid-CAC (30/10 mcg), Cefepime-CPM (30 mcg), Imipenem-IPM (10 mcg). Disk 2: Cefotaxime-CTX (30 mcg), Cetriaxone-CTR (30 mcg), Cefoxitin-CX (30 mcg), Meropenem-MRP (10 mcg), Piperacillin/Tazobactam-PIT (100/10 mcg), Aztreonam-AT (30 mcg), Gatifloxacin-GAT (5 mcg), Ampicillin/Sulbactam-A/S (10/10 mcg), Cefoperazone-CPZ (75 mcg), Levofloxacin-LE (5 mcg), Ceftizoxime-CZX (30 mcg), Ticarcillin/Clavulanic acid-TCC (75/10 mcg).*

#### Hemocompatibility of Silver Nanoparticles

Extent of hemolysis of red blood cells was determined to check hemocompatibility of silver nanoparticles. It was observed that AgNPs at concentrations of 1, 3 and 6 μg/ml, exhibited only 0.063, 0.31, and 0.63% of hemolysis, respectively (**Figure 2**). At higher concentrations of AgNP (i.e., 9 and 12 μg/ml) hemolysis was approximately 2%. Nanoparticles exhibiting hemolysis below 5% are considered hemocompatible (Jana et al., 2016). Hence, our results indicated that AgNPs to be hemocompatible.

#### Effect of Ag-MCNPs on Cell Viability

We had previously shown that AgNP's were non-toxic to mammalian cells (Sanyasi et al., 2016). Here, we have assessed the cytotoxic effect of Ag-MCNPs on macrophage RAW 264.7 cell line using MTT assay. The MTT assay is rapid, sensitive, and inexpensive method to determine cell viability. The dose dependent viability of RAW 264.7 cells in different concentration of the Ag-MCNPs is shown in **Figure 3**. Cell viability result revealed that 99% cells were viable in presence of Ag-MCNPs at concentration of up to 3 μg/ml, while at 4 μg/ml concentration of Ag-MCNPs, 82% cells remained viable (**Figure 3**). However, at higher concentration (6 μg/ml) of Ag-MCNP, cell viability was reduced to 55% suggesting that Ag-MCNP was toxic to mammalian cells at this dosage. This indicated that Ag-MCNPs below concentrations of 6 μg/ml are non-toxic to mammalian cells. Notably, the concentration of Ag-MCNPs that was antibacterial in nature (i.e., 1.5 and 3 μg/ml), are non-toxic to mammalian cells and hence could be suitable for biomedical applications.

### Antimicrobial Efficacy of AgNP and Ag-MCNP

We determined the MIC breakpoints for sliver nanoparticle (AgNP) and Ag-MCNP. We observed that both the nanoparticles tested significantly inhibited bacterial growth in a dose dependent manner (**Table 2** and Supplementary Figure S1). However, MIC

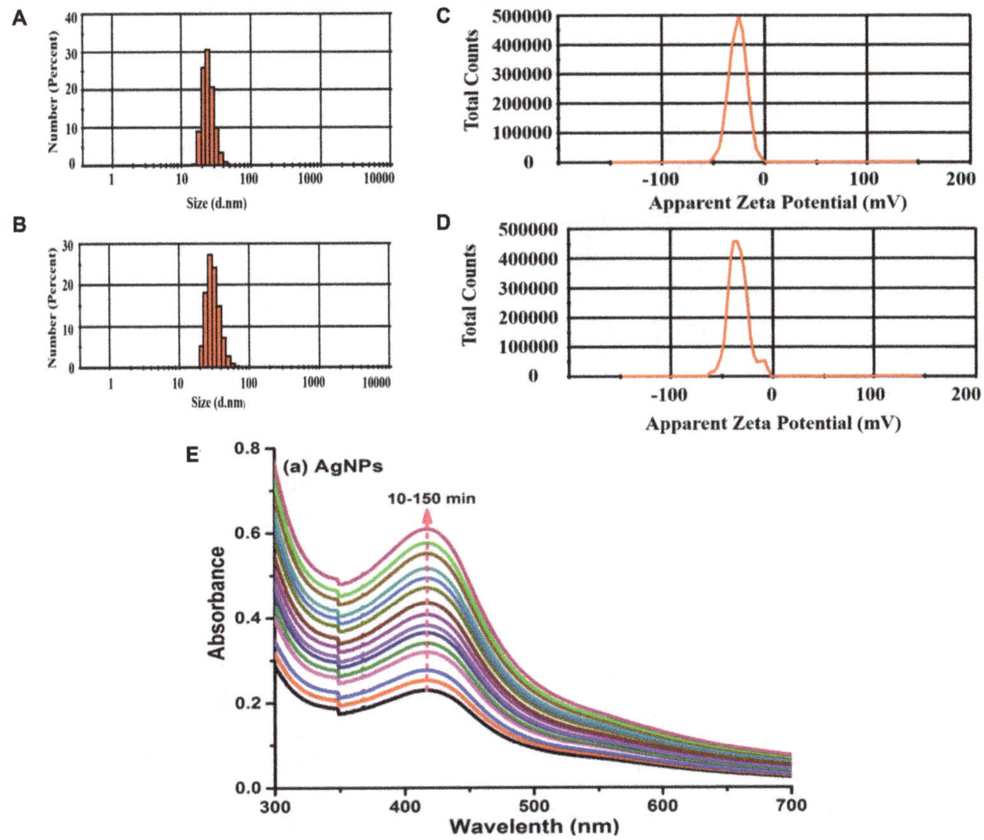


**FIGURE 1 |** Characterization of silver nanoparticles. Size of AgNps was determined by photon correlation spectroscopy immediately after synthesis **(A)** and 6 months post-synthesis **(B)**. Stability of AgNPs in terms of Zeta potential (–34 mV) was measured immediately after synthesis **(C)** and 6 months post-synthesis **(D)**. Determination of stability of AgNPs by SPR was conducted at λmax 420 over 10–150 min **(E)**.

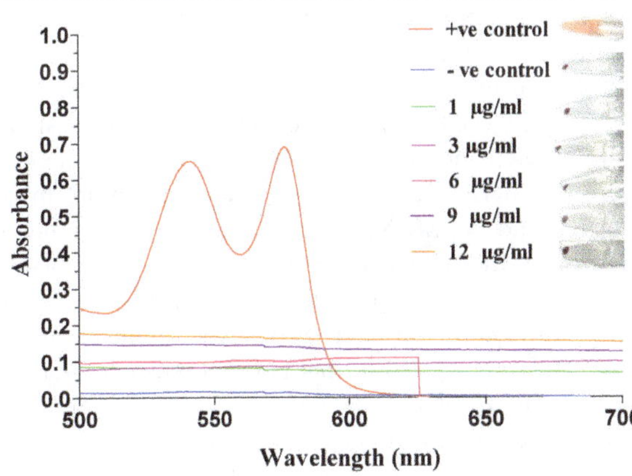


**FIGURE 2 |** Hemolysis activity of silver nanoparticle. Determination of hemolytic activity at different concentrations (1, 3, 6, 9, and 12 μg/ml) of Ag-NPs, along with positive and negative control, recorded at 541 nm by UV-Vis spectrophotometer.

breakpoint for AgNPs was 12 μg/ml for both EspIMS6 and *E. cloacae* ATCC 13047. Interestingly, Ag-MCNPs had a much lower MIC breakpoint of 1.5 and 3 μg/ml for isolates EspIMS6 and *E. cloacae* ATCC 13047, respectively. The results clearly indicated that Ag-MCNPs was more efficient in killing the MDR *E. cloacae* compared to AgNPs alone.

## Effect of Silver Nanoparticles on AcrAB-TolC Efflux Pump Protein Expression

As reported from the literature, success of potential antibacterial agents rested upon their efficacy to be retained in the cell vis-à-vis being effluxed out. We investigated this by studying the effect of silver nanoparticles on expression of multidrug efflux pump proteins AcrAB-TolC.

Overall immunoblotting results revealed that presence of silver nanoparticles did not significantly affect AcrA and TolC efflux pump protein expression (**Figures 4A,C**). However, in the *E. cloacae* ATCC 13047, AcrB, and TolC protein expression showed slight albeit insignificant decrease in presence of Ag-MCNPs (**Figures 4B,C** and Supplementary Figure S2). Inhibition of AcrB monomeric protein expression was more prominent in clinical isolate EspIMS6, where only 38 kDa AcrB protein was consistently expressed at all the time points of exposure to AgNP (at 6 μg/ml) as well as Ag-MCNP (at 0.75 μg/ml) (**Figure 4B** and Supplementary Figure S2). Though, ~112 kDa

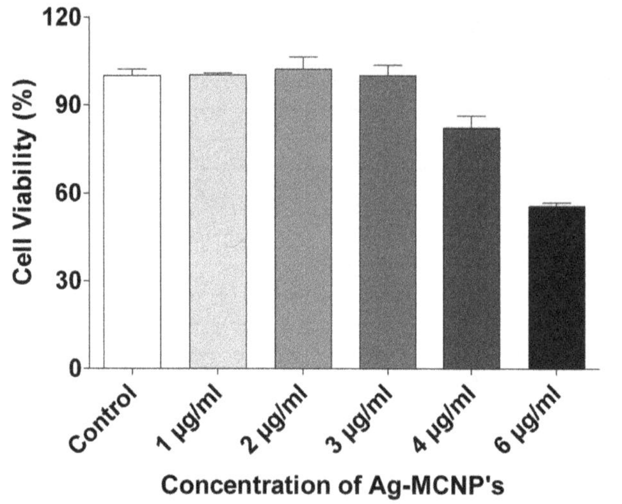


**FIGURE 3** | Cytotoxicity assay of silver nanoparticle. Effect of Ag-MCNP on cell viability was determined by MTT assay with RAW 264.7 cells with increasing concentrations (1, 2, 3, 4, and 6 µg/ml) of the nanoparticle. Percentage of cell viability was calculated with respect to untreated cells.

**TABLE 2** | Antibacterial activity of silver and silver-metal composite nanoparticles.

| Isolates ID | MIC (in µg/ml) | |
|---|---|---|
| | AgNP | Ag-MCNP |
| EspIMS6 | 12 | 1.5 |
| ATCC-13047 | 12 | 3 |

band was less expressed in *E. cloacae* ATCC 13047 in response to AgNP (at 6 µg/ml), a 38 kDa band of AcrB was observed post 30 min of treatment with Ag-MCNP at a concentration of 0.75 µg/ml in *E. cloacae* ATCC 13047 (**Figure 4B**, panels 3 and 4 and Supplementary Figure S2). It is pertinent to mention here that, AcrB is a transmembrane RND transporter protein of the tripartite efflux pump assembly. The functional membrane embedded protein is a homotrimer with molecular masses of ~380 kDa, with each monomer of approximately 112 kDa (Tikhonova et al., 2011). However, in both isolates EspIMS6 and *E. cloacae* ATCC 13047 treated with the AgNP nanoparticles, it was shown to inhibit monomeric 112 kDa bands, and showed bands corresponding to ~38 kDa (Supplementary Figure S2). This ~38 kDa band perhaps represents the truncated by product of the AcrB protein complex. It is pertinent to mention that the antibodies used were beyond doubt.

Expression of outer membrane protein TolC decreased post 120 min in *E. cloacae* ATCC 13047, in presence both the silver nanoparticles tested *viz.* AgNPs and Ag-MCNPs (**Figure 4C**, panels 3 and 4). Here too we did not observe any significant changes in TolC expression for the wild type isolate EspIMS6 in presence of either of the nanoparticles (**Figure 4C**, panels 1 and 2).

## DISCUSSION

The present study reports no decrease in antibacterial efficacy of silver nanoparticles *viz.* AgNP and Ag-MCNP, despite expression of AcrAB-TolC efflux protein in MDR bacteria. This finding is significant as it reports no noticeable effect of nanoparticles on AcrAB-TolC efflux pump protein expression that are implicated in MDR phenotype. Secondly, the results corroborate with our previous report and confirm sustainability of using the said silver nanoparticles as antibacterial agents.

During the past decade, silver nanoparticles owing to their low toxicity, antibacterial and wound healing properties, have emerged as promising therapeutic alternatives (Ambrožová et al., 2017). To ensure feasibility of large-scale use of nanoparticles for medicinal purposes, eco-friendly approaches have been widely adapted to generate silver nanoparticles. Such approaches circumvent the use of toxic chemicals and hazardous equipment. Eco-friendly green synthesis approach utilizes natural cost-effective reductants such as microorganisms and plant products (Rao and Tang, 2017). We had earlier reported utilization of green synthesis approach to generate polysaccharide-capped AgNPs (Sanyasi et al., 2016).

Few of the important physical parameters essential for development of nanoparticles include size and surface charge that affects their stability (Lamprecht et al., 2001). In the present study, photon correlation spectroscopy results revealed that the CMT-capped AgNPs were smaller in size and are monodispersed in nature (Chandni et al., 2013). The mean zeta potential of AgNPs used was measured to be $-34.5 \pm 2.2$ mV, suggesting higher electrical charge on their surface and thus, approved their long-term stability (Yue et al., 2008). SPR characterization of AgNPs demonstrated their size to be around 30–40 nm, which corroborated well with previous report (Oldenburg, 2012). Biocompatibility is extremely important feature for nanoparticles to be used as therapeutic agents. For this, we performed hemolysis assay that described the AgNPs to be non-hemolytic. We had previously reported AgNPs to be less cytotoxic toward mammalian cells even at higher concentrations (Sanyasi et al., 2016). The newly developed Ag-MCNPs reported here, too displayed minimal cytotoxic activity toward mammalian cells. Both AgNPs and Ag-MCNPs revealed excellent antimicrobial activity against multiple drug resistant *E. cloacae* isolates at low dose. Our results corroborated well with previous reports suggesting antimicrobial properties of silver nanoparticles (Kim et al., 2007; Chen et al., 2014), that boosted their candidature as potential antimicrobial agents. Durán et al. (2016) proposed cell membrane disruption by the silver ions as a plausible mechanism of antibacterial activity by silver nanoparticles.

However, one of the less addressed aspect has been the effect of AgNPs on bacterial efflux systems. Kovács et al. (2016) reported AgNPs to inhibit activity of *p*-glycoproteins efflux pump (belonging to ABC transporter family) in MDR cancer cells, thereby enhancing effectiveness of chemotherapy. Christena et al. (2015) have established the efflux inhibitory properties of copper nanoparticles (CuNPs) in tackling MDR *Staphylococcus aureus* and *Pseudomonas aeruginosa* isolates. However, effect of AgNPs on expression of bacterial

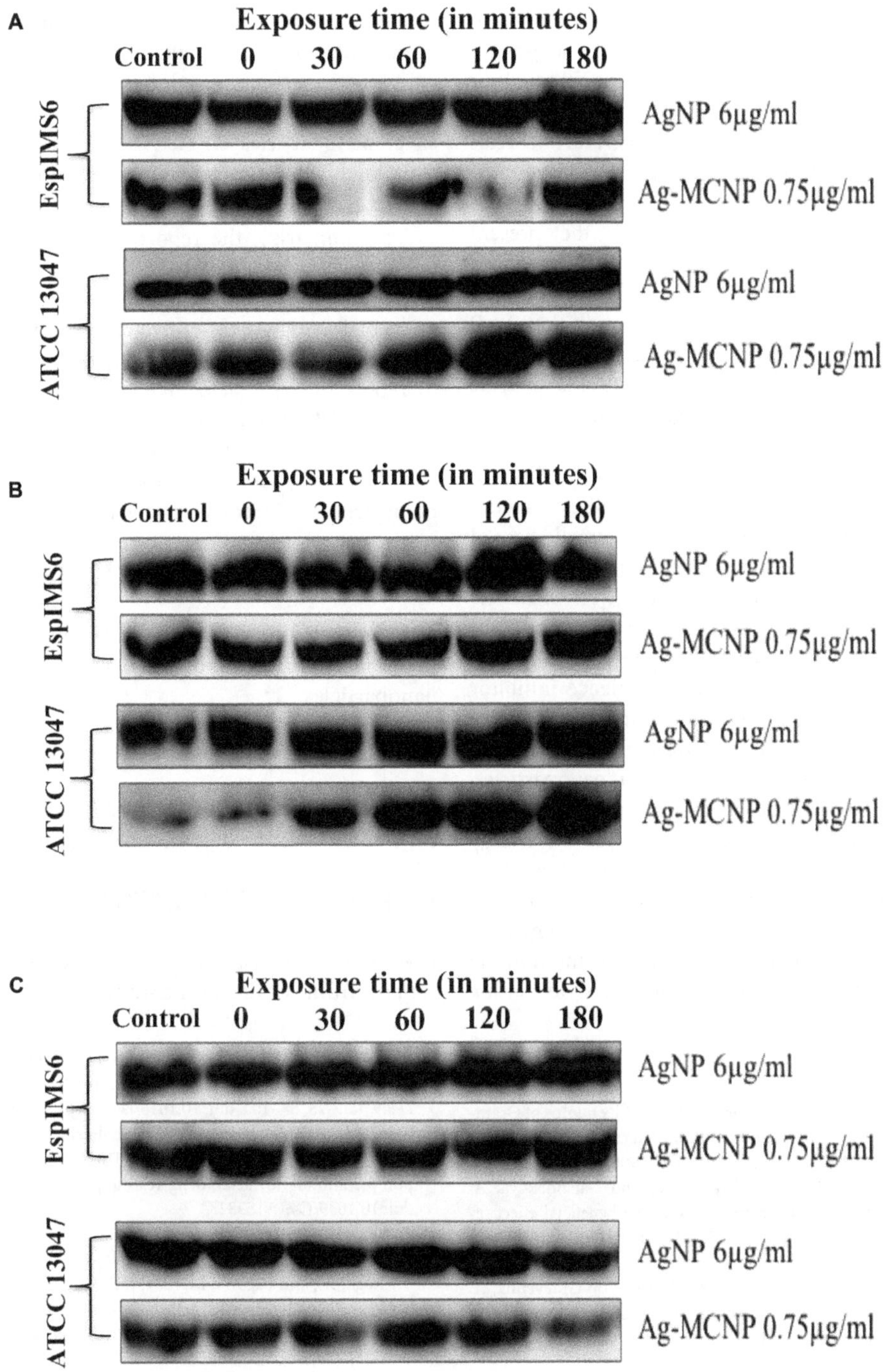


**FIGURE 4 |** Effect of silver and silver-metal composite nanoparticles on AcrAB-TolC expression. **(A)** AcrA (42 kDa) protein expression in EspIMS6 (top panel) and *Enterobacter cloacae* ATCC 13047 (bottom panel); **(B)** AcrB (~38 kDa) protein expression in EspIMS6 (top panel) and *E. cloacae* ATCC 13047 (bottom panel); **(C)** TolC (55 kDa) protein expression in EspIMS6 (top panel) and *E. cloacae* ATCC 13047 (bottom panel).

MDR efflux pumps has not been elucidated. AcrAB-TolC efflux pumps have been found to mediate MDR phenotype in many clinically significant gram-negative pathogens including *E. cloacae* (Piddock, 2006; Pérez et al., 2012; Amaral et al., 2013). These efflux systems efficiently extrude out of the bacterial cell, structurally divergent classes of drugs, resulting in multiple antibiotic resistance phenotype (Poole, 2005; Sun et al., 2014). This prompted us to study the effect of AgNPs and Ag-MCNPs on AcrAB-TolC efflux pump protein expression. Our results indicated that AgNPs affected the expression of AcrB transporter protein to a greater extent as compared to AcrA and TolC. Functional AcrB is a trimeric RND transporter protein with each monomer of ~112 kDa (Du et al., 2015). Review of literature reveals antimicrobial drugs to induce over expression of AcrAB-TolC efflux pump protein, which in turn facilitates their rapid extrusion (Rosenberg et al., 2003). In the present study, expression of functional AcrB protein was reduced in *E. cloacae* isolates upon addition of silver nanoparticles (Supplementary Figure S2). It is pertinent to mention that AcrB protein is responsible for substrate recognition and binding of diverse structures (Sun et al., 2014). The results provide circumstantial evidence indicative of AgNPs functioning as efflux inhibitor. Efflux inhibitory role of metal nanoparticles have been hypothesized to be either by direct binding to active site of the efflux pumps or hindering efflux kinetics (Gupta et al., 2017). However, owing to the small size of nanoparticles and substrate non-specific nature of efflux pumps proteins these explicit mechanisms still remain elusive. Earlier studies have shown that expression of AcrB transporter is affected by cellular metabolites (Ruiz and Levy, 2014) and hence forms an ideal target for efflux and virulence inhibitor design (Blair et al., 2015). Also, AcrB is a proton motive force (PMF) dependent RND transporter. Interestingly, Dibrov et al. (2002) in a study on mechanism of action of nanoparticles, observed that metal nanoparticles such as AgNPs, dissipate PMF by interfering with bacterial respiration. Hence, energy required for this tripartite efflux system may be hindered by the addition of AgNPs. In the present study, in presence of AgNPs, though TolC and AcrA protein expression remained more or less unaffected, the absence of a functional monomeric AcrB perhaps renders the bacterial cells impaired for efflux activity. Change in efflux activity in *Enterobacter* spp. by AgNPs has been reported in context of EmmDR efflux pump [belonging to multiple antibiotic and toxic extrusion (MATE) superfamily] (Gui et al., 2013). However, to the best of our knowledge, this is the first report on effect of silver nanoparticles on AcrAB-TolC efflux protein expression. This study indicates potential efflux inhibitor property of the AgNPs.

To summarize, the reported silver nanoparticles generated by green synthesis method, are highly stable, small in size, non-hemolytic with minimal cytotoxic effect. Further, their antimicrobial activity is not affected by expression of AcrAB-TolC efflux proteins. Such versatile repertoire of qualities enables us to report the said silver nanoparticles as strong candidates as antibacterial agents. The results of the present study support further development of silver nanoparticle formulations as alternate therapeutic agents to combat infections caused by MDR gram-negative Enterobacterial pathogens.

## AUTHOR CONTRIBUTIONS

The present study was conceived by HM and executed by MM. SK, LG, RM, and CG developed and characterized the nanoparticles.

## FUNDING

MM received INSPIRE fellowship from the Department of Science and Technology, New Delhi (Grant No. IF110739).

## ACKNOWLEDGMENTS

HM and MM thankfully acknowledge intramural financial support from NISER for the study.

## REFERENCES

Amaral, L., Martins, A., Spengler, G., and Molnar, J. (2013). Efflux pumps of Gram-negative bacteria: What they do, how they do it, with what and how to deal with them. *Front. Pharmacol.* 4:168. doi: 10.3389/fphar.2013.0900168

Ambrožová, N., Zálešák, B., Ulrichová, J., Čížková, K., and Galandáková, A. (2017). Low concentrations of silver nanoparticles have a beneficial effect on wound healing in vitro. *J. Nanoparticle Res.* 19:108. doi: 10.1007/s11051-017-3809-7

Bauer, A. W., Kirby, W. M., Sherris, J. C., Turck, A. M., and Von Graevenitz, A. (1966). 40 Microbiology:a centenary perspective 1966 antibiotic susceptibility testing by a standardized single disk method. *Am. J. Clin. Pathol.* 45, 493–496. doi: 10.1093/ajcp/45.4_ts.493

Blair, J. M., Smith, H. E., Ricci, V., Lawler, A. J., Thompson, L. J., and Piddock, L. J. V. (2015). Expression of homologous RND efflux pump genes is dependent upon AcrB expression: implications for efflux and virulence inhibitor design. *J. Antimicrob. Chemother.* 70, 424–431. doi: 10.1093/jac/dku380

Boucher, W. H., Talbot, G. H., Bradley, J. S., Edwards, J. E., Gilbert, D., Rice, L. B., et al. (2009). Bad bugs, no drugs: no ESKAPE! An update from the infectious diseases society of America. *Clin. Infect. Dis.* 48, 1–12. doi: 10.1086/595011

Chandni, Andhariya, N., Pandey, O., and Chudasama, B. (2013). A growth kinetic study of ultrafine monodispersed silver nanoparticles. *RSC Adv.* 3, 1127–1136. doi: 10.1039/C2RA21912C

Chen, C. W., Hsu, C. Y., Lai, S. M., Syu, W. J., Wang, T. Y., and Lai, P. S. (2014). Metal nanobullets for multidrug resistant bacteria and biofilms. *Adv. Drug Deliv. Rev.* 78, 88–104. doi: 10.1016/j.addr.2014.08.004

Christena, L. R., Mangalagowri, V., Pradheeba, P., Ahmed, K. B. A., Shalini, B. I. S., Vidyalakshmi, M., et al. (2015). Copper nanoparticles as an efflux pump inhibitor to tackle drug resistant bacteria. *RSC Adv.* 5, 12899–12909. doi: 10.1039/C4RA15382K

CLSI (2016). *M100S: Performance Standards for Antimicrobial Susceptibility Testing.* Wayne, PA: CLSI.

Davin-Regli, A., and Pagès, J. M. (2015). *Enterobacter* aerogenes and *Enterobacter cloacae*; Versatile bacterial pathogens confronting antibiotic treatment. *Front. Microbiol.* 6:392. doi: 10.3389/fmicb.2015.00392

Dibrov, P., Dzioba, J., Gosink, K. K., Häse, C. C., and Ha, C. C. (2002). Chemiosmotic mechanism of antimicrobial activity of Ag+ in *Vibrio cholerae. Antimicrob. Agents Chemother.* 46, 2668–2670. doi: 10.1128/AAC.46.8.2668

Du, D., Wang, Z., James, N. R., Voss, J. E., Klimont, E., Ohene-, T., et al. (2015). Structure of the AcrAB-TolC multidrug efflux pump. *Nature* 509, 512–515. doi: 10.1038/nature13205

Durán, N., Durán, M., de Jesus, M. B., Seabra, A. B., Fávaro, W. J., and Nakazato, G. (2016). Silver nanoparticles: a new view on mechanistic aspects on antimicrobial activity. *Nanomedicine* 12, 789–799. doi: 10.1016/j.nano.2015.11.016

Fraser, S. L., and Arnett, M. (2010). *Enterobacter* infections. *J. WebM D* 7, 114–120.

Gelperina, S., Kisich, K., Iseman, M. D., and Heifets, L. (2005). The potential advantages of nanoparticle drug delivery systems in chemotherapy of tuberculosis. *Am. J. Respir. Crit. Care Med.* 172, 1487–1490. doi: 10.1164/rccm.200504-613PP

Grimont, F., and Grimont, P. (2006). The genus *Enterobacter. Prokaryotes* 6, 197–214. doi: 10.1007/0-387-30746-x_9

Gui, H., Wei, Z., Huizhong, C., Sam, S., Conner, T., Eugene, R., et al. (2013). Impacts of silver nanoparticles on bacterial multidrug efflux pump. *FASEB J.* 27. Available at: https://www.fasebj.org/doi/abs/10.1096/fasebj.27.1_supplement.575.12

Gupta, D., Singh, A., and Khan, A. U. (2017). Nanoparticles as efflux pump and biofilm inhibitor to rejuvenate bactericidal effect of conventional antibiotics. *Nanoscale Res. Lett.* 12:454. doi: 10.1186/s11671-017-2222-6

Jana, S. K., Mandal, A. K., Kumar, A., Puschmann, H., Hossain, M., and Dalai, S. (2016). Sensing of tryptophan by a non-toxic cobalt(II) complex. *RSC Adv.* 6, 95888–95896. doi: 10.1039/c6ra16086g

Kerantzas, C. A., and Jacobs, W. R. (2017). Origins of combination therapy for tuberculosis: lessons for future antimicrobial development and application. *mBio* 8:e01586-16. doi: 10.1128/mBio.01586-16

Kim, J. S., Kuk, E., Yu, K. N., Kim, J. H., Park, S. J., Lee, H. J., et al. (2007). Antimicrobial effects of silver nanoparticles. *Nanomedicine* 3, 95–101. doi: 10.1016/j.nano.2006.12.001

Kovács, D., Szoke, K., Igaz, N., Spengler, G., Molnár, J., Tóth, T., et al. (2016). Silver nanoparticles modulate ABC transporter activity and enhance chemotherapy in multidrug resistant cancer. *Nanomedicine* 12, 601–610. doi: 10.1016/j.nano.2015.10.015

Lamprecht, A., Schäfer, U., and Lehr, C. M. (2001). Size-dependent bioadhesion of micro- and nanoparticulate carriers to the inflamed colonic mucosa. *Pharm. Res.* 18, 788–793. doi: 10.1023/A:1011032328064

Mahlapuu, M., Håkansson, J., Ringstad, L., and Björn, C. (2016). Antimicrobial peptides: an emerging category of therapeutic agents. *Front. Cell. Infect. Microbiol.* 6:194. doi: 10.3389/fcimb.2016.00194

Mangalaraj, D., and Devi, D. N. (2017). "Ag/TiO2 (Metal/Metal Oxide) core shell nanoparticles for biological applications," in *Recent Trends in Materials Science and Applications*, ed. J. Ebenezar (Cham: Springer International Publishing), 9–17. doi: 10.1007/978-3-319-44890-9_2

Martins, M., and McCusker, M. P. (2016). Editorial: Alternative therapeutics against MDR bacteria - "Fighting the epidemic of antibiotic resistance." *Front. Microbiol.* 7:1559. doi: 10.3389/fmicb.2016.01559

Mezzatesta, M. L., Gona, F., and Stefani, S. (2012). *Enterobacter cloacae* complex: clinical impact and emerging antibiotic resistance. *Future Microbiol.* 7, 887–902. doi: 10.2217/fmb.12.61

Oldenburg, S. J. (2012). *Silver Nanoparticles: Properties and Applications. Sigma-Aldrich.* Available at: https://www.sigmaaldrich.com/technical-documents/articles/materials-science/nanomaterials/silver-nanoparticles.html

Pelgrift, R. Y., and Friedman, A. J. (2013). Nanotechnology as a therapeutic tool to combat microbial resistance. *Adv. Drug Deliv. Rev.* 65, 1803–1815. doi: 10.1016/j.addr.2013.07.011

Pendleton, J. N., Gorman, S. P., and Gilmore, B. F. (2013). Clinical relevance of the ESKAPE pathogens. *Expert Rev. Anti Infect. Ther.* 11, 297–308. doi: 10.1586/eri.13.12

Pérez, A., Poza, M., Fernández, A., Del Carmen Fernández, M., Mallo, S., Merino, M., et al. (2012). Involvement of the AcrAB-TolC efflux pump in the resistance, fitness, and virulence of *Enterobacter cloacae. Antimicrob. Agents Chemother.* 56, 2084–2090. doi: 10.1128/AAC.05509-11

Piddock, L. J. (2006). Clinically relevant chromosomally encoded multidrug resistance efflux pumps in bacteria. *Clin. Microbiol. Rev.* 19, 382–402. doi: 10.1128/CMR.19.2.382

Poole, K. (2005). Efflux-mediated antimicrobial resistance. *J Antimicrob Chemother.* 56, 20–51. doi: 10.1093/jac/dki171

Rangel-Vega, A., Bernstein, L. R., Mandujano-Tinoco, E. A., García-Contreras, S. J., and García-Contreras, R. (2015). Drug repurposing as an alternative for the treatment of recalcitrant bacterial infections. *Front. Microbiol.* 6:282. doi: 10.3389/fmicb.2015.00282

Rao, B., and Tang, R.-C. (2017). Green synthesis of silver nanoparticles with antibacterial activities using aqueous Eriobotrya japonica leaf extract. *Adv. Nat. Sci. Nanosci. Nanotechnol.* 80:015014. doi: 10.1088/2043-6254/aa5983

Rosenberg, E. Y., Bertenthal, D., Nilles, M. L., Bertrand, K. P., and Nikaido, H. (2003). Bile salts and fatty acids induce the expression of *Escherichia coli* AcrAB multidrug efflux pump through their interaction with Rob regulatory protein. *Mol. Microbiol.* 48, 1609–1619. doi: 10.1046/j.1365-2958.2003.03531.x

Ruiz, C., and Levy, S. B. (2014). Regulation of acrAB expression by cellular metabolites in *Escherichia coli. J. Antimicrob. Chemother.* 69, 390–399. doi: 10.1093/jac/dkt352

Salata, O. (2004). Applications of nanoparticles in biology and medicine. *J. Nanobiotechnol.* 2:3.

Sanders, W. E., and Sanders, C. C. (1997). *Enterobacter* spp.: Pathogens poised to flourish at the turn of the century. *Clin. Microbiol. Rev.* 10, 220–241.

Sanyasi, S., Majhi, R. K., Kumar, S., Mishra, M., Ghosh, A., Suar, M., et al. (2016). Polysaccharide-capped silver Nanoparticles inhibit biofilm formation and eliminate multi-drug-resistant bacteria by disrupting bacterial cytoskeleton with reduced cytotoxicity towards mammalian cells. *Sci. Rep.* 6:24929. doi: 10.1038/srep24929

Singh, R., and Lillard, J. W. (2009). Nanoparticle-based targeted drug delivery. *Exp. Mol. Pathol.* 86, 215–223. doi: 10.1016/j.yexmp.2008.12.004

Sun, J., Deng, Z., and Yan, A. (2014). Bacterial multidrug efflux pumps: Mechanisms, physiology and pharmacological exploitations. *Biochem. Biophys. Res. Commun.* doi: 10.1016/j.bbrc.2014.05.090

Tamma, P. D., Cosgrove, S. E., and Maragakis, L. L. (2012). Combination therapy for treatment of infections with gram-negative bacteria. *Clin. Microbiol. Rev.* 25, 450–470. doi: 10.1128/CMR.05041-11

Tikhonova, E. B., Yamada, Y., and Zgurskaya, H. I. (2011). Sequential mechanism of assembly of multidrug efflux pump AcrAB-TolC. *Chem. Biol.* 18, 454–463. doi: 10.1016/j.chembiol.2011.02.011

Tran, P. A., and Webster, T. J. (2011). Selenium nanoparticles inhibit *Staphylococcus aureus* growth. *Int. J. Nanomedicine* 6, 1553–1558. doi: 10.2147/IJN.S21729

WHO (2014). *ANTIMICROBIAL RESISTANCE Global Report on Surveillance 2014.* Geneva: WHO.

Yang, H., Yu, J., and Wei, H. (2014). Engineered bacteriophage lysins as novel anti-infectives. *Front. Microbiol.* 5:542. doi: 10.3389/fmicb.2014.00542

Yue, P. F., Yuan, H. L., Yang, M., You, R. H., Cong, L. B., Zhu, J., et al. (2008). Preparation, characterization, and pharmacokinetic evaluation of puerarin submicron emulsion. *PDA J. Pharm. Sci. Technol.* 62, 32–45.

Zgurskaya, H. I. (2009). Multicomponent drug efflux complexes: architecture and mechanism of assembly. *Future Microbiol.* 4, 919–932. doi: 10.2217/fmb.09.62. Multicomponent

# Permissions

All chapters in this book were first published by Frontiers; hereby published with permission under the Creative Commons Attribution License or equivalent. Every chapter published in this book has been scrutinized by our experts. Their significance has been extensively debated. The topics covered herein carry significant findings which will fuel the growth of the discipline. They may even be implemented as practical applications or may be referred to as a beginning point for another development.

The contributors of this book come from diverse backgrounds, making this book a truly international effort. This book will bring forth new frontiers with its revolutionizing research information and detailed analysis of the nascent developments around the world.

We would like to thank all the contributing authors for lending their expertise to make the book truly unique. They have played a crucial role in the development of this book. Without their invaluable contributions this book wouldn't have been possible. They have made vital efforts to compile up to date information on the varied aspects of this subject to make this book a valuable addition to the collection of many professionals and students.

This book was conceptualized with the vision of imparting up-to-date information and advanced data in this field. To ensure the same, a matchless editorial board was set up. Every individual on the board went through rigorous rounds of assessment to prove their worth. After which they invested a large part of their time researching and compiling the most relevant data for our readers.

The editorial board has been involved in producing this book since its inception. They have spent rigorous hours researching and exploring the diverse topics which have resulted in the successful publishing of this book. They have passed on their knowledge of decades through this book. To expedite this challenging task, the publisher supported the team at every step. A small team of assistant editors was also appointed to further simplify the editing procedure and attain best results for the readers.

Apart from the editorial board, the designing team has also invested a significant amount of their time in understanding the subject and creating the most relevant covers. They scrutinized every image to scout for the most suitable representation of the subject and create an appropriate cover for the book.

The publishing team has been an ardent support to the editorial, designing and production team. Their endless efforts to recruit the best for this project, has resulted in the accomplishment of this book. They are a veteran in the field of academics and their pool of knowledge is as vast as their experience in printing. Their expertise and guidance has proved useful at every step. Their uncompromising quality standards have made this book an exceptional effort. Their encouragement from time to time has been an inspiration for everyone.

The publisher and the editorial board hope that this book will prove to be a valuable piece of knowledge for researchers, students, practitioners and scholars across the globe.

# List of Contributors

**Li Guo, Dingxin Liu, Zhijie Liu and Xiaohua Wang**
State Key Laboratory of Electrical Insulation and Power Equipment, Center for Plasma Biomedicine, Xi'an Jiaotong University, Xi'an, China

**Ruobing Xu and Yiming Zhao**
School of Life Science and Technology, Xi'an Jiaotong University, Xi'an, China

**Hailan Chen**
Frank Reidy Center for Bioelectrics, Old Dominion University, Norfolk, VA, United States

**Michael G. Kong**
State Key Laboratory of Electrical Insulation and Power Equipment, Center for Plasma Biomedicine, Xi'an Jiaotong University, Xi'an, China
Frank Reidy Center for Bioelectrics, Old Dominion University, Norfolk, VA, United States
Department of Electrical and Computer Engineering, Old Dominion University, Norfolk, VA, United States

**Dairong Wang**
Department of Infectious Diseases, Sir Run Run Shaw Hospital, College of Medicine, Zhejiang University, Hangzhou, China
Blood Center of Zhejiang Province, Hangzhou, China

**Xinli Mu, Ying Chen, Dongdong Zhao, Yan Jiang, Yiwei Zhu, Jingjing Quan, Xiaoting Hua and Yunsong Yu**
Department of Infectious Diseases, Sir Run Run Shaw Hospital, College of Medicine, Zhejiang University, Hangzhou, China
Key Laboratory of Microbial Technology and Bioinformatics of Zhejiang Province, Zhejiang Institute of Microbiology, Hangzhou, China

**Ying Fu**
Key Laboratory of Microbial Technology and Bioinformatics of Zhejiang Province, Zhejiang Institute of Microbiology, Hangzhou, China
Department of Clinical Laboratory, Sir Run Run Shaw Hospital, College of Medicine, Zhejiang University, Hangzhou, China

**Cui-Ting Peng, Li Liu and Luo-Ting Yu**
Pharmaceutical and Biological Engineering Department, School of Chemical Engineering, Sichuan University, Chengdu, China
Center of Infectious Diseases, State Key Laboratory of Biotherapy, West China Hospital, Sichuan University and Collaborative Innovation Center, Chengdu, China

**Guofeng Mao**
Department of Laboratory Medicine, Shaoxing People's Hospital, Shaoxing, China

**Xi Li**
Centre of Laboratory Medicine, Zhejiang Provincial People's Hospital, People's Hospital of Hangzhou Medical College, Hangzhou, China

**Julang Li**
Department of Animal Biosciences, University of Guelph, Guelph, ON, Canada
College of Life Science and Engineering, Foshan University, Foshan, China

**Viviam de Oliveira Silva**
Department of Veterinary Medicine, Federal University of Lavras, Lavras, Brazil
Division of Periodontology, Diagnostic Sciences, Dental Hygiene and Biomedical Science, Herman Ostrow School of Dentistry, University of Southern California, Los Angeles, CA, United States

**Luciano José Pereira**
Department of Health Sciences, Federal University of Lavras, Lavras, Brazil

**Silvana Pasetto and Maike Paulino da Silva**
Division of Periodontology, Diagnostic Sciences, Dental Hygiene and Biomedical Science, Herman Ostrow School of Dentistry, University of Southern California, Los Angeles, CA, United States

**Jered Cope Meyers**
Department Foundational Sciences, School of Dental Medicine, East Carolina University, Greenville, NC, United States

**Ramiro Mendonça Murata**
Department Foundational Sciences, School of Dental Medicine, East Carolina University, Greenville, NC, United States
Department of Microbiology and Immunology, Brody School of Medicine, East Carolina University, Greenville, NC, United States

**Chang-Cheng Li, Li-Hui He, Tao Li, Ya-Lin Shen, Chao Gao, Yong Xia, Yi-Bo Zhu, Ying-Jie Song, Qian Lei and Rui Bao**
Center of Infectious Diseases, State Key Laboratory of Biotherapy, West China Hospital, Sichuan University and Collaborative Innovation Center, Chengdu, China

**Evanna Huynh and Nadeem Akhtar**
Department of Animal Biosciences, University of Guelph, Guelph, ON, Canada

**Ning-Yu Wang**
Center of Infectious Diseases, State Key Laboratory of Biotherapy, West China Hospital, Sichuan University and Collaborative Innovation Center, Chengdu, China
School of Life Sciences and Engineering, Southwest Jiaotong University, Chengdu, China

**Yixin Chen, Weifen Zhu, Hanxin Zhao and Lin Li**
Department of Endocrinology, Zhejiang University School of Medicine Sir Run Run Shaw Hospital, Hangzhou, China

**Ya Shi**
Hangzhou Digital Micro Biotech Co. Ltd., Hangzhou, China

**Jiaxing You, Jie Yang, Hongye Li Shunwu Fan and Chao Liu**
Department of Orthopedics, Zhejiang University School of Medicine Sir Run Run Shaw Hospital, Hangzhou, China

**Yaping Xie**
Department of Hematology, Affiliated Hangzhou First People's Hospital, Zhejiang University School of Medicine, Hangzhou, China

**Varsha Shriram**
Department of Botany, Prof. Ramkrishna More College, Savitribai Phule Pune University, Pune, India

**Tushar Khare**
Department of Biotechnology, Modern College of Arts, Science and Commerce (Savitribai Phule Pune University), Pune, India

**Rohit Bhagwat**
Department of Environmental Science, Savitribai Phule Pune University, Pune, India

**Ravi Shukla**
Centre for Advanced Materials and Industrial Chemistry, School of Science, RMIT University, Melbourne, VIC, Australia

**Vinay Kumar**
Department of Biotechnology, Modern College of Arts, Science and Commerce (Savitribai Phule Pune University), Pune, India
Department of Environmental Science, Savitribai Phule Pune University, Pune, India

**Yong-Guy Kim, Jin-Hyung Lee, Chaitany J. Raorane and Jintae Lee**
School of Chemical Engineering, Yeungnam University, Gyeongsan, South Korea

**Seong T. Oh**
College of Pharmacy, Yeungnam University, Gyeongsan, South Korea

**Jae G. Park**
Advanced Bio Convergence Center, Pohang Technopark Foundation, Pohang, South Korea

**Yan Li, Qian Wang and Kai Peng**
College of Veterinary Medicine, Yangzhou University, Yangzhou, China

**Yuan Liu and Ruichao Li**
College of Veterinary Medicine, Yangzhou University, Yangzhou, China
Institute of Comparative Medicine, Yangzhou University, Yangzhou, China
Jiangsu Co-innovation Center for Prevention and Control of Important Animal Infectious Diseases and Zoonoses, Yangzhou University, Yangzhou, China

**Zhiqiang Wang**
College of Veterinary Medicine, Yangzhou University, Yangzhou, China
Jiangsu Co-innovation Center for Prevention and Control of Important Animal Infectious Diseases and Zoonoses, Yangzhou University, Yangzhou, China

**Hua-le Chen**
Department of Clinical Laboratory, The First Affiliated Hospital of Wenzhou Medical University, Wenzhou, China
Department of Laboratory Medicine, The Second Affiliated Hospital of Wenzhou Medical University, Wenzhou, China

**Yan Jiang and Mei-mei Li**
Department of Infectious Diseases, Sir Run Run Shaw Hospital, Zhejiang University School of Medicine, Hangzhou, China

**Yao Sun, Cui Zhou, Xiao-xiao Zhang and Tie-li Zhou**
Department of Clinical Laboratory, The First Affiliated Hospital of Wenzhou Medical University, Wenzhou, China

**Jian-ming Cao**
School of Laboratory Medicine and Life Science, Wenzhou Medical University, Wenzhou, China

**Yue Qu**
Biomedicine Discovery Institute, Department of Microbiology, Faculty of Medicine, Nursing and Health Sciences, Monash University, Clayton, VIC, Australia

**Gurmeet Kaur, P. Balamurugan, Sahana Vasudevan, Saikiran Jadav and S. A. Princy**
Quorum Sensing Laboratory, Centre for Research in Infectious Diseases, School of Chemical and Biotechnology, SASTRA University, Thanjavur, India

**Dale N. Gerding**
Research Service, Edward Hines Jr. VA Hospital, Hines, IL, United States

**Susan P. Sambol and Stuart Johnson**
Research Service, Edward Hines Jr. VA Hospital, Hines, IL, United States
Department of Medicine, Loyola University Chicago Medical Center, Maywood, IL, United States

**Wantana Paveenkittiporn and Watcharaporn Kamjumphol**
National Institute of Health, Department of Medical Sciences, Ministry of Public Health, Nonthaburi, Thailand

**Ratchadaporn Ungcharoen and Anusak Kerdsin**
Faculty of Public Health, Kasetsart University, Nakhon, Thailand

**Yuet Ying Loo, Yaya Rukayadi and Mahmud-Ab-Rashid Nor-Khaizura**
Department of Food Science, Faculty of Food Science and Technology, Universiti Putra Malaysia, Selangor, Malaysia

**Chee Hao Kuan**
Department of Agricultural and Food Science, Faculty of Science, Universiti Tunku Abdul Rahman, Kampar, Malaysia

**Buong Woei Chieng**
Department of Chemistry, Faculty of Science, Universiti Putra Malaysia, Selangor, Malaysia
Materials Processing and Technology Laboratory, Institute of Advanced Technology, Universiti Putra Malaysia, Selangor, Malaysia

**Mitsuaki Nishibuchi**
Center for Southeast Asian Studies, Kyoto University, Kyoto, Japan

**Qiucheng Shi**
Department of Clinical Laboratory, National Clinical Research Center for Child Health, The Children's Hospital, Zhejiang University School of Medicine, Hangzhou, China

**Son Radu**
Department of Food Science, Faculty of Food Science and Technology, Universiti Putra Malaysia, Selangor, Malaysia
Laboratory of Food Safety and Food Integrity, Institute of Tropical Agriculture and Food Security (ITAFoS), Universiti Putra Malaysia, Selangor, Malaysia

**Perumal Karthick and Raju Mohanraju**
Department of Ocean Studies and Marine Biology, Pondicherry University, Port Blair, India

**Dongdong Zhao, Dandan Hu, Li Fang, Yihan Mao, Peng Lan, Xinhong Han, Ping Zhang, Huangdu Hu, Yanfei Wang, Jingjing Quan, Yunsong Yu and Yan Jiang**
Department of Infectious Diseases, Sir Run Run Shaw Hospital, Zhejiang University School of Medicine, Hangzhou, China
Key Laboratory of Microbial Technology and Bioinformatics of Zhejiang Province, Hangzhou, China
Regional Medical Center for National Institute of Respiratory Diseases, Sir Run Run Shaw Hospital, Zhejiang University School of Medicine, Hangzhou, China

**Deepti P. Karumathil, Meera Surendran Nair and Kumar Venkitanarayanan**
Department of Animal Science, University of Connecticut, Storrs, CT, United States

**James Gaffney**
College of Veterinary Medicine, Cornell University, Ithaca, NY, United States

**Anup Kollanoor-Johny**
Department of Animal Science, University of Minnesota, Saint Paul, MN, United States

**Hongxia Ma**
Department of Health Management Medicine, Shanghai East Hospital, Tongji University School of Medicine, Shanghai, China

**Xuemei Zhang**
Department of Oncology, Shanghai East Hospital, Tongji University School of Medicine, Shanghai, China

**Xiaoxing Shi**
Department of Clinical Laboratory, Shanghai Provincial Crops Hospital of Chinese People's Armed Police Forces, Shanghai, China

**Jun Zhang**
Department of Clinical Laboratory, Sir Run Run Shaw Hospital Zhejiang University School of Medicine, Hangzhou, China

**Yunheng Zhou**
Department of Clinical Laboratory, Zhabei Central Hospital of Jing'an District, Shanghai, China

**Ling Jia, Lu Han, Ze-Hua Cui, Run-Shi Yang, Rong-Min Zhang, Shuan-Cheng Bai, Xu-Wei Liu, Ran Wei, Xiao-Ping Liao and Jian Sun**
National Risk Assessment Laboratory for Antimicrobial Resistance of Animal Original Bacteria, South China Agricultural University, Guangzhou, China
Guangdong Provincial Key Laboratory of Veterinary Pharmaceutics Development and Safety Evaluation, South China Agricultural University, Guangzhou, China

**He-Xin Cai and Xi-Ming Li**
College of Mathematics and Informatics, South China Agricultural University, Guangzhou, China

**Liang Chen**
Public Health Research Institute Tuberculosis Center, New Jersey Medical School, Rutgers University, Newark, NJ, United States

**Ya-Hong Liu**
National Risk Assessment Laboratory for Antimicrobial Resistance of Animal Original Bacteria, South China Agricultural University, Guangzhou, China
Guangdong Provincial Key Laboratory of Veterinary Pharmaceutics Development and Safety Evaluation, South China Agricultural University, Guangzhou, China
Jiangsu Co-Innovation Center for Prevention and Control of Important Animal Infectious Diseases and Zoonoses, Yangzhou, China

**Pooja Singh and Selvakumar Subbian**
Public Health Research Institute at New Jersey Medical School, Rutgers Biomedical and Health Sciences Rutgers, The State University of New Jersey, Newark, NJ, United States

**Vladimir Gostev and Sergey Sidorenko**
Department of Medical Microbiology and Molecular Epidemiology, Pediatric Research and Clinical Center for Infectious Diseases, Saint Petersburg, Russia,
Department of Medical Microbiology, North-Western State Medical University Named After I. I. Mechnikov, Saint Petersburg, Russia

**Semen Leyn**
Infectious and Inflammatory Disease Center, Sanford Burnham Prebys Medical Discovery Institute, La Jolla, CA, United States

**Alexander Kruglov and Marina Baykina**
Laboratory of Clinical Microbiology, National Agency for Clinical Pharmacology and Pharmacy, Moscow, Russia

**Daria Likholetova**
Department of Medical Microbiology and Molecular Epidemiology, Pediatric Research and Clinical Center for Infectious Diseases, Saint Petersburg, Russia
Saint Petersburg State University, Saint Petersburg, Russia

**Olga Kalinogorskaya**
Department of Medical Microbiology and Molecular Epidemiology, Pediatric Research and Clinical Center for Infectious Diseases, Saint Petersburg, Russia

**Natalia Dmitrieva and Zlata Grigorievskaya**
Department of Microbiology, N. N. Blokhin Russian Cancer Research Center, Moscow, Russia

**Tatiana Priputnevich, Lyudmila Lyubasovskaya and Alexey Gordeev**
Department of Microbiology, Clinical Pharmacology and Epidemiology, National Medical Research Center for Obstetrics, Gynecology and Perinatology, Moscow, Russia

**Shi Wu, Yonggui Zheng, Yan Guo, Dandan Yin, Demei Zhu and Fupin Hu**
Institute of Antibiotics, Huashan Hospital, Fudan University, Shanghai, China
Key Laboratory of Clinical Pharmacology of Antibiotics, Ministry of Health, Shanghai, China

**Mitali Mishra, Rakesh K. Majhi, Chandan Goswami and Harapriya Mohapatra**
School of Biological Sciences, National Institute of Science Education and Research, Homi Bhabha National Institute, Bhubaneswar, India

**Satish Kumar and Luna Goswami**
School of Biotechnology, Kalinga Institute of Industrial Technology, Bhubaneswar, India

# Index

## N



## O



## P



## R



## S



## T



## U



## V

www.ingramcontent.com/pod-product-compliance
Lightning Source LLC
LaVergne TN
LVHW082131200926
848484LV00008B/2040